TRENDS IN PERSONALIZED NUTRITION

TRENDS IN PERSONALIZED NUTRITION

Edited by

CHARIS M. GALANAKIS

Research & Innovation Department, Galanakis Laboratories, Chania, Greece
Food Waste Recovery Group, ISEKI Food Association, Vienna, Austria

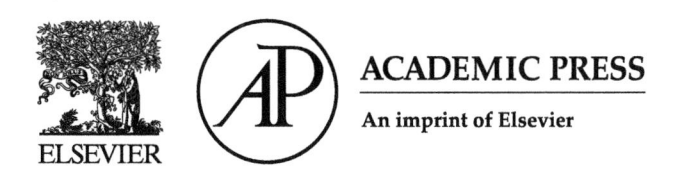

ACADEMIC PRESS

An imprint of Elsevier

Academic Press is an imprint of Elsevier
125 London Wall, London EC2Y 5AS, United Kingdom
525 B Street, Suite 1650, San Diego, CA 92101, United States
50 Hampshire Street, 5th Floor, Cambridge, MA 02139, United States
The Boulevard, Langford Lane, Kidlington, Oxford OX5 1GB, United Kingdom

Copyright © 2019 Elsevier Inc. All rights reserved.

No part of this publication may be reproduced or transmitted in any form or by any means, electronic or mechanical, including photocopying, recording, or any information storage and retrieval system, without permission in writing from the publisher. Details on how to seek permission, further information about the Publisher's permissions policies and our arrangements with organizations such as the Copyright Clearance Center and the Copyright Licensing Agency, can be found at our website: www.elsevier.com/permissions.

This book and the individual contributions contained in it are protected under copyright by the Publisher (other than as may be noted herein).

Notices
Knowledge and best practice in this field are constantly changing. As new research and experience broaden our understanding, changes in research methods, professional practices, or medical treatment may become necessary.

Practitioners and researchers must always rely on their own experience and knowledge in evaluating and using any information, methods, compounds, or experiments described herein. In using such information or methods they should be mindful of their own safety and the safety of others, including parties for whom they have a professional responsibility.

To the fullest extent of the law, neither the Publisher nor the authors, contributors, or editors, assume any liability for any injury and/or damage to persons or property as a matter of products liability, negligence or otherwise, or from any use or operation of any methods, products, instructions, or ideas contained in the material herein.

British Library Cataloguing-in-Publication Data
A catalogue record for this book is available from the British Library

Library of Congress Cataloging-in-Publication Data
A catalog record for this book is available from the Library of Congress

ISBN: 978-0-12-816403-7

For Information on all Academic Press publications
visit our website at https://www.elsevier.com/books-and-journals

Publisher: Charlotte Cockle
Acquisition Editor: Megan R. Ball
Editorial Project Manager: Katerina Zaliva
Production Project Manager: Omer Mukthar
Cover Designer: Matthew Limbert

Typeset by MPS Limited, Chennai, India

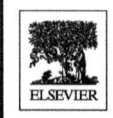

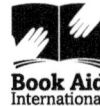

Contents

List of Contributors ix
Preface xiii

SECTION A
INSIGHTS OF PERSONALIZED NUTRITION

1. An Introduction to Personalized Nutrition
DANIELA BRACONI, VITTORIA CICALONI, OTTAVIA SPIGA AND ANNALISA SANTUCCI

Introduction 4
Biological Variability: From Genomics to Systems Biology 7
Role of Behavior, Limitations, and Ethical Issues 13
Future Perspectives 16
Acknowledgments 25
References 25

2. Guidelines to Evaluate the Scientific Validity for Genotype-Based Dietary Advice
KEITH ANTHONY GRIMALDI

Introduction 34
Nutrigenetics and Nutrigenomics 35
How Should We Assess the Evidence in Nutrigenetics? 36
What Needs to be Assessed? 37
Utility and Randomized Controlled Trials 38
Conclusions 41
Where are We Today About Validating Personal Nutrition? 41
To Summarize—Some Components of a Personalized Nutrition 42
Appendix 43
Framework for Evidence Assessment 43
Scientific Validity Assessment of a Putative Gene × Diet Interaction 46
References 48

3. Personalized Nutrition by Predicting Glycemic Responses
VAIA KATSAROU AND MAGDALINI TSOLAKI

Introduction 55
Current Methods for Glucose Response Prediction 57
Variability in Glucose Responses 58
Method 59
Results 59
Conclusions 74
References 76

4. The Role of Bacteria in Personalized Nutrition
SIM K. SINGHRAO, SARITA ROBINSON AND ALICE HARDING

Introduction 81
References 96
Further Reading 104

5. Cognitive Dissonance in Food and Nutrition
ANDY S.J. ONG

Introduction 105
Cognitive Dissonance Theory in Food and Nutrition 107
The Food Cognition Dissonance (FCD) Conceptual Framework 116

Locating Cognitive Dissonance (and Its Role) in the Overall Scheme of Food and Nutrition Research   124
Conclusion   127
References   128
Further Reading   133

SECTION B
APPLICATIONS OF PERSONALIZED NUTRITION

6. Trends, Insights, and Approaches to Diet and Obesity
I. IGLESIA, P. DE MIGUEL-ETAYO, T. BATTELINO AND L.A. MORENO

General Concepts   138
Diagnosis Criteria   138
Epidemiology   139
Causes   141
Associated Comorbidities   145
Prevention Obesity Strategies   146
Future Approaches   151
Obesity Treatment   151
Conclusion   158
References   159

7. Personalized Nutrition for Women, Infants, and Children
ELIZABETH WAMBUI KIMANI-MURAGE, CAROLYN K. NYAMASEGE, SANDRINE MUTONI, TERESIA MACHARIA, MILKA WANJOHI, EVA W. KAMANDE, ELIZABETH MWANIKI, PETER G. MURIUKI, FREDERICK MURUNGA WEKESAH, CAROLINE WAINAINA, MAURICE MUTISYA AND TADDESE ALEMU ZERFU

Introduction   170
Personalized Nutrition for Women: Maternal and Adolescent Nutrition   172
Personalized Nutrition for Infants and Children   174
Economic and Social Returns on Investments of Personalized Nutrition Interventions for Women, Infants, and Children   186
Impending Implementation Research of Personalized Nutrition Programs for Women, Infants, and Children in LMICs   187

Conclusion   189
References   189

8. Modern Technologies for Personalized Nutrition
MIKE BOLAND, FAKHRUL ALAM AND JOHN BRONLUND

Introduction   196
Modern Technologies and Food Acquisition   200
Modern Technologies, Nutrition, and Health   202
Modern Technologies and Food Intake   204
Modern Technologies and Energy Expenditure (Exercise)   206
Modern Technologies and Food Preparation   207
Modern Technologies and Food Composition   209
Bringing It All Together   211
Areas That Need to be Addressed   216
Future Perspective   218
Conclusion   218
References   219
Further Reading   222

SECTION C
POLICY AND COMMERCIALIZATION OF PERSONALIZED NUTRITION

9. Consumer Acceptance of Personalized Nutrition
ZOLTÁN SZAKÁLY, ANDRÁS FEHÉR AND MARIETTA KISS

Introduction   226
Concept, Areas, and Applications of Personalized Nutrition   226
Consumer Judgment of Personalized Nutrition and Nutrigenomics   228
Factors Influencing the Consumer Acceptance of Personalized Nutrition   230
Comprehensive Models of Factors Influencing the Consumer Acceptance of Genetic-Based Personalized Nutrition   241
Consumer Acceptance of Personalized Nutrition in Central Europe: The Case of Hungary   245
The Future of Personalized Nutrition   250
References   253

Chapter 10 Personalized Nutrition: Making It Happen
BARBARA STEWART-KNOX, EILEEN R. GIBNEY, MARIETTE ABRAHAMS, AUDREY RANKIN, ELEANOR BRYANT, BRUNO M.P.M. OLIVEIRA AND RUI POÍNHOS

Current Evidence, What it Means and How Reliable is It? 262
What Does the Consumer Want From Personalized Nutrition? 266
Implementation of Personalized Nutrition in Practice: Implications for Nutrition/Health Professionals 270
Conclusions 272
References 273

11. Personalized Nutrition Education to the Adherence to Dietary and Physical Activity Recommendations
LILIANA GUADALUPE GONZÁLEZ-RODRÍGUEZ, JOSÉ MIGUEL PEREA-SÁNCHEZ, PABLO VEIGA-HERREROS AND ÁFRICA PERAL SUÁREZ

Health and Nutrition Education Challenges 278
Current Dietary and Physical Activity Guidelines 280
Determinants of Food Choice 283
Personalized Nutrition Education Interventions 288

Effectiveness of Personalized Nutrition Education Intervention 290
Methodology for Personalized Nutrition Education 295
Nutrition Education Design Procedure in the Personalized Nutrition Education 299
Other Aspects to Take into Account in Personalized Nutritional Education 303
Conclusion 303
References 304

12. Personalized Expert Recommendation Systems for Optimized Nutrition
CHIH-HAN CHEN AND CHRISTOFER TOUMAZOU

Introduction 309
Nutrients and Genes Correlation Data 311
Scalable Food Categorization 313
Personalized Recommendation System 327
Framework Personalized Expert Recommendation System for Optimized Nutrition 334
Conclusion and Outlook 335
Acknowledgment 336
References 336
Further Reading 338

Index 339

List of Contributors

Mariette Abrahams Department of Psychology, University of Bradford, Bradford, United Kingdom
Fakhrul Alam Massey University, Auckland, New Zealand
T. Battelino Department of Pediatric Endocrinology, Diabetes and Metabolism, University Children's Hospital (UMC), Ljubljana, Slovenia; Faculty of Medicine, University of Ljubljana, Ljubljana, Slovenia
Mike Boland Riddet Institute, Massey University, Palmerston North, New Zealand
Daniela Braconi Department of Biotechnology, Chemistry, and Pharmacy, University of Siena, Siena, Italy
John Bronlund Riddet Institute, Massey University, Palmerston North, New Zealand
Eleanor Bryant Department of Psychology, University of Bradford, Bradford, United Kingdom
Chih-Han Chen IEEE, Imperial College London, London, United Kingdom
Vittoria Cicaloni Department of Biotechnology, Chemistry, and Pharmacy, University of Siena, Siena, Italy
P. De Miguel-Etayo Growth, Exercise, NUtrition and Development (GENUD) Research Group, Faculty of Health Sciences, Agri-food Institute of Aragón (IA2), University of Zaragoza, Zaragoza, Spain; Health Research Institute of Aragón (IIS Aragón), Zaragoza, Spain; Biomedical Research Center in the Physiopathology of Obesity and Nutrition network (CIBERObn), Carlos III Health Institute, Madrid, Spain
András Fehér University of Debrecen, Debrecen, Hungary
Eileen R. Gibney UCD Institute of Food and health, University College Dublin, Dublin, Ireland
Liliana Guadalupe González-Rodríguez Department of Nutrition and Dietetics, Universidad Alfonso X El Sabio, Madrid, Spain
Keith Anthony Grimaldi Eurogenetica Ltd, Sliema, Malta
Alice Harding Research Group: Dementia & Neurodegenerative Diseases Research Group, Faculty of Clinical and Biomedical Sciences, School of Dentistry, University of Central Lancashire, Preston, United Kingdom
I. Iglesia Growth, Exercise, NUtrition and Development (GENUD) Research Group, Faculty of Health Sciences, Agri-food Institute of Aragón (IA2), University of Zaragoza, Zaragoza, Spain; Health Research Institute of Aragón (IIS Aragón), Zaragoza, Spain; Maternal and child health and development network (SAMID), Carlos III Health Institute, Madrid, Spain
Eva W. Kamande Maternal and Child Wellbeing Unit, African Population and Health Research Center, Nairobi, Kenya

Vaia Katsarou Greek Association of Alzheimer's Disease and Related Disorders, Thessaloniki, Greece

Elizabeth Wambui Kimani-Murage Maternal and Child Wellbeing Unit, African Population and Health Research Center, Nairobi, Kenya; Wellcome Trust, London, United Kingdom

Marietta Kiss University of Debrecen, Debrecen, Hungary

Teresia Macharia Maternal and Child Wellbeing Unit, African Population and Health Research Center, Nairobi, Kenya

L.A. Moreno Growth, Exercise, NUtrition and Development (GENUD) Research Group, Faculty of Health Sciences, Agri-food Institute of Aragón (IA2), University of Zaragoza, Zaragoza, Spain; Health Research Institute of Aragón (IIS Aragón), Zaragoza, Spain; Biomedical Research Center in the Physiopathology of Obesity and Nutrition network (CIBERObn), Carlos III Health Institute, Madrid, Spain

Peter G. Muriuki Maternal and Child Wellbeing Unit, African Population and Health Research Center, Nairobi, Kenya; University of Global Health Equity, Kigali, Rwanda

Maurice Mutisya Maternal and Child Wellbeing Unit, African Population and Health Research Center, Nairobi, Kenya

Sandrine Mutoni School of Human Nutrition, McGill University, Montreal, Canada

Elizabeth Mwaniki Maternal and Child Wellbeing Unit, African Population and Health Research Center, Nairobi, Kenya

Carolyn K. Nyamasege Graduate School of Comprehensive Human Sciences, University of Tsukuba, Tsukuba, Japan

Bruno M.P.M. Oliveira Faculty of Nutrition and Food Sciences, University of Porto, Porto, Portugal

Andy S.J. Ong School of Health & Social Sciences, Nanyang Polytechnic, Singapore, Singapore

África Peral Suárez Department of Nutrition and Food Science, Universidad Complutense de Madrid, Madrid, Spain

José Miguel Perea-Sánchez Department of Nutrition and Dietetics, Universidad Alfonso X El Sabio, Madrid, Spain

Rui Poínhos Faculty of Nutrition and Food Sciences, University of Porto, Porto, Portugal

Audrey Rankin School of Pharmacy, Queen's University, Belfast, United Kingdom

Sarita Robinson Faculty of Science and Technology, School of Psychology, University of Central Lancashire, Preston, United Kingdom

Annalisa Santucci Department of Biotechnology, Chemistry, and Pharmacy, University of Siena, Siena, Italy

Sim K. Singhrao Research Group: Dementia & Neurodegenerative Diseases Research Group, Faculty of Clinical and Biomedical Sciences, School of Dentistry, University of Central Lancashire, Preston, United Kingdom

Ottavia Spiga Department of Biotechnology, Chemistry, and Pharmacy, University of Siena, Siena, Italy

Barbara Stewart-Knox Department of Psychology, University of Bradford, Bradford, United Kingdom

Zoltán Szakály University of Debrecen, Debrecen, Hungary

Christofer Toumazou IEEE, Imperial College London, London, United Kingdom

Magdalini Tsolaki Greek Association of Alzheimer's Disease and Related Disorders, Thessaloniki, Greece; 1st Department of Neurology, Medical school, Aristotle University of Thessaloniki, Thessaloniki, Greece

Pablo Veiga-Herreros Department of Nutrition and Dietetics, Universidad Alfonso X El Sabio, Madrid, Spain

Caroline Wainaina Maternal and Child Wellbeing Unit, African Population and Health Research Center, Nairobi, Kenya

Milka Wanjohi Maternal and Child Wellbeing Unit, African Population and Health Research Center, Nairobi, Kenya

Frederick Murunga Wekesah Maternal and Child Wellbeing Unit, African Population and Health Research Center, Nairobi, Kenya; Julius Global Health, Julius Center for Health Sciences and Primary Care, University Medical Center Utrecht, Utrecht, The Netherlands

Taddese Alemu Zerfu Maternal and Child Wellbeing Unit, African Population and Health Research Center, Nairobi, Kenya

Preface

Nowadays, nutrition trends do not only concern the well-known and well respected "dietary guidelines" since the concept of "one-size-fits-all" belongs to the previous century. Nutrition in the 21st century is driven by the need of individuals for tailor-made products and diets that fit their personal needs. To this end, personalized nutrition has been introduced in order to reflect that each person is unique and each one responds differently to the same food. This modern approach is a key growth opportunity for food companies to develop innovations based on consumers' diets.

Nevertheless, despite the fact that personalized nutrition is gaining more and more attention, there is no target reference for this urgent topic. Nowadays, modern nutritionists and food technologists often deal with personalized diets, new product development, and functional foods, and therefore integral information is needed upon this topic. These specialists are interested in the development of commercialization strategies for personalized nutrition, for example, who will adopt it and why, how do commercialization strategies link to public health policies, etc. This book fills the gap existing in the current literature by providing target information of personalized nutrition that covers both characteristics and potential applications. The ultimate goal is to support the scientific community, professionals, and enterprises that aspire to develop the relevant commercialized products and applications of personalized nutrition.

The book consists of three sections and 12 chapters. Section A (Insights of Personalized Nutrition) includes five chapters. Chapter 1, Introduction to Personalized Nutrition, provides an introduction to the book by giving an overview of strategies to deliver personalized nutrition and future perspectives in the field. Generalized dietary recommendations have a limited impact and often lead to modest improvements in food intake. The personalization of dietary recommendations, by taking into account specific characteristics of the recipients, may thus increase the motivation toward dietary changes. On the other hand, genotype-based dietary advice, commonly known as nutrigenetics, uses individual genetic information to contribute to personalized nutrition. Currently, like most applied genetics approaches, nutrigenetics is unregulated and there are no defined standards beyond some commercially adopted codes of practice. Therefore, Chapter 2, Guidelines to Evaluate the Scientific Validity for Genotype-Based Dietary Advice, reviews the recent work in this area and focuses on the guidelines developed within a project funded by the EU (Food4Me). Chapter 3, Personalized Nutrition by Predicting Glycemic Responses, presents recent studies in the field of personalized nutrition in relation to blood glucose responses, focusing on individual responses to lifestyle interventions. Although some of these findings support the suggestion that personalized dietary interventions can predict blood glucose responses accurately, we are still at the beginning.

Chapter 4, The Role of Bacteria in Personalized Nutrition, aims to enable the reader to make informed decisions on how best to improve their gut health by promoting the colonization of the gastrointestinal tract by commensals. Although diet plays an important role in supporting general health, its efficacy in restoring symbiosis remains to be fully investigated. In addition, professional interventions are important, because factors such as genetics, certain medications, and lifestyles also contribute to dysbiosis. As our knowledge grows regarding how best to maintain a healthy oral/gastrointestinal tract microbiome, dieticians will be able to formulate personalized nutrition plans to better support general health throughout life. Chapter 5, Cognitive Dissonance in Food and Nutrition, examines cognitive dissonance in food and nutrition by addressing the current gaps and critical issues as well as following the context of public health promotion, with practical illustrations. Guidelines pertaining to instrumentation of the framework's novel attitudinal dimensions of cognitive dissonance are provided and demonstrated within the parameters of the above practical illustrations for clarity.

Section B (Applications of Personalized Nutrition) includes three chapters. Chapter 6, Trends, Insights, and Approaches to Diet and Obesity, deals with trends, insights, and approaches to diet and obesity. Obesity, which is a multifactorial disease, is defined by an excess of fat deposits, which may lead to alterations in the functioning of the body. Genetic, phychological, and lifestyle factors can be considered as the main reasons for developing the disease that may later be linked with other comorbidities such as hypertension, dyslipidemia, type 2 diabetes, or cardiovascular disease. In recent years science has been focused in discerning what the influences of lifestyle factors (e.g., dietary factors, physical activity or sleeping habits) are in obesity. Omics technologies are today contributing to the modification and improvements of obesity treatment, but the use of genetic tools in public health nutrition policy is not prevalent and requires an evidence-based approach to validate that the personalized recommendations result in health benefits.

Malnutrition remains a problem globally, with at least one in three people experiencing it. It is linked, either directly or indirectly, to the major causes of death and disability. In Africa, more than one-third of children under the age of 5 are stunted, while close to half of the women are underweight. There is, however, no single personalized approach toward solving the high malnutrition rates. Therefore Chapter 7, Personalized Nutrition for Women, Infants, and Children, discusses these and other issues of personalized nutrition for women, infants, and children.

Personal wearable devices (including smartphones) are tracking levels of energy expenditure and other aspects of health, and in turn can allow device-supported advice about dietary needs. Devices will soon be able to record the consumption of different foods by an individual in nonintrusive ways, and artificial intelligence will be deployed to provide decisions (or decision support) about food purchasing and meal planning, based on food preferences, long-term personal nutrition planning, and other applications. These advances and possible future developments are discussed in Chapter 8, Modern Technologies for Personalized Nutrition.

The final Section C (Policy and Commercialization) is compiled of four chapters. Consumer acceptance of personalized nutrition is discussed in Chapter 9, Consumer Acceptance of Personalized Nutrition. The efforts made to reduce the occurrence of nutrition-related diseases over the last few decades have not been effective. A move from population-based nutrition guidance toward personalized nutrition (including nutrigenomics) may offer a new way of changing nutrition habits, but it still awaits widespread consumer acceptance, despite the mainly positive consumer attitude toward the concept itself. In another approach, Chapter 10, Personalized Nutrition: Making It Happen, discusses how dieticians can make personalized nutrition happen in the future, for which specialized training and guidelines for practice will be required. When setting up the provision of personalized nutrition services across Europe, intercountry differences should be considered in terms of perceived barriers to uptake associated with personalized nutrition and the wider eating context. Irrespective of the European country, potential consumers trusted health professionals such as doctors and dietitians over commercial agents to provide personalized nutrition.

In recent years, there has been a significant increase worldwide in the prevalence and incidence of noncommunicable diseases both in children and adults. Food choice is a complex process that is influenced by different determinants that must be taken into account in the design of a nutrition education intervention. The traditional nutrition education approach has been considered ineffective. Therefore there is a need to design and apply new models to support people to adhere to the dietary and physical guidelines. Chapter 11, Personalized Nutrition Education to the Adherence to Dietary and Physical Activity Recommendations, highlights how personalized nutrition education plays a key role in the promotion of healthy eating habits, an active lifestyle, and related health behaviors. Finally, Chapter 12, Personalized Expert Recommendation Systems for Optimized Nutrition, covers the correlation between nutrients and genes, the data categorization of food products, modeling with a type of machine learning model called deep neural network, a recommendation system with a genetic algorithm, and the overall operation of the whole framework. The framework aims to categorize products automatically with the ability to scale with unknown new data, and then be able to recommend products through filtering with a model based on individual genetic data with associated phenotypic information. A case study with databases from three different sources is carried out to confirm the system.

Conclusively, the book provides a reference addressing all nutritionists, food chemists, food scientists, new product developers, and other relevant professionals in a direct, integrated, and holistic way. It covers the cutting edge topics of personalized nutrition for researchers, postgraduate students, interested academics seeking to obtain a broader view of the issues, as well as stakeholders in the industry (including small start-ups) interested in developing nutrition-based tests or products. It could be utilized as a handbook and/or ancillary reading in undergraduate and postgraduate level multidiscipline courses dealing with nutritional chemistry.

I would also like to thank and acknowledge all authors of this book for accepting my invitation, as well as showing dedication to the book's concept, editorial guidelines, and timeline. Their collaboration and creative work are highly appreciated. I consider myself fortunate to have had the opportunity to collaborate with so many experts from Canada, Greece, Hungary, Italy, Ireland, Malta, New Zealand, Portugal, Rwanda, Singapore, Slovenia, Spain, the Netherlands, and the United Kingdom. In addition, I would like to thank the acquisition editor Megan Ball and the book manager Katerina Zaliva for their assistance during editing, and all the team at Elsevier during the production process. Finally, a message for each individual reader separately. Such a collaborative project contains typically minor errors. If you find any mistakes, or have any objections to the content of the current book, you are very welcome to contact me.

Charis M. Galanakis

Research & Innovation Department, Galanakis Laboratories, Chania, Greece;
Food Waste Recovery Group, ISEKI Food Association, Vienna, Austria

SECTION A

INSIGHTS OF PERSONALIZED NUTRITION

CHAPTER 1

An Introduction to Personalized Nutrition

Daniela Braconi, Vittoria Cicaloni, Ottavia Spiga and Annalisa Santucci

Department of Biotechnology, Chemistry, and Pharmacy, University of Siena, Siena, Italy

OUTLINE

Introduction	4	Role of Behavior, Limitations, and Ethical Issues	13
What, How, and Why	4		
Where It Comes From?	5	Future Perspectives	16
Strategies to Deliver Personalized Dietary Advice	5	From Knowledge to Practice	16
		"Omic" Technologies	18
Biological Variability: From Genomics to Systems Biology	7	Big Data and Machine Learning	19
		What Is Needed for the Future?	23
Genes	7	Acknowledgments	25
Gut Microbiota	9		
Foodomics	10	References	25
Other "Omics" Repertoires and Systems Biology Approaches	11		

In memory of Duccio Calamandrei, a man of science and a friend

INTRODUCTION

What, How, and Why

Dietary factors are known to play a role in health and diseases, and there is already convincing evidence that adopting a correct lifestyle (diet included) can be more effective than drug treatment in the prevention of diseases in susceptible subjects (Knowler et al., 2002). Generalized dietary and lifestyle recommendations are delivered as a common practice in an attempt to motivate people toward healthy choices. Yet these recommendations have a limited impact; in fact, we are still witnessing a pandemic raise in noncommunicable, complex metabolic diseases. According to the World Health Organization (WHO), noncommunicable diseases (NCDs), which include heart disease, stroke, cancer, diabetes, and chronic lung disease, collectively account for almost 70% of all deaths worldwide and have relevant socioeconomic costs (http://www.who.int/ncds/introduction/en/). This implies that the one-size-fits-all diet approach is not efficacious and not able to address interindividual variability. In this framework, personalization of diet emerged as a strategy relying on the use of individual information to deliver finely customized nutritional advice, products, or services (Ordovas, Ferguson, Tai, & Mathers, 2018). Such an approach could be able to *assist individuals in achieving a lasting dietary behavior change that is beneficial for health* (Gibney, Walsh & Goosens).

The overall goal of personalized nutrition is to preserve or increase health by collecting individual information at the genetic, phenotypic, medical, and nutritional level, and to use such information to deliver customized nutritional guidance, an approach that could prove more efficacious not only for disease management, but especially for disease prevention. Even if the traditional focus is on health, other personal goals such as reshaping the body or preparing for sport competitions might be envisaged; also, personal preferences might be taken into account. Targets for personalized nutrition are both healthy and diseased subjects, as well as genetically susceptible individuals. Yet although easy to be conceptualized, an agreed definition of "personalized nutrition" is lacking still. Even the term "personalized" can be replaced by other terms such as "stratified," "tailored," or "individually-tailored," although these descriptors imply subtly different meanings (Ordovas et al., 2018).

Individuals are far from standardized specimens: an absolute normal does not exist, but rather multiple diverse entities do exist. Furthermore, different population groups (such as children, elderly, pregnant women, athletes, subjects with inborn errors of metabolism where a specific nutrition component can be found) might require specific dietary guidelines. Hence, we should not think of health only in terms of disease prevention/treatment, but rather embrace the concept of well-being in the sense of ameliorating mood, attention, endurance, weight management, or control of specific biochemical parameters. These are the reasons why one-size-fits-all approaches in nutrition often lead to modest improvements in food intake. Personalization, by taking into account specific characteristics of the recipients, may thus increase motivation toward dietary changes. In order for these changes to be effective, personalization can be based on biological evidence and/or personal behaviors, preferences, or objectives, as discussed later on.

Where It Comes From?

The idea of adapting our diet according to "personal" factors such as age, gender, physiological state, or physical activity, as well as to special conditions such as pregnancy or risk of disease, is common today. The same holds true when thinking of different diets in terms of individual, social, cultural, and traditional preferences: food goes beyond the mere concept of nutrition, being a shaper of social relationships and part of cultural and personal identity (Kohlmeier et al., 2016). However, there is more than this. The concept of "personalization" dates back to more than one century ago with the observations made by Garrod in the study of inborn errors of metabolism, which highlighted how biological individuality could be reflected by different chemistries of body fluids. Garrod wrote "...*just as no two individuals of a species are absolutely identical in bodily structure neither are their chemical processes carried out on exactly the same lines...*" (Garrod, 1996). Some years later, stemming largely from research on bacteria, a clearer understanding of the relationships between genotype and nutrition was obtained (Roper, 1960) but it was only with the completion of the Human Genome Project that completely new approaches to the study of the interaction between genes and diet were provided. It is from such studies that two main disciplines emerged: "nutrigenetics," which studies how genetic background affects response to dietary components, nutrient requirement, and predisposition to certain diseases; and "nutrigenomics," which provides information on how diet affects gene transcription, protein expression, and metabolism (Kussmann, Raymond, & Affolter, 2006; Peregrin, 2001). Both these disciplines are aimed at deciphering the molecular mechanisms by which nutrients and dietary components interact to maintain or disturb cellular homeostasis and health outcomes (Peregrin, 2001).

Strategies to Deliver Personalized Dietary Advice

Early definitions of personalized nutrition relied mainly on a gene-focused (i.e., "individually-tailored," often used as a synonym of "personalized") approach (Ordovas et al., 2018). However, this concept was soon revised in order to include the idea of "levels." According to the analysis of different sets of data, three levels of customization can in fact be provided to deliver personalized nutrition (Fig. 1.1) (Gibney & Walsh, 2013; O'Donovan et al., 2017), as exemplified by the recent Food4me pan-European study, the largest randomized controlled trial to have investigated the efficacy of personalized nutrition (Celis-Morales et al., 2017). The study was designed as a four-arm, multicenter, web-based randomized clinical trial conducted across seven European countries. Approximately 1600 participants were randomly assigned to one of the following intervention groups for a 6-month period:

1. Level 0, Control group, receiving conventional, nonpersonalized advice;
2. Level 1, receiving personalized advice based on *dietary intake* alone;
3. Level 2, receiving personalized advice based on *dietary intake* and *phenotype*;
4. Level 3, receiving personalized advice based on *dietary intake*, *phenotype*, and *genotype*.

The above three-levels classification still deals with delivering dietary advice at a personal level; however, there is an emerging approach, called metabotyping, shifting from individuals to groups. Approaches delivering nutritional intervention/advice to groups of individuals are referred to as "stratified" or "tailored" (Ordovas et al., 2018). They rely on

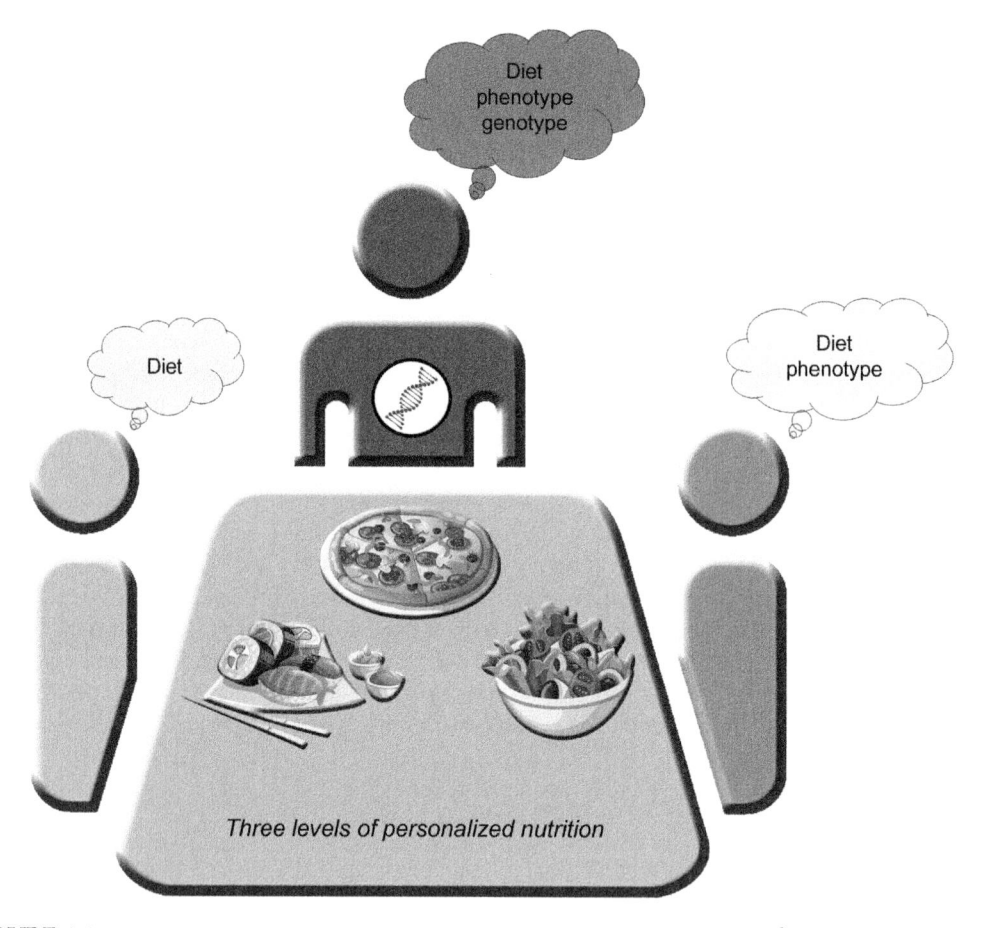

FIGURE 1.1 Strategies to deliver personalized nutrition: the "three levels" approach.[1]

metabolic profiling and clustering tools to group subjects that share a common metabolic profile or dietary intervention (Gibney & Walsh, 2013; O'Donovan et al., 2017). The most common clustering methods are K-nearest neighbors (K-NN) and K-means. The first one is a simple, nonparametric classifier often used for its flexibility and reasonable accuracy; the second one allows subdividing a set of objects into K groups based on their attributes (Hartigan & Wong, 1979).

The success of the metabotyping approach is mainly due to its ability to encompass several biological processes, since genes, environmental factors, and gut microbiota contribute to the final metabotype (Brennan, 2017). However, in the context of nutrition, there are so far more examples of clustering techniques than developing personalized interventions for such clusters (Fenech et al., 2011; Gibney & Walsh, 2013; O'Donovan, Walsh, Gibney, Gibney, & Brennan, 2016; O'Donovan et al., 2017; Stover, 2004). For instance, metabotyping

[1] Original artwork by F. Pettini available at: https://commons.wikimedia.org/wiki/File:Levels_nutrition.jpg.

could successfully identify responders to vitamin D supplementation (O'Sullivan et al., 2011), or segregate subjects into distinct groups according to their response to an oral glucose tolerance test, identifying also those with a more severe metabolic dysfunction and thus at higher risk (Morris et al., 2013). Another example showed how metabotyping could identify responders to fenofibrate treatment according to lipoprotein profiles, an approach that was more effective than conventional ones (van Bochove et al., 2012). One of the few examples where metabotyping is coupled to delivery of targeted dietary advice, offering a potential tool to be easily translated into healthcare settings, was proposed recently on a large cohort of healthy Irish subjects who underwent routine biochemical analyses for four markers of metabolic health (triacylglycerols, total cholesterol, direct HDL cholesterol, and glucose). Clustering analysis and a decision tree approach were undertaken based on biochemical parameters, anthropometry, and blood pressure to deliver dietary advice, whose appropriateness was compared to manually compiled individualized advice, revealing good agreement (O'Donovan et al., 2014). In a European framework, the Food4me study was also the first to identify metabotypes among participants, and demonstrate that such metabotypes were related to nutrient intake, supporting their use. Also in this study, recommendations provided through a decision tree approach were in good agreement with advice provided by nutritionists (O'Donovan et al., 2017).

BIOLOGICAL VARIABILITY: FROM GENOMICS TO SYSTEMS BIOLOGY

Genes

Public dietary recommendations (like the common "eat five servings of fruits and vegetables per day") rely on average population data and nutritional epidemiology studies. However, individuals respond differently to lifestyle and diet modifications, which is due to their own genetic makeup and interactions with their environment. The human genome contains many genetic variants that are involved in nutrition-related processes, some of which through mechanisms not fully understood yet (van Ommen et al., 2017). This implies that a diet suitable for one genotype is unlikely to be suitable for individuals with different genotypes, and hence that establishing common dietary recommendations might not be an optimal approach (Kohlmeier et al., 2016; Stover, 2004). Different genetic polymorphisms might (El-Sohemy, 2007):

1. Affect specific metabolic pathways, eventually leading to diseases requiring very specific dietary adjustments.
2. Disturb metabolism in terms of absorption, transport, digestion, excretion of nutrients, and bioactive compounds.
3. Induce alterations in the response to diet and nutrients.

An increased genetic knowledge could help health interventions by identifying polymorphisms increasing the risk of developing certain diseases or conditions that require specific dietary interventions (Kohlmeier et al., 2016). A number of single-nucleotide polymorphisms (SNPs) are known to alter nutrient metabolism, but assessments are complicated due to the fact the metabolism of a single nutrient can be affected by SNPs in the same gene or in different genes within the same metabolic pathway. Interestingly, in the context of multifactorial diseases, a cumulative genetic risk score (GRS) taking into account the cumulative theoretical contribution of genetics to a specific condition was proposed recently (Fall & Ingelsson, 2014). GRS is usually obtained as an average value from large studies, thus is not ideal for an aim of personalization; furthermore, it does not bring along mechanistic information, and single genetic variants may be part of multiple GRSs at the same time. Nevertheless, existing gene–diet and gene–environment catalogs may represent useful resources to build process-based GRSs (Parnell et al., 2014).

The use of genomics to deliver dietary guidelines and control diseases is exemplified easily in monogenic disorders, such as the rare disease phenylketonuria (requiring restriction in phenylalanine and supplementation in tyrosine due to deficiency in the phenylalanine–tyrosine converting enzyme), or galactosemia (grouping three different conditions with enzyme deficiencies in galactose metabolism, requiring galactose restriction). A genetic component is also found in lactose intolerance, where the ability to digest lactose is progressively lost with aging due to a decreased lactase biosynthesis, which is managed through a lactose-free diet (Deng, Misselwitz, Dai, & Fox, 2015). A more complicated case involves carriers of the methylenetetrahydrofolate reductase (*MTHFR*) C677T gene polymorphism (rs1801133), where "T" is the allele associated with reduced enzyme activity, who may require supplementation with folate (substrate) and/or riboflavin (cofactor). Homozygotes can show in fact up to a 30% enzyme activity reduction, possible lowering of folate bioavailability (associated and mechanistically related to neural tube defects) and hyperhomocysteinemia (a risk factor for cardiovascular diseases). However, despite the knowledge of folate-related genetics and health consequences, still no genetics-based dietary recommendation exists on folate intake during pregnancy (Levin & Varga, 2016).

Differently from diseases following classical Mendelian inheritance, where a single gene variant is involved, diet-related diseases are more complex and often due to a number of genes that can belong to multiple pathways or be related to different aspects of metabolism (Mathers, 2017). For such multifactorial, complex diseases, tailoring diets with prevention/intervention aims has been proven to be much more complicated and, so far, to have limited value (Bashiardes, Godneva, Elinav, & Segal, 2018). For instance, an interaction among a functional *APOA2* polymorphism, food intake, and body mass index (BMI) was shown in three independent populations (Corella, Peloso, & Arnett, 2009). The synergistic effect between the Mediterranean diet and *GSTP1* or *NAT2* SNPs (involved in xenobiotic metabolism pathway) was found to decrease breast cancer risk (Kakkoura et al., 2017). The effects of the Mediterranean diet were also studied related to the presence of polymorphisms of *TCF7L2* (Corella et al., 2009, 2013) and *CLOCK* genes (Corella et al., 2016), which are both linked to the development of type 2 diabetes. In particular, Corella et al. (2013) have observed in the randomized PREDIMED study that the Mediterranean diet can reduce the incidence of stroke in genetically susceptible subjects. Relevant strengths of the study are the large population ($n = 7018$) and the long follow-up period (4.8 years). Significant evidence was obtained on the association between *TCF7L2* polymorphisms and fasting glucose/lipid profiles, underscoring the need for assessing the effects of complete dietary patterns rather than single components.

Other conflicting or less consistent results are found in the literature dealing with gene—diet interaction studies. As an example, a metaanalysis by Pavlidis et al. focusing on 38 genes tested in commercially available nutrigenomics kits failed to highlight any significant association with several diet-related diseases, implying that at present such tests cannot be recommended, although holding some potential (Pavlidis et al., 2015; Pavlidis, Patrinos, & Katsila, 2015). Similarly, a review by Li et al. (2017) analyzed studies reporting gene—macronutrient interactions and type 2 diabetes and identified eight unique gene—macronutrient interactions, although none of them could be replicated in the large-scale EPIC-Interact study.

It has also been acknowledged that the effects of a diet on human health can be related to the specific gene makeup of a population, and not be transferred to other populations. An interesting example comes from observations in the traditional Inuit population that, despite a diet rich in polyunsaturated fatty acids (PUFA), shows a low rate of cardiovascular diseases. This observation was linked to different variants of the fatty acids desaturase (*FADS*) gene that are rarely found in the European population. These variants can lower the production of $n=3$ and $n=6$ fatty acids, which is likely to counteract the high dietary intake of PUFA (Fumagalli et al., 2015). Similarly, the Inuit population shows variants of the fructosamine 3 kinase-related protein (*FN3KRP*) gene that are associated with increased protection from oxidative stress, which might be related to PUFA (Mathieson et al., 2015).

Gut Microbiota

Recent evidence shed light onto the biological basis of interindividual variability pointing toward not only our genome, but also to our commensal gut microbiota as another important key player in the response to diet and nutrients. In fact, we host millions of commensals, symbiotic, and pathogenic microorganisms, which makes us "superorganisms" (Greer, Dong, Morgun, & Shulzhenko, 2016); such microorganisms play a fundamental role in essential physiological (Guven-Maiorov, Tsai, & Nussinov, 2017; Moco, Martin, & Rezzi, 2012) and pathological (Goto, Kurashima, & Kiyono, 2015; Kelly, Minuto, Cryan, Clarke, & Dinan, 2017; Maguire & Maguire, 2017; Uniken Venema, Voskuil, Dijkstra, Weersma, & Festen, 2017; Weiss et al., 2004) processes.

Along with lifestyle and genetic factors, gut microbiota is an important modulator of response to diet; vice versa, diet can shape the microbial environment at both the taxonomic and gene expression level (David et al., 2014; Hadrich, 2018). Although relatively stable in adulthood (Faith et al., 2013), rapid and short-term alterations of gut microbiota are seen upon diet changes (David et al., 2014; Wu et al., 2011), and long-term dietary modifications may produce even more profound alterations (Faith et al., 2013; Wu et al., 2011). Incorporating knowledge of the gut microbiota and its modifications into a holistic, personalized dietary approach may be an effective way to address health challenges that holds great potential (Bashiardes et al., 2018). An interesting example was provided recently by Korem et al. (2017) who highlighted through a randomized crossover trial that microbiome-based parameters could predict response to dietary interventions based only on prior knowledge of microbiome data, suggesting that understanding the effects of diet requires the integration of individual factors.

The growing awareness of the relevance of gut microbiota for health also led to the metaomics approaches, which mean the high-throughput global analysis (often in an untargeted fashion) of genes, transcripts, proteins, or metabolites of a community of organisms (Rowland et al., 2017). Integrated metaomics datasets linking diseases to gut microbiota are being produced (Putignani & Dallapiccola, 2016) integrating information provided through metagenomics, metaproteomics, and phenomics (link to clinical conditions). Focus has been so far the understanding of metabolic pathways to discriminate healthy and diseased subjects (Santoru et al., 2017). By contrast, only a few dietary ingredients have been systematically investigated for their effects toward the gut microbiota. This is the case, for instance, of a crossover study where metaomics techniques were combined to provide a mechanistic understanding of the effects of resistant starch (Maier et al., 2017).

Foodomics

The growing interest on food has led recently to a novel discipline called *foodomics* (Braconi, Bernardini, Millucci, & Santucci, 2018). This term was coined in 2009 to describe *"a discipline that studies the Food and Nutrition domains through the application of advanced omics technologies to improve consumer's well-being, health, and confidence"* (Cifuentes, 2009; Herrero, Simo, Garcia-Canas, Ibanez, & Cifuentes, 2012; Simo et al., 2010). Hence, foodomics is a holistic approach integrating information from several working areas: nutrition, omics technologies (possibly coupled to in vitro, in vivo, and clinical studies), and bioinformatics. Such a new discipline holds the potential to improve our (so far) limited understanding of the role of food in health, diseases, and individual performances, possibly identifying bioactive molecules, helping to dissect the mechanisms through which such molecules induce changes in cells, tissues, or organs, and demonstrate their efficacy (Badimon, Vilahur, & Padro, 2017; Kussmann et al., 2006).

Foodomics can thus provide optimal tools to identify personalized dietary lifestyles (Remely, Stefanska, Lovrecic, Magnet, & Haslberger, 2015) and help in deciphering how food can interact with genes, proteins, or metabolites, leading to the identification of biomarkers to monitor dietary interventions and the implementation of strategies to manipulate cell functioning through diet. Furthermore, by identifying and characterizing bioactive compounds from various sources (e.g., plant kingdom, algae), foodomics might provide relevant information for the development of *nutraceuticals* and *functional foods* (Herrero et al., 2012; Ibanez, Simo, Garcia-Canas, Cifuentes, & Castro-Puyana, 2013) for which modern nutrition research is highlighting potential positive effects for human health (Badimon et al., 2017). Nutraceuticals are "diet supplements that deliver a concentrated form of a presumed bioactive agent from a food, presented in a non-food matrix, and used to enhance health in dosages that exceed those that could be obtained from normal foods" (Zeisel, 1999). Conversely, a definition of functional food is still lacking. A functional food can be natural or processed, but should be consumed regularly in its original matrix in normal, defined, nontoxic amounts as a part of standard diets. It should also have a documented health benefit that goes beyond basic nutritional functions, for example, prevention, management, or treatment of chronic diseases (Bernal, Mendiola, Ibanez, & Cifuentes, 2011; Doyon & Labrecque, 2008; Martirosyan & Singh, 2015).

In addition, foodomics can play a role in the identification of potentially hazardous compounds such as food allergens (https://www.fda.gov/Food/ResourcesForYou/Consumers/ucm079311.htm) or contaminants (Martinović, Andjelković, Gajdošik, Rešetar, & Josić, 2016), which represent issues of great economic and public health relevance. Overall, foodomics can respond to the producers' and consumers' increasing demand for biomarkers assessing food quality and authenticity (Arena, Salzano, & Scaloni, 2016; Cuadros-Rodríguez, Ruiz-Samblás, Valverde-Som, Pérez-Castaño, & González-Casado, 2016).

Foodomics might also help in unraveling the effects of complex food matrices, where bioactive molecules are mixed with synergistic or antagonist molecules. For instance, Danesi and colleagues were able to highlight slight modifications in the cholesterol-lowering effect of dill and kale, matrices that share the same major bioactive component but significantly differ in their composition (Danesi, Govoni, D'Antuono, & Bordoni, 2016). Other foodomics approaches have been used to understand how food matrices are metabolized and bio-transformed (Bordoni et al., 2011, 2014; Lopez-Rubio, Flanagan, Shrestha, Gidley, & Gilbert, 2008; Picariello, Mamone, Nitride, Addeo, & Ferranti, 2013), which is essential information in order to achieve progress toward a better understanding of how diet affects human health (Scalbert et al., 2014).

Other "Omics" Repertoires and Systems Biology Approaches

Translation from genotype to phenotype is not straightforward, since physiological systems respond and adapt continuously to a variety of stimuli, diet included (Hesketh, 2012; Mathers, 2017; Thomas, 2010). Downstream processes such as epigenetics (i.e., the study of modifications of the genetic material), miRNA interference, and other forms of posttranslational modifications (PTMs) of proteins can affect the proteome (i.e., the entire set of expressed proteins) and metabolome (i.e., the entire set of metabolites), contributing substantially to the phenotype. The importance of these events is just starting to emerge from large-scale cohort studies also in the context of nutrition (de Roos & Brennan, 2017).

In the postgenomic era, the opportunity to combine and integrate cutting-edge analytical platforms and data processing systems can promote the understanding of the health-promoting effects of food and customized dietary interventions. "Omic" technologies could represent valuable tools for disease diagnosis, enabling the implementation of customized effective dietary interventions. They might also provide valuable tools to monitor the efficacy of the interventions by analyzing appropriate biomarkers (e.g., proteins, metabolites) and dietary components, also in terms of bioactive compounds, thus allowing a better understanding of human nutrition and diet customization (Braconi et al., 2018). "Omic" technologies offer natural synergies that could help overcoming reproducibility of food-related studies, as active components in food can vary notably, thus introducing uncertainties in assessing interactions between nutrition and genome. Furthermore, they address biological variations that are downstream from structural genomic differences, which is important in order to develop more robust customization of nutrition, and for validation purposes.

Transcriptomics and proteomics can provide a global view of active genes and expressed proteins with their PTMs, respectively; hence, they can be useful tools to identify efficacy and intervention markers (Ibanez et al., 2013), biological contaminants, and to assess the impact of genetic manipulation (Valdés et al., 2013; Valdés, Simó, Ibáñez, & García-Cañas, 2013). Proteomics can offer further applications in the characterization of food composition (Nazzaro, Orlando, Fratianni, Di Luccia, & Coppola, 2012) and the detection of allergens (Boschetti & Righetti, 2012; Gallo & Ferranti, 2016; Ibanez et al., 2013; Ibanez, Simo, Garcia-Canas, Acunha, & Cifuentes, 2015). Metabolomics, by characterizing the whole set of metabolites, their dynamics, and interactions, emerged mainly for its ability to deliver functional data (Whitfield, German, & Noble, 2004) and today represents probably the most active and growing field of investigation (Robinette, Bruschweiler, Schroeder, & Edison, 2012). Assessment of the whole set of metabolites in a biological sample through an untargeted analysis (*metabolomics* or *metabolic fingerprinting*) might represent an optimal strategy to analyze the interplay between food and host in nutritional intervention studies (Claus, 2014). The quantitative measurement of the metabolic response to nutritional changes (*nutrimetabonomics*) might be used to screen and identify metabolic markers of a healthy lifestyle and food-modulated endogenous metabolic pathways (Claus, 2014). As an example, the INTERMAP study highlighted the possibility to link the nutrimetabonome profile of urine to food intake and cardiovascular health (Stamler et al., 2013).

Since nutrition can markedly modulate biochemical pathways through epigenetic modifications, the nascent *nutriepigenomics* field has the potential to advance the understanding of interactions between food and epigenome (i.e., chemical changes to the DNA and histone proteins) in the development of human diseases (de Luca et al., 2017). Recent examples of the role of epigenetics have been provided in obesity (Bordoni & Capozzi, 2014; Capozzi & Bordoni, 2013) and in the susceptibility to develop type 2 diabetes, metabolic syndrome, and cardiovascular diseases as a consequence of perinatal malnutrition (de Luca et al., 2017; Remely et al., 2015). Interestingly, diet polyphenols were proposed as potential agents to address insulin resistance and dyslipidemia related to metabolic syndrome for their ability to modulate miRNAs expression (de Luca et al., 2017). Similarly, certain nutrients (mainly fatty acids) may hold the potential to modify the genetic predisposition to metabolic syndrome, although functional studies are needed to evaluate biological significance and clinical utility (Phillips, 2013). There is also evidence of epigenetic changes induced by weight loss interventions that might pave the way to personalized recommendations for weight control programs (Goni, Milagro, Cuervo, & Martinez, 2014).

Four "omics" domains related to agriculture (*agrigenomics*) and nutrition (*nutrigenomics*, *nutriproteomics*, and *nutrimetabolomics*) have been suggested as valuable tools to understand interindividual variability in response to food-related environmental exposure (Özdemir & Kolker, 2016). As discussed, nutrigenomics is already a well-established study domain in food nutrition; by contrast, the study of other complementary "omics" domains still lags behind.

We have already provided examples underpinning the complexity of personalizing dietary advice even when considering "only" genomic variability. The overarching complexity of doing the same for complex systems that have multiple pathways working in concert at the same time and interact continuously with the gut microbiota and the environment can be easily imagined (van Ommen et al., 2017). In this context, the concept of

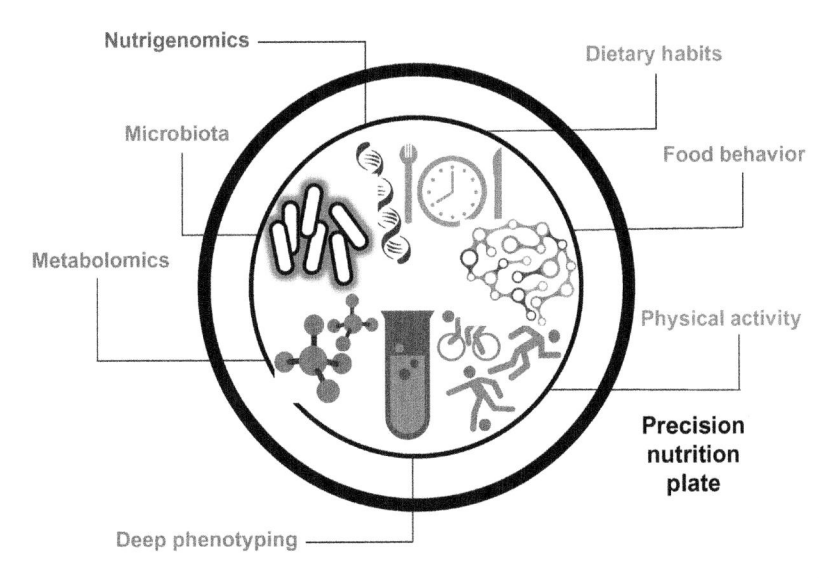

FIGURE 1.2 The precision nutrition plate. A schematic representation of the main factors worth considering when approaching precision nutrition (available from de Toro-Martín et al., 2017, https://doi.org/10.3390/nu9080913, https://creativecommons.org/licenses/by/4.0/).[2]

"systems flexibility" has emerged to introduce a systems biology-based approach taking into account the most relevant interacting biological mechanisms in order to deliver personalized dietary recommendations (van Ommen & Wopereis, 2016) (Fig. 1.2). Although associated to major analytical challenges, only the proper integration of multiomic studies and the implementation of bioinformatics tools and databases will help translate findings from clinical practice into effective personalized dietary strategies (Braconi et al., 2018). Once fully exploited and integrated in a systems biology perspective, "omics" repertoires could be central to the so-called Precision Nutrition 4.0 approach, which holds the potential for relevant innovations (Özdemir & Kolker, 2016).

ROLE OF BEHAVIOR, LIMITATIONS, AND ETHICAL ISSUES

Together with other lifestyle modifications, improving diet could represent a way to significantly reduce the burden of diseases and increase well-being. To this aim, most of the efforts have been so far dedicated to measuring and characterizing biological repertoires and metabolic diversity: the underlying idea is that a deeper characterization of biological diversity would allow for more effective personalized interventions (Riedl, Gieger, Hauner, Daniel, & Linseisen, 2017). However, it is increasingly realized that dietary changes could be hard to achieve and maintain, as they require a constant and

---

[2] This is an open access article distributed under the Creative Commons Attribution License, which permits unrestricted use, distribution, and reproduction in any medium, provided the original work is properly cited. (CC BY 4.0).

thorough collaboration of participants, who are asked to make each time the right choice (Ordovas et al., 2018). Furthermore, dietary restrictions can have societal and cultural implications that go beyond mere nutritional considerations. Delivering appropriate information on how to make good dietary choices that will be beneficial for our health may be not enough, since knowledge alone is typically insufficient to change behavior. Although most people know what is "good" or "not good" to eat, turning intentions into action is notoriously difficult; this is especially relevant for those conditions where diet plays a role as an etiological factor, like in metabolic diseases (de Roos & Brennan, 2017).

In order to develop informed communication strategies based on consumers' priorities and concerns, an online survey was carried out to study how food choice motives could be related to an intention to adopt personalized nutrition. The general concept is that people may have different needs and goals that should be addressed adequately to enhance motivation. Those individuals for whom health is an important driver of food choice may already believe they eat a healthy diet; they might think that a personalized diet would not provide them with additional benefits. By contrast, determinants such as weight control, mood, and pricing of food are critical motivators that should be taken into account in tailoring communications (Rankin et al., 2018).

Acceptance and adherence to dietary guidelines seem to be better achieved if participants are engaged in a shared decision-making context (Ordovas et al., 2018), as exemplified by the Food4me pan-European study (Celis-Morales et al., 2017). The main aims of Food4me were to assess whether personalization could impact subjects' motivation to follow a healthy diet compared to conventional one-size-fits-all population-based advice, and whether providing phenotypic/genotypic information could provide further motivation and being more effective in assisting/motivating study participants compared to personalization alone (Celis-Morales et al., 2015). Results clearly showed that personalization led to an increased Heathy Eating Index (used as an overall measure of "healthfulness" of diet patterns), motivating and assisting participants in making appropriate choices more than conventional approaches (Celis-Morales et al., 2017). However, there was no clear additional benefit from delivering more sophisticated and expensive phenotypic and genotypic information. The study demonstrated that digitally delivered personalized dietary interventions could represent valuable tools as far as they could enhance intervention efficacy and be able to collect relevant data to be analyzed through intelligent and cost-effective systems (Celis-Morales, Lara, & Mathers, 2014). Furthermore, once study participants were clustered according to whether their baseline food intake met European dietary recommendations, those with the least adequate diet were found to benefit most from personalized diet intervention (Livingstone et al., 2016).

Positive behavior changes and motivation seem to be more likely when higher susceptibility to diseases is perceived. It is possible to facilitate such changes by using genetic testing as the catalyst (Bouwman & Koelen, 2007; Horne, Madill, O'Connor, Shelley, & Gilliland, 2018). Although genetic testing may lead to increased anxiety and distress (Lippi, Favaloro, & Plebani, 2011) or unnecessarily burden the healthcare system (McGuire & Burke, 2008), it has been suggested that individuals with personal experience of chronic diseases are more likely to undergo genetic testing and engage a nutrigenomics-based personalized dietary intervention (Fallaize, Macready, Butler, Ellis, & Lovegrove, 2013; Stewart-Knox, 2008; Ahlgren, 2013). However, knowledge of the genotype can have no effect in terms of lifestyle and dietary changes, as demonstrated in the case of *MTHFR* 677C→T polymorphism and folate intake within the Food4me study (O'Donovan et al., 2016). Similarly, diabetes genetic risk counseling (based on evaluation of 36 SNPs) was not found to alter significantly self-reported motivation and intention to adopt a prevention program in overweight individuals at risk (Grant et al., 2013). Additionally, communication of risk for Crohn's disease (based on family history and smoking status alone, or with additional DNA analysis for the *NOD2* genotype) was not related to an intention to stop smoking (Hollands et al., 2012).

There are several companies offering genetic testing and providing results directly to consumers, bypassing healthcare professionals through a Direct-To-Consumer (DTC) approach. This has been suggested to promote health behavior change (Bloss, Madlensky, Schork, & Topol, 2011), but conflicting evidence is available (Covolo, Rubinelli, Ceretti, & Gelatti, 2015; O'Donovan, Walsh, Gibney, Brennan, & Gibney, 2017; Stewart, Wesselius, & Schreurs, 2018). Upon reception of DTC results, examples of either positive lifestyle changes (Egglestone, Morris, & O'Brien, 2013; Kaufman, Bollinger, Dvoskin, & Scott, 2012) or no changes (Bloss, Schork, & Topol, 2011; Bloss, Wineinger, Darst, Schork, & Topol, 2013; Hollands et al., 2016; Smerecnik, Grispen, & Quaak, 2012) are reported.

The use of sensitive personal data is central to personalized nutrition: not only genetic, but also phenotypic and lifestyle data need to be disclosed to service providers, which implies potential negative consequences caused by privacy loss (Mothersbaugh, Foxx, Beatty, & Wang, 2011). It appears that health is the most important determinant to undergo genetic tests; personal experience of diseases (even in terms of affected relatives) or perceived increased susceptibility to disease are the most important motivators (Fallaize et al., 2013). Although the general public hold a positive view of nutrigenomics and personalized nutrition, still reservations persist on the ability to securely handle and use the data collected by the service providers (Stewart-Knox et al., 2015). Consumers' genetic data is sensitive information with far-reaching implications and ease of misuse. Public acceptance is a direct consequence of the estimation of benefits, costs, and risks. Transparent information on the potential benefits and the protection of consumers' personal data are likely to affect the adoption, the delivery of public health benefits, and the commercialization of personalized nutrition (Poínhos et al., 2014). Thus in order to consolidate adoption, service providers are asked to address specific concerns that have been raised by both researchers and consumers. These concerns are mainly related to:

1. The safety/reliability of the way information is collected and service delivered (through personal interaction with healthcare professionals or DTC approach).
2. Breaches of privacy, since inappropriate disclosure of genetic information to insurance companies, employers, or other public groups might raise the risk of discrimination (Shi & Wu, 2017).
3. Fear of results, since unwanted information may be found and delivered, causing unnecessary concerns and anxiety (Fallaize et al., 2013).

Consumers' trust in and preference for personalized nutrition services are significant predictors of the intention to adopt them (Poínhos et al., 2017). Service providers should take into account the serious consideration of privacy issues, reduce the perception of risks, and increase the perception of benefits (Berezowska, Fischer, Ronteltap, van der Lans, & van Trijp, 2015). This is especially relevant for novel communication tools, marketing approaches, online services, and apps, which are frequently used tools although doubts have been raised in terms of their efficacy and safety compared to the advice of health professionals (Kohlmeier et al., 2016). Privacy issues might keep consumers from engaging; this means that service providers should reduce consumers' perceived risks by using the least intrusive types of personal information and adequately anonymizing data (Berezowska et al., 2015). Concerns about inadequate procedures to guarantee data privacy, and distrust in commercial service providers may reduce the willingness to pay for such services regardless of perceived acceptance of personalized nutrition per se (Fischer et al., 2016).

FUTURE PERSPECTIVES

From Knowledge to Practice

Great expectations have arisen for personalized nutrition, stemming mainly from the idea that nutritional genomics could provide insights into the relationships among genes, diet, and environment. However, concerns about overpromising have been expressed (Ferguson et al., 2016; Kohlmeier et al., 2016) and more research is needed for personalized nutrition to achieve its expected goals (Camp & Trujillo, 2014). Despite significant advancements, personalized nutrition is not available for delivery at the population level yet (O'Donovan et al., 2016). The so far limited success of personalized nutrition may be due to three main reasons (Schork & Goetz, 2017):

1. More time is needed to identify definite connections between dietary interventions and specific individual profiles.
2. Molecular and physiological processes underlying these connections are complex to be deciphered.
3. Assessing the efficacy of interventions require different, nontrivial approaches based on different study design/analytical methods compared to classical population-based studies in order to collect enough data on a single subject and to allow for unequivocal inference about the unique response obtained.

Nutrigenetics is a promising field, but it is challenged by the methodological limitations associated with clinical research; underscoring the importance of such limitations might stimulate biohype (Stenne, Hurlimann, & Godard, 2012, 2013). Additionally, advances in the annotation of the human genome have not been paralleled by a concomitant shift in refined treatments, nor by the identification of genetic predictors able to discriminate between responders and nonresponders to treatments (Cardon & Harris, 2016; de Roos & Brennan, 2017). Most nutrigenetics studies assessing how dietary interventions can modify disease risk are based on associations only, being specifically focused on a specific genotype at a candidate gene locus; they often lack reproducibility and have limited statistical power, with findings not confirmed by others (de Roos & Brennan, 2017). The FINGEN study (Caslake et al., 2008) and a study on *MTHFR* polymorphisms and blood pressure (Wilson et al., 2012) are notable exceptions; apart from these, no other study provided conclusive evidence of how dietary changes or nutrient intake can affect the role of single SNPs. In general, our ability to define valid associations among genes, pathways and disease risk is limited (Hesketh, 2012), although the field is expanding rapidly.

There is an enormous number of genetic tests available on the market today (Hogarth & Saukko, 2017), which reflects not only the heterogeneity of the analyzed polymorphisms, but also specific population- or ethnic-related information sometimes lacking sufficient validation. Convincing evidence is available on how single gene variants may affect biological response to nutrients, but their predictive value on risk or risk factor levels for complex diseases is not well established (Kohlmeier et al., 2016). The complexity of the interactions among gene, nutrition, and health is an enormous challenge for healthcare professionals to keep track, manage, analyze, interpret, and apply personalized nutrition on a patient scale. Experts from both genomics and nutrition fields are urgently asked to provide summaries and working guidelines based on the available evidence (Murgia & Adamski, 2017). A multilevel organization of data able to capture knowledge from the type of intervention, the molecular/biological components and the final phenotype, as well as to describe how they are related, could help the design of decision trees and the delivery of customized recommendations (van Ommen et al., 2017), as exemplified in the Food4me study (Forster et al., 2016).

Complexity is an issue in assessing the efficacy of personalized nutrition interventions. Classical approaches through large, randomized controlled trials have demonstrated that only a minority of individuals in a cohort might respond to dietary interventions (Tierney et al., 2011), and lifestyle measures that reduce disease risk in an entire population may offer little benefit to specific individuals (de Roos & Brennan, 2017; Manach et al., 2017). However, assessing effects on single individuals through randomized controlled trials is an impractical task due to the vast number of genome—phenome—exome combinations that should be addressed (van Ommen et al., 2017). Clinical trials are usually designed to minimize variation across study population groups, which is by contrast the fundamental paradigm of personalization. In this framework, biological variability should not be dismissed as confounding, nor minimized through stratification. Tools to bring this genotypic and phenotypic variability into clinical research have been proposed and have gained momentum, such as the n-of-1 paradigm for clinical studies (Schork & Goetz, 2017) whose importance has been recognized also by regulatory agencies (e.g., FDA) (de Roos & Brennan, 2017). These n-of-1 trials collect data over a time course on a single subject undergoing different interventions. Study design, methods, and statistical issues of n-of-1 studies are nicely reviewed in Schork and Goetz (2017); notably, these studies can also be aggregated allowing for a generalization of results for other individuals or subpopulations sharing the same genetic or phenotypic factors (Schork & Goetz, 2017). A number of studies support the use of n-of-1 trials in the context of nutrition. For instance, it was recently described that changes in eating patterns of two subjects were reflected onto their microbiome on a daily timescale over a 1-year time course (David et al., 2014). Similarly, high variability in blood glucose levels after identical meals in an 800-person cohort (week-long monitoring of response to nearly 47,000 meals) was described, suggesting that individual dietary needs should be identified based on individuals' responses to dietary changes, as they are hard to be anticipated by any prior information on these individuals (Zeevi et al., 2015).

"Omic" Technologies

In the future, personalized nutrition approaches could significantly affect the way dietary advices are formulated. Nevertheless, in order to move from population-based, general guidelines to dietary customization for single individuals or population subgroups, several implementations are required. In this context, a deeper understanding of the interindividual variability in response to diet has been recently indicated by the American Society of Nutrition (ASN) as one of the main important points to be addressed in nutrition to face the imminent challenges in population health managing (Ohlhorst et al., 2013). Several goals and tools to achieve this aim were identified, such as (de Toro-Martín, Arsenault, Després, & Vohl, 2017):

- Enable an accurate prediction of the impact of nutrition on health through "omic" technologies and biomarker identification.
- Enhance patient information surveys through bioinformatics and database management.
- Assess disease progression and patient response to nutritional interventions through "omic" technologies and biomarker identification.

In the rapidly expanding era of "omic" technologies, a key point will be the fine phenotyping of individuals through nutrigenomics, nutriproteomics, and nutrimetabolomics at a systems biology perspective in order to identify specific biomarker signatures. Currently, biomarkers are mainly used to assess the effects of interventions, evaluating the impact of either diets or single nutrients, as indicators or predictors of pathological conditions. Although some nutritional biomarkers are now successfully used (e.g., serum retinol, zinc, ferritin, and folate), a comprehensive set of biomarkers to assess the nutritional status and metabolic conditions of nutritional relevance is not available yet (Rubio-Aliaga, Kochhar, & Silva-Zolezzi, 2012). Moreover, our current knowledge of biomarkers may not be adequate to understand complex diseases, which have the potential to start developing in the first decades of life (Mensink et al., 2003; Riccardi et al., 2004; Vasan, 2006) and biomarkers may not be able to reflect subtle dietary modifications (de Roos & Brennan, 2017). Yet, significant advances in the identification of novel biomarkers in nutrition have been made through the development of human intervention studies where transcriptomics, proteomics, metabolomics, and nutrigenetics approaches have been applied supported by robust bioinformatics and statistical methods (Rubio-Aliaga et al., 2012). Significant technological advancements have led us to a point where unraveling a variety of "omics" repertoires is feasible, providing a solid framework for a systems biology approach and a deeper understanding of dynamic changes in molecular components and biological pathways. The elucidation of an individual's "omics" profiles through iPOP (integrative personal omic profiling) was proposed as a tool to diagnose, manage. and treat diseases (Li-Pook-Than & Snyder, 2013). By allowing a deeper characterization of various "omics" repertoires, systems biology approaches could also increase the robustness of customized dietary interventions. Yet questions remain on how they could be incorporated into personalized nutrition interventions in order to achieve specific performance/health goals. Methods to share, analyze, integrate, and interpret data need further implementation, and still there are no examples of such an integrated approach in the context of personalized nutrition, which would offer the possibility to finely customize personalized interventions (van Ommen et al., 2017).

Progression in "omics" techniques is steadily pushing customized lifestyle medicine toward reality (Bland, Minich, & Eck, 2017). High-throughput platforms have allowed the powerful and comprehensive analysis of complex biological systems upon ingestion of a single phytochemical compound or following a new dietary and exercise regimen (Badimon et al., 2017). Transcriptomics, proteomics, metabolomics, and novel "omics" such as epigenomics, exposomics, interactomics, lipidomics, regulomics, and exosomics offer valuable tools to allow a comprehensive view of the effects of nutritional interventions on health (Badimon et al., 2017). For instance, they might allow a better understanding of nutrient bioactivity, bioefficacy, metabolic individuality, and ultimately help the search of nutritional biomarkers (Rubio-Aliaga et al., 2012).

Big Data and Machine Learning

Nutrition is central to health, social, and cultural contexts; understanding how nutrition can evolve in the era of big data from the scientific and technological point of view is a relevant research task on a worldwide scale (Ferguson, 2016; Pavlidis et al., 2015; Pavlidis, Nebel, Katsila, & Patrinos, 2016). Machine learning (ML) is bioinformatics approach capable of creating data-driven models that can "learn" information about a system directly from observed big data. ML algorithms improve their performance with each new data sample. Tasks of ML are typically classified into three categories (Russell & Norvig, 2003):

1. Supervised learning, in which the system infers a function from labeled training data. The system "learns" inductively a function (target function), which is an expression of a model describing the dataset. Such a function is used to predict the value of a variable, called a dependent or output variable, from a set of features, which are independent or input variables. A subset of all cases, for which the output variable value is known (labeled), is called training data or examples. In order to infer the best target function, the learning system, given a training set, takes into consideration alternative functions and selects the best one of them (Kavakiotis et al., 2017).
2. Unsupervised learning, in which the learning system tries to infer the structure of unlabeled data. The system tries to discover the hidden structure of data or associations between variables. In this case, training data consists of a set of input values without any corresponding labels. The used algorithms can vary, but the one most often used is clustering, that is dividing a whole dataset into groups that differ from each other, with each group containing similar objects (input data) (Jiawei, Micheline, & Jian, 2011).
3. Reinforcement learning, a general term given to a family of techniques, in which the system attempts to learn through direct interaction with the environment to maximize some notions of cumulative reward (Alpaydin, 2004).

Up to now, ML has become the main technology for several real-world applications from weather forecasting to DNA sequencing (Kavakiotis et al., 2017). One of the first steps in the ML algorithm development is the features selection. This is defined as the process of selecting a subset of features from the feature space, which is more relevant to and informative for the construction of a model. The advantages of feature selection are many, especially in a complex investigation like nutritional personalization, and relate to

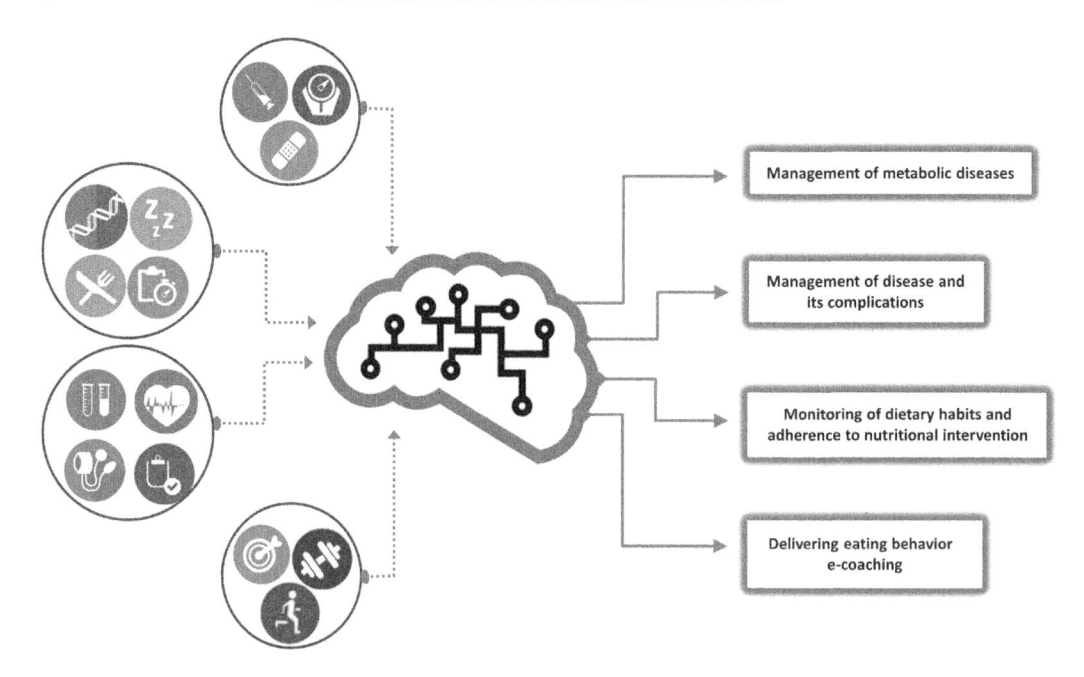

FIGURE 1.3 Personalized nutrition by prediction. Graphical representation of a machine learning approach from person profiling toward computational tools in health studies.[3]

different aspects of data analysis, such as better understanding of data, reduction of computational duration of analysis, and better prediction accuracy (Guyon & Elisseeff, 2003; Witten, Frank, & Hall, 2011).

Remarkable advances in biotechnology and health sciences have led to a significant production of data, so that the application of ML and data mining methods in biosciences has become vital and indispensable in efforts to transform intelligently all available information into valuable knowledge. Concerted efforts combining "omics," bioinformatics, ML approaches, big data mining/analysis, and computational modeling are needed in order to overcome challenges and exploit the full potential of personalized nutrition, developing highly customized dietary recommendations (Bashiardes et al., 2018; Maher, Pooler, Kaput, & Kussmann, 2016; Pranavchand & Reddy, 2016). Similarly, strong efforts will be needed in order to create a comprehensive framework allowing the application of these new findings at the population level. In a world characterized by an enhancement of obesity cases and associated metabolic disturbances, customized nutrition represents a promising approach for both the prevention and management of metabolic syndrome (de Toro-Martín et al., 2017).

Examples of the application of ML and computational tools in health studies are already available, as in the following contexts (Fig. 1.3):

1. *Management of metabolic diseases.* Diabetes mellitus is an ensemble of metabolic disorders widespread on a worldwide scale. Extensive research in all aspects of diabetes has led

---

[3] Original artwork by F. Pettini available at: https://commons.wikimedia.org/wiki/File:Machine_learning.jpg.

to the generation of huge amounts of data. In this framework, ML could help (Kavakiotis et al., 2017):
   a. The identification of diagnostic and prognostic markers (biomarker discovery). In this framework, a feature selection step is used at first, and then a classification algorithm is used to assess the prediction accuracy of the selected features.
   b. Prediction of disease, with a number of algorithms and approaches that have been applied to increase classification accuracy.
   c. The selection of the most effective drugs and therapy regimens (personalization). In the era of postgenomic drug development, data mining techniques can represent optimal tools to extract knowledge from large datasets (chemical, biological, clinical) offering stimulating challenges for the pharmaceutical industry. They can be used to recommend dietary approaches, medications, drug schedules, overall implementing drug administration in a more personalized fashion.
   d. Understanding the role of genetic background and environmental factors in disease development. Both type 1 and type 2 diabetes are due to a combination of genetic and environmental factors, and they are inherited with complex patterns. Significant advances in genotyping technology have facilitated large-scale genetic studies and offered the opportunity to associate genetic information with clinical practice, with possible relapse for risk prediction.
2. *Management of disease and its complications.* The main pathophysiological feature of diabetes is hyperglycemia, whose complications are of great concern. In their study, Zeevi et al. (2015) first highlighted huge interindividual variability in blood glucose levels after identical meals. Then they devised a ML algorithm integrating blood parameters, dietary habits, anthropometrics, physical activity, and gut microbiota data, that was able to accurately predict postprandial glycemic response. Results were independently validated in a smaller cohort; then, a blinded randomized controlled trial was carried out, demonstrating the efficacy of the algorithm to develop short-term personalized dietary interventions to successfully lower postmeal glycemic responses. Albers et al. (2017) were also able to generate a computational machinery approach relying on data assimilation and model development. Forecasts were empirically evaluated against both actual postprandial glucose measurements and predictions generated by experienced diabetes educators after reviewing a set of historical nutritional records and glucose measurements for the same individual. Interestingly, forecasts compared well with specific glucose measurements, and matched or even exceeded the accuracy of experts' forecasts. Such innovative prediction algorithms, which use clinical, nutritional, and lifestyle variables, exemplify the great possibilities offered by these sophisticated methods for further implementations in the field of personalized nutrition (de Toro-Martín et al., 2017).
3. *Monitoring of dietary habits and adherence to nutritional intervention.* Sophisticated statistical approaches may help in monitoring adherence to a nutritional intervention, which would lead to a more precise detection of the probable associations between dietary interventions and metabolic improvements (de Toro-Martín et al., 2017). In this context, it has been recently reported that adherence evaluation through trajectory analysis could allow researchers to understand how study participants evolve during a nutritional intervention depending upon their assigned nutritional group (Sevilla-Villanueva, Gibert,

Sanchez-Marre, Fito, & Covas, 2017). An artificial intelligence-based approach was proposed working on the classification of individuals according to 65 parameters divided into two blocks: one describing the health condition (biometric measures, tobacco and drug consumption, sociodemographic characteristics, diseases, and biomarkers); the other for food habits and physical activity. Clustering was performed before and after the study, creating trajectory maps showing changes in diet indicators (Sevilla-Villanueva et al., 2017). By using this approach, researchers could be able to unmask dietary changes within a given group, and to discriminate participants according to their particular diet trajectories during the study. This type of study could allow for a more accurate evaluation of adherence and characterization of the impact of the intervention.

4. *Delivering eating behavior e-coaching.* Eating behavior is a field that can benefit from the improvement of psychological theories and data science techniques. ML could efficiently be used to exploit data collected from mobile applications designed to assess eating behavior using experience-sampling methods. The final aim is to analyze individual person status (emotions, location, activity, etc.) and assess its impact on eating. In this framework, a classification algorithm was proposed to advise people prior to a possible unhealthy eating event. Results from this study revealed that participants could be clustered into six robust groups (the "evening at home" eaters, the "outdoors/social" eaters, the "circumstances-driven" eaters, the "very-occasional" eaters, the "after-activity" snackers, and the "unhealthy-cravings satisfaction" eaters) based on their eating behavior, and that there were specific rules discriminating which conditions lead to healthy or unhealthy eating. The effectiveness of the approach was confirmed by observing a decreasing trend in rule activation toward the end of the intervention period (Spanakis, Weiss, Boh, Lemmens, & Roefs, 2017).

Several challenges are likely to be faced by nutrition science in the coming years, especially in view of an increasing prevalence of obesity and associated metabolic disorders resulting largely from the adoption of unhealthy feeding behaviors in an obesogenic food environment where adherence to healthy dietary patterns has become increasingly difficult (de Toro-Martín et al., 2017). Central questions in the nutrition field include, for instance, what are the fundamental elements for a nutritionally balanced diet and what are the consequences of the failure to achieve a diet balance. Answering such questions is not an easy task. One is required to take into account the multidimensionality and dynamic nature of nutritional requirements, foods, and diets, and the intricate relationships between nutrition and health, but their inherent complexity can be overwhelming. How to face this complexity? An approach called the Geometric Framework for Nutrition (GFN) was proposed recently (Simpson et al., 2017) as a tool to understand the ways that nutrients, other dietary constituents, and their interactions influence physiology and health. Based both on observational and experimental studies, GFN has been used to shed light into the dietary determinants of chronic diseases associated with obesity and aging (David & Stephen, 2016; Gosby et al., 2011; Gosby, Conigrave, Raubenheimer, & Simpson, 2014; Le Couteur, Solon-Biet, Cogger, et al., 2016; Le Couteur, Solon-Biet, Wahl, et al., 2016; Simpson & Raubenheimer, 2005). It could be useful to design experiments that powerfully explore not only the main effects of a particular dietary intervention, but also the relationships with other dietary factors, therefore improving their overall reliability (Simpson et al., 2017).

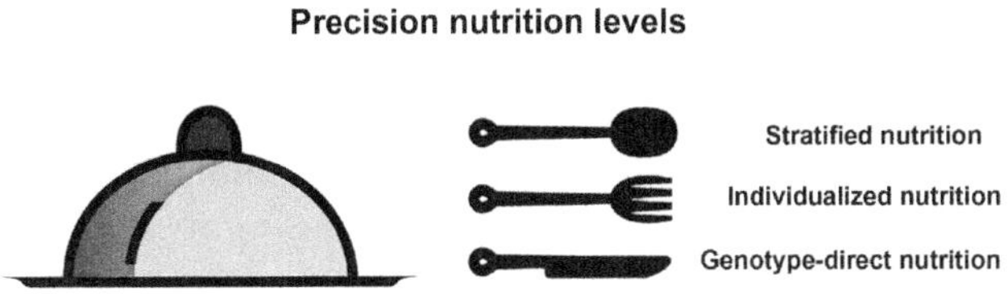

Precision nutrition levels

- Stratified nutrition
- Individualized nutrition
- Genotype-direct nutrition

FIGURE 1.4 The three levels of precision nutrition according to the International Society of Nutrigenetics/Nutrigenomics.[4]

What Is Needed for the Future?

According to the International Society of Nutrigenetics/Nutrigenomics (ISNN), the future of personalized nutrition could be discussed at different steps: stratification of conventional nutritional guidelines into population subgroups by age, gender, and other social determinants; individual approaches issued from a deep and refined phenotyping; and, in conclusion, a genetic-directed nutrition based on rare genetic variants having high penetrance and impact on individuals' responses to particular foods (Fig. 1.4) (Ferguson et al., 2016).

In order to exploit the potential of personalized nutrition, several challenges need to be faced in the near future, such as:

- The establishment of a strong and solid theoretical basis for personalized dietary approaches, with the identification of the most critical factors to be identified in the personalization process (Ordovas et al., 2018).
- The development of novel and more reliable tools to monitor food intake, enabling nutrient-related studies to be more accurate (Kohlmeier et al., 2016). Novel digital tools have been developed to replace Food Frequency Questionnaires (FFQs) and 24-hour dietary recall diaries. These tools are based on online, mobile, and sensor-based technologies, which are preferred over traditional methods mainly for their feasibility, scalability, and reduced burden to researchers and users. In particular, smartphones and apps have a huge potential, as they can reach large population groups and be more effective than traditional methods, although in some cases with limited validity and accuracy (Forster, Walsh, Gibney, Brennan, & Gibney, 2016). In this context, tracking food intake through mobile technology is increasingly exploited and expanding fast. For instance, tools to capture images of food and beverages to be sent to an analytical center where they can be identified and quantified are available, offering intuitive opportunities for technology-friendly users (Chae et al., 2011; Daugherty et al., 2012). In spite of these advancements, by contrast, analytical tools to *generate* the advice are far less described in the literature. The majority of studies relying on technology-based dietary assessment tools have been developed to provide personalized advice on specifically relevant nutrients or groups of foods. The already mentioned Food4me study stands out as one of the few exceptions, since decision trees were developed to provide personalized feedback according to online FFQs and nutrient-related goals (Celis-Morales et al., 2015). However, even if recent technologies have a huge potential to deliver personalized nutrition at a wider level, more work is still needed in order to include critical factors (feedback content, frequency, target population, personalization

---

[4] Original artwork by F. Pettini available at: https://commons.wikimedia.org/wiki/File:Precision_nutrition.jpg

of contents and feedback) able to increase efficacy and promote sustained dietary changes (Forster et al., 2016). Similarly, it will be fundamental to develop novel tools to assess dietary intake and nutrition status through a multipronged approach able to capture the multidimensional nature of diet (Bhupathiraju & Hu, 2017), and efforts will be necessary for their implementation and validation (de Roos & Brennan, 2017).

- The development and implementation of tools to collect and analyze biological samples. Dried blood spots represent useful tools to measure a number of analytes, as they can be easily used by consumers and then sent to analytical centers (Gibney & Walsh, 2013). In this context, there is a growing interest in developing monitoring devices coupled with mobile technology (e.g., to measure urinary or blood analytes, track physical activity or sleep, etc.). The growing interest in n-of-1 trial underscores the need for reliable and cost-effective data collection devices for self-monitoring, and for large databases and mining tools (Schork & Goetz, 2017).

- The quantification and modeling of multiple biomarkers to characterize a robust individual's metabolic signature through different "omic" technologies (Hesketh, 2012) and an integrative personal "omic" profiling. This would help to assess the efficacy of interventions, to enable a better follow-up of disease progression, and to better monitor metabolic interventions. Bioinformatics approaches should be developed too, providing appropriate tools for big data management, integration, and analysis. Although associated to major analytical challenges, only thanks to the integration of cutting-edge "omics" and robust bioinformatics tools through system biology approaches, a better understanding of diseases and translation of personalized nutrition into clinical practice might be achieved.

- The development of metaomics approaches that, although coupled to significant analytical and intrinsic challenges, could shed more light onto the intricate relationships connecting the host, its microbiota, and diet-related effects.

- The development of business models and the implementation of ethical rules for sensitive data (Kohlmeier et al., 2016). There is a strong need for guidelines and legal regulations both to protect individuals from unwanted relapses of genetic testing and to guarantee that analytical and clinical factors (validity and utility) are adequately taken into account (Kohlmeier et al., 2016). Informed consent represents a relevant tool for consumers rather than a mere formality, and efforts are needed to make consumers aware of the importance of such a document. The Food4me study showed that legal instruments specifically dealing with personalized nutrition are often lacking in Europe (Celis-Morales et al.).

- The assessment of the validity of nutrigenetics, which is an unregulated research field lacking definite standards, except for a few commercially adopted codes of practice. To overcome this, a draft framework of criteria to establish the validity of genes and diet interactions and to determine the likelihood that predicted outcomes will be consistent and reproducible was proposed recently (Grimaldi et al., 2017). Future work will be needed in order to regularly revise these criteria and use them as a basis for developing transparent and scientifically sound advice related to nutrigenetic tests.

- Addressing socioeconomic and ethical issues. A recent survey showed that higher socioeconomic classes had the highest willingness to pay for personalized nutrition services. A direct implication is that commercial markets may explicitly target this population, which is acknowledged to have better health already (Cohen, Rai, Rehkopf, & Abrams, 2013), to maximize incomes. This would not only have the least positive effect on public health, but also raise relevant socioeconomic and ethical issues (Fischer et al., 2016).

- Integrate personalized nutrition into routine clinical care, by increasing interest and providing adequate training of key personnel (Kohlmeier et al., 2016), as well as by increasing consumers' trust and confidence. To this aim, evidence for efficacy and cost-effectiveness is required, implying the more robust design of studies (n-of-1 or aggregated n-of-1 trials) and multidisciplinary research study teams (Ordovas et al., 2018).

To drive nutrition into a new era, it is necessary to commit the resources essential to undertake well-powered studies. Academic and commercial efforts are gathering huge volumes of data that will be crucial to understand which measurements are significant, what resolution is needed, and whether patterns in the data can be correlated to disease, wellness, or behavioral phenotypes. Even if the challenges must not be underestimated, it is becoming obvious that systems medicine really can change lives (McDonald, Glusman, & Price, 2016).

Acknowledgments

The authors would like to thank Francesco Pettini.

This work was supported by Regione Toscana grant OPENRICCIO (PSR 2014–2020) and grant BEERBONE (Nutraceutica 2015). The Department of Biotechnology, Chemistry and Pharmacy has been granted by the Minister of Education, University and Research (MIUR) as "Department of Excellence 2018–2022."

References

Ahlgren, J., Nordgren, A., Perrudin, M., Ronteltap, A., Savigny, J., van Trijp, H., Nordström, K., & Görman, U. (2013). Consumers on the Internet: ethical and legal aspects of commercialization of personalized nutrition. *Genes & Nutrition*, 8, 349–355.

Albers, D. J., Levine, M., Gluckman, B., Ginsberg, H., Hripcsak, G., & Mamykina, L. (2017). Personalized glucose forecasting for type 2 diabetes using data assimilation. *PLoS Computational Biology* (13), e1005232.

Alpaydin, E. (2004). *Introduction to machine learning*. The MIT Press.

Arena, S., Salzano, A. M., & Scaloni, A. (2016). Identification of protein markers for the occurrence of defrosted material in milk through a MALDI-TOF-MS profiling approach. *Journal of Proteomics*, 147, 56–65.

Badimon, L., Vilahur, G., & Padro, T. (2017). Systems biology approaches to understand the effects of nutrition and promote health. *British Journal of Clinical Pharmacology*, 83, 38–45.

Bashiardes, S., Godneva, A., Elinav, E., & Segal, E. (2018). Towards utilization of the human genome and microbiome for personalized nutrition. *Current Opinion in Biotechnology*, 51, 57–63.

Berezowska, A., Fischer, A. R. H., Ronteltap, A., van der Lans, I. A., & van Trijp, H. C. M. (2015). Consumer adoption of personalised nutrition services from the perspective of a risk-benefit trade-off. *Genes & Nutrition*, 10, 42.

Bernal, J., Mendiola, J. A., Ibanez, E., & Cifuentes, A. (2011). Advanced analysis of nutraceuticals. *Journal of Pharmaceutical and Biomedical Analysis*, 55, 758–774.

Bhupathiraju, S. N., & Hu, F. B. (2017). One (small) step towards precision nutrition by use of metabolomics. *The Lancet Diabetes & Endocrinology*, 5, 154–155.

Bland, J. S., Minich, D. M., & Eck, B. M. (2017). A systems medicine approach: Translating emerging science into individualized wellness. *Advances in Medicine*, 5. Available from http://dx.doi.org/10.1155/2017/1718957.

Bloss, C. S., Madlensky, L., Schork, N. J., & Topol, E. J. (2011). Genomic information as a behavioral health intervention: Can it work? *Personalized Medicine, 8*, 659−667.

Bloss, C. S., Schork, N. J., & Topol, E. J. (2011). Effect of direct-to-consumer genomewide profiling to assess disease risk. *New England Journal of Medicine, 364*, 524−534.

Bloss, C. S., Wineinger, N. E., Darst, B. F., Schork, N. J., & Topol, E. J. (2013). Impact of direct-to-consumer genomic testing at long term follow-up. *Journal of Medical Genetics, 50*, 393−400.

Bordoni, A., & Capozzi, F. (2014). Foodomics for healthy nutrition. *Current Opinion in Clinical Nutrition and Metabolic Care, 17*, 418−424.

Bordoni, A., Laghi, L., Babini, E., Di Nunzio, M., Picone, G., Ciampa, A., et al. (2014). The foodomics approach for the evaluation of protein bioaccessibility in processed meat upon in vitro digestion. *Electrophoresis, 35*, 1607−1614.

Bordoni, A., Picone, G., Babini, E., Vignali, M., Danesi, F., Valli, V., et al. (2011). NMR comparison of in vitro digestion of Parmigiano Reggiano cheese aged 15 and 30 months. *Magnetic Resonance in Chemistry, 49*, S61−S70.

Boschetti, E., & Righetti, P. G. (2012). Breakfast at Tiffany's? Only with a low-abundance proteomic signature!. *Electrophoresis, 33*, 2228−2239.

Bouwman, L. I., & Koelen, M. A. (2007). Communication on personalised nutrition: Individual-environment interaction. *Genes & Nutrition, 2*, 81−83.

Braconi, D., Bernardini, G., Millucci, L., & Santucci, A. (2018). Foodomics for human health: Current status and perspectives. *Expert Review of Proteomics, 15*, 153−164.

Brennan, L. (2017). Use of metabotyping for optimal nutrition. *Current Opinion in Biotechnology, 44*, 35−38.

Camp, K. M., & Trujillo, E. (2014). Position of the academy of nutrition and dietetics: Nutritional genomics. *Journal of the Academy of Nutrition and Dietetics, 114*, 299−312.

Capozzi, F., & Bordoni, A. (2013). Foodomics: A new comprehensive approach to food and nutrition. *Genes & Nutrition, 8*, 1−4.

Cardon, L. R., & Harris, T. (2016). Precision medicine, genomics and drug discovery. *Human Molecular Genetics, 25*, R166−R172.

Caslake, M. J., Miles, E. A., Kofler, B. M., Lietz, G., Curtis, P., Armah, C. K., et al. (2008). Effect of sex and genotype on cardiovascular biomarker response to fish oils: The FINGEN Study. *The American Journal of Clinical Nutrition, 88*, 618−629.

Celis-Morales, C., Lara, J., & Mathers, J. C. (2014). Personalising nutritional guidance for more effective behaviour change. *Proceedings of the Nutrition Society, 74*, 130−138.

Celis-Morales, C., Livingstone, K. M., Marsaux, C. F. M., Forster, H., O'Donovan, C. B., Woolhead, C., et al. (2015). Design and baseline characteristics of the Food4Me study: A web-based randomised controlled trial of personalised nutrition in seven European countries. *Genes & Nutrition, 10*, 450.

Celis-Morales, C., Livingstone, K. M., Marsaux, C. F. M., Macready, A. L., Fallaize, R., O'Donovan, C. B., et al. (2017). Effect of personalized nutrition on health-related behaviour change: Evidence from the Food4Me European randomized controlled trial. *International Journal of Epidemiology, 46*, 578−588.

Celis-Morales, C., Mathers, J., Gibney, M., Walsh, M., Eufics, Gibney, E., et al. White paper on personalised nutrition - paving a way to better population health. doi: 10.13140/RG.2.2.13147.16166.

Chae, J., Woo, I., Kim, S., Maciejewski, R., Zhu, F., Delp, E. J., et al. (2011). Volume estimation using food specific shape templates in mobile image-based dietary assessment. *Proceedings of SPIE - The International Society for Optical Engineering, 7873*, 78730K.

Cifuentes, A. (2009). Food analysis and foodomics. *Journal of Chromatography A, 1216*, 7109.

Claus, S. P. (2014). Development of personalized functional foods needs metabolic profiling. *Current Opinion in Clinical Nutrition and Metabolic Care, 17*, 567−573.

Cohen, A. K., Rai, M., Rehkopf, D. H., & Abrams, B. (2013). Educational attainment and obesity: A systematic review. *Obesity Reviews: An Official Journal of the International Association for the Study of Obesity, 14*, 989−1005.

Corella, D., Asensio, E. M., Coltell, O., Sorlí, J. V., Estruch, R., Martínez-González, M. Á., et al. (2016). CLOCK gene variation is associated with incidence of type-2 diabetes and cardiovascular diseases in type-2 diabetic subjects: Dietary modulation in the PREDIMED randomized trial. *Cardiovascular Diabetology, 15*, 4.

Corella, D., Carrasco, P., Sorlí, J. V., Estruch, R., Rico-Sanz, J., Martínez-González, M. Á., et al. (2013). Mediterranean diet reduces the adverse effect of the TCF7L2-rs7903146 polymorphism on cardiovascular risk factors and stroke incidence. A randomized controlled trial in a high-cardiovascular-risk population. *Diabetes Care, 36*, 3803−3811.

Corella, D., Peloso, G., Arnett, D. K., et al. (2009). Apoa2, dietary fat, and body mass index: Replication of a gene-diet interaction in 3 independent populations. *Archives of Internal Medicine, 169*, 1897–1906.

Covolo, L., Rubinelli, S., Ceretti, E., & Gelatti, U. (2015). Internet-based direct-to-consumer genetic testing: A systematic review. *Journal of Medical Internet Research, 17*, e279.

Cuadros-Rodríguez, L., Ruiz-Samblás, C., Valverde-Som, L., Pérez-Castaño, E., & González-Casado, A. (2016). Chromatographic fingerprinting: An innovative approach for food 'identitation' and food authentication − A tutorial. *Analytica Chimica Acta, 909*, 9–23.

Danesi, F., Govoni, M., D'Antuono, L. F., & Bordoni, A. (2016). The molecular mechanism of the cholesterol-lowering effect of dill and kale: The influence of the food matrix components. *Electrophoresis, 37*, 1805–1813.

Daugherty, B. L., Schap, T. E., Ettienne-Gittens, R., Zhu, F. M., Bosch, M., Delp, E. J., et al. (2012). Novel technologies for assessing dietary intake: Evaluating the usability of a mobile telephone food record among adults and adolescents. *Journal of Medical Internet Research, 14*, e58.

David, L. A., Materna, A. C., Friedman, J., Campos-Baptista, M. I., Blackburn, M. C., Perrotta, A., et al. (2014). Host lifestyle affects human microbiota on daily timescales. *Genome Biology, 15*, R89.

David, L. A., Maurice, C. F., Carmody, R. N., Gootenberg, D. B., Button, J. E., Wolfe, B. E., et al. (2014). Diet rapidly and reproducibly alters the human gut microbiome. *Nature, 505*, 559–563.

David, R., & Stephen, J. S. (2016). Nutritional ecology and human health. *Annual Review of Nutrition, 36*, 603–626.

de Luca, A., Hankard, R., Borys, J. M., Sinnett, D., Marcil, V., & Levy, E. (2017). Nutriepigenomics and malnutrition. *Epigenomics, 9*, 893–917.

de Roos, B., & Brennan, L. (2017). Personalised interventions-precision approach for the next generation of dietary intervention studies. *Nutrients, 9*, 847.

de Toro-Martín, J., Arsenault, B., Després, J.-P., & Vohl, M.-C. (2017). Precision nutrition: A review of personalized nutritional approaches for the prevention and management of metabolic syndrome. *Nutrients, 9*, 913.

Deng, Y., Misselwitz, B., Dai, N., & Fox, M. (2015). Lactose intolerance in adults: Biological mechanism and dietary management. *Nutrients, 7*, 8020–8035.

Doyon, M., & Labrecque, J. (2008). Functional foods: A conceptual definition. *British Food Journal, 110*, 1133–1149.

Egglestone, C., Morris, A., & O'Brien, A. (2013). Effect of direct-to-consumer genetic tests on health behaviour and anxiety: A survey of consumers and potential consumers. *Journal of Genetic Counseling, 22*, 565–575.

El-Sohemy, A. (2007). Nutrigenetics. *Forum of Nutrition, 60*, 25–30.

Faith, J. J., Guruge, J. L., Charbonneau, M., Subramanian, S., Seedorf, H., Goodman, A. L., et al. (2013). The long-term stability of the human gut microbiota. *Science, 341*, 1237439.

Fall, T., & Ingelsson, E. (2014). Genome-wide association studies of obesity and metabolic syndrome. *Molecular and Cellular Endocrinology, 382*, 740–757.

Fallaize, R., Macready, A. L., Butler, L. T., Ellis, J. A., & Lovegrove, J. A. (2013). An insight into the public acceptance of nutrigenomic-based personalised nutrition. *Nutrition Research Reviews, 26*, 39–48.

Fenech, M., El-Sohemy, A., Cahill, L., Ferguson, L. R., French, T. A. C., Tai, E. S., et al. (2011). Nutrigenetics and nutrigenomics: Viewpoints on the current status and applications in nutrition research and practice. *Lifestyle Genomics, 4*, 69–89.

Ferguson, L. R. (2016). The value of nutrigenomics science. *OMICS: A Journal of Integrative Biology, 20*, 122.

Ferguson, L. R., De Caterina, R., Görman, U., Allayee, H., Kohlmeier, M., Prasad, C., et al. (2016). Guide and position of the International Society of Nutrigenetics/Nutrigenomics on personalised nutrition: Part 1 - Fields of precision nutrition. *Lifestyle Genomics, 9*, 12–27.

Fischer, A. R. H., Berezowska, A., van der Lans, I. A., Ronteltap, A., Rankin, A., Kuznesof, S., et al. (2016). Willingness to pay for personalised nutrition across Europe. *European Journal of Public Health, 26*, 640–644.

Forster, H., Walsh, M. C., Gibney, M. J., Brennan, L., & Gibney, E. R. (2016). Personalised nutrition: The role of new dietary assessment methods. *Proceedings of the Nutrition Society, 75*, 96–105.

Forster, H., Walsh, M. C., O'Donovan, C. B., Woolhead, C., McGirr, C., Daly, E. J., et al. (2016). A dietary feedback system for the delivery of consistent personalized dietary advice in the web-based multicenter Food4Me study. *Journal of Medical Internet Research, 18*, e150.

Fumagalli, M., Moltke, I., Grarup, N., Racimo, F., Bjerregaard, P., Jørgensen, M. E., et al. (2015). Greenlandic Inuit show genetic signatures of diet and climate adaptation. *Science, 349*, 1343–1347.

Gallo, M., & Ferranti, P. (2016). The evolution of analytical chemistry methods in foodomics. *Journal of Chromatography A, 1428*, 3–15.

Garrod, A. E. (1996). The incidence of alkaptonuria: A study in chemical individuality. 1902. *Molecular Medicine, 2*, 274–282.

Gibney, M., Walsh, M., & Goosens, J. (2016). Personalized nutrition: Paving the way to better population health. In M. Eggersdorfer, K. Kraemer, J. B. Cordaro, J. Fanzo, M. Gibney, E. Kennedy, A. Labrique, & J. Steffen (Eds.), *Good nutrition: Perspectives for the 21st century* (pp. 235–248). Basel: Karger.

Gibney, M. J., & Walsh, M. C. (2013). The future direction of personalised nutrition: My diet, my phenotype, my genes. *Proceedings of the Nutrition Society, 72*, 219–225.

Goni, L., Milagro, F. I., Cuervo, M., & Martinez, J. A. (2014). Single-nucleotide polymorphisms and DNA methylation markers associated with central obesity and regulation of body weight. *Nutrition Review, 72*, 673–690.

Gosby, A. K., Conigrave, A. D., Lau, N. S., Iglesias, M. A., Hall, R. M., Jebb, S. A., et al. (2011). Testing protein leverage in lean humans: A randomised controlled experimental study. *Public Library of Science One, 6*, e25929.

Gosby, A. K., Conigrave, A. D., Raubenheimer, D., & Simpson, S. J. (2014). Protein leverage and energy intake. *Obesity Reviews, 15*, 183–191.

Goto, Y., Kurashima, Y., & Kiyono, H. (2015). The gut microbiota and inflammatory bowel disease. *Current Opinion of Rheumatology, 27*, 388–396.

Grant, R. W., O'Brien, K. E., Waxler, J. L., Vassy, J. L., Delahanty, L. M., Bissett, L. G., et al. (2013). Personalized genetic risk counseling to motivate diabetes prevention. A randomized trial. *Diabetes Care, 36*, 13–19.

Greer, R., Dong, X., Morgun, A., & Shulzhenko, N. (2016). Investigating a holobiont: Microbiota perturbations and transkingdom networks. *Gut Microbes, 7*, 126–135.

Grimaldi, K. A., van Ommen, B., Ordovas, J. M., Parnell, L. D., Mathers, J. C., Bendik, I., et al. (2017). Proposed guidelines to evaluate scientific validity and evidence for genotype-based dietary advice. *Genes & Nutrition, 12*, 35.

Guven-Maiorov, E., Tsai, C. J., & Nussinov, R. (2017). Structural host-microbiota interaction networks. *PLoS Computational Biology, 13*, e1005579.

Guyon, I., & Elisseeff, A. (2003). An introduction to variable and feature selection. *Journal of Machine Learning Research, 3*, 1157–1182.

Hadrich, D. (2018). Microbiome research is becoming the key to better understanding health and nutrition. *Frontiers in Genetics, 9*, 212.

Hartigan, J. A., & Wong, M. A. (1979). Algorithm AS 136: A K-means clustering algorithm. *Journal of the Royal Statistical Society. Series C (Applied Statistics), 28*, 100–108.

Herrero, M., Simo, C., Garcia-Canas, V., Ibanez, E., & Cifuentes, A. (2012). Foodomics: MS-based strategies in modern food science and nutrition. *Mass Spectrometry Reviews, 31*, 49–69.

Hesketh, J. (2012). Personalised nutrition: How far has nutrigenomics progressed? *European Journal of Clinical Nutrition, 67*, 430.

Hogarth, S., & Saukko, P. (2017). A market in the making: The past, present and future of direct-to-consumer genomics. *New Genetics and Society, 36*, 197–208.

Hollands, G. J., French, D. P., Griffin, S. J., Prevost, A. T., Sutton, S., King, S., et al. (2016). The impact of communicating genetic risks of disease on risk-reducing health behaviour: Systematic review with meta-analysis. *The British Medical Journal, 352*, i1102.

Hollands, G. J., Whitwell, S. C. L., Parker, R. A., Prescott, N. J., Forbes, A., Sanderson, J., et al. (2012). Effect of communicating DNA based risk assessments for Crohn's disease on smoking cessation: Randomised controlled trial. *The British Medical Journal, 345*, e4708.

Horne, J., Madill, J., O'Connor, C., Shelley, J., & Gilliland, J. (2018). A systematic review of genetic testing and lifestyle behaviour change: Are we using high-quality genetic interventions and considering behaviour change theory?. *Lifestyle Genomics, 11*(1), 49–63.

Ibanez, C., Simo, C., Garcia-Canas, V., Acunha, T., & Cifuentes, A. (2015). The role of direct high-resolution mass spectrometry in foodomics. *Analytical and Bioanalytical Chemistry, 407*, 6275–6287.

Ibanez, C., Simo, C., Garcia-Canas, V., Cifuentes, A., & Castro-Puyana, M. (2013). Metabolomics, peptidomics and proteomics applications of capillary electrophoresis-mass spectrometry in Foodomics: A review. *Analytica Chimica Acta, 802*, 1–13.

Jiawei, H., Micheline, K., & Jian, P. (2011). *Data mining: Concepts and techniques*. Morgan Kaufmann Publishers Inc.

Kakkoura, M. G., Loizidou, M. A., Demetriou, C. A., Loucaides, G., Daniel, M., Kyriacou, K., et al. (2017). The synergistic effect between the Mediterranean diet and GSTP1 or NAT2 SNPs decreases breast cancer risk in Greek-Cypriot women. *European Journal of Nutrition, 56*, 545–555.

REFERENCES

Kaufman, D. J., Bollinger, J. M., Dvoskin, R. L., & Scott, J. A. (2012). Risky business: Risk perception and the use of medical services among customers of DTC personal genetic testing. *Journal of Genetic Counseling, 21*, 413–422.

Kavakiotis, I., Tsave, O., Salifoglou, A., Maglaveras, N., Vlahavas, I., & Chouvarda, I. (2017). Machine learning and data mining methods in diabetes research. *Computational and Structural Biotechnology Journal, 15*, 104–116.

Kelly, J. R., Minuto, C., Cryan, J. F., Clarke, G., & Dinan, T. G. (2017). Cross talk: The microbiota and neurodevelopmental disorders. *Frontiers in Neuroscience, 11*, 490.

Knowler, W., Barrett-Connor, E., Fowler, S., Hamman, R., Lachin, J., Walker, E., et al. (2002). Reduction in the incidence of type 2 diabetes with lifestyle intervention or metformin. *New England Journal of Medicine, 346*, 393–403.

Kohlmeier, M., De Caterina, R., Ferguson, L. R., Gorman, U., Allayee, H., Prasad, C., et al. (2016). Guide and position of the International Society of Nutrigenetics/Nutrigenomics on personalized nutrition: Part 2 - Ethics, challenges and endeavors of precision nutrition. *Journal of Nutrigenetics and Nutrigenomics, 9*, 28–46.

Korem, T., Zeevi, D., Zmora, N., Weissbrod, O., Bar, N., Lotan-Pompan, M., et al. (2017). Bread affects clinical parameters and induces gut microbiome-associated personal glycemic responses. *Cell Metabolism, 25*, 1243–1253, e1245.

Kussmann, M., Raymond, F., & Affolter, M. (2006). OMICS-driven biomarker discovery in nutrition and health. *Journal of Biotechnology, 124*, 758–787.

Le Couteur, D. G., Solon-Biet, S., Cogger, V. C., Mitchell, S. J., Senior, A., de Cabo, R., et al. (2016). The impact of low-protein high-carbohydrate diets on aging and lifespan. *Cellular and Molecular Life Sciences, 73*, 1237–1252.

Le Couteur, D. G., Solon-Biet, S., Wahl, D., Cogger, V. C., Willcox, B. J., Willcox, D. C., et al. (2016). New horizons: Dietary protein, ageing and the Okinawan ratio. *Age and Ageing, 45*, 443–447.

Levin, B. L., & Varga, E. (2016). MTHFR: Addressing genetic counseling dilemmas using evidence-based literature. *Journal of Genetic Counseling, 25*, 901–911.

Li, S. X., Imamura, F., Ye, Z., Schulze, M. B., Zheng, J., Ardanaz, E., et al. (2017). Interaction between genes and macronutrient intake on the risk of developing type 2 diabetes: Systematic review and findings from European Prospective Investigation into Cancer (EPIC)-InterAct. *The American Journal of Clinical Nutrition, 106*, 263–275.

Li-Pook-Than, J., & Snyder, M. (2013). iPOP goes the world: Integrated personalized omics profiling and the road towards improved health care. *Chemistry & Biology, 20*, 660–666.

Lippi, G., Favaloro, E. J., & Plebani, M. (2011). Direct-to-consumer testing: More risks than opportunities. *International Journal of Clinical Practice, 65*, 1221–1229.

Livingstone, K. M., Celis-Morales, C., Lara, J., Woolhead, C., O'Donovan, C. B., Forster, H., et al. (2016). Clustering of adherence to personalised dietary recommendations and changes in healthy eating index within the Food4Me study. *Public Health Nutrition, 19*, 3296–3305.

Lopez-Rubio, A., Flanagan, B. M., Shrestha, A. K., Gidley, M. J., & Gilbert, E. P. (2008). Molecular rearrangement of starch during in vitro digestion: Toward a better understanding of enzyme resistant starch formation in processed starches. *Biomacromolecules, 9*, 1951–1958.

Maguire, M., & Maguire, G. (2017). The role of microbiota, and probiotics and prebiotics in skin health. *Archives of Dermatological Research, 309*, 411–421.

Maher, M., Pooler, A. M., Kaput, J., & Kussmann, M. (2016). A systems approach to personalised nutrition: Report on the keystone symposium "Human nutrition, environment and health. *Applied & Translational Genomics, 10*, 16–18.

Maier, T. V., Lucio, M., Lee, L. H., VerBerkmoes, N. C., Brislawn, C. J., Bernhardt, J., et al. (2017). Impact of dietary resistant starch on the human gut microbiome, metaproteome, and metabolome. *MBio, 8*. Available from https://doi.org/10.1128/mBio.01343-17.

Manach, C., Milenkovic, D., Van de Wiele, T., Rodriguez-Mateos, A., de Roos, B., Garcia-Conesa, M. T., et al. (2017). Addressing the inter-individual variation in response to consumption of plant food bioactives: Towards a better understanding of their role in healthy aging and cardiometabolic risk reduction. *Molecular Nutrition & Food Research, 61*, 1600557.

Martinović, T., Andjelković, U., Gajdošik, M. Š., Rešetar, D., & Josić, D. (2016). Foodborne pathogens and their toxins. *Journal of Proteomics, 147*, 226–235.

Martirosyan, D. M., & Singh, J. (2015). A new definition of functional food by FFC: What makes a new definition unique? *Functional Foods in Health and Diseases, 5*(6), 209–223.

Mathers, J. C. (2017). Nutrigenomics in the modern era. *Proceedings of the Nutrition Society, 76*, 265–275.

Mathieson, I., Lazaridis, I., Rohland, N., Mallick, S., Patterson, N., Roodenberg, S. A., et al. (2015). Genome-wide patterns of selection in 230 ancient Eurasians. *Nature, 528*, 499–503.

McDonald, D., Glusman, G., & Price, N. D. (2016). Personalized nutrition through big data. *Nature Biotechnology, 34*, 152.

McGuire, A. L., & Burke, W. (2008). An unwelcome side effect of direct-to-consumer personal genome testing: Raiding the medical commons. *Journal of American Medical Society, 300*, 2669–2671.

Mensink, R. P., Aro, A., Den Hond, E., German, J. B., Griffin, B. A., ten Meer, H. U., et al. (2003). PASSCLAIM - Diet-related cardiovascular disease. *European Journal of Nutrition, 42*(Suppl. 1), I6–27.

Moco, S., Martin, F. P., & Rezzi, S. (2012). Metabolomics view on gut microbiome modulation by polyphenol-rich foods. *Journal of Proteome Research, 11*, 4781–4790.

Morris, C., O'Grada, C., Ryan, M., Roche, H. M., Gibney, M. J., Gibney, E. R., et al. (2013). Identification of differential responses to an oral glucose tolerance test in healthy adults. *Public Library of Science One, 8*, e72890.

Mothersbaugh, D. L., Foxx, W. K., Beatty, S. E., & Wang, S. (2011). Disclosure antecedents in an online service context: The role of sensitivity of information. *Journal of Service Research, 15*, 76–98.

Murgia, C., & Adamski, M. M. (2017). Translation of nutritional genomics into nutrition practice: The next step. *Nutrients, 9*, 366.

Nazzaro, F., Orlando, P., Fratianni, F., Di Luccia, A., & Coppola, R. (2012). Protein analysis-on-chip systems in foodomics. *Nutrients, 4*, 1475–1489.

O'Donovan, C. B., Walsh, M. C., Forster, H., Woolhead, C., Celis-Morales, C., Fallaize, R., et al. (2016). The impact of MTHFR 677C→T risk knowledge on changes in folate intake: Findings from the Food4Me study. *Genes & Nutrition, 11*, 25.

O'Donovan, C. B., Walsh, M. C., Gibney, M. J., Brennan, L., & Gibney, E. R. (2017). Knowing your genes: Does this impact behaviour change? *Proceedings of the Nutrition Society, 76*, 182–191.

O'Donovan, C. B., Walsh, M. C., Gibney, M. J., Gibney, E. R., & Brennan, L. (2016). Can metabotyping help deliver the promise of personalised nutrition? *Proceedings of the Nutrition Society, 75*, 106–114.

O'Donovan, C. B., Walsh, M. C., Nugent, A. P., McNulty, B., Walton, J., Flynn, A., et al. (2014). Use of metabotyping for the delivery of personalised nutrition. *Molecular Nutrition & Food Research, 59*, 377–385.

O'Donovan, C. B., Walsh, M. C., Woolhead, C., Forster, H., Celis-Morales, C., Fallaize, R., et al. (2017). Metabotyping for the development of tailored dietary advice solutions in a European population: The Food4Me study. *British Journal of Nutrition, 118*, 561–569.

Ohlhorst, S. D., Russell, R., Bier, D., Klurfeld, D. M., Li, Z., Mein, J. R., et al. (2013). Nutrition research to affect food and a healthy life span. *The American Journal of Clinical Nutrition, 98*, 620–625.

Ordovas, J. M., Ferguson, L. R., Tai, E. S., & Mathers, J. C. (2018). Personalised nutrition and health. *The British Medical Journal, 361*. Available from https://doi.org/10.1136/bmj.k2173.

O'Sullivan, A., Gibney, M. J., Connor, A. O., Mion, B., Kaluskar, S., Cashman, K. D., et al. (2011). Biochemical and metabolomic phenotyping in the identification of a vitamin D responsive metabotype for markers of the metabolic syndrome. *Molecular Nutrition & Food Research, 55*, 679–690.

Özdemir, V., & Kolker, E. (2016). Precision Nutrition 4.0: A big data and ethics foresight analysis--Convergence of agrigenomics, nutrigenomics, nutriproteomics, and nutrimetabolomics. *OMICS: A Journal of Integrative Biology, 20*, 69–75.

Parnell, L. D., Blokker, B. A., Dashti, H. S., Nesbeth, P.-D., Cooper, B. E., Ma, Y., et al. (2014). CardioGxE, a catalog of gene-environment interactions for cardiometabolic traits. *BioData Mining, 7*, 21.

Pavlidis, C., Lanara, Z., Balasopoulou, A., Nebel, J. C., Katsila, T., & Patrinos, G. P. (2015). Meta-analysis of genes in commercially available nutrigenomic tests denotes lack of association with dietary intake and nutrient-related pathologies. *Omics, 19*, 512–520.

Pavlidis, C., Nebel, J.-C., Katsila, T., & Patrinos, G. P. (2016). Nutrigenomics 2.0: The need for ongoing and independent evaluation and synthesis of commercial nutrigenomics tests' scientific knowledge base for responsible innovation. *OMICS: A Journal of Integrative Biology, 20*, 65–68.

Pavlidis, C., Patrinos, G. P., & Katsila, T. (2015). Nutrigenomics: A controversy. *Applied & Translational Genomics, 4*, 50–53.

Peregrin, T. (2001). The new frontier of nutrition science: Nutrigenomics. *Journal of the American Dietetic Association, 101*, 1306.

Phillips, C. M. (2013). Nutrigenetics and metabolic disease: Current status and implications for personalised nutrition. *Nutrients, 5*, 32–57.

REFERENCES

Picariello, G., Mamone, G., Nitride, C., Addeo, F., & Ferranti, P. (2013). Protein digestomics: Integrated platforms to study food-protein digestion and derived functional and active peptides. *TrAC Trends in Analytical Chemistry, 52*, 120−134.

Poínhos, R., Oliveira, B. M. P. M., van der Lans, I. A., Fischer, A. R. H., Berezowska, A., Rankin, A., et al. (2017). Providing personalised nutrition: Consumers' trust and preferences regarding sources of information, service providers and regulators, and communication channels. *Public Health Genomics, 20*, 218−228.

Poínhos, R., van der Lans, I. A., Rankin, A., Fischer, A. R. H., Bunting, B., Kuznesof, S., et al. (2014). Psychological determinants of consumer acceptance of personalised nutrition in 9 European countries. *Public Library of Science One, 9*, e110614.

Pranavchand, R., & Reddy, B. M. (2016). Genomics era and complex disorders: Implications of GWAS with special reference to coronary artery disease, type 2 diabetes mellitus, and cancers. *Journal of Postgraduate Medicine, 62*, 188−198.

Putignani, L., & Dallapiccola, B. (2016). Foodomics as part of the host-microbiota-exposome interplay. *Journal of Proteomics, 147*, 3−20.

Rankin, A., Bunting, B. P., Poínhos, R., van der Lans, I. A., Fischer, A. R. H., Kuznesof, S., et al. (2018). Food choice motives, attitude towards and intention to adopt personalised nutrition. *Public Health Nutrition*, 1−11.

Remely, M., Stefanska, B., Lovrecic, L., Magnet, U., & Haslberger, A. G. (2015). Nutriepigenomics: The role of nutrition in epigenetic control of human diseases. *Current Opinion in Clinical Nutrition and Metabolic Care, 18*, 328−333.

Riccardi, G., Aggett, P., Brighenti, F., Delzenne, N., Frayn, K., Nieuwenhuizen, A., et al. (2004). PASSCLAIM--Body weight regulation, insulin sensitivity and diabetes risk. *European Journal of Nutrition, 43*(Suppl. 2), II7−II46.

Riedl, A., Gieger, C., Hauner, H., Daniel, H., & Linseisen, J. (2017). Metabotyping and its application in targeted nutrition: An overview. *British Journal of Nutrition, 117*, 1631−1644.

Robinette, S. L., Bruschweiler, R., Schroeder, F. C., & Edison, A. S. (2012). NMR in metabolomics and natural products research: Two sides of the same coin. *Accounts of Chemical Research, 45*, 288−297.

Roper, J. A. (1960). Genetic determination of nutritional requirements. *Proceedings of the Nutrition Society, 19*, 39−45.

Rowland, I., Gibson, G., Heinken, A., Scott, K., Swann, J., Thiele, I., et al. (2017). Gut microbiota functions: Metabolism of nutrients and other food components. *European Journal of Nutrition, 57*, 1−24.

Rubio-Aliaga, I., Kochhar, S., & Silva-Zolezzi, I. (2012). Biomarkers of nutrient bioactivity and efficacy: A route toward personalized nutrition. *Journal of Clinical Gastroenterology, 46*, 545−554.

Russell, S., & Norvig, P. (2003). *Artificial intelligence: A modern approach* (2nd ed.). Prentice Hall.

Santoru, M. L., Piras, C., Murgia, A., Palmas, V., Camboni, T., Liggi, S., et al. (2017). Cross sectional evaluation of the gut-microbiome metabolome axis in an Italian cohort of IBD patients. *Scientific Reports, 7*, 9523.

Scalbert, A., Brennan, L., Manach, C., Andres-Lacueva, C., Dragsted, L. O., Draper, J., et al. (2014). The food metabolome: A window over dietary exposure. *The American Journal of Clinical Nutrition, 99*(6), 1286−1308.

Schork, N. J., & Goetz, L. H. (2017). Single-subject studies in translational nutrition research. *Annual Review of Nutrition, 37*, 395−422.

Sevilla-Villanueva, B., Gibert, K., Sanchez-Marre, M., Fito, M., & Covas, M. I. (2017). Evaluation of adherence to nutritional intervention through trajectory analysis. *IEEE Journal of Biomedical and Health Informatics, 21*, 628−634.

Shi, X., & Wu, X. (2017). An overview of human genetic privacy. *Annals of the New York Academy of Sciences, 1387*, 61−72.

Simo, C., Dominguez-Vega, E., Marina, M. L., Garcia, M. C., Dinelli, G., & Cifuentes, A. (2010). CE-TOF MS analysis of complex protein hydrolyzates from genetically modified soybeans--A tool for foodomics. *Electrophoresis, 31*, 1175−1183.

Simpson, S. J., Le Couteur, D. G., James, D. E., George, J., Gunton, J. E., Solon-Biet, S. M., et al. (2017). The geometric framework for nutrition as a tool in precision medicine. *Nutrition and Healthy Aging, 4*, 217−226.

Simpson, S. J., & Raubenheimer, D. (2005). Obesity: The protein leverage hypothesis. *Obesity Reviews, 6*, 133−142.

Smerecnik, C., Grispen, J. E. J., & Quaak, M. (2012). Effectiveness of testing for genetic susceptibility to smoking-related diseases on smoking cessation outcomes: A systematic review and meta-analysis. *Tobacco Control, 21*, 347−354.

Spanakis, G., Weiss, G., Boh, B., Lemmens, L., & Roefs, A. (2017). Machine learning techniques in eating behavior e-coaching. *Personal and Ubiquitous Computing, 21*, 645−659.

Stamler, J., Brown, I. J., Yap, I. K., Chan, Q., Wijeyesekera, A., Garcia-Perez, I., et al. (2013). Dietary and urinary metabonomic factors possibly accounting for higher blood pressure of black compared with white Americans: Results of International Collaborative Study on macro-/micronutrients and blood pressure. *Hypertension, 62*, 1074−1080.

Stenne, R., Hurlimann, T., & Godard, B. (2012). Are research papers reporting results from nutrigenetics clinical research a potential source of biohype? *Accountability in Research, 19*, 285−307.

Stenne, R., Hurlimann, T., & Godard, B. (2013). Benefits associated with nutrigenomics research and their reporting in the scientific literature: Researchers' perspectives. *Accountability in Research, 20*, 167−183.

Stewart, K. F. J., Wesselius, A., Schreurs, M. A. C., Schols, A. M. W. J. C., & Zeegers, M. P. (2018). Behavioural changes, sharing behaviour and psychological responses after receiving direct-to-consumer genetic test results: A systematic review and meta-analysis. *Journal of Community Genetics, 9*, 1−18.

Stewart-Knox, B. J., Bunting, B. P., Gilpin, S., Parr, H. J., Pinhão, S., Strain, J. J., de Almeida, M. D. V., & Gibney, M. (2008). Attitudes toward genetic testing and personalised nutrition in a representative sample of European consumers. *British Journal of Nutrition, 101*, 982−989.

Stewart-Knox, B., Rankin, A., Kuznesof, S., Poinhos, R., Vaz de Almeida, M. D., Fischer, A., et al. (2015). Promoting healthy dietary behaviour through personalised nutrition: Technology push or technology pull? *Proceedings of the Nutrition Society, 74*, 171−176.

Stover, P. J. (2004). Nutritional genomics. *Physiological Genomics, 16*, 161−165.

Thomas, D. (2010). Gene--Environment-wide association studies: Emerging approaches. *Nature Review Genetics, 11*, 259−272.

Tierney, A. C., McMonagle, J., Shaw, D. I., Gulseth, H. L., Helal, O., Saris, W. H. M., et al. (2011). Effects of dietary fat modification on insulin sensitivity and on other risk factors of the metabolic syndrome--LIPGENE: A European randomized dietary intervention study. *International Journal of Obesity, 35*, 800.

Uniken Venema, W. T., Voskuil, M. D., Dijkstra, G., Weersma, R. K., & Festen, E. A. (2017). The genetic background of inflammatory bowel disease: From correlation to causality. *Journal of Pathology, 241*, 146−158.

Valdés, A., García-Cañas, V., Rocamora-Reverte, L., Gómez-Martínez, A., Ferragut, J. A., & Cifuentes, A. (2013). Effect of rosemary polyphenols on human colon cancer cells: Transcriptomic profiling and functional enrichment analysis. *Genes & Nutrition, 8*, 43−60.

Valdés, A., Simó, C., Ibáñez, C., & García-Cañas, V. (2013). Foodomics strategies for the analysis of transgenic foods. *TrAC Trends in Analytical Chemistry, 52*, 2−15.

van Bochove, K., van Schalkwijk, D. B., Parnell, L. D., Lai, C.-Q., Ordovás, J. M., de Graaf, A. A., et al. (2012). Clustering by plasma lipoprotein profile reveals two distinct subgroups with positive lipid response to fenofibrate therapy. *Public Library of Science One, 7*, e38072.

van Ommen, B., van den Broek, T., de Hoogh, I., van Erk, M., van Someren, E., Rouhani-Rankouhi, T., et al. (2017). Systems biology of personalized nutrition. *Nutrition Reviews, 75*, 579−599.

van Ommen, B., & Wopereis, S. (2016). Next-generation biomarkers of health. *Nestle Nutrition Institute Workshop Series, 84*, 25−33.

Vasan, R. S. (2006). Biomarkers of cardiovascular disease: Molecular basis and practical considerations. *Circulation, 113*, 2335−2362.

Weiss, R., Dziura, J., Burgert, T. S., Tamborlane, W. V., Taksali, S. E., Yeckel, C. W., et al. (2004). Obesity and the metabolic syndrome in children and adolescents. *New England Journal of Medicine, 350*, 2362−2374.

Whitfield, P. D., German, A. J., & Noble, P. J. (2004). Metabolomics: An emerging post-genomic tool for nutrition. *British Journal of Nutrition, 92*, 549−555.

Wilson, C. P., Ward, M., McNulty, H., Strain, J. J., Trouton, T. G., Horigan, G., et al. (2012). Riboflavin offers a targeted strategy for managing hypertension in patients with the MTHFR 677TT genotype: A 4-y follow-up. *The American Journal of Clinical Nutrition, 95*, 766−772.

Witten, I. H., Frank, E., & Hall, M. A. (2011). *Data mining: Practical machine learning tools and techniques*. Morgan Kaufmann Publishers Inc.

Wu, G. D., Chen, J., Hoffmann, C., Bittinger, K., Chen, Y. Y., Keilbaugh, S. A., et al. (2011). Linking long-term dietary patterns with gut microbial enterotypes. *Science, 334*, 105−108.

Zeevi, D., Korem, T., Zmora, N., Israeli, D., Rothschild, D., Weinberger, A., et al. (2015). Personalized nutrition by prediction of glycemic responses. *Cell, 163*, 1079−1094.

Zeisel, S. H. (1999). Regulation of "nutraceuticals.". *Science, 285*, 1853−1855.

CHAPTER 2

Guidelines to Evaluate the Scientific Validity for Genotype-Based Dietary Advice

Keith Anthony Grimaldi
Eurogenetica Ltd, Sliema, Malta

OUTLINE

Introduction	34
Nutrigenetics and Nutrigenomics	35
How Should We Assess the Evidence in Nutrigenetics?	36
What Needs to be Assessed?	37
Utility and Randomized Controlled Trials	38
Randomized Clinical Trials	39
Primary Prevention in High-Risk Groups	39
Secondary Prevention in Subjects with Pathology	40
Conclusions	41
Where are We Today About Validating Personal Nutrition?	41
To Summarize—Some Components of a Personalized Nutrition	42
Appendix	43
The Global Nutrigenetics Knowledge Network Guidelines (from the Food4Me Project)	43
Framework for Evidence Assessment	43
Scientific Validity Assessment of a Putative Gene × Diet Interaction	46
Convincing	46
Probable	47
Possible	47
Not Demonstrated	47
References	48

INTRODUCTION

What exactly is genotype-based dietary advice? It refers to nutrigenetics (sometimes also called nutrigenomics but see later) and the main purpose is to use genetic variations to modify, where possible, the "standard healthy eating" guidelines and make them more relevant for the individual. It is a part of personalized nutrition (PN), small changes are made, it is not possible to design a diet or way of eating based only on genetics. The genetics does not lead to a "highly personalized" diet—but the changes are important for long-term good health. It was tentatively proposed over 15 years ago that:

> With the identification of polymorphisms, or common mutations, in vitamin metabolism, large percentages of the population may have higher requirements for specific vitamins (Rozen, 2002)

Research since then has resulted in significant progress and has identified some well-defined "gene × diet" interactions, supporting the concept that diets tailored to the individual's genotype might result in long-term health benefits (Corella et al., 2013; Görman, Mathers, Grimaldi, Ahlgren, & Nordström, 2013; Huo et al., 2015).

The general objective of PN in healthy individuals is the maintenance of health by optimizing diet and lifestyle—which may involve genotype, phenotype (including metabolomics), epigenetics, and the microbiome. Regarding genotype and PN, for decades PN has been part of daily life for people with inborn errors of metabolism, such as glucosemia, hereditary fructose intolerance, and phenylketonuria (Bouteldja & Timson, 2010; de Baulny, Abadie, Feillet, & de Parscau, 2007; Novelli & Reichardt, 2000), which are rare metabolic diseases arising from gene mutations. It happens also in more common disorders, for example, lactose intolerance, celiac disease (Heap & van Heel, 2009; IOM, 2018; NIH, 2018). More recently, interest has grown in the wider application of PN for the general public through using information about (common) genetic variants as the basis for targeted dietary and lifestyle recommendations. The scientific literature of the last 15–20 years contains reproducible evidence of several gene × diet interactions. Indeed Lee et al. (2011) and Parnell et al. (2014) describe the creation of a database of over 550 gene × environment interactions related to lipids, cardiovascular disease (CVD), and type 2 diabetes. In this chapter we look at the questions: When can a genetic variation × diet component be regarded as scientifically valid? What are the evidence requirements and the context in which that evidence should be assessed?

Nutrition research is complex and this chapter explores the ways to establish scientific validity, which is essential for dietary recommendations. Another question that should be addressed regards *utility*. It is explained why that is a much more difficult question and it is often different for different people. A scientifically valid study may have outcomes that are positive, negative, or neutral, as far as health is concerned, on the other hand utility can be seen as a measure of the health *benefit*.

> *Scientific validity*—concerns the accuracy of the interpretation, i.e. the accuracy with which a test predicts an outcome. For example, a certain genetic variant may be predicated to influence LDL cholesterol levels according to dietary saturated fat levels.

Clinical/Health/Personal utility—the measure of the likelihood that the recommended intervention will lead to a beneficial outcome. E.g. does reducing saturated fats in the diet of individuals with specific genetic variant(s) reduce and/or maintain LDL cholesterol levels?

This chapter mainly deals with the framework, or guidelines, for evidence evaluation from the Food4Me EU research project (Grimaldi et al., 2017). A "Global Nutrigenetics Knowledge Network (GNKN)" was established involving experts in different areas of PN, to collate all relevant information on genetic variations involved in the nutrient−health relationships and to deliver guidelines for the evaluation of evidence for diet−gene interactions.

While the guidelines have been developed for nutrigenetics, they are not limited to this field, but are also applicable to other areas of nutrigenomics, including metabolite profiling, gene expression analysis, and epigenetics (Afman & Müller, 2011; Bondia-Pons et al., 2013; Radonjic, van Erk, Pasman, Wortelboer, Hendriks, & van Ommen, 2009), as these begin to be translated into applications for use in personalizing diet and lifestyle.

The guidelines stop at the assessment of scientific validity. Their objectives are to help dieticians, nutritionists, doctors, and genetic counselors (and customers too) to judge the soundness of gene(s)−diet interactions. The recommendations are to provide clear and enough detail so that any opinion on health (or clinical) utility can be derived by the user (including the individual, dietician/nutritionist/medical doctor, companies, claim regulation bodies, etc.). Ultimately, the use of evidence-based nutrigenetic and other PN tools should be the basis for dietary advice aimed not only to reduce the risk of disease but as a tool to optimize diet to promote long-term health.

NUTRIGENETICS AND NUTRIGENOMICS

Nutrigenetics involves the study of how individual genetic variation affects interaction with components of the diet, including micro- and macronutrients and toxins. Genetic variation has been demonstrated to affect uptake, transport, metabolism, and elimination of food components and affects individual daily requirements for some essential nutrients. It is sometimes also referred to as nutrigenomics which actually is an umbrella term for all aspects of gene and diet interactions, including the effects of dietary molecules on gene expression and metabolic profiles (Corella & Ordovas, 2009). Nutrigenetic studies assess how genes and diet (and sometimes lifestyle) interact, where the effect of one component is dependent on the status of the other. A classic example is that involving lactose intolerance. In most humans, the enzyme lactase is only produced for the first few years of life when the infant is dependent on milk for nutrition, after which production of the enzyme reduces almost completely. Milk is the only naturally occurring source of lactose and since milk and dairy products have only recently, in evolutionary terms, been common components of the human diet, there was no requirement for the enzyme throughout adult life. A few thousand years ago in Central Europe a mutation appeared upstream of the lactase gene and the effect was continued production of the enzyme lactase throughout adult life. The mutation proliferated through the generations, presumably because of a survival advantage, and is now a very common polymorphism in Europe (range 30%−95%) (Enattah, Sahi, Savilahti,

Terwilliger, Peltonen, & Järvelä, 2002; Itan, Powell, Beaumont, Burger, & Thomas, 2009). Another example of genetics affecting nutrition is seen in taste reception. The perception of bitter taste varies among individuals and the population is divided into "super"tasters, tasters, and nontasters. The phenotypes are almost completely accounted for by three common SNPs (single nucleotide polymorphism) in the gene of the bitter taste receptor *TAS2R38* (Kim, Jorgenson, Coon, Leppert, Risch, & Drayna, 2003).

HOW SHOULD WE ASSESS THE EVIDENCE IN NUTRIGENETICS?

Nutrigenetics, and PN itself, should be evaluated in the context of conventional "standard healthy eating" advice which forms the basis of public health recommendations aimed at guiding diet and lifestyle habits in populations. Nutrigenetic information can be used to modify existing standard guidelines and provide an element of personalization to the otherwise "one size fits all" advice. Genetic information can be beneficial when it is *added* to other information such as sex, height, weight, age, state of health, etc.; it is not used in isolation nor does it override other parameters. Nutrigenetics is part of everyday nutrition—it is not specifically therapeutic and does not depend on the use of nutraceuticals or supplements. In general use it is not intended for specific disease prevention but as an aid in optimizing diet and lifestyle for promoting long-term health based on the best evidence that is available. Nutrigenetic, and indeed nutritional advice in general, is useful for *maintaining health* and its primary purpose is not for treating disease. All these points are important for determining the threshold of evidence required to support nutrigenetic advice and in this context the appropriate level of evidence should be the same as that applied to existing nutritional guidelines in the first place.

From the point of view of evidence assessment, nutrigenetic information should not be separate or treated differently in any way from the standard nutritional guidelines. There is no reason or justification to require a higher evidence threshold simply because genetic information is included. It is worth pointing out here that no component of standard nutritional guidelines (recommended vitamin intakes, salt and saturated fat reductions, fruit and vegetables, etc.) has been assessed and "proven" to prevent disease in randomized clinical trials (RCTs) in healthy individuals (see later for discussion on RCT). It is unlikely that such a level of evidence will ever be reached. RCTs may have demonstrated that reducing salt in hypertensive individuals can reduce blood pressure but there are no RCTs on the effects of decades-long low salt diets and the reduction of heart disease (Furberg, 2012). While the *therapeutic* applications of nutrition might be amenable to RCT, the proposed benefits of general nutritional guidelines cannot be tested in this way (see Blumberg et al., 2010 for extended discussion). Thus nutrigenetics should not be held to a higher (unreachable) standard as has sometimes been suggested (Haga, Khoury, & Burke, 2003; Wood, 2008). It should be supported by the type of evidence used, for example, to set vitamin, salt, and saturated fat recommendations in healthy people, which is mainly epidemiological and interventional in nature (Görman et al., 2013).

Current nutrition guidelines are formulated by a variety of organizations at various levels (e.g., Food Standards Agency (FSA) of the United Kingdom and the Institute of Medicine (IOM) in the United States). This information is used by scientists, dieticians, and other health professionals to communicate nutritional advice to the public through scientific publications, the mass media, and personal consultation. In formulating the guidelines, the expert committees have to make decisions based on the best evidence available, it is clear that there are gaps in the evidence but it is acknowledged that a scientific judgment of some sort has to be made, that "no decision is not an option" as we all have to consume nutrients daily (Taylor, 2008). The correct application of nutrigenetics, or PN in general, is to use these guidelines as the starting point and to examine where there is evidence that incorporating genetic information to modify intakes of specific nutrients may be beneficial. To validate nutrigenetic advice for a nutrient the question should be: Is the evidence of the same or higher standard compared to that used to justify the standard recommendations? For example, if there is evidence that a genetic variation increases daily requirements for a specific vitamin the quality of the evidence should be compared to that used to formulate the standard RDA for that vitamin for the general population. Nutrigenetic evidence can be formally assessed to determine if the required criteria, scientific validity, and health utility are met.

WHAT NEEDS TO BE ASSESSED?

There is currently a growing commercial market for nutrigenetic tests which claim to interpret and translate gene × diet information into benefits for the consumer. These tests, just like other routine laboratory tests, could be potentially useful for the individual or health professional but, as with any test, before they should be used it is necessary to know how reliable the evidence is and how useful is the result for the individual. These questions are encapsulated in the ACCE (Analytical and Clinical Validity, Clinical Utility and Ethics) definitions of "scientific validity" and "clinical utility" (CDC - Public Health Genomics | Genetic Testing | ACCE, 2010) which were developed for the evaluation of medical tests. ACCE is an appropriate starting point—with the caveat that it should be modified to account for the different settings, that is, diet and lifestyles versus medical diagnostics. According to ACCE, a medical genetic test should fulfill requirements regarding:

1. Analytical validity—a measure of the accuracy of the genotyping.
2. Scientific validity—concerns the strength of the evidence linking a genetic variant with a specific outcome.
3. Clinical utility—the measure of the likelihood that the recommended advice or therapy will lead to a beneficial outcome beyond the current state of the art.
4. Ethical, legal, and social implications that may arise in the context of using the test.

The regulation of analytical validity is relatively straightforward, and many countries have their own laboratory accreditation procedures that cover accuracy and reproducibility (EuroGentest, 2018). Ethical and legal aspects are beyond the scope of this chapter and are discussed elsewhere (Ahlgren et al., 2013; San-Cristobal, Milagro, & Martínez, 2013). Scientific validity is less clear-cut, in some cases the validity of a gene × diet interaction is generally accepted but often this is not the case, hence the requirements for the framework we describe here. Utility is the final requirement; however, this is a more difficult concept to precisely define. Clinical utility has strict criteria in the medical sense, demanding strong evidence that a given therapy "will lead to an improved health outcome" (Directors, 2015). Determining clinical utility works well for assessing specific disease prevention measures but has limitations when applied to nutrition and health maintenance. The positive and negative effects of nutrition usually act over years and decades and may even begin before birth, therefore different criteria need to be applied to the assessment of the health utility of gene × nutrition interactions. In this context "personal health utility" is the preferred term as the alternative to clinical utility. There are also cases where this may be limited to simply "personal utility," where the nutrigenetic information may be interesting and useful to the individual but has no actual demonstrated health benefit.

In the case of lactose/lactase it is relatively straightforward to talk about person health utility. To the approximately 70% of the world's population without the lactase persistent polymorphism (e.g., in southern Europe) the dietary advice to reduce exposure to lactose will almost certainly lead to the disappearance of the related unpleasant effects caused by lactose fermentation—a definite health benefit. Bitter taste receptor SNPs provide another example, but with no definite *health* benefits. It is accepted as validated that SNPs in the *TAS2R38* gene largely determine the extent to which an individual can taste bitter flavors, which are common in many green vegetables (Duffy et al., 2010; Gorovic, Afzal, Tjønneland, Overvad, Vogel, Albrechtsen, & Poulsen, 2011). Whilst there is a hypothesis that bitter tasters often do not meet the recommended vegetable intake and could benefit from increasing their consumption, the studies are inconsistent, and the evidence is not good enough to recommend testing for this "health" reason. It is acceptable though to propose that testing may be interesting from a personal information point of view—the test has a certain utility in this sense. It is important to convey the extent and the limit of the utility and this is one purpose of the guideline's framework discussed here.

If scientific validity is established, it would be possible to claim that a nutrigenetic test can be used to predict a specific outcome according to genotype and diet. This does not signify utility though and the next step is to determine whether the test results are in any way useful. Upon receipt of the results is there an action that can be taken (e.g., some diet or lifestyle change) that is likely to be beneficial for the individual health utility? Or is the knowledge likely to be useful to the individual in some other way, not necessarily related to a direct impact on health personal utility?

UTILITY AND RANDOMIZED CONTROLLED TRIALS

Clinical utility is the most controversial aspect: it is often difficult to define and must take into consideration many factors including positive or negative psychological or motivational effects on the end user (Roberts, Gornick, Carere, Uhlmann, Ruffin, & Green, 2017). Others contend that clinical utility can only be thoroughly established through RCTs but these are challenging for the personal nutrition environment: diet, lifestyle, and behavioral changes, which have small cumulative effects over decades [see Gulcher & Stefansson, 2010 and Ransohoff & Khoury, 2010 for an example of the, still current, debate]. A further problem is the precise definition of a clinical benefit. A gene—diet interaction may not be associated directly with disease risk, such as CVD, but with intermediate phenotypes, for example, lipid levels, hypertension, homocysteine, etc., which are independent risk factors for disease. Some commentators require that clinical utility is demonstrated as a reduction in disease incidence. The majority view accepts that lowering of intermediate risk factors is acceptable [as is the case for phytosterols and their cholesterol lowering properties (Ostlund, 2004; Smith & Ordovás, 2010)].

Randomized Clinical Trials

In PN research, or any nutrition research for that matter, RCTs with disease incidence as the endpoint are not practically feasible as they will require long-lasting nutritional changes, making compliance difficult and very expensive, at least in terms of primary prevention in healthy people—apart from any ethical problems. RCTs that address disease incidence reduction in middle-aged or elderly high-risk subjects, secondary prevention in individuals with disease, and/or on effects on intermediate biomarkers or risk factors can be useful, but care is required in drawing conclusions. RCTs in nutrition and genetics are often complex, difficult to design, and challenging to conduct in a reasonable time frame. Some examples given below illustrate this and may be helpful when interpreting RCT data for personalized diet and lifestyle evidence advice.

Primary Prevention in High-Risk Groups

Genetics × diet × T2DM (Type 2 Diabetes Mellitus) —The T allele of the *TCF7L2* rs7903146 SNP has been associated repeatedly with an increased risk of T2DM [twofold in homozygotes (Tong, Lin, Zhang, Yang, Zhang, Liu, & Zhang, 2009)]. Compared with nonrisk allele carriers, individuals who carry the risk allele and who are at high risk phenotypically (glucose intolerance, prediabetes diagnosis) require a longer lasting and a more intense dietary and lifestyle recommendation to divert the trajectory from disease over a period of 12 months, and to maintain health gains over a 4-year period (Bo et al., 2009). Although useful, these findings have been obtained in clinical trials of unhealthy people, who typically were older. Thus to be precise, it does not demonstrate, and cannot be used to claim, that specific dietary modifications in younger, healthier people will prevent the development of glucose intolerance or T2D in those carrying the risk allele. However, this evidence of gene × diet interactions in prediabetics is consistent with the evidence from other types of studies in healthy subjects (epidemiological, cohort, effects on biomarkers) and can provide supporting evidence, but not conclusive evidence, that specific dietary guidelines would be appropriate for healthy carriers of this *TCF7L2* risk allele. This example shows how difficult it is to validate a gene−diet interaction but suggests that adjusting the environment will improve the individuals' health.

The same *TCF7L2* genetic variant was assessed in the study from the PREDIMED project (Corella et al., 2013), a large randomized trial in 7018 high-cardiovascular-risk individuals comparing two Mediterranean (Med) diets and a control diet. *TCF7L2* TT homozygotes at SNP rs7903146 had higher blood glucose levels, total cholesterol, LDL-cholesterol, and triglycerides but only when adherence to the Med diet was low. Furthermore, incidence of stroke was almost three times higher in TT homozygotes as in the control group, but this increased risk was completely dissolved in the Med diet group

(Hazard Ratio, HR = 0.96). Thus compared to the control diet, both Med diets were effective at reducing both risk biomarkers and disease incidence itself in a genotype specific manner. While this is a strong endorsement of the Mediterranean diet, it is also relevant that the age range was 55–80 years. This RCT supports the epidemiological evidence for health benefits of the Med diets for older persons who are at increased risk of CVD and can only suggest such benefits for other age groups who carry the *TCF7L2* TT genotype at rs7903146.

Secondary Prevention in Subjects with Pathology

MTHFR × folate × homocysteine on CVD risk—Results of several large homocysteine-lowering clinical trials have been published over the last decade and none reported any benefit in the prevention of secondary CVD by folate supplementation. These results have been used widely to declare that there is no evidence that elevated plasma homocysteine levels are relevant for CVD and that there is no benefit in homocysteine-lowering in primary prevention (Clarke et al., 2010; Lonn, 2008; Tice, 2010). However, these were all short-term trials in older people already suffering from (mainly) CVD and taking several medications, where incidence of further cardiovascular events was measured. None of the trials were performed in healthy people. Thus the conclusion from these studies states that over the trial periods there was no apparent benefit in lowering homocysteine in ill people, that is, as in secondary prevention. However, lowering homocysteine by using folate still may reduce risks of CVD in healthy people with high risk (Selhub, 2006; Wald, Wald, Morris, & Law, 2006; Wald, Morris, & Wald, 2011). For instance, the China Stroke Primary Prevention Trial (Huo et al., 2015; Stampfer & Willett, 2015) reported on a total of 20,702 adults with hypertension without history of stroke or myocardial infarction who participated in the study. That study compared a single-pill combination containing 10 mg of enalapril and 0.8 mg of folic acid with a tablet containing 10 mg of enalapril only. Among adults with hypertension, the combined use of enalapril and folic acid, compared with enalapril alone, significantly reduced the risk of first stroke (HR = 0.79). Analysis of the *MTHFR* 677 genotype showed further that the TT genotype had the largest risk reduction in the highest folate quartile (HR = 0.24), suggesting that individuals with the TT genotype may have a greater folate requirement.

MTHFR × riboflavin × hypertension—Several RCTs have demonstrated that riboflavin supplementation contributes to blood pressure-lowering specifically in hypertensive carriers of the 677 T allele (Horigan, McNulty, Ward, Strain, Purvis, & Scott, 2010; Ward, Wilson, Strain, Horigan, Scott, & McNulty, 2011; Wilson et al., 2012, 2013). The trials do not prove primary prevention (i.e., they do not demonstrate that increasing riboflavin in 677 T normotensives prevents development of hypertension) and they do not prove the ultimate health benefit of riboflavin to reduce incidence of heart disease. However, reducing blood pressure is a health benefit in itself and although the results cannot be used to establish a genotype specific role of riboflavin in primary prevention of hypertension, they can be used to support other types of studies.

Overall, outcomes of RCTs can be useful for nutrition/lifestyle advice but they need to be interpreted with care. Furthermore, it must be accepted that conducting an RCT in young healthy people with the aim of investigating the effect of nutrition on actual reduction of disease incidence over the long term is not feasible either ethically, economically, or scientifically [see also Blumberg et al., (2010) for discussion]. On the other hand, the use of RCTs to study the effects on biomarkers that quantify health (i.e., not simple risk markers of impending disease) is a promising new approach (van Ommen, van der Greef, Ordovas, & Daniel, 2014).

CONCLUSIONS

Nutrigenetics has value and can make a definite contribution to individual health and well-being provided it is used in the right way. Gene × diet evidence should be assessed at the same level as other nutritional evidence that is used to formulate advice and guidelines and for continued progress it will be important to develop reliable information resources giving access to such assessments and to help professionals to provide good quality nutrigenetic services.

Nutrigenetics represents right now a valuable tool in the hands of the health professional, especially for dieticians and nutritionists who should incorporate evidence-based gene/diet information when devising nutrition programs for their clients. Health professionals routinely evaluate a range of biological data (biomarkers, height, weight, gender, ethnicity, health issues, etc.) when formulating personalized diets and it is entirely logical that genotype should also be included where the evidence is enough. This is the case for several gene × diet interactions and there is evidence that nutrigenetic advice is better understood and more likely to be followed compared to general dietary advice (Nielsen & El-Sohemy, 2014), plus it can be beneficial for example in long-term weight control (Arkadianos, Valdes, Marinos, Florou, Gill, & Grimaldi, 2007).

WHERE ARE WE TODAY ABOUT VALIDATING PERSONAL NUTRITION?

We are faced with the commercial introduction of greater or lesser validated means to give PN advice, for example, from nutrigenetics, by other biochemical tests, microbiome analysis, and self-tracking wearables for exercise, heart rate, blood pressure, and others. By following the guidelines highlighted in the appendix of this chapter we can make judgments about these other types of PN measurements, not just nutrigenetics. Commercial testing is flowing ever faster from the lab to the market. The shape of the market itself is changing—because of the many ways to test, track, and report individual data, through smartphone apps, the world is becoming a laboratory. This is interesting—a test which is determined to be "not yet validated" no longer means that it should not be sold, but it defines the way it should be marketed, that is as part of a research endeavor to validate it in the process. We can see this in two examples: the microbiome and the "metabolome."

The microbiome is potentially interesting—can we really sample an individual's microbiome and add information to personalized diet? Maybe. A smart study was published in 2015 in Cell that described that glucose responses depended on the components of the microbiome and the diet, suggesting that what is good for one person is not necessarily good for another (Zeevi et al., 2015). For example, eating a banana caused spikes in postprandial glucose levels in one individual but in another glucose remain stable. The method has not been replicated by others and it was only tested directly in a few people for the clinical study (26 people for the 2-week clinical trial). It cannot be judged as scientifically valid, but must be viewed as still very experimental. Some companies are already selling such tests, some are clearly designating them as research testing, which is reasonable—it would be a good way to reproduce the results in a real-world environment—but the emphasis should be on the experimental aspect. It should be sold as a research endeavor rather than promising better health with personalized nutrition.

Another example of what some have decided is too early is the idea of phenotype flexibility. This is actually better validated than the microbiome test but has not yet been tested in a published randomized trial. It is phenotypic flexibility as a measure of health—the optimal nutritional stress response test is directed toward "biomarkers of health" rather than "biomarkers of disease" (van Ommen et al., 2014). To measure a person's phenotypic flexibility, the homeostasis of that person must be perturbed, followed by determining the response of a single or multiple markers during a limited period of time. This has now become commercial—a challenge test, based on carbohydrates, lipids, and proteins, has been designed to temporarily disturb the body's homeostasis and the extent of the disruption and the speed of recovery to homeostasis are health indicators. Is it too early? No, but it depends on what is said and what is claimed.

We have to remember that we are talking about food, not medicine; almost all of the standard dietary guidelines have not been validated, certainly not in RCTs—with good reason (see above and Grimaldi, 2014). So we can applaud these initiatives to get away from the academic test environment into real-life studies and to get over the universal advice of 5-a-day for everyone with whole grain, low fat, etc., diets. The new technologies will bring successes and failures and it is up to the companies (which often are university start-ups) to fail quickly and move on with the successes.

TO SUMMARIZE—SOME COMPONENTS OF A PERSONALIZED NUTRITION

Valid:
1. Genetic variation is essential for PN—it cannot be ignored either in PN research or application to the individual. It could be seen as the operating system in a smart phone (iOS, Android OS), the fixed genetic background on which the "apps" would be everything else that measures the constantly varying biophysical biomarkers.
2. Phenotype assessments—based on validated tests such as cholesterol, glucose, and some vitamins.
   To be determined:
3. The experimental nutrition stress drink for phenotypic flexibility.
4. The highly experimental microbiome system to predict good and bad foods.
5. Wearable technology—measure activity, heart rate, etc.

1 and 2 are validated, easy to process and measure, and are ready for use. 3, 4, and 5 are in the experimental stages, as are other efforts, no doubt with many more to come—some or all may become fixed validated aspects for PN.

The PN field, both in research and application, can benefit from evidence guidelines to encourage commercial good practice and to stimulate interest and learning among the relevant health professionals. The GNKN Food4Me guidelines are a good starting point.

APPENDIX

The Global Nutrigenetics Knowledge Network Guidelines (from the Food4Me Project)

The GNKN reviewed guidelines for genetics, medical genetic tests, and nutritional recommendations [Evaluation of Genomic Applications in Practice and Prevention (EGAPP), Strengthening the Reporting of Genetic Association Studies (STREGA), Grading of Recommendations Assessment, Development, and Evaluation (GRADE), European Food Safety Authority (EFSA) (Brozek et al., 2009; EFSA Panel on Dietetic Products, 2010; EGAPP, 2016; Little et al., 2009; Schünemann et al., 2008)] and concluded that these did not fully cover the needs for assessing the evidence for genetics-based personalized dietary advice. EGAPP assesses the clinical utility of a gene, or genes, in conjunction with their variants as predictors of disease and EFSA assesses the evidence for the potential nutritional or health benefits of specific foods or food components. However, none of these guidelines addresses the evidence from studies that investigate the combined effect of genotype plus diet on health outcomes, which is essential for establishing evidence-based nutrigenetic advice.

FRAMEWORK FOR EVIDENCE ASSESSMENT

The components relevant to this assessment are summarized in Table 2.1. Scientific validity may be graded as (the percentages are based on the Guidance on Uncertainty in EFSA Scientific Assessment (EFSA, 2018)):

TABLE 2.1 Grading Scientific Validity Based on the Guidance on Uncertainty in EFSA Scientific Assessment (EFSA, 2018)

Probability Term	Subjective Probability Range (%)
A. Convincing	>90
B. Probable	66–90
C. Possible	33–66
D. Insufficient	<33

A. INSIGHTS OF PERSONALIZED NUTRITION

"Convincing" should be based on several (at least three) strong studies with high subject numbers showing the relationship and/or mechanistic knowledge; "probable" should be based on several studies showing the relationship and/or some mechanistic understanding; and "possible" should be based on a few studies showing the relation. See below in the text for a fuller explanation.

Scientific validation determines the strength of the evidence for an interaction between a specific genetic marker or set of markers and a dietary component or pattern on a health outcome of interest (such as disease or risk factors for disease). The scientific validity criteria for genetic-based dietary advice include (1) study design and quality and (2) biological mechanism including the nature of the genetic variant(s) and biological plausibility, as discussed below. The probability term is the overall judgment of the evidence provided and in this sense "it is possible for an evidentiary conclusion based on many papers, each of which may be relatively weak, to be graded as 'moderate' [probable] or even 'strong' [convincing], if there are multiple small case reports or studies that are all supportive with no contradictory studies" (Caudle et al., 2014).

1. Study design and quality

    The evaluation of the study quality considers several aspects including:
    a. Interventional or observational design.
    b. Prospective or retrospective approach.
    c. Study power (including numbers of participants with "effect" allele).
    d. Effect magnitude*.
    e. *P*-Values, false discover rate, multiple testing**.
    f. Is the interaction replicated in different populations or systematically reviewed?

    *The "effect magnitude" required depends on the type of study. For example, the effect of folate on high homocysteine in carriers of the effect allele in *MTHFR* should be a return to normal within a few weeks of stopping the intervention. The magnitude of reduction of blood pressure would be acceptable for as little as 1 mmHg, and any risk reduction, however small, for CVD would be adequate.

    **P*-Values must be at least 0.05 to be significant. The *P*-value must remain within 0.05 after correcting for multiple testing, for example Bonferroni.

2. Biological plausibility

    "a gene–environment interaction will only be accepted if it can be reproduced in two or more studies and also seems plausible at the biological level." (Hunter, 2005)

Biological plausibility is a judgment based on the collected evidence of a gene × diet interaction on a phenotype. For example smoking introduces carcinogens into the body, which could cause DNA damage, increased mutational events, and consequently increasing the risk of cancer (Alexandrov et al., 2016). Thus a validated gene × nutrition interaction such as *GSTM1* × cruciferous vegetable consumption leading to reduction of DNA (Lam et al., 2009; Palli et al., 2004) is consistent with an association between *GSTM1* × cruciferous and reduced cancer risk (Brennan et al., 2005).

Gene × diet interactions, the scientific underpinning of this paper, are defined here as the physiological response to a dietary component which occurs only—or is more pronounced—in persons with a specific version of a gene (or genes). For example, a certain genotype may be associated with increased concentrations of LDL cholesterol and increased risk of cardiovascular complications, but only in the case of long-term, higher-than-average saturated fat consumption (Ordovas, 2006; Smith & Ordovás, 2010). Evidence of this type of interaction may be used to develop an appropriate dietary recommendation (e.g., consuming lower than average intake of saturated fats) which may reduce or eliminate the potential negative consequences associated with the specific genotype and may be targeted to specific groups of people.

1. *Gene × diet interaction*

    We identify three broad types of gene × diet interactions: direct, intermediate, and complex.
    a. A "direct" interaction is a mechanistic interaction between the genetic variant and the dietary component on the health biomarker. This type of interaction is most similar to the metabolism of a drug by the gene encoding the enzyme that directly metabolizes the drug.
    b. An intermediate interaction is a mechanistic interaction between the genetic variant and the dietary component on the health biomarker, but other processes also affect the level of the biomarker.
    c. An indirect interaction is the case where a mechanistic interaction between the genetic variant and the dietary component on a health biomarker, including disease, is affected to some extent by the gene × diet interaction, but is also influenced by many other, possibly unknown, processes and it may take years for symptoms to manifest. This type of interaction may not be fully explained physiologically or may be only demonstrated statistically.

A well-researched example is the case of supplementation with folate (substrate) and/or riboflavin (cofactor) in persons who are carriers or noncarriers of the methylenetetrahydrofolate reductase (*MTHFR*) C677T polymorphism (rs1801133) where "T" is the allele associated with reduced enzymatic activity. Examples with the folate related enzyme MTHFR are:

a. Direct: for example, *MTHFR* × folate → levels of homocysteine (Ashfield-Watt et al., 2002)
b. Intermediate: for example, *MTHFR* × riboflavin → blood pressure (Wilson et al., 2013)
c. Indirect: for example,*MTHFR* × folate /riboflavin → cardiovascular disease (Wald et al., 2006)

2. *Nature of the genetic variant*

    This framework considers three major classes of genetic variants, with differing strengths of evidence.
    a. The genetic variant has a demonstrated causal effect on the function of the gene product, for example, on enzyme activity or protein abundance, which provides a biologically plausible explanation for the gene–diet interaction.
    b. The genotyped variant may not itself affect the protein of interest but it may be in linkage disequilibrium (LD) with another relevant functional variant—one SNP is said to "tag" the other (Bush & Moore, 2012; Reich et al., 2001). Evidence would be required to validate both the LD score and the putative gene × diet interaction. In addition, the results also would be applicable only to the population(s) in which high LD has been established.

    c. The effect of the SNP on function of the gene product is unknown and is based only on a statistical association for the gene × diet effect (Bush & Moore, 2012; Reich et al., 2001).

Examples of these three types of genetic variants are:

    i. *Causative*: SNP rs1801133 (TT) reduces the activity of the MTHFR enzyme (Frosst et al., 1995).
    ii. *In LD with known causative variant*: the SNP rs4341, which is in LD with an InDel variant (rs4646994) in the same gene, angiotensin converting enzyme (*ACE*), that affects the plasma ACE levels (Glenn, Du, Eisenmann, & Rothschild, 2009; Tanaka, Kamide, Takiuchi, Miwa, Yoshii, Kawano, & Miyata, 2003).
    iii. *Unknown*: for example, rs7903146 (CT and TT) intron SNP in the *TCF7L2* gene is linked to type 2 diabetes risk. An interaction with carbohydrate and diet has been demonstrated but the effect of this polymorphism, if any, on function of the corresponding gene product has not been characterized. This SNP may be in LD with a functional SNP, or has an as yet uncharacterized function (Cornelis, Qi, Kraft, & Hu, 2009; Lyssenko et al., 2007).

SCIENTIFIC VALIDITY ASSESSMENT OF A PUTATIVE GENE × DIET INTERACTION

Assessing the validity of a putative gene × diet interaction is generally complex, and as knowledge deepens in nutrigenetics, assessment of its validity will develop. We propose a pragmatic way to assess the validity by relying initially on semiquantitative measures that can be improved with additional data. The numbers used below to assess the validity should be considered an arbitrary but coherent guideline based on suggested power calculations and the precision of measurements of diet exposure and outcome (Hunter, 2005; Luan, Wong, Day, & Wareham, 2001; Reddon, Guéant, & Meyre, 2016), plus experience based on successfully repeated gene × diet studies published to date.

The assessment should explicitly specify for which subgroup (e.g., sex, ancestral background, and other relevant subgroups) the evidence is collected.

Convincing

- Two independent studies that have shown the relationship between the gene—diet interaction and the specific health outcome. Together those studies should include at least 100 subjects carrying the effect allele (i.e., the presumed functional variant or in LD with the functional variant) for intervention studies and at least 500 subjects for observational studies. Specifically, if the frequency of the effect allele is 10% that means a total of at least 1000 and 5000 subjects for intervention and observational studies, respectively.
- Biological mechanism fully understood or largely explained, or
- Biological mechanism partly explained and having one correlative study that at least includes 50 (intervention) or 250 (observational) subjects carrying the effect allele.

Probable

- Two independent studies that have shown the correlation between the gene—diet and health outcome [together <100 (intervention) or <500 (observational) subjects carrying the effect allele]
- One study that has shown the correlation between the gene—diet and health outcome including at least 100 (intervention) or 500 (observational) subjects carrying the effect allele.
- Biological mechanism partly explained and having one small correlative study [<50 (intervention) or <250 (observational) subjects carrying the effect allele].

Possible

- One study has shown the correlation between the gene—diet and health outcome [<100 (intervention) or <500 (observational) subjects carrying the effect allele].
- Biological mechanism partly explained and having one small correlative study [<50 (intervention) or <250 (observational) subjects carrying the effect allele].

Not Demonstrated

- Any other studies, excluding the abovementioned studies.

Based on the factors described above, an overall assessment of all evidence can be made to arrive at a combined score on the scientific validity, and our degree of confidence in that assessment, of the gene × diet interaction being predictive of the outcome of interest. Some examples include:

- *Convincing – very high confidence*: MTHFR and homocysteine concentrations which are influenced by dietary folate: a large numbers of studies including randomized trials, very consistent results, direct effect of the genetic variation on enzyme activity, high biological plausibility (Homocysteine Lowering Trialists' Collaboration, 2005; West & Caudill, 2010).
- *Probable – high confidence*: SOD2 × antioxidants and prostate and breast cancer risk has been demonstrated consistently in gene × diets studies. Some large studies show a reduction in cancer risk when antioxidant intake is high. The biological plausibility is high but all available evidence comes from prospective or retrospective observation trials and not randomized trials (Ambrosone et al., 1999; Kang et al., 2007; Li, Kantoff, Giovannucci, Leitzmann, Gaziano, Stampfer, & Ma, 2005).
- *Possible*: BCMO1 × carotenoid and retinal levels. The BCMO1 gene product is an enzyme that converts β-carotene to vitamin A (retinal). Certain BCMO1 alleles are associated with higher plasma β-carotene levels, and such allele variants may result in lower enzyme activity. However, no clear demonstration on the effect of dietary advice has been reported (Ferrucci et al., 2009; Lietz, Oxley, Leung, & Hesketh, 2012).
- *Not demonstrated*: FADS2 × breastfeeding and IQ: three published studies, with three conflicting results:
  - In 3269 children, in two cohorts (UK and New Zealand), an increase in IQ but only in breastfed infants who were carriers of the C-allele for the FADS2 rs174575 SNP,

TABLE 2.2 Framework for Stepwise Assessment of the Evidence Relating to Gene × Diet Interactions

---

STUDY QUALITY RATING (A, B, C, D):

- Interventional or observational design
- Prospective, retrospective approach
- Randomized, placebo controlled, blinded
- Study power (high subject number with "effect" allele)
- Effect magnitude
- *P*-values, false discover rate (FDR), multiple testing
- Replication study in different populations, metaanalysis

TYPE OF GENE × DIET INTERACTION

- Direct phenotype
- Intermediate phenotype
- Indirect phenotype

NATURE OF THE GENETIC VARIANT

- Causal
- In LD with functional variant
- Associated but unknown function

BIOLOGICAL PLAUSIBILITY

- Rated as high/medium/low/unknown

SCIENTIFIC VALIDITY SCORE FOR GENE × DIET INTERACTION

- Convincing
- Probable
- Possible
- Not demonstrated

---

which is the major allele intronic tag SNP associated with higher docosahexaenoic acid (DHA) (Caspi et al., 2007).
- Second study examined 5934 British children—breastfed children with the GG genotype were actually associated with higher IQ (Steer, Davey Smith, Emmett, Hibbeln, & Golding, 2010).
- Third study of 1431 Australian children—there were no differences in IQ either for breastfeeding or genotype at the FADS2 rs174575 SNP (Martin, Benyamin, Hansell, Montgomery, Martin, Wright, & Bates, 2011). (Table 2.2)

References

Afman, L. A., & Müller, M. (2011). Human nutrigenomics of gene regulation by dietary fatty acids. *Progress in Lipid Research*, 1–8. Available from https://doi.org/10.1016/j.plipres.2011.11.005.

Ahlgren, J., Nordgren, A., Perrudin, M., Ronteltap, A., Savigny, J., van Trijp, H., … Görman, U. (2013). Consumers on the Internet: Ethical and legal aspects of commercialization of personalized nutrition. *Genes & Nutrition*, 8(4), 349–355. Available from https://doi.org/10.1007/s12263-013-0331-0.

REFERENCES

Alexandrov, L. B., Ju, Y. S., Haase, K., Van Loo, P., Martincorena, I., Nik-Zainal, S., ... Stratton, M. R. (2016). Mutational signatures associated with tobacco smoking in human cancer. *Science, 354*, 6312.

Ambrosone, C. B., Freudenheim, J. L., Thompson, P. A., Bowman, E., Vena, J. E., Marshall, J. R., ... Shields, P. G. (1999). Manganese superoxide dismutase (MnSOD) genetic polymorphisms, dietary antioxidants, and risk of breast cancer 1. *Cell*, 602–606.

Arkadianos, I., Valdes, A. M., Marinos, E., Florou, A., Gill, R. D., & Grimaldi, K. A. (2007). Improved weight management using genetic information to personalize a calorie controlled diet. *Nutrition Journal, 6*, 29. Available from https://doi.org/10.1186/1475-2891-6-29.

Ashfield-Watt, P. A. L., Pullin, C. H., Whiting, J. M., Clark, Z. E., Moat, S. J., Newcombe, R. G., ... McDowell, I. F. W. (2002). Methylenetetrahydrofolate reductase 677C-->T genotype modulates homocysteine responses to a folate-rich diet or a low-dose folic acid supplement: A randomized controlled trial. *The American Journal of Clinical Nutrition, 76*(1), 180–186. Available at http://www.ncbi.nlm.nih.gov/pubmed/12081832.

Blumberg, J., Heaney, R. P., Huncharek, M., Scholl, T., Stampfer, M., Vieth, R., ... Zeisel, S. (2010). Evidence-based criteria in the nutritional context. *Nutrition Reviews, 68*(8), 478–484. Available from https://doi.org/10.1111/j.1753-4887.2010.00307.x.

Bo, S., Gambino, R., Ciccone, G., Rosato, R., Milanesio, N., Villois, P., ... Cavallo-perin, P. (2009). Effects of TCF7L2 polymorphisms on glucose values after a lifestyle. *American Journal of Clinical Nutrition*(C), 1–7. Available from https://doi.org/10.3945/ajcn.2009.28379.

Bondia-Pons, I., Cañellas, N., Abete, I., Rodríguez, M. Á., Perez-Cornago, A., Navas-Carretero, S., ... Martínez, J. A. (2013). Nutri-metabolomics: Subtle serum metabolic differences in healthy subjects by NMR-based metabolomics after a short-term nutritional intervention with two tomato sauces. *Omics: A Journal of Integrative Biology, 17*(12), 611–618. Available from https://doi.org/10.1089/omi.2013.0027.

Bouteldja, N., & Timson, D. J. (2010). The biochemical basis of hereditary fructose intolerance. *Journal of Inherited Metabolic Disease, 33*(2), 105–112. Available from https://doi.org/10.1007/s10545-010-9053-2.

Brennan, P., Hsu, C. C., Moullan, N., Szeszenia-Dabrowska, N., Lissowska, J., Zaridze, D., ... Canzian, F. (2005). Effect of cruciferous vegetables on lung cancer in patients stratified by genetic status: A mendelian randomisation approach. *Lancet, 366*(9496), 1558–1560. Available from https://doi.org/10.1016/S0140-6736(05)67628-3.

Brozek, J. L., Akl, E. A., Jaeschke, R., Lang, D. M., Bossuyt, P., Glasziou, P., ... Schünemann, H. J. (2009). Grading quality of evidence and strength of recommendations in clinical practice guidelines: Part 2 of 3. The GRADE approach to grading quality of evidence about diagnostic tests and strategies. *Allergy, 64*(8), 1109–1116. Available from https://doi.org/10.1111/j.1398-9995.2009.02083.x.

Bush, W. S., & Moore, J. H. (2012). Chapter 11: Genome-wide association studies. *Public Library of Sciences Computational Biology, 8*(12), e1002822. Available from http://dx.doi.org/10.1371/journal.pcbi.1002822.

Caspi, A., Williams, B., Kim-Cohen, J., Craig, I. W., Milne, B. J., Poulton, R., ... Moffitt, T. E. (2007). Moderation of breastfeeding effects on the IQ by genetic variation in fatty acid metabolism. *Proceedings of the National Academy of Sciences of the United States of America, 104*(47), 18860–18865. Available from https://doi.org/10.1073/pnas.0704292104.

Caudle, K. E., Klein, T. E., Hoffman, J. M., Muller, D. J., Whirl-Carrillo, M., Gong, L., ... Johnson, S. G. (2014). Incorporation of pharmacogenomics into routine clinical practice: The Clinical Pharmacogenetics Implementation Consortium (CPIC) guideline development process. *Current Drug Metabolism, 15*(2), 209–217. Available at http://www.ncbi.nlm.nih.gov/pubmed/24479687 (Accessed: 05.06.17).

CDC - Public Health Genomics|Genetic Testing|ACCE (2010). Available at <http://www.cdc.gov/genomics/gtesting/ACCE/index.htm> (Accessed 06.05.18).

Clarke, R., Halsey, J., Lewington, S., Lonn, E., Armitage, J., Manson, J. E., ... Collins, R. (2010). Effects of lowering homocysteine levels with B vitamins on cardiovascular disease, cancer, and cause-specific mortality: Meta-analysis of 8 randomized trials involving 37 485 individuals. *Archives of Internal Medicine, 170*(18), 1622–1631. Available from https://doi.org/10.1001/archinternmed.2010.348.

Corella, D., Carrasco, P., Sorlí, J. V., Estruch, R., Rico-Sanz, J., Martínez-González, M. Á., ... Ordovás, J. M. (2013). Mediterranean diet reduces the adverse effect of the TCF7L2-rs7903146 polymorphism on cardiovascular risk factors and stroke incidence: A randomized controlled trial in a high-cardiovascular-risk population. *Diabetes Care, 36*(11), 3803–3811. Available from https://doi.org/10.2337/dc13-0955.

Corella, D., & Ordovas, J. M. (2009). Nutrigenomics in cardiovascular medicine. *Circulation. Cardiovascular Genetics, 2*(6), 637–651. Available from https://doi.org/10.1161/CIRCGENETICS.109.891366.

Cornelis, M. C., Qi, L., Kraft, P., & Hu, F. B. (2009). TCF7L2, dietary carbohydrate, and risk of type 2 diabetes in US women. *The American Journal of Clinical Nutrition, 89*(4), 1256–1262. Available from https://doi.org/10.3945/ajcn.2008.27058.

de Baulny, H. O., Abadie, V., Feillet, F., & de Parscau, L. (2007). Management of phenylketonuria and hyperphenylalaninemia. *The Journal of Nutrition, 137*(6 Suppl 1), 1561S–1563S. discussion 1573S–1575S. Available at http://www.ncbi.nlm.nih.gov/pubmed/17513425 (Accessed 12.10.14).

Directors, A. B. (2015). of., Clinical utility of genetic and genomic services: A position statement of the American College of Medical Genetics and Genomics. *Genetics in Medicine: Official Journal of the American College of Medical Genetics, 17*(6), 505–507. Available from https://doi.org/10.1038/gim.2015.41.

Duffy, V. B., Hayes, J. E., Davidson, A. C., Kidd, J. R., Kidd, K. K., & Bartoshuk, L. M. (2010). Vegetable intake in college-aged adults is explained by oral sensory phenotypes and TAS2R38 genotype. *Chemosensory Perception, 3*(3–4), 137–148. Available from https://doi.org/10.1007/s12078-010-9079-8.

EFSA (2018) *Uncertainty assessment I European Food Safety Authority*. Available at https://www.efsa.europa.eu/en/topics/topic/uncertainty-assessment (Accessed 30.10.18).

EFSA Panel on Dietetic Products, N. and A. (NDA). (2010). Scientific opinion on principles for deriving and applying dietary reference values. *EFSA Journal 2010, 8*(3). Available at http://www.efsa.europa.eu/it/efsajournal/pub/1458.htm (Accessed 15.01.15).

EGAPP (2016) *The Evaluation of Genomic Applications in Practice and Prevention (EGAPP) initiative: Methods of the EGAPP Working Group*. Available at https://www.cdc.gov/egappreviews/ (Accessed 30.10.18).

Enattah, N. S., Sahi, T., Savilahti, E., Terwilliger, J. D., Peltonen, L., & Järvelä, I. (2002). Identification of a variant associated with adult-type hypolactasia. *Nature Genetics, 30*(2), 233–237. Available from https://doi.org/10.1038/ng826.

EuroGentest (2018) *EuroGentest: Genetic Laboratories*. Available at http://www.eurogentest.org/index.php?id = 139 (Accessed 30.10.18).

Ferrucci, L., Perry, J. R. B., Matteini, A., Perola, M., Tanaka, T., Silander, K., ... Frayling, T. M. (2009). Common variation in the beta-carotene 15,15'-monooxygenase 1 gene affects circulating levels of carotenoids: A genome-wide association study. *American Journal of Human Genetics, 84*(2), 123–133. Available from https://doi.org/10.1016/j.ajhg.2008.12.019.

Frosst, P., Blom, H. J., Milos, R., Goyette, P., Sheppard, C. A., Matthews, R. G., ... van den Heuvel, L. P. (1995). A candidate genetic risk factor for vascular disease: A common mutation in methylenetetrahydrofolate reductase. *Nature Genetics, 10*(1), 111–113. Available from https://doi.org/10.1038/ng0595-111.

Furberg, C. D. (2012). Public health policies: No place for surrogates. *American Journal of Hypertension, 25*(1), 21. Available from https://doi.org/10.1038/ajh.2011.203.

Glenn, K. L., Du, Z.-Q., Eisenmann, J. C., & Rothschild, M. F. (2009). An alternative method for genotyping of the ACE I/D polymorphism. *Molecular Biology Reports, 36*(6), 1305–1310. Available from https://doi.org/10.1007/s11033-008-9313-5.

Görman, U., Mathers, J. C., Grimaldi, K. A., Ahlgren, J., Nordström, K., et al. (2013). Do we know enough? A scientific and ethical analysis of the basis for genetic-based personalized nutrition. *Genes & Nutrition, 8*(4), 373–381. Available from https://doi.org/10.1007/s12263-013-0338-6.

Gorovic, N., Afzal, S., Tjønneland, A., Overvad, K., Vogel, U., Albrechtsen, C., & Poulsen, H. E. (2011). Genetic variation in the hTAS2R38 taste receptor and brassica vegetable intake. *Scandinavian Journal of Clinical and Laboratory Investigation, 71*(4), 274–279. Available from https://doi.org/10.3109/00365513.2011.559553.

Grimaldi, K. A. (2014). Nutrigenetics and personalized nutrition: Are we ready for DNA-based dietary advice?. *Personalized Medicine, 11*(3), 297–307. Available from http://dx.doi.org/10.2217/pme.14.2.

Grimaldi, K. A., van Ommen, B., Ordovas, J. M., Parnell, L. D., Mathers, J. C., Bendik, I., ... Bouwman, J. (2017). Proposed guidelines to evaluate scientific validity and evidence for genotype-based dietary advice. *Genes & Nutrition, 12*(1). Available from https://doi.org/10.1186/s12263-017-0584-0.

Gulcher, J., & Stefansson, K. (2010). Genetic risk information for common diseases may indeed be already useful for prevention and early detection. *European Journal of Clinical Investigation, 40*(1), 56–63. Available from https://doi.org/10.1111/j.1365-2362.2009.02233.x.

Haga, S. B., Khoury, M. J., & Burke, W. (2003). Genomic profiling to promote a healthy lifestyle: Not ready for prime time. *Nature Genetics, 34*(4), 347–350. Available from https://doi.org/10.1038/ng0803-347.

Heap, G. A., & van Heel, D. A. (2009). Genetics and pathogenesis of coeliac disease. *Seminars in Immunology, 21*(6), 346–354. Available from https://doi.org/10.1016/j.smim.2009.04.001.

Homocysteine Lowering Trialists' Collaboration. (2005). Dose-dependent effects of folic acid on blood concentrations of homocysteine: A meta-analysis of the randomized trials. *The American Journal of Clinical Nutrition*, 82 (4), 806–812. Available at http://www.ncbi.nlm.nih.gov/pubmed/16210710 (Accessed 05.01.12).

Horigan, G., McNulty, H., Ward, M., Strain, J. J., Purvis, J., & Scott, J. M. (2010). Riboflavin lowers blood pressure in cardiovascular disease patients homozygous for the 677C-->T polymorphism in MTHFR. *Journal of Hypertension*, 28(3), 478–486. Available from https://doi.org/10.1097/HJH.0b013e328334c126.

Hunter, D. J. (2005). Gene-environment interactions in human diseases. *Nature Reviews. Genetics*, 6(4), 287–298. Available from https://doi.org/10.1038/nrg1578.

Huo, Y., Li, J., Qin, X., Huang, Y., Wang, X., Gottesman, R. F., ... Hou, F. F. (2015). Efficacy of folic acid therapy in primary prevention of stroke among adults with hypertension in China. *The Journal of the American Medical Association*, 313(13), 1325–1335. Available from https://doi.org/10.1001/jama.2015.2274.

IOM (2018) *Food and Nutrition - Institute of Medicine*. Available at http://nationalacademies.org/hmd/Global/Topics/Food-Nutrition.aspx (Accessed 30.10.18).

Itan, Y., Powell, A., Beaumont, M. A., Burger, J., & Thomas, M. G. (2009). The origins of lactase persistence in Europe. *PLoS Computational Biology*, 5(8), e1000491. Available from https://doi.org/10.1371/journal.pcbi.1000491.

Kang, D., Lee, K.-M., Park, S. K., Berndt, S. I., Peters, U., Reding, D., ... Hayes, R. B. (2007). Functional variant of manganese superoxide dismutase (SOD2 V16A) polymorphism is associated with prostate cancer risk in the prostate, lung, colorectal, and ovarian cancer study.' *Cancer Epidemiology, Biomarkers & Prevention*, 16(8), 1581–1586. Available from https://doi.org/10.1158/1055-9965.EPI-07-0160.

Kim, U., Jorgenson, E., Coon, H., Leppert, M., Risch, N., & Drayna, D. (2003). Positional cloning of the human quantitative trait locus underlying taste sensitivity to phenylthiocarbamide. *Science*, 299(5610), 1221–1225. Available from https://doi.org/10.1126/science.1080190.

Lam, T. K., Gallicchio, L., Lindsley, K., Shiels, M., Hammond, E., Tao, X. G., ... Alberg, A. J. (2009). Cruciferous vegetable consumption and lung cancer risk: A systematic review. *Cancer Epidemiology, Biomarkers & Prevention*, 18(1), 184–195. Available from https://doi.org/10.1158/1055-9965.EPI-08-0710.

Lee, Y.-C., Lai, C.-Q., Ordovas, J. M., & Parnell, L. D. (2011). A database of gene-environment interactions pertaining to blood lipid traits, cardiovascular disease and type 2 diabetes. *Journal of Data Mining in Genomics & Proteomics*, 2(1). Available from https://doi.org/10.4172/2153-0602.1000106.

Li, H., Kantoff, P. W., Giovannucci, E., Leitzmann, M. F., Gaziano, J. M., Stampfer, M. J., & Ma, J. (2005). Manganese superoxide dismutase polymorphism, prediagnostic antioxidant status, and risk of clinical significant prostate cancer. *Cancer Research*, 6, 2498–2504.

Lietz, G., Oxley, A., Leung, W., & Hesketh, J. (2012). Single nucleotide polymorphisms upstream from the β-carotene 15,15′-monoxygenase gene influence provitamin A conversion efficiency in female volunteers. *The Journal of Nutrition*, 142(1), 161S–165SS. Available from https://doi.org/10.3945/jn.111.140756.

Little, J., Higgins, J. P. T., Ioannidis, J. P. a, Moher, D., Gagnon, F., von Elm, E., ... Birkett, N. (2009). STrengthening the REporting of Genetic Association studies (STREGA)--an extension of the STROBE statement. *European Journal of Clinical Investigation*, 39(4), 247–266. Available at http://www.pubmedcentral.nih.gov/articlerender.fcgi?artid=2730482&tool=pmcentrez&rendertype=abstract.

Lonn, E. (2008). Homocysteine-lowering B vitamin therapy in cardiovascular prevention--wrong again? *the journal of the American Medical Association*, 299(17), 2086–2087. Available from https://doi.org/10.1001/jama.299.17.2086.

Luan, J. A., Wong, M. Y., Day, N. E., & Wareham, N. J. (2001). Sample size determination for studies of gene-environment interaction. *International Journal of Epidemiology*, 30(5), 1035–1040. Available at http://www.ncbi.nlm.nih.gov/pubmed/11689518 (Accessed 08.09.16).

Lyssenko, V., Lupi, R., Marchetti, P., Del Guerra, S., Orho-Melander, M., Almgren, P., ... Groop, L. (2007). Mechanisms by which common variants in the TCF7L2 gene increase risk of type 2 diabetes. *The Journal of Clinical Investigation*, 117(8), 2155–2163. Available from https://doi.org/10.1172/JCI30706.

Martin, N. W., Benyamin, B., Hansell, N. K., Montgomery, G. W., Martin, N. G., Wright, M. J., & Bates, T. C. (2011). Cognitive function in adolescence: Testing for interactions between breast-feeding and FADS2 polymorphisms. *Journal of the American Academy of Child and Adolescent Psychiatry*, 50(1), 55–62. e4. https://doi.org/10.1016/j.jaac.2010.10.010.

Nielsen, D. E., & El-Sohemy, A. (2014). Disclosure of genetic information and change in dietary intake: A randomized controlled trial. *Public Library of Science ONE*, 9(11), e112665. Available from https://doi.org/10.101610.1016:10.1371/journal.pone.0112665.

NIH (2018) *Lactose intolerance: Your guide to understanding genetic conditions, genetics home reference*. Available at https://ghr.nlm.nih.gov/condition/lactose-intolerance (Accessed 30.10.18).

Novelli, G., & Reichardt, J. K. (2000). Molecular basis of disorders of human galactose metabolism: Past, present, and future. *Molecular Genetics and Metabolism*, 71(1−2), 62−65. Available from https://doi.org/10.1006/mgme.2000.3073.

Ordovas, J. M. (2006). Nutrigenetics, plasma lipids, and cardiovascular risk. *Journal of the American Dietetic Association*, 106(7), 1074−1081. Available from https://doi.org/10.1016/j.jada.2006.04.016, quiz 1083.

Ostlund, R. E. (2004). Phytosterols and cholesterol metabolism. *Current Opinion in Lipidology*, 15(1), 37−41. Available at http://www.ncbi.nlm.nih.gov/pubmed/15166807 (Accessed 04.07.16).

Palli, D., Masala, G., Peluso, M., Gaspari, L., Krogh, V., Munnia, A., ... Garte, S. (2004). The effects of diet on DNA bulky adduct levels are strongly modified by GSTM1 genotype: A study on 634 subjects. *Carcinogenesis*, 25(4), 577−584. Available from https://doi.org/10.1093/carcin/bgh033.

Parnell, L. D., Blokker, B. A., Dashti, H. S., Nesbeth, P.-D., Cooper, B. E., Ma, Y., ... Ordovás, J. M., et al. (2014). CardioGxE, a catalog of gene-environment interactions for cardiometabolic traits. *BioData Mining*, 7, 21. Available from https://doi.org/10.1186/1756-0381-7-21.

Radonjic, M., van Erk, M. J., Pasman, W. J., Wortelboer, H. M., Hendriks, H. F. J., & van Ommen, B. (2009). Effect of body fat distribution on the transcription response to dietary fat interventions. *Genes & Nutrition*, 4(2), 143−149. Available from https://doi.org/10.1007/s12263-009-0122-9.

Ransohoff, D. F., & Khoury, M. J. (2010). Personal genomics: Information can be harmful. *European Journal of Clinical Investigation*, 40, 64−68. Available from https://doi.org/10.1111/j.1365-2362.2009.02232.x.

Reddon, H., Guéant, J.-L., & Meyre, D. (2016). The importance of gene-environment interactions in human obesity. *Clinical Science*, 130(18), 1571−1597. Available from https://doi.org/10.1042/CS20160221.

Reich, D. E., Cargill, M., Bolk, S., Ireland, J., Sabeti, P. C., Richter, D. J., ... Lander, E. S. (2001). Linkage disequilibrium in the human genome. *Nature*, 411(6834), 199−204. Available from http://dx.doi.org/10.1038/35075590.

Roberts, J. S., Gornick, M. C., Carere, D. A., Uhlmann, W. R., Ruffin, M. T., & Green, R. C. (2017). Direct-to-consumer genetic testing: User motivations, decision making, and perceived utility of results. *Public Health Genomics*, 20(1), 36−45. Available from https://doi.org/10.1159/000455006.

Rozen, R. (2002). Methylenetetrahydrofolate reductase: A link between folate and riboflavin? *The American Journal of Clinical Nutrition*, 76(2), 301−302. Available at http://www.ncbi.nlm.nih.gov/pubmed/12144998 (Accessed 11.11.13).

San-Cristobal, R., Milagro, F. I., & Martínez, J. A. (2013). Future challenges and present ethical considerations in the use of personalized nutrition based on genetic advice. *Journal of the Academy of Nutrition and Dietetics*, 113(11), 1447−1454. Available from https://doi.org/10.1016/j.jand.2013.05.028.

Schünemann, H. J., Schünemann, A. H. J., Oxman, A. D., Brozek, J., Glasziou, P., Jaeschke, R., ... Guyatt, G. H. (2008). Grading quality of evidence and strength of recommendations for diagnostic tests and strategies. *The British Medical Journal*, 336(7653), 1106−1110. Available from https://doi.org/10.1136/bmj.39500.677199.AE.

Selhub, J. (2006). The many facets of hyperhomocysteinemia: Studies from the Framingham cohorts. *The Journal of Nutrition*, 136(6 Suppl), 1726S−1730S. Available at http://www.ncbi.nlm.nih.gov/pubmed/16702347 (Accessed 11.11.13).

Smith, C. E., & Ordovás, J. M. (2010). Fatty acid interactions with genetic polymorphisms for cardiovascular disease. *Current Opinion in Clinical Nutrition and Metabolic Care*, 13(2), 139−144. Available from https://doi.org/10.1097/MCO.0b013e3283357287.

Stampfer, M., & Willett, W. (2015). Folate supplements for stroke prevention: Targeted trial trumps the rest. *the Journal of the American Medical Association*, 313(13), 1321−1322. Available from https://doi.org/10.1001/jama.2015.1961.

Steer, C. D., Davey Smith, G., Emmett, P. M., Hibbeln, J. R., & Golding, J. (2010). FADS2 polymorphisms modify the effect of breastfeeding on child IQ. *Public Library of Science one*, 5(7), e11570. Available from https://doi.org/10.1371/journal.pone.0011570.

Tanaka, C., Kamide, K., Takiuchi, S., Miwa, Y., Yoshii, M., Kawano, Y., & Miyata, T. (2003). An alternative fast and convenient genotyping method for the screening of angiotensin converting enzyme gene polymorphisms. *Hypertension Research: Official Journal of the Japanese Society of Hypertension*, 26(4), 301−306. Available at http://www.ncbi.nlm.nih.gov/pubmed/12733698 (Accessed 13.08.14).

Taylor, C.L. (2008) *Framework for DRI development: Components "known" and components "to be explored,"* 2008. Available at https://www.nal.usda.gov/sites/default/files/fnic_uploads/Framework_DRI_Development.pdf (Accessed 05.06.18).

Tice, J. A. (2010). The vital amines: Too much of a good thing?: Comment on "Effects of lowering homocysteine levels with B vitamins on cardiovascular disease, cancer, and cause-specific mortality. *Archives of Internal Medicine, 170*(18), 1631–1633. Available from https://doi.org/10.1001/archinternmed.2010.338.

Tong, Y., Lin, Y., Zhang, Y., Yang, J., Zhang, Y., Liu, H., & Zhang, B. (2009). Association between TCF7L2 gene polymorphisms and susceptibility to type 2 diabetes mellitus: A large Human Genome Epidemiology (HuGE) review and meta-analysis. *BMC Medical Genetics, 10*, 15. Available from https://doi.org/10.1186/1471-2350-10-15.

van Ommen, B., van der Greef, J., Ordovas, J. M., & Daniel, H. (2014). Phenotypic flexibility as key factor in the human nutrition and health relationship. *Genes & Nutrition, 9*(5), 423. Available from https://doi.org/10.1007/s12263-014-0423-5.

Wald, D. S., Wald, N. J., Morris, J. K., & Law, M. (2006). Folic acid, homocysteine, and cardiovascular disease: Judging causality in the face of inconclusive trial evidence. *British Medical Journal, 333*(7578), 1114–1117. Available from http://doi.org/10.1136/bmj.39000.486701.68.

Wald, D. S., Morris, J. K., & Wald, N. J. (2011). Reconciling the evidence on serum homocysteine and ischaemic heart disease: A meta-analysis. *Public Library of Science One, 6*(2), e16473. Available from https://doi.org/10.1371/journal.pone.0016473.

Ward, M., Wilson, C. P., Strain, J. J., Horigan, G., Scott, J. M., & McNulty, H. (2011). B-vitamins, methylenetetrahydrofolate reductase (MTHFR) and hypertension. *International Journal for Vitamin and Nutrition Research, 81*(4), 240–244. Available from https://doi.org/10.1024/0300-9831/a000069.

West, A. A., & Caudill, M. A. (2010). Genetic variation: Impact on folate (and choline) bioefficacy. *International Journal for Vitamin and Nutrition Research, 80*(4–5), 319–329. Available from https://doi.org/10.1024/0300-9831/a000040.

Wilson, C. P., Ward, M., McNulty, H., Strain, J. J., Trouton, T. G., Horigan, G., ... Scott, J. M. (2012). Riboflavin offers a targeted strategy for managing hypertension in patients with the MTHFR 677TT genotype: A 4-y follow-up. *The American Journal of Clinical Nutrition, 95*(3), 766–772. Available from https://doi.org/10.3945/ajcn.111.026245.

Wilson, C. P., McNulty, H., Ward, M., Strain, J. J., Trouton, T. G., Hoeft, B. A., ... Scott, J. M. (2013). 'Blood pressure in treated hypertensive individuals with the MTHFR 677TT genotype is responsive to intervention with riboflavin: Findings of a targeted randomized trial.'. *Hypertension*. Available from https://doi.org/10.1161/HYPERTENSIONAHA.111.01047.

Wood, P. A. (2008). Potential of nutrigenetics in the treatment of metabolic disorders. *Expert Review of Endocrinology & Metabolism*, 705–713.

Zeevi, D., Korem, T., Zmora, N., Israeli, D., Rothschild, D., Weinberger, A., ... Segal, E. (2015). Personalized nutrition by prediction of glycemic responses. *Cell, 163*(5), 1079–1094. Available from https://doi.org/10.1016/j.cell.2015.11.001.

CHAPTER 3

Personalized Nutrition by Predicting Glycemic Responses

Vaia Katsarou[1] and Magdalini Tsolaki[1,2]

[1]Greek Association of Alzheimer's Disease and Related Disorders, Thessaloniki, Greece
[2]1st Department of Neurology, Medical school, Aristotle University of Thessaloniki, Thessaloniki, Greece

OUTLINE

Introduction	55
Current Methods for Glucose Response Prediction	**57**
Meal Carbohydrate Content	57
Glycemic Index	57
Fiber Content	57
Physical Activity	58
Variability in Glucose Responses	**58**
Method	**59**
Search Strategy	59
Selection Process and Data Extraction	59
Results	**59**
Personalized Nutrition	59
Gut Microbiota	61
Eating Behavior	64
Phenotype	66
Genotype	70
Physical Activity	72
Conclusions	**74**
References	**76**

INTRODUCTION

When we eat a meal that contains carbohydrates, they are broken down into glucose. Glucose passes into the bloodstream and insulin is released. If blood glucose (BG) is not managed efficiently by insulin, glucose reaches a high level and this condition increases the risk of diabetes.

Hyperglycemia is the excess of glucose in the bloodstream. Postprandial hyperglycemia (PPG) is defined as the peak value of BG caused by diabetes, which is measured 2 hours after the start of a meal. Postprandial hyperglycemia has been linked to several chronic diseases such as obesity, type 2 diabetes mellitus (T2DM), and cardiovascular disease (CVD) (Augustin, Franceschi, Jenkins, Kendall, & La Vecchia, 2002; Jenkins et al., 2002).

More specifically, it is associated with long-term damage, dysfunction, and failure of some organs, especially the eyes, the kidneys, the nerves, the heart, and the blood vessels. Hyperglycemia causes symptoms such as polyuria, polydipsia, and weight loss and in some cases polyphagia and blurred vision. Uncontrolled hyperglycemia can cause ketoacidosis, a buildup of acids in the blood that could be life-threatening, or nonketotic hyperosmolar syndrome (American Diabetes Association, 2014).

Type 2 diabetes is associated with atherosclerosis, and thus with mortality and morbidity (Ceriello et al., 2004). It seems that improving glycemic control can reduce the risk of heart diseases. Glycosylated hemoglobin (HbA1c) and postprandial hyperglycemia seem to play key roles in this process. There are two paths for the effect of postprandial glucose. One is the possible toxic effect on the vascular endothelium mediated by oxidative stress. Another is its contribution to total glycemic exposure. What is important is that if we interfere and manage postprandial glucose levels then we can reduce or prevent the cardiovascular complications caused by diabetes.

Postprandial hyperglycemia is associated with an increased risk of death from CVD, even if HbA1c is normal. Also, postprandial hyperglycemia may cause abnormal HbA1c. Thus glucose levels after meals should be monitored in diabetic patients in addition to their HbA1c. Nondiabetic patients with known cardiovascular risk factors should also check their postprandial glucose levels (Gerich, 2003). It has been proposed that patients with normal or near-normal fasting plasma glucose levels that have elevated HbA1c levels should aim to monitor postprandial glucose levels. This is explained by the fact that fasting and postprandial glucose levels are interrelated.

Prediabetes is a case in which early intervention can reduce the risk of progression to diabetes. DeJesus et al., 2017 assessed data of 10,796 people with prediabetes. According to their findings, reducing fasting BG can reduce the risk of diabetes and the reduction was greater in a subgroup of patients with baseline glucose of 100–119 mg/dL. It is very important that people with prediabetes control their BG levels as soon as possible in order to be able to delay the onset of diabetes.

Hyperglycemia is one of the most usual symptoms of metabolic syndrome. Metabolic syndrome includes three of the following symptoms: obesity, hyperglycemia, hypercholesterolemia, and hypertension. Since metabolic syndrome has devastating consequences to people and the global economy, it is of high importance to find ways to improve glycemic control. The current strategies used to improve glycemic control are pharmacological approaches and surgery, such as bariatric surgery. These strategies have a number of side effects. The alternative approach with minimal side effects compared to the strategies mentioned above are lifestyle interventions with dietary approach to be the most effective. Weight loss and reducing carbohydrate intake can lead to an improvement of glycemic control (Dumas, 2016).

Diet plays a major role in glucose responses but factors other than food can affect BG levels as well (Mahan & Escott-Stump, 2004). Factors that increase BG can be insufficient insulin, too much food, and increases in glucagon and other hormones that are increased during stress, illness, or infection. Factors that decrease BG include too much insulin, not enough food, excessive exercise, and skipped or delayed meals.

There are a number of methods that are traditionally used in order to predict glucose responses in the majority of the population. But all of these methods have mixed results in their efficacy as predictive methods.

CURRENT METHODS FOR GLUCOSE RESPONSE PREDICTION

Nutritional factors that affect the glycemic response to foods include the amount of carbohydrate that is consumed and the composition of the carbohydrate, such as the content of glucose or resistant starch it contains. Physical activity is also an important lifestyle factor that can affect glucose responses.

Meal Carbohydrate Content

The amount of carbohydrates that a food or a meal contains could possibly be used in order to predict how much postprandial glucose increases. But foods rich in carbohydrates are important for all people's diets, including those with diabetes. Simple sugars, such as sucrose, are rapidly digested and absorbed. For this reason, in the past it was suggested that food with simple sugars should be excluded from the diet of a person with hyperglycemia. However, today this is considered as a false belief, and it is suggested that the glycemic effect of foods that contain high doses of carbohydrates cannot be predicted based on their structure, for example, starch or sugar (Mahan & Escott-Stump, 2004).

Glycemic Index

The glycemic index is a useful tool in managing blood sugar levels. But it is not without disadvantages, since the amount of carbohydrates that a meal contains affects glucose levels more than the types of carbohydrates a person consumes (Gibney, Elia, Ljungqvist, & Dowsett, 2005). Glycemic index for a given food seems to have low reliability (Hirsch, Barrera, Leiva, de la Maza, & Bunout, 2013). Glucose and insulin responses of a standard meal seem to have a high interindividual variation but it is lower than the intraindividual variation.

Fiber Content

It seems that diets rich in fiber—in large amounts of approximately 50 g per day—have a beneficial effect on glycemia. However, the consumption of such high levels of fiber is difficult for people to consume and it is uncertain if this amount is acceptable to most people. Therefore, increasing fiber consumption to levels higher than the recommended ones (25 g per day) (Mahan & Escott-Stump, 2004).

Physical Activity

In persons with T2DM, exercise generally improves BG control. This happens either through decreased insulin resistance or increased insulin sensitivity (IS), through decreasing the effects of counterregulatory hormones (Mahan & Escott-Stump, 2004).

VARIABILITY IN GLUCOSE RESPONSES

Special diets are recommended in the general hyperglycemic population but it is hard to predict how these people will respond to these dietary interventions.

A number of studies have suggested that there is an increased interpersonal variability in postmeal glucose from identical meals (Vega-López, Ausman, Griffith, & Lichtenstein, 2007; Vrolix & Mensink, 2010). It seems that there is a high variation of glucose response to a reference food both between and within individuals (Hirsch et al., 2013). This might be explained by the fact that the glucose and insulin response is not only influenced by the meal composition and the carbohydrate content, but also other factors.

A highly effective intervention for an individual should consider all the other factors that can affect glucose responses. Today, specific nutritional recommendations are suggested to all people with hyperglycemia or prediabetes in order to reduce the risk or to delay the incidence of diabetes. Although the dietetic approach is still considered as a primary management strategy of glucose impaired responses and diabetes mellitus (DM) prevention, it has been observed that for a minority of individuals these recommendations are not enough (De Roos, 2013). There is a substantial interindividual variation in response to dietary interventions. An individual may express a unique response to a certain food or nutrient that is influenced not only by their physiological status but also by genetic or environmental factors. And this is how the need for a personalized approach to individuals' diets seems to emerge, although the concept of personalized nutrition is not new.

A personalized diet is based on the idea that personal data should be collected for every single individual in order to identify their specific needs or traits and to design a unique intervention for them. Human biology is so complex and unique that if we want to provide an effective therapy to everyone, we should first assess the genetic and environmental parameters of diseases.

Price et al. (2017) suggest that the data that need to be collected should be in a form of "personal, dense and dynamic data clouds: personal, because each data cloud is unique to an individual; dense, because of the high number of measurements; and dynamic, because we monitor longitudinally." For example, in their study they analyzed the data of 108 individuals that were collected in a 9-month period. They collected data from clinical tests, metabolomes, proteomes, and microbiomes, and activity measurements. They were able to generate a correlation network and identify communities of related analytes that were associated with physiology and disease. They also provided participants with behavioral coaching based on personalized data in order to improve clinical biomarkers.

The research in the field of personalized nutrition by predicting glucose responses is still taking its first steps. So far a number of studies have been conducted and the results seem to be promising.

METHOD

Search Strategy

A systematic search of literature was carried out in the following databases: Pubmed, Sciencedirect, and EBSCOhost. The search strategy was conducted by using the following terms: "personalized OR precision AND nutrition AND glucose," "exercise OR activity AND personalized AND glucose," "gut AND microbiota AND glucose," "personalized AND nutrition AND genotype OR phenotype."

Selection Process and Data Extraction

All articles were retrieved until October 2018. Articles were screened by articles, abstract, and relevance. Full texts of articles that seemed to be relevant were screened. The following criteria were implemented:

1. studies aiming to assess glucose responses
2. studies were relevant to factors that affect response variability
3. studies were written in English language

Studies which met the following criteria were excluded:

1. no association to glucose or diabetes
2. case studies
3. studies in languages other than English

RESULTS

Personalized Nutrition

For those few individuals for whom the general dietary guidelines for the prevention of DM that aim to normalize BG levels may be inappropriate, prediction methods are being tested. So far there is no tool that can efficiently predict glucose responses in order to identify the minority of people that react reversely to certain foods.

The current methods that are used to predict glucose responses, as has already been stated, do not seem to be accurate since the results usually are characterized by high variability. Confounders inducing this variability might be baseline BG, body mass index, gender, interpersonal variation, intrapersonal variation, gut microbiome, and also factors like meal frequency, speed of eating, amount of chewing, size of meal, rate of gastric emptying, physical fitness of the person, and previous meals (Latulippe et al., 2013).

There is a clear need for methods that can be used in order to help people with DM predict their glucose responses to their food choices. This could lead to a better management of their glucose levels and to the limitation of the consequences of hyperglycemia.

Factors that associate with the variability of postprandial glucose responses (PPGRs) are separated and discussed below by category. The latest advances on the effects of dietary habits, food behaviors, physical activity, phenotyping, nutrigenomics, metabolomics, and microbiota on glucose levels are included. The results of published studies will be presented in an attempt to highlight the currently available information about the potentiality of using personalized nutrition as a predictive tool for glucose responses.

Trying to use personalized nutrition as a means to predict glucose postprandial responses is not an easy task. A number of requirements has to be fulfilled in order for the possible method to be appropriate. According to Albers et al. (2017), an appropriate predictive method for glucose responses, in the form of a personalized modeling engine, that is capable of predicting postprandial glucose in real time should satisfy four requirements: "(1) use the minimally invasive data that diabetes patients collect in routine care, up to a maximum of 6–10 measurements a day, (2) personalize to the individual and adapt to changes in behavior and health-state, (3) work in real time, and (4) be accurate enough to produce a forecast that can differentiate glucose values that correspond to between 0.5%–2% differences in HbA1c values."

Albers et al. (2017) used a method that satisfied all four of the requirements. The method is called data assimilation (DA) and is a "data science machine that unifies models with data to reconstruct the model state and provide forecasts." Researchers used this method to reconstruct the state of the human endocrine system relevant to glucose–insulin dynamics regulation using the BG measurements that a patient with DM is expected to have. In order to develop this forecasting machinery, they gathered DA that provided real-time glucose predictions for each individual. This machinery was able to adapt and identify the changes of a person's state over time. It was also validated with data from five people with DM. The results of the study support the idea that this computational machinery could be applied more directly to predict PPGRs in order to help people make appropriate nutritional choices.

Frequent and regular monitoring of BG levels is difficult and may cause discomfort in patients. Many diabetes patients, especially those on insulin treatment, may not be able to measure their BG four times a day as is usually recommended. For those patients, models that are not invasive to daily life and can accurately predict BG levels are very important. In recent years the research on automatic BG measurement machines has been expanding. These machines are based on algorithms that are constructed using population and personal data.

A unique study in the field of personalized nutrition in relation to PPGRs was carried out by Zeevi et al. (2015). Their work showed that it might be feasible to predict glucose responses of individuals using personalized nutrition. In this study they created a computer algorithm using a basket of information from 800 participants. They combined information derived from the assessment of dietary habits, physical activity, blood tests, and gut microbiota (GM).

The process was divided into two phases. In the first discovery phase the algorithm was developed on the main cohort of 800 participants, and the second phase was the validation phase which included 100 participants. The algorithm was then used to predict what physical characteristics and behavior can induce different reactions to different food. Based on the algorithm, they created personalized diets for the participants whom they followed and, as expected, they had lowered BG responses after meals.

What was surprising was that which food was good for each individual was not the same for all of them, as a traditional approach for glucose response would suggest.

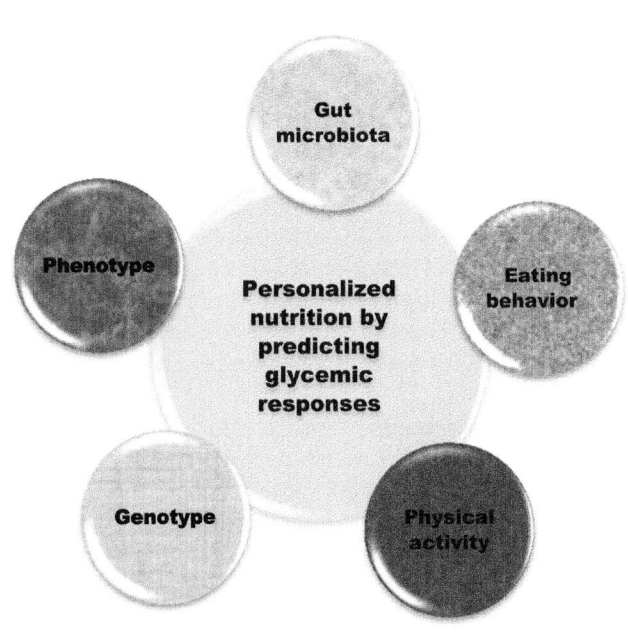

FIGURE 3.1 Personalized Nutrition by predicting glycemic responses. A schematic representation of the main parameters considered to play an important role in designing a personalized nutrition in relation to glycemic responses.

Foods that tended to increase BG levels in most people had adverse results in some of the subjects and vice versa. For example, bread increased postprandial glucose levels dramatically in some people but had no effect on others. This study was an attempt to support the idea that tailored diets could help in the prevention of DM and other noncommunicable diseases, by personalizing each persons' daily meals and food choices. Diets based on the unique characteristics of people support the idea that general recommendations about healthy food choices are not suitable for everyone.

Since the response to diet is affected by a number of epigenetic and metabolic factors, the differential responses on diet elements need to be investigated. Thus it could be possible to define distinct metabolic groups within a population.

The study discussed above assessed many factors that affect the variability in glucose responses at the same time. Other studies have assessed these factors separately, and it is very interesting to analyze the possible effects of each factor.

The analysis of parameters that need to be considered in order to predict glycemic responses is a priority in the field of personalized nutrition. The various contributing factors are illustrated in Fig. 3.1.

Gut Microbiota

Any two humans will share nearly 99.9% of their genes, but the GM contains about 100 times more genes than any individual human genome. This could allow us to assume that differences in the GM system could play a significant role in the explanation of the high interpersonal variations of phenotypes (Ejtahed, Soroush, Angoorani, Larijani, & Hasani-Ranjbar, 2016).

The GM community contains about 500−1000 species of gut microorganisms in humans. It has the ability to interact with the host and it can have a beneficial role on an individual's immune system and metabolism. The GM is modifiable, and this could be achieved by the use of probiotics and probiotics that have a therapeutic effect (Sommer & Backhed, 2013).

Environmental changes, such as dietary habits and sedentary time, have had a negative impact on the increase of the prevalence of diabetes. The GM is affected by not only genetics but also environmental factors (Brunkwall & Orho-Melander, 2017). Interestingly, it has been observed that interindividual variation in GM is high. The composition of GM is regulated by a number of factors such as diet habits or drugs. In addition to the fact that GM contributes to diabetes development, changing the GM synthesis is a target area for diabetes prevention and treatment.

An association of the gut with host health and disease (Han et al., 2018) has been observed. Gut bacterial composition is highly associated with insulin impairment and type 1 DM (T1DM). It would be useful to be able to intervene in GM synthesis of individuals in order to help them manage their glucose levels. The GM composition differs between individuals with or at risk of T1DM. This association relies on different mechanisms. The abundance, stability, and connectivity have an important impact. It seems that a low diversity and smaller numbers of the GM might lead to a difficulty in digesting a diverse diet. Thus the limiting of gut microbial fermentation products increases the risk of T1DM. Other factors that can influence the intestinal microbial composition and activity include altering the intestinal permeability, the immune response, sex hormones, and diet parameters, such as conventional diets, minor food components, and food additives.

With regards to the GM as a parameter that could be used to predict glucose responses, the study of Zeevi et al. (2015) showed very interesting results. Stool samples of 800 participants were analyzed in order to assess their microbiomes, that is, the collection of bugs that live in the gut. It was found that the types of microbes present in their gut could affect how their BG responded to particular meals. Bacterial taxa were either beneficial, showing a lower PPGR, or nonbeneficial, showing the opposite reaction. Also Enterobacteriaceae and Actinobacteria were found to be nonbeneficial as they were positively correlated with postprandial hyperglycemia. Moreover, beneficial microbiome factors were also negatively associated with glycosylated hemoglobin (HbA1c). These findings might provide some answers to the question of why people have different reactions to the same food and also highlight the potential of the GM to play an important role in personalized nutrition.

In another study, Korem et al. (2017) also aimed to show that the GM can be used to predict glycemic responses. It was a randomized crossover trial with two 1-week interventions separated by a 2-week long washout period. The researchers assessed the effect of two types of bread on glucose and on the GM. An industrial whole bread made from refined wheat flour and a whole grain wheat flour bread made through traditional methods were used in the study and 50 g of bread was consumed by each participant every day. The GM composition remained generally stable and person specific. There was a highly significant interpersonal variation in the glucose response to the two types of bread. It was very interesting that microbiome data alone could predict the type of bread that induced high glycemic responses. This study also supports the suggestion that universal dietary recommendations may have limited efficacy as the comparison of breads considered healthy or unhealthy have personal effects on PPGRs.

The fact that the GM analysis could allow us to predict how an individual responds to a food, in addition to the possibility of intervening in our GM synthesis to change it, indicates that designing a personalized approach to monitor glucose responses seems to be realistic. We could then help individuals make beneficial food choices in order to have PPGRs within the normal ranges. Hasani-Ranjbar and Larijani (2017) suggest that this could happen through strategies such as personalized probiotic and prebiotic supplements, dietary interventions, and fecal microbiota transplantation.

A comparison of the effect of personalized nutrition with or without probiotics supplementation showed that personalized diet did decrease glucose levels, but the addition of probiotics in the diet did not show any effect on glucose (Valentini et al., 2015). The diet was provided through the web to 62 healthy people aged 65–85 years for 7 weeks. It was based on their local food customs and preferences, and followed WHO recommendations for nutrient intake. Blood and stool samples were assessed before and after the intervention. The baseline levels of the probiotics *Clostridium* and *Bifidobacterium* were similar between the two groups with an evident high interindividual variability. Although the levels of these probiotics had no significant changes in the fecal abundances observed after the intervention, the proportion of subjects with changes in bifidobacteria concentrations after the intervention tended to be different between the two groups.

Palacios et al. (2017), in a randomized controlled trial that started in 2015, hypothesized that changing the GM synthesis using multispecies probiotics would decrease metabolic and inflammatory markers and improve BG management. Sixty adults with prediabetes or early T2DM participated. They were provided with either a multispecies probiotics capsule or a placebo for 12 weeks. The researches hoped that this study would result in novel treatments able to reduce the metabolic disturbances associated with prediabetes and T2DM.

Although probiotics intake seems to have a beneficial effect on BG, some studies failed to support this suggestion. In one study (Mazloom, Yousefinejad, & Dabbaghmanesh, 2013), 34 patients with T2DM were divided into two groups: an intervention group, who received 1500 mg probiotics capsules twice a day for 6 weeks, and a placebo group. The lactobacillus probiotics contained *L. acidophilus*, *L. bulgarium*, *L. bifidum*, and *L. casei*. This single-blinded trial showed that the fasting blood sugar did not change significantly after probiotics treatment. But the study had the limitations of a small sample size and short duration.

In the same context, another study (Ivey et al., 2014) could not support the hypothesis that probiotics are of benefit for short-term glycemic control. In this randomized control study 156 overweight men and women were divided into four intervention groups that received (1) probiotics yogurt plus probiotics capsules, (2) probiotics yogurt plus placebo capsules, (3) control milk plus probiotics capsules, and (4) control milk plus placebo capsules. The probiotics used were *L. acidophilus* La5 and *Bifidobacterium animalis* subsp *lactics* Bb12, either isolated or as part of a whole food, and they were offered for 6 weeks. Another randomized double-blinded placebo-controlled clinical trial (Ostadrahimi et al., 2015) showed similar results. In this study 60 diabetic patients were divided into two groups. One group received probiotic fermented milk (kefir) that contained *L. casei*, *L. acidophilus*, and Bifidobacteria, and the other one received conventional fermented milk.

Fasting BG was decreased in the kefir group but the decrease was not statistically significant. For both the studies, the researchers suggest that the effect of probiotics bacteria on the metabolism is complex, partly due to the complexity of the host—microbiome interactions.

A meta-analysis of 11 randomized placebo-controlled trials (Sun & Buys, 2016) assessed the effect of probiotic intake on the postprandial glucose and also other risk factors of 614 subjects in total. The results highlighted a statistically significant difference between the control and the intervention group, showing a reduction in glucose levels. A meta-regression analysis showed the same results but only in subjects with DM, in contrast with subjects with other risk factors.

Although some parameters that affect GM synthesis are modifiable, some others are not. These refer to age and sex, parameters that have a big impact in the human GM (Singh & Manning, 2016), thus they might play an important role in different glucose responses. Sex seems to be associated with the GM composition overall (Dominianni et al., 2015). Women tend to have a lower abundance of Bacteroidetes than men.

A number of studies support the statement that the GM is associated with host health and disease. Diet and food components affect the GM and especially its composition, stability, and connectivity. Moreover, the GM influences immune response and through this path it can affect the development of diabetes. More research is needed in order to shed light on the underlying mechanisms.

Analysis of the GM for diabetes purposes would be very useful in personalized treatments. Although it is expensive and thus may not be applicable to all populations, there is no doubt that this will change in the future. Further advances in technology will decrease the cost of GM analysis and it will become more accessible. The ultimate goal is to improve the efficacy of the treatment of diabetes. There is still a lot to be understood about the role of the GM on glucose responses but it might not take too long for new opportunities in therapeutic approaches to open up. Advances in this area would help with the aim of achieving a better control of glucose responses and furthermore help in diabetes management.

Eating Behavior

Eating behaviors such as mastication, chewing style, and number of bites can affect PPGRs. Mastication is the start point of digestion. It breaks down the food into small particles and helps enzymes to release nutrients and absorb them into bloodstream. Mastication enables complex carbohydrates, proteins, and lipids to be broken down into simple forms. Then insulin is released to help with glucose absorption. Taste cells and receptors that exist on the tongue take part in a process where more insulin is released independent of glucose values. The mastication process differs between individuals and its characteristics such as frequency and thoroughness may affect the feeling of satiety or weight management. Traditionally it has been suggested that proper mastication (of high frequency) helps to control body weight. Some studies have investigated the role of mastication on carbohydrate metabolism, BG, and serum insulin on postprandial glucose levels. It is very interesting to assess the effect of specific chewing styles on postprandial glucose levels both in dysglycemic and normoglycemic individuals.

A method designed to test all relevant digestion parameters of realistic food has been developed in order to test a wide variety of food and meals. Bellmann, Minekus, Sanders, Bosgra, and Havenaar (2018) described a combined in vitro and in silico (input data for mathematical computer modeling) technology that can predict the glycemic response curves in individuals. This method tested 22 food products and has taken into account the major determinants of the glycemic response, such as the glucose the incremental area under the curve (iAUC) and the maximum glucose concentration between the predicted glycemic response curves (Cmax). It seems to be able to accurately measure the digestibility of foods and the availability of glycemic carbohydrates for absorption. According to the research, the advantages are that it is time- and cost-efficient, and an effective alternative to invasive human studies.

Another study (Tan et al., 2016) investigated the key digestive parameters that influence and impact interindividual differences in glucose response. Mastication is a potential digestive parameter that may contribute to the variability of postprandial glucose. Chewing style is another possible digestive parameter that was tested in the same study. The number of chews per mouthful and chewing time per mouthful characterize the chewing style. The results showed a positive relationship between the number of chews at each mouthful and glucose increase. Also, the mastication parameters predicted glucose response. The authors suggested that eating quickly could lead us to consume larger amounts of food in a shorter period of time and this will increase glucose responses. For this reason, eating slowly and chewing less is recommended to help control PPGRs.

The number of bites is important for glycemic responses. Chewing 15 times compared with 30 times significantly reduced glycemic response, peak glycemic response, and the glycemic index of rice (Ranawana, Leow, & Henry, 2014). The potential of mastication to affect postprandial plasma glucose is attributed to the improved digestibility and absorption of nutrients.

Mastication seems to affect people with normal glucose tolerance and people with a predisposition to T2DM differently. A crossover trial (Suzuki et al., 2005) of 52 test meals showed that in people with normal glucose tolerance the postprandial plasma glucose concentration was significantly lower after thorough mastication. This might be attributed to the potentiation of early-phase insulin secretion. In contrast, thorough mastication increased plasma glucose and serum insulin significantly compared to usual mastication in people with a predisposition to DM. In this group, thorough mastication did not potentiate early-phase insulin secretion.

Another similar but bigger crossover trial (Madhu et al., 2016) found significant differences in the postprandial BG levels between routine and thorough mastication in a normoglycemic group. The authors suggested that this simple lifestyle modification of thorough mastication could be used by people with increased risk factors for DM as a preventive strategy.

It seems that eating behavior plays an important role in glucose responses, but it is of high importance that we are able to assess accurately food behavior to account for interindividual differences. In order for the measurements to be accurate, we have to rely on methods that are able to provide unbiased interpretations.

In a recent review (de Toro-Martín, Arsenault, Després, & Vohl, 2017) a number of assessment methods were presented, such as innovative tools. One tool of this category that can be used in free-living conditions is the Automatic Ingestion Monitor. It is a wearable device and uses three different sensors: jaw motion, hand gesture, and accelerometer. It can assess snacking habits and also night eating or weekend overeating. Another tool is the Universal Eating Monitor, a table-embedded scale that can measure the amount of food an individual eats during the day. It is a useful device that has the ability to assess different eating behavior parameters such as eating rate, bite size, and food-to-drink ratio. Being able to give information about the food frequency and snacking habits of individuals makes it a precious tool. This monitor has the disadvantage that it requires restricted conditions on the foods someone consumes and the behaviors that he or she is allowed to express during eating, such as stirring and manipulating foods or placing napkins on the scale, because that would change the scale weight and give false measurements.

A new algorithm was developed in order to detect and measure the weight or individual bites consumed outside laboratory or clinical settings (Mattfeld, Muth, & Hoover, 2017). This algorithm has the ability to analyze the surrounding weight changes and has been tested on 271 subjects with satisfying results.

Future work on mastication must establish the extent to which a chewing style affects postprandial BG levels. It could also assess the possibility to use chewing habits in order to reduce glycemic effects of food.

Phenotype

It is important that an alternative to the traditional methods for predicting glucose responses to food should be developed, since the currently available glycemic measures were found to be inadequate. The use of the phenotype has shown potential in being effective in the process of glucose prediction.

In order to construct an effective algorithm for predicting glucose responses, personalization has to be based on an individual's personal characteristics. Capel et al., 2014 in a randomized crossover clinical study used an artificial pancreas for this purpose. In this study a closed-loop system consisting of a personalized predictive rule-based algorithm was compared with a usual continuous subcutaneous insulin infusion of 10 people with T1DM. The algorithm was based on patients' personal data and was superior concerning the ability to achieve better nocturnal normoglycemia (90% of the time during nocturnal period) without significant hypoglycemia as only one hypoglycemic event took place with the algorithm compared to nine events that manifested by following their usual method. Although the use of the algorithm seemed to be beneficial by this aspect, no clear benefit appeared over prandial bolus on the postprandial glycemia and it did not avoid an excessive glycemic excursion in some patients. The use of the algorithm provides us with the possibility of predicting glucose excursion with a maximum around 90 minutes after meal intake. However, its usefulness is still unclear.

Fasting metabolic profile may be possibly used to predict postprandial insulin demands in individuals with normal glucose metabolism, as has been shown in the study of Moazzami et al., 2014. They tried not only to predict hyperglycemia or hypoglycemia, but also to determine an accepted stability in glucose fluctuations. The metabolic profiles of 19 postmenopausal women with normal fasting glucose and normal glucose tolerance were assessed. Three bread types (refined wheat, whole-meal rye, and refined rye) providing 50 g of carbohydrates were given to the participants as a single meal and their postprandial metabolic profiles were measured. The results showed that women with higher fasting concentrations of leucine and isoleucine and lower fasting concentrations of sphingomyelins and phosphatidylcholines had higher insulin responses despite consuming the same grams of carbohydrates. Differences were observed in the postprandial responses of amino acids, and were not attributed to the fiber content of each bread type or enhanced insulin response. This predictive rule-based algorithm can be used in the concept of personalized nutrition for the stratification of individuals.

In a different study (Rozendaal et al., 2018), the PPGR dynamics were described using a systems approach, and it considered heterogeneity in both composition and amount of food, and also the metabolic status, for example, the IS of the subject. After the evaluation of the glycemic index of 53 common food products and mixed meals, the physiology-based dynamic approach was used to reconstruct postprandial response profiles of glucose and insulin. The researchers suggest that this method can systematically and accurately analyze PPGRs and it can be adjusted to account for the metabolic status of an individual.

In another study (Morris et al., 2013) a metabolic phenotyping approach was developed in order to identify which people responded differently to an oral glucose tolerance test (OGTT). This study combined data from three cohorts. Data of 214 subjects aged 18–60 years were evaluated. The researchers collected data on fasting glucose, triacylglycerols, high density lipoproteins (HDL), low density lipoproteins (LDL), and hemoglobin concentrations. Subjects were then divided randomly into three groups: a group that received an OGTT and an oral lipid tolerance test (OLTT), an OGTT only, and an OLTT only. In addition to blood and urine samples other data were included such as anthropometrics, body composition information, fitness tests, and data on biochemical and immune parameters. Data of the OGTT was collected for 116 subjects and their analysis led to the identification of 4 distinct metabotypes. Cluster 1 had the highest BMI, the highest percentage of body fat, and the lowest VO_{2max}. Cluster 2 had the highest mean VO_{2max}, and cluster 3 had the lowest BMI and lowest percentage of body fat. Cluster 1 displayed a very different response for glucose insulin and c-peptide compared to the other clusters, having the highest baseline glucose, peak glucose, and glucose score at 120 minutes. It also had the highest insulin concentration and a reduced beta cell function during the test. With the method used in this study, at-risk phenotypes could be identified. This study showed that it might be possible to identify people who are at risk for T2DM by predicting glucose response. This is a typical example of how a personalized diet could help prevent the disease.

Another case of the use of phenotyping in personalized nutrition is the Maastricht Study (Schram et al., 2014), an observational prospective population-based cohort study which aimed to investigate the etiology of T2DM, its classic complications, and associated disturbances. In this study, imaging techniques and extensive biobanking such as body composition by dual energy X-ray absorptiometry, electrophysiology of the heart, and spirometry were used to determine health status in a cohort of 10,000 individuals with a high prevalence of T2DM. The study population was enriched with T2DM to increase the statistical power to identify differences between individuals with and without DM. Glucose metabolism was assessed by a standardized 7-point OGTT after an overnight fast. The subjects had a 75 g glucose drink and their BG was measured at baseline and 15, 30, 45, 60, 90, and 120 minutes after ingestion. When the results of this study concerning glucose response are derived, important information about how phenotyping can be used in personalized nutrition will be obtained.

Postprandial glycemic responses seem to be associated with multiple risk factors and the assessment of this association may give some insight into their role when designing a personalized diet. In the study by Zeevi et al. (2015), risk factors such as BMI, glycosylated hemoglobin (HbA1c), wake up glucose, and age were found to persist along the entire range of PPGR values. Lower values of glucose response were associated with lower levels of risk factors even within the normal value ranges. Also, using the monitor for continuous glucose measurements, researchers examined the associations between risk factors and glucose level at different percentiles of each participant. The results showed that the correlation was higher for different percentiles with particular risk factors. Thus the entire range of glucose levels of an individual may have clinical relevance.

Using meal challenges and statistical exploratory tools could stratify metabolic phenotypes that have different PPGRs. Krishnan et al., 2012 have been able to identify individuals that have metabolic responses that are dissimilar to the majority of the normal healthy population's responses based on their metabolic characteristics. In this crossover design study, 24 overweight women provided data for their glucose, insulin, leptin, and nonesterified fatty acids. The subjects consumed low (LGI) and high glycemic index (HGI) meals in the following pattern: they were tested either with a HGI meal followed by an LGI meal, or an LGI meal followed by an HGI meal. Researchers assessed their glucose, insulin, and leptin responses and clustered subjects into three groups. The first group with the majority of subjects displayed the expected glucose and insulin responses. The second group had lower postprandial leptin, higher insulin, and higher glucose relative responses to the two meal challenges. The third group had high leptin and glucose with similar insulin responses to the first group. Thus the second and third group displayed alternate physiological responses, in contrast to the first group. The researchers hypothesize that these alternate response profiles depend on the metabolic phenotypes of individuals and can be identified using their postprandial response to a single meal test. This study analyzed the variance in the meal challenge responses using a phenotyping approach and showed that it could be possible to detect subclinical metabolic dysfunctions and thus apply personalized nutrition management approaches.

Another measurement tool was developed in a recent study (Hall et al., 2018). Using a wearable CGM device, the researchers developed a new method to measure glucose variability. In order to characterize detailed glycemic patterns they used standardized meals and pattern analysis to define individual glucotypes. They categorized 57 individuals into three glucotypes of increasing variability in glucose measurements: low (L), moderate (M), or severe (S). This categorization explained 73% of the observed variance in glucose. They were able to identify individuals with impaired glucose metabolism or prediabetes, even though they were supposed to have normal BG levels. This could be attributed to insulin resistance and relative insulin secretion defects. In addition, the individual variability in glycemic responses was highlighted in this study, as well as the ability to detect hyperglycemia when this was not possible using other traditional tests such as fasting glucose, OGTT, and HbA1c.

A 12-month, prospective, controlled, cluster-randomized program was implemented to 907 patients with insulin treated T2D (Kulzer et al., 2018). In this study, the researchers examined HbA1c levels, therapy changes, hypoglycemic events, and other parameters relevant to diabetes. The method included (1) structured assessment; (2) self-measured blood glucose (SMBG) data; (3) use of data management software to systemically document, process, and visualize SMBG data; (4) systemic analytics and change of therapy; and (5) collaborative communication. The results showed that the group of patients in the intervention group, in comparison with patients in the control group to which treatment according to their customary medical routine was provided, demonstrated an improved glycemic control. Specifically, HbA1c was reduced significantly at the 3-month follow-up and this reduction remained nearly constant for the remaining study period. This study showed demonstrated that an integrated, structured, and personalized approach is beneficial for patients with insulin treated T2DM. The low cost approach that was used was easy to implement and integrated a software solution. The researchers suggest that since it is compatible with novel diagnostic tools, such as the continuous glucose monitoring (CGM), it can be implemented in a broad range of health care systems in order to achieve better glycemic control, more timely treatment adjustments, and better patient adherence and treatment satisfaction from both patients and physicians.

Contreras and his colleagues (Contreras, Oviedo, Vettoretti, Visentin, & Vehí, 2017) designed a hybrid model that uses grammatical evolution (GE), insulin on board, and glucose rate of absorption methods to predict BG values. It is a combination of physiological models for insulin and grammatical evolution. A penalizing fitness function was used to control the clinical harm caused by deviations from the target BG. In order to construct the prediction models they invented an algorithm that used data of 100 virtual patients generated by a T1DM simulator. The data collection lasted for 14 days and included insulin, carbohydrate, and CGM. By using personalized models and different scenarios they managed to make reliable BG predictions. The results of the study were promising. They supported the suggestion that the use of a glucose-specific cost function that takes into account the possible errors makes the prediction model more reliable. Also using individual specific dynamics, lifestyle, and other parameters can improve the performance and safety of the alternative prediction methods. This study described an alternative method for predicting BG and customized patients' treatments. The researchers suggested that this approach could be used to predict short-term BG values to identify errors in glucose monitoring.

Another personalized diabetes prediction mechanism used mobile technology in order to collect diabetes patient data and population data (Li & Fernando, 2016). This method is personalized for every individual and its goal is to improve the prediction accuracy and reduce the negative impact of sparse data of traditional prediction approaches. The data was collected through smartphones and included insulin, meals, exercise, and sleep. A three-stage evolution model used to obtain more accurate and personalized predictions included (1) a time-series prediction model based on patient data, (2) a pooled panel data regression model, and (3) a preclustered personalized regression model. The results of the study support the suggestion that this model improves the prediction accuracy and controls the problems of data accuracy of the traditional methods. It could be a useful tool for personalized treatment of impaired BG.

HbA1c is important in glycemic control and affects glucose responses. From the perspective of personalization, it has been proposed that personalized care plans (PCPs) and HbA1c levels are mediated by BMI and physical activity. 3894 responders to the 2014 Health Survey for England were used in the study of Umeh (2017). The data they provided for assessment included HbA1c levels, PCP, BMI, and physical activity. The subjects were 16 to 90 years old and were included regardless of their diabetes status. A PCP usually consists of written documented recommendations that aim to help patients achieve specific goals. They are personalized and essential for effective self-management. It was expected that patients with PCPs will have lower HbA1c levels than those who had not agreed to be provided with a care plan. Also it was expected that BMI and physical activity would affect this relationship between PCPs and HbA1c and could at least partly explain it. The results showed that patients with a PCP had higher HbA1c levels than those without a care plan. The mediation effect of BMI was more severe among patients aged 40–60 years. What was interesting was that physical activity did not seem to affect the relationship between PCPs and glucose control. It seemed that BMI was important as a mediator in contrast to physical activity. Also a higher BMI might explain higher HbA1c levels in patients with a PCP.

Variation in human data can be observed in a number of ways. Identifying the characteristics of individuals that play a key role in this variation can reduce the complexity and the "noise" of data sets. More research is needed in this field. Ethnic diversity is an important study area in this field and so are a wide range of parameters that are relevant to phenotype.

Genotype

Diabetes management can sometimes be inappropriate and fail to control hyperglycemic events. A personalized diabetes treatment that is based on the genetic background of an individual may allow a more successful disease progression and reduce the complications. Genetic testing could identify not only those who are at risk, but may also identify those with diabetes or prediabetes who could benefit from tailor-made interventions based on their genetic profile.

There are two approaches that focus on the interaction between genes and diet (Gaboon, 2011). Nutrigenetics focuses on how the genetic background of an individual affects their responses to various dietary nutrients. This research area could give answers about why and how people have different responses to the same nutrient intake, thus it could explain interindividual variability. Diabetes with its glucose fluctuations is known to have genetic and/or nutritional components, thus it is an area of investigation into whether dietary intervention can affect the glucose responses. Nutrigenomics focuses on the effects of the ingested nutrients on gene expression. Nutrigenomics can provide important information that will be used in the identification of the dietetic components that can benefit or damage health, thus it could help in the design of an optimal diet for an individual.

Diet plays a major role in insulin resistance by interacting with genetic variants (López-Miranda et al., 2007). Some individuals appear to be relatively insensitive to dietary interventions and some others are more sensitive. Thus general dietetic recommendations are not necessarily good for all individuals. An example of gene-diet interaction is Apolipoprotein E (ApoE) which is a structural component of several lipoproteins. The effect of this polymorphism on peripheral IS was examined for the consumption of three diets: a high monounsaturated fatty acids diet, a high saturated fatty acids diet, and a high carbohydrate diet on 43 volunteers with the ApoE3/E3 genotype (8 GG, 25 GT, and 10 TT) (Moreno et al., 2004). The steady-state plasma glucose (SSPG) concentration was lower in GG subjects than in GT and TT individuals, regardless of the diet consumed. Significant diet by genotype interactions were found for SSPG and plasma FFA concentrations.

A diet rich in carbohydrates may not be suitable for all genotypes. Two groups, a control and a group of 235 patients with metabolic syndrome, participated in an intervention study which aimed to test how the genetic polymorphisms of the lipoprotein lipase (LPL) would modulate the effects of a diet high in carbohydrate in metabolic syndrome adults (Zhang, Ma, Guo, Wan, & Xue, 2015). The dietetic intervention included increased whole grain food, deep colored vegetables and fruits, and low intake of sodium, simple sugars, and dietary fat. The haplotype rs328G located within the LPL locus is associated with insulin resistance. The study showed that after a diet high in carbohydrates, fasting glucose was improved in subjects of rs328CC homozygotes, in contrast to the group of rs328G carriers. These results highlight the need for personalized nutrition for this group of patients.

There is no doubt that genotyping plays an important role for a personalized approach to diet. But for complex polygenic traits such as diabetes, it is very difficult to separate the effects of specific genes on the development of the disease characteristics (De Roos, 2013). It is difficult to assess the susceptibility of an individual to impaired glucose responses and even more complex to develop and implement a personalized diet in order to change the effects of his or her genes on glucose function.

The interaction of food behavior with the circadian system may also account for interindividual variability in metabolic processes (de Toro-Martín et al., 2017). The circadian biological clock is maintained endogenously by a number of genes and it affects numerous aspects of human physiology including feeding behavior, the sleep/wake cycle, and metabolism. In a study (Dashti et al., 2014) the interactions between CRY1 polymorphism, rs2287161, and carbohydrate intake on insulin resistance were tested. 1548 participants from two independent populations (Mediterranean and North American) were investigated for this study. The findings showed that an increase in carbohydrate intake was associated with a significant increase in homeostasis model assessment of insulin resistance, fasting insulin, and a decrease in quantitative insulin sensitivity check index (QUICKI), only among individuals homozygous for the minor C allele. This study supports the link between the circadian system and glucose metabolism and suggests the importance of this CRY1 locus in developing personalized nutrition interventions in people at risk of diabetes.

A review of 15 cohort studies and 28,190 participants has observed significant associations between relative macronutrient intakes and glycemic traits and short sleep duration and higher fasting glucose. Also, in this review, known MTNR1B (circadiant variants) associations with glycemic traits were replicated (Dashti et al., 2015). Specifically, significant interactions between carbohydrate intake and the variant MTNR1B-rs1387153 for fasting glucose have been revealed. It is concluded that lower carbohydrate intake and normal sleep duration may help metabolic abnormalities that are influenced by common circadian-related genetic variants. Identifying dietary components that could modulate the risk of diabetes together with clock genetic variants could help in the design of personalized nutrition interventions for individuals at risk.

In recent years, major advances have been made in the young science of Nutrigenomics. The paths by which genetics contribute in diseases such as diabetes make up a research area of high interest. However, there is still much to be investigated and explored as to how diet elements and genotypes interact. The application of Nutrigenomics research provides an opportunity to implement personalized nutrition interventions that will improve the health not only of some individuals but also subgroups of people and improve overall public health.

Physical Activity

If we could identify the determinants that contribute to individual variability in response to exercise, we could approach the idea of providing individuals with personalized lifestyle-based treatments. There is a high variability in measurements of glucose responses to physical activity. However, it is of high importance to assess whether the glucose responses to exercise are beyond the day-to-day variability.

de Lannoy, Clarke, Stotz, and Ross (2017) investigated the individual and combined effects of the amount and intensity of exercise on glucose and insulin levels of 171 sedentary, middle-aged adults with obesity. The researchers suggest that when considering the individual response to treatment, it is important to take into account the day-to-day variability in measurement. The participants were separated randomly into four exercise groups with different levels of intensity: no exercise, low amount/low intensity, high amount/low intensity, and high amount/high intensity. In this study the day-to-day variability of glucose and insulin was calculated and taken into account. The results showed that 80% of the subjects did now show any significant improvement in glucose and insulin levels independently of the level of physical activity intensity. Analyzing the day-to-day variability, it has been shown that this kind of variability for insulin and glucose variables was extremely large. According to the researchers, this variability consists of biological variability, meaning variability due to fluctuations in free-living habits such as dietary composition, sleep patterns, and stress level, and also of analytical variability. The findings of this study suggest that although recommendations for increasing physical activity and following a balanced diet remain a cornerstone of diabetes prevention, it is uncertain that the use of exercise to improve glucose control is an effective strategy for every person.

In the same context, Shambrook et al. (2018) investigated the effect of different levels of physical activity intensity on glucose response. Ten males underwent interventions of low, moderate, and high intensity exercise or no exercise. Glucose response was assessed with a continuous glucose monitor under free-living conditions. The results showed that glucose response to exercise 30 minutes after a meal is independent of exercise intensity in healthy insufficiently active males. This study could not support the idea that the intensity of exercise could possibly predict changes in glucose responses.

On the other hand, an algorithm for carbohydrate and insulin adjustment could predict glucose responses after exercise. Kilbride et al. (2011) tested the use of an algorithm in a quasiexperimental study with 14 subjects with T1DM. They compared the reproducibility of glucose response to the algorithm with that of their self-management strategies. The results showed that despite the interpersonal variability of glucose responses, there was a good reproducibility rate after 40 minutes of moderate intensity exercise either using the algorithm or using self-management strategies.

Bouchard et al. (2012) suggested that searching for potential physiological and molecular predictors for adverse response of risk factors to exercise is of high importance. Some of the 1687 adults from six previous studies that were analyzed experienced changes in an opposite direction to the expected effects, thus increasing their risk factor. The researchers investigated the differences between individuals in the response to regular exercise. Concerning the risk for DM, an adverse response was recorded if an increase in insulin reached 24 pmol/L or more. The results showed that 8.4% of the subjects had an adverse change in insulin response. Another interesting finding of the study was that approximately 7% of the participants experienced adverse responses to exercise for at least two risk factors for cardiometabolic diseases and DM and less than 1% for three or more. On the question of whether those who responded adversely for a given risk factor were also those who experienced the least improvement in cardiorespiratory fitness with regular exercise the answer was no. Also the three levels of exercise energy expenditure tested showed no significant differences. This study highlights the interpersonal variability in insulin response and other cardiovascular and diabetes risk factors and suggests that this variability should be identified in order to design personalized exercise prescriptions.

In another randomized three period, three treatment crossover trial (Dunstan et al., 2012), participants underwent three laboratory conditions which followed the consumption of food:

1. uninterrupted sitting;
2. sitting interrupted every 20 minutes by 2 minutes light intensity activity breaks; and
3. sitting interrupted every 20 minutes by 2 minutes moderate intensity activity breaks.

The study showed that it is possible to attenuate acute postprandial plasma glucose and serum insulin response during prolonged sitting, with small breaks of light to moderate intensity physical activity.

Further research is needed in order to identify predictors of the inability to benefit from exercise that is generally recommended. Adverse or no effects of exercise need to be addressed. Mediators of the relationship between physical activity and BG should be identified and assessed. The roles of health status, age, amount and intensity of exercise are key areas of focus. All these and also other potential physiological predictors need to be identified in order to provide a personalized physical activity plan that could correct adverse response patterns.

CONCLUSIONS

This chapter has focused on multiple environmental and genetic factors that affect interpersonal variability in glycemic responses. There are still many questions about the relationships between these parameters and glucose responses. Until more light is shed on this field, it is very difficult to design a personalized diet for individuals that could help them to control their glucose levels.

Personalized nutrition for glucose response prediction is equally applicable to people with impaired glucose control and to healthy people with a genetic susceptibility to diabetes. The fact that the focus is on individuals enhances the limited impact on populations. However, it is considered a huge advantage for those individuals that cannot benefit from general recommendations and wish to have tools to achieve personal goals.

Whether environmental or genetic factors are more important, we do not know. 353 overweight and obese adults participated in a 12-month weight loss program (Walker et al., 2015) that looked at the integrated effect of a number of lifestyle changes such as weight, diet, and physical activity, taking account the genetic susceptibility of developing T2DM on changes in glycemic traits. The results of this study showed that the paths through modifiable components relating to body weight, diet, and physical activity had a greater impact than genetic predisposition on change in glycemic characteristics. Diabetes is a complex disease and there are a number of genetic and environmental factors that contribute to its appearance and progression. Many studies do not consider the contribution of these factors and this fact is responsible for the interpersonal variability in glucose responses and the T2DM development.

Interventions that aim to control glycemic control can be more effective if attention is shifted to the large variability observed in glucose responses. If interventions focus on additional information that differentiates responses between individuals, then personalized diets can be designed. This area of focus used to be considered as "noise" in the results of older studies and the participants who did not demonstrate the outcomes of the majority were labeled as "nonresponders" or of "low sensitivity." Is it feasible that personalized diets can be put into clinical practice?

There is already some strong evidence that personalized nutrition is feasible and one of the most supportive studies of this idea is the intervention trials by Zeevi et al. (2015). The findings provide proof that indeed personalized nutrition can be used as a predictor of PPGRs. They designed a two-arm blinded randomized controlled trial with 26 subjects. Dietitians designed diets for the participants according to their regular dietary habits. They provided all the data (microbiome, blood tests, etc.) needed for the calculation of the algorithm of the main body of the study mentioned above. Then they were blindly divided into two arms. The first one was the "prediction arm" where the algorithm was applied. Based on the algorithm they designed two diets, a good and a bad diet that contained food that induced low or high PPGRs, respectively. The participants followed each diet for a week and glucose and microbiota were assessed. The second arm was called the "expert arm" and was used as a gold standard for comparison. The results of the intervention showed that the personalized approach used in both is effective, with the predictor-based approach to be preferable as it is more applicable. This study suggests that the algorithm used can be a useful tool for improving PPGRs.

On the other hand, Betts and Gonzalez (2016) suggested that although we are not all the same and that interindividual differences between us do exist, they are a rare minority and day-to-day variance within us is more important. Studies on the importance of microbiota on glucose response highlight its promising role when designing a personalized nutrition plan for individuals with impaired glucose function. It might be possible that the heterogeneity of glucose responses is influenced by interindividual variability in GM composition and diversity (Suez, Shapiro, & Elinav, 2016). In the future, the GM will be a target for intervention from a personalized aspect, in order to differentiate glucose responses of individuals with hyperglycemia.

On the road to identifying individual different responses, a lot of caution should be taken on how statistical analysis is made and how the study is designed in order for the results to be realistic. Atkinson and Batterham (2015) argued that trying to identify individual differences in response to an intervention may lead to false results if popular methods are used. The differences are contaminated by random within-subject variation. Changes in the intervention group can not be used alone to identify responders and non responders but a sample group for comparison is needed. If the researcher neglects to analyze data from a comparator sample group when assessing the individual differences in response, interferential errors are inevitable. Standard deviations of individual responses have to be derived and if they are not substantially larger than those in the comparison sample group then the changes after the intervention cannot be attributed to the interindividual variability. They also suggested that the magnitude of true individual responses should be appraised in terms of clinical importance and not statistical significance. Finally, they highlighted the importance of an intervention study design including data from a comparison sample, because otherwise it would be assigned a very low quality score.

Postprandial glucose prediction methods need to evolve because this would give us the ability to provide a better impaired BG treatment by identifying ineffective treatment points that lead to hyperglycemic or hypoglycemic episodes. These episodes can be prevented and BG can be controlled if we intervene early after the first signs are present.

The goal of studying the importance of personalized nutrition in glucose prediction is to help individuals control their glucose responses and improve their glucose levels by reducing fluctuations, thus reducing the risk of DM. Tailor-made diets can be applicable not only to patients but also to healthy people with genetic susceptibility to diabetes development. The focus is on the individual and not on the general population. The fact that personalized diets are based on genotypic or phenotypic characteristics of individuals and also on their behavior such as diet, eating patterns, physical activities, currently sheds light on the research in these areas.

Personalized nutrition has a number of strengths. First of all, there is no doubt that interindividual variability in response to dietary factors is a reality. Also, tailor-made diets have better results for some individuals compared to the recommendations that refer to the general population. Moreover, it is possible for some individuals to show higher levels of adherence if the treatment or diet plan is designed especially for them. Thus they can maintain the personalized recommendations. Finally, the personalized approach in nutrition for glucose responses is in alignment with the increased interest in the field of personalized approach in health in general.

On the other hand, personalized nutrition has also some weaknesses. Specifically referring to glucose responses, the parameters that are important in the relevant research are assessed mostly through observational studies, although there are a small number of randomized controlled trials. In addition, personalized nutrition plans are already available in the market, although there is not yet enough evidence for their use.

In conclusion, implementing personalized nutrition in clinical practice is possible for the future, but the underlying pathways are yet to be identified. Although in some rare genetic disorders genetic screening is already implemented, in DM genetics or other omic biomarkers have a long way to go until they can be used routinely. Factors that affect glucose response prediction and are responsible for interindividual variability have to be identified and assessed accurately (Mutie, Giordano, & Franks, 2017).

References

Albers, D. J., Levine, M., Gluckman, B., Ginsberg, H., Hripcsak, G., & Mamykina, L. (2017). Personalized glucose forecasting for type 2 diabetes using data assimilation. *PLoS Computational Biology*, 13(4), e1005232.

American Diabetes Association. (2014). Diagnosis and classification of diabetes mellitus. *Diabetes Care*, 37 (Supplement 1), S81–S90.

Atkinson, G., & Batterham, A. M. (2015). True and false interindividual differences in the physiological response to an intervention. *Experimental Physiology*, 100(6), 577–588.

Augustin, L. S., Franceschi, S., Jenkins, D. J., Kendall, C. W., & La Vecchia, C. (2002). Glycemic index in chronic disease: A review. *European Journal of Clinical Nutrition*, 56(11), 1049–1071.

Bellmann, S., Minekus, M., Sanders, P., Bosgra, S., & Havenaar, R. (2018). Human glycemic response curves after intake of carbohydrate foods are accurately predicted by combining in vitro gastrointestinal digestion with in silico kinetic modeling. *Clinical Nutrition Experimental*, 17, 8–22.

Betts, J. A., & Gonzalez, J. T. (2016). Personalised nutrition: What makes you so special? *Nutrition Bulletin*, 41(4), 353–359.

Bouchard, C., Blair, S. N., Church, T. S., Earnest, C. P., Hagberg, J. M., Häkkinen, K., Karavirta, L., ... Rankinen, T. (2012). Adverse metabolic response to regular exercise: Is it a rare or common occurrence. *PLoS One*, 7(5), e37887.

Brunkwall, L., & Orho-Melander, M. (2017). The gut microbiome as a target for prevention and treatment of hyperglycaemia in type 2 diabetes: From current human evidence to future possibilities. *Diabetologia*, 60(6), 943–951.

Capel, I., Rigla, M., García-Sáez, G., Rodríguez-Herrero, A., Pons, B., Subías, D., ... Gomez, E. J. (2014). Artificial pancreas using a personalized rule-based controller achieves overnight normoglycemia in patients with type 1 diabetes. *Diabetes Technology & Therapeutics*, 16(3), 172–179.

Ceriello, A., Hanefeld, M., Leiter, L., Monnier, L., Moses, A., Owens, D., ... Tuomilehto, J. (2004). Postprandial glucose regulation and diabetic complications. *Archives of Internal Medicine*, 164(19), 2090–2095.

Contreras, I., Oviedo, S., Vettoretti, M., Visentin, R., & Vehí, J. (2017). Personalized blood glucose prediction: A hybrid approach using grammatical evolution and physiological models. *PLoS One*, 12(11), e0187754.

Dashti, H. S., Follis, J. L., Smith, C. E., Tanaka, T., Garaulet, M., Gottlieb, D. J., ... Scheer, F. A. (2015). Gene-environment interactions of circadian-related genes for cardiometabolic traits. *Diabetes Care*, 38(8), 1456–1466, dc142709.

Dashti, H. S., Smith, C. E., Lee, Y. C., Parnell, L. D., Lai, C. Q., Arnett, D. K., ... Garaulet, M. (2014). CRY1 circadian gene variant interacts with carbohydrate intake for insulin resistance in two independent populations: Mediterranean and North American. *Chronobiology International*, 31(5), 660–667.

DeJesus, R. S., Breitkopf, C. R., Rutten, L. J., Jacobson, D. J., Wilson, P. M., & Sauver, J. S. (2017). Incidence rate of prediabetes progression to diabetes: Modeling an optimum target group for intervention. *Population Health Management*, 20(3), 216–223.

de Lannoy, L., Clarke, J., Stotz, P. J., & Ross, R. (2017). Effects of intensity and amount of exercise on measures of insulin and glucose: Analysis of inter-individual variability. *PLoS One*, 12(5), e0177095.

De Roos, B. (2013). Personalised nutrition: Ready for practice? *Proceedings of the Nutrition Society, 72*(1), 48–52.

de Toro-Martín, J., Arsenault, B. J., Després, J. P., & Vohl, M. C. (2017). Precision nutrition: A review of personalized nutritional approaches for the prevention and management of metabolic syndrome. *Nutrients, 9*(8), 913.

Dominianni, C., Sinha, R., Goedert, J. J., Pei, Z., Yang, L., Hayes, R. B., & Ahn, J. (2015). Sex, body mass index, and dietary fiber intake influence the human gut microbiome. *PLoS One, 10*(4).

Dumas, M. E. (2016). Is the way we're dieting wrong? *Genome Medicine, 8*(1), 7.

Dunstan, D. W., Kingwell, B. A., Larsen, R., Healy, G. N., Cerin, E., Hamilton, M. T., ... Owen, N. (2012). Breaking up prolonged sitting reduces postprandial glucose and insulin responses. *Diabetes Care, 35*(5), 976–983, DC_111931.

Ejtahed, H. S., Soroush, A. R., Angoorani, P., Larijani, B., & Hasani-Ranjbar, S. (2016). Gut microbiota as a target in the pathogenesis of metabolic disorders: A new approach to novel therapeutic agents. *Hormone and Metabolic Research, 48*(06), 349–358.

Gaboon, N. E. (2011). Nutritional genomics and personalized diet. *Egyptian Journal of Medical Human Genetics, 12*(1).

Gerich, J. E. (2003). Clinical significance, pathogenesis, and management of postprandial hyperglycemia. *Archives of Internal Medicine, 163*(11), 1306–1316.

Gibney, M. J., Elia, M., Ljungqvist, O., & Dowsett, J. (2005). *Clinical nutrition*. Oxford: Blackwell Science.

Hall, H., Perelman, D., Breschi, A., Limcaoco, P., Kellogg, R., McLaughlin, T., & Snyder, M. (2018). Glucotypes reveal new patterns of glucose dysregulation. *PLoS Biology, 16*(7).

Han, H., Li, Y., Fang, J., Liu, G., Yin, J., Li, T., & Yin, Y. (2018). Gut microbiota and type 1 diabetes. *International Journal of Molecular Sciences, 19*(4), 995.

Hasani-Ranjbar, S., & Larijani, B. (2017). Human microbiome as an approach to personalized medicine. *Alternative Therapies in Health and Medicine, 23*(6), 8–9.

Hirsch, S., Barrera, G., Leiva, L., de la Maza, M. P., & Bunout, D. (2013). Variability of glycemic and insulin response to a standard meal, within and between healthy subjects. *Nutricion Hospitalaria, 28*(2).

Ivey, K. L., Hodgson, J. M., Kerr, D. A., Lewis, J. R., Thompson, P. L., & Prince, R. L. (2014). The effects of probiotic bacteria on glycaemic control in overweight men and women: A randomised controlled trial. *European Journal of Clinical Nutrition, 68*(4), 447.

Jenkins, D. J., Kendall, C. W., Augustin, L. S., Franceschi, S., Hamidi, M., Marchie, A., et al. (2002). Glycemic index: Overview of implications in health and disease. *The American Journal of Clinical Nutrition, 76*(1), 266S–273S.

Kilbride, L., Charlton, J., Aitken, G., Hill, G. W., Davison, R. C., & McKnight, J. A. (2011). Managing blood glucose during and after exercise in type 1 diabetes: Reproducibility of glucose response and a trial of a structured algorithm adjusting insulin and carbohydrate intake. *Journal of Clinical Nursing, 20*(23-24), 3423–3429.

Korem, T., Zeevi, D., Zmora, N., Weissbrod, O., Bar, N., Lotan-Pompan, M., ... Suez, J. (2017). Bread affects clinical parameters and induces gut microbiome-associated personal glycemic responses. *Cell Metabolism, 25*(6), 1243–1253.

Krishnan, S., Newman, J. W., Hembrooke, T. A., & Keim, N. L. (2012). Variation in metabolic responses to meal challenges differing in glycemic index in healthy women: Is it meaningful? *Nutrition & Metabolism, 9*(1), 26.

Kulzer, B., Daenschel, W., Daenschel, I., Schramm, W., Messinger, D., Weissmann, J., ... Heinemann, L. (2018). Integrated personalized diabetes management improves glycemic control in patients with insulin-treated type 2 diabetes: Results of the PDM-ProValue study program. *Diabetes Research and Clinical Practice, 144*, 200–212.

Latulippe, M., Meheust, A., Augustin, L., Benton, D., Berčík, P., Birkett, A., ... Kendall, C. (2013). ILSI Brazil International Workshop on Functional Foods: A narrative review of the scientific evidence in the area of carbohydrates, microbiome, and health. *Food & Nutrition Research, 57*(1), 19214.

Li, J., & Fernando, C. (2016). Smartphone-based personalized blood glucose prediction. *ICT Express, 2*(4), 150–154.

López-Miranda, J., Pérez-Martínez, P., Marin, C., Fuentes, F., Delgado, J., & Pérez-Jiménez, F. (2007). Dietary fat, genes and insulin sensitivity. *Journal of Molecular Medicine, 85*(3), 213–226.

Madhu, V., Shirali, A., Pawaskar, P. N., Madi, D., Chowta, N., & Ramapuram, J. T. (2016). Mastication frequency and postprandial blood sugar levels in normoglycaemic and dysglycaemic individuals: A cross-sectional comparative study. *Journal of Clinical and Diagnostic Research: JCDR, 10*(7), OC06.

Mahan, L. K., & Escott-Stump, S. (2004). *Krause's food, nutrition & diet therapy*. Elsevier Health Sciences.

Mattfeld, R. S., Muth, E. R., & Hoover, A. (2017). Measuring the consumption of individual solid and liquid bites using a table-embedded scale during unrestricted eating. *IEEE Journal of Biomedical and Health Informatics, 21*(6), 1711–1718.

Mazloom, Z., Yousefinejad, A., & Dabbaghmanesh, M. H. (2013). Effect of probiotics on lipid profile, glycemic control, insulin action, oxidative stress, and inflammatory markers in patients with type 2 diabetes: A clinical trial. *Iranian Journal of Medical Sciences, 38*(1), 38.

Moazzami, A. A., Shrestha, A., Morrison, D. A., Poutanen, K., & Mykkänen, H. (2014). Metabolomics reveals differences in postprandial responses to breads and fasting metabolic characteristics associated with postprandial insulin demand in postmenopausal women−3. *The Journal of Nutrition, 144*(6), 807–814.

Moreno, J. A., Pérez-Jiménez, F., Marín, C., Gómez, P., Pérez-Martínez, P., Moreno, R., ... López-Miranda, J. (2004). Apolipoprotein E gene promoter −219G→T polymorphism increases LDL-cholesterol concentrations and susceptibility to oxidation in response to a diet rich in saturated fat. *The American Journal of Clinical Nutrition, 80*(5), 1404–1409.

Morris, C., O'Grada, C., Ryan, M., Roche, H. M., Gibney, M. J., Gibney, E. R., & Brennan, L. (2013). Identification of differential responses to an oral glucose tolerance test in healthy adults. *PLoS One, 8*(8).

Mutie, P. M., Giordano, G. N., & Franks, P. W. (2017). Lifestyle precision medicine: The next generation in type 2 diabetes prevention? *BMC Medicine, 15*(1), 171.

Ostadrahimi, A., Taghizadeh, A., Mobasseri, M., Farrin, N., Payahoo, L., Gheshlaghi, Z. B., & Vahedjabbari, M. (2015). Effect of probiotic fermented milk (kefir) on glycemic control and lipid profile in type 2 diabetic patients: A randomized double-blind placebo-controlled clinical trial. *Iranian Journal of Public Health, 44*(2), 228.

Palacios, T., Vitetta, L., Coulson, S., Madigan, C. D., Denyer, G. S., & Caterson, I. D. (2017). The effect of a novel probiotic on metabolic biomarkers in adults with prediabetes and recently diagnosed type 2 diabetes mellitus: Study protocol for a randomized controlled trial. *Trials, 18*(1), 7.

Price, N. D., Magis, A. T., Earls, J. C., Glusman, G., Levy, R., Lausted, C., ... Qin, S. (2017). A wellness study of 108 individuals using personal, dense, dynamic data clouds. *Nature Biotechnology, 35*(8), 747.

Ranawana, V., Leow, M. K., & Henry, C. J. K. (2014). Mastication effects on the glycaemic index: Impact on variability and practical implications. *European Journal of Clinical Nutrition, 68*(1), 137.

Rozendaal, Y. J., Maas, A. H., van Pul, C., Cottaar, E. J., Haak, H. R., Hilbers, P. A., & van Riel, N. A. (2018). Model-based analysis of postprandial glycemic response dynamics for different types of food. *Clinical Nutrition Experimental, 19*, 32–45.

Schram, M. T., Sep, S. J., van der Kallen, C. J., Dagnelie, P. C., Koster, A., Schaper, N., ... Stehouwer, C. D. (2014). The Maastricht Study: An extensive phenotyping study on determinants of type 2 diabetes, its complications and its comorbidities. *European Journal of Epidemiology, 29*(6), 439–451.

Shambrook, P., Kingsley, M. I., Wundersitz, D. W., Xanthos, P. D., Wyckelsma, V. L., & Gordon, B. A. (2018). Glucose response to exercise in the post-prandial period is independent of exercise intensity. *Scandinavian Journal of Medicine & Science in Sports, 28*(3), 939–946.

Singh, P., & Manning, S. D. (2016). Impact of age and sex on the composition and abundance of the intestinal microbiota in individuals with and without enteric infections. *Annals of Epidemiology, 26*(5), 380–385.

Sommer, F., & Backhed, F. (2013). The gut microbiota—Masters of host development and physiology. *Nature Reviews Microbiology, 11*, 227–238.

Suez, J., Shapiro, H., & Elinav, E. (2016). Role of the microbiome in the normal and aberrant glycemic response. *Clinical Nutrition Experimental, 6*, 59–73.

Sun, J., & Buys, N. J. (2016). Glucose- and glycaemic factor-lowering effects of probiotics on diabetes: A meta-analysis of randomised placebo-controlled trials. *British Journal of Nutrition, 115*(7), 1167–1177.

Suzuki, H., Fukushima, M., Okamoto, S., Takahashi, O., Shimbo, T., Kurose, T., ... Fukui, T. (2005). Effects of thorough mastication on postprandial plasma glucose concentrations in nonobese Japanese subjects. *Metabolism, 54*(12), 1593–1599.

Tan, V. M. H., Ooi, D. S. Q., Kapur, J., Wu, T., Chan, Y. H., Henry, C. J., & Lee, Y. S. (2016). The role of digestive factors in determining glycemic response in a multiethnic Asian population. *European Journal of Nutrition, 55*(4), 1573–1581.

Umeh, K. (2017). Personal care plans and glycaemic control: The role of body mass index and physical activity. *British Journal of Nursing, 26*(10), 543–551.

Valentini, L., Pinto, A., Bourdel-Marchasson, I., Ostan, R., Brigidi, P., Turroni, S., ... Leoncini, E. (2015). Impact of personalized diet and probiotic supplementation on inflammation, nutritional parameters and intestinal microbiota—the "RISTOMED project": Randomized controlled trial in healthy older people. *Clinical Nutrition*, *34*(4), 593–602.

Vega-López, S., Ausman, L. M., Griffith, J. L., & Lichtenstein, A. H. (2007). Inter-individual variability and intra-individual reproducibility of glycemic index values for commercial white bread. *Diabetes Care*, *30*(6), 1412–1417.

Vrolix, R., & Mensink, R. P. (2010). Variability of the glycemic response to single food products in healthy subjects. *Contemporary Clinical Trials*, *31*(1), 5–11.

Walker, C. G., Solis-Trapala, I., Holzapfel, C., Ambrosini, G. L., Fuller, N. R., Loos, R. J., ... Jebb, S. A. (2015). Modelling the interplay between lifestyle factors and genetic predisposition on markers of type 2 diabetes mellitus risk. *PLoS One*, *10*(7), e0131681.

Zeevi, D., Korem, T., Zmora, N., Israeli, D., Rothschild, D., Weinberger, A., ... Suez, J. (2015). Personalized nutrition by prediction of glycemic responses. *Cell*, *163*(5), 1079–1094.

Zhang, S. X., Ma, Y. Y., Guo, H. W., Wan, W. T., & Xue, K. (2015). Diets high in carbohydrate may not be appropriate for rs328 G carriers with the metabolic syndrome. *Asia Pacific Journal of Clinical Nutrition*, *24*(3), 546–554.

CHAPTER 4

The Role of Bacteria in Personalized Nutrition

Sim K. Singhrao[1], Sarita Robinson[2] and Alice Harding[1]

[1]Research Group: Dementia & Neurodegenerative Diseases Research Group, Faculty of Clinical and Biomedical Sciences, School of Dentistry, University of Central Lancashire, Preston, United Kingdom [2]Faculty of Science and Technology, School of Psychology, University of Central Lancashire, Preston, United Kingdom

OUTLINE

Introduction	81	Conclusions on the Role of Bacteria in Personalized Nutrition	96
The Gastrointestinal Tract Microbiome Establishment	82	References	96
Why is Dysbiosis of the Gut Microbiota Detrimental to General Health?	88	Further Reading	104
Future Perspectives	95		

INTRODUCTION

The gastrointestinal (GI) tract is the system of organs that is responsible for the digestion of food and removal of waste from the body. The GI tract encompasses the upper/middle/lower anatomical regions of the alimentary canal, covered throughout by mucosae. The upper area of the GI tract consists of the oral cavity and stomach extending to the duodenum; the middle GI tract refers to the beginning to the end of the small intestine; and the lower GI tract is the area of the colon to the anus. Commensal bacteria and host mucosal surfaces of the GI tract harbor a mutualistic, resilient symbiotic relationship during health (Rosier, Marsh, & Mira, 2018). The Human Microbiome Project consortium (2012) estimated that the human GI tract contains around 10^{14} microorganisms, outnumbering the cells of the host by 100 to 1 (Bhattacharjee & Lukiw, 2013; Lukiw, 2016).

This means humans harbor significantly more bacterial cells in their bodies than their own cells. In addition, these organisms contain more than 3 million genes, implying that commensal microbes contribute 150-fold more genes than the total number of genes in a person. This simply means that both bacteria and the host employ host/bacterial genes for their harmonious (symbiotic) relationship during good health. The oral/gut symbiotic microbiome (Aas, Paster, Stokes, Olsen, & Dewhirst, 2005; The Human Microbiome Project consortium studies, 2012) therefore acts as a "surrogate human organ."

The gut microbiota has important physiological functions including digesting certain foods, producing important neuroactive proteins that shape a person's social behavior, producing vitamins for essential biochemical and metabolic pathway activities, and establishing a functional immune system to help fight infections. This chapter outlines our current understanding of how the GI tract microbiota is delicately balanced, and acts as an efficient sensor to environmental/behavioral changes via microbial community shifts. It also informs the reader about specific nutritional interventions that may have value in improving their gut and general health. Starting by briefly outlining the origins of the harmonious relationship between the host and their GI tract microbiota, the health problems related to dysbiosis (microbial imbalance) are discussed in the context of specific diseases before outlining any of the dietary interventions to correct imbalances between the host and their GI tract microbiota. The chapter focuses also on culturable bacterial-based dietary products, in the form of probiotics and prebiotics, which may act as a useful intervention to promote gut health. However, there is currently little proof of our long-term ability to repopulate the gut with commensals, which maintain oral/gut health at optimal levels. Our understanding of the role of bacteria in the maintenance of physical and mental health is still in its infancy. Therefore further research is essential in order to fill gaps in our knowledge, and to establish which prebiotics and probiotics will slow down and/or halt the pathogenicity and/or manage symptoms of the chronic complex diseases discussed here.

The Gastrointestinal Tract Microbiome Establishment

Establishment of the GI tract microbial ecology occurs early in life as a result of exposure to maternal microbiota following vaginal childbirth (Ebersole, Holt, & Delaney, 2014; Reid, 2004; https://hmpdacc.org/), through breast-feeding and weaning (liquid to solid foods) stages (Kussmann & Fay, 2008). Thus nature provides the newborn with specific start-up microbes for the digestive system, which then becomes delicately balanced with immune and emotional development throughout life (Honda & Littman, 2016; Kennedy, Cryan, Dinan, & Clarke, 2014; Thaiss, Zmora, Levy, & Elinav, 2016; Yoo & Mazmanian, 2017). Conversely children who are born by cesarean section, or who are formula fed, experience a reduction in microbial exposure, which could result in disturbances in their intestinal microbiota later in life (Bokulich et al., 2016). Furthermore, a study conducted by Ebersole et al. (2014) on nonhuman primates, suggests that it is possible for a newborn to acquire the dysbiotic microbiome pathogens associated with periodontal disease from their mothers. Since periodontal pathogens are anaerobic, how they survive in the human edentate neonate is puzzling. A plausible suggestion is that the opportunistic bacteria may persist in the younger healthy hosts within nutrient retaining areas of the oral cavity (Papaioannou et al., 2009). Since the keystone pathogen of periodontal disease is a master of immune subversion (Hajishengallis, Darveau, & Curtis, 2012), the early colonization, while the host's innate immune system is still developing, may help the pathogen to evade detection in the neonate's whole life span.

Recent studies suggest that exposing the neonate to maternal vaginal fluids can partially restore the microbiota so that it more closely matches the microbiota of conventionally born infants (Dominguez-Bello et al., 2016). However, nutritional interventions to support GI tract microbial ecology in formula fed infants are currently lacking. In the future, it is possible that microbiome analysis of mother's vaginal fluid or breast milk could be undertaken. It is plausible to suggest that identification of beneficial bacteria from the vaginal fluid and/or breast milk could lead to their isolation and culture for supplementing as food for babies who may lack natural exposure to those missing bacteria.

How Has Evolution Shaped and Protected the Continuity of the GI Tract Microbial Ecology Within the Human Host?

Host enzymes digest some of the foods we eat, however certain foods need specific enzymes found within specific genera of bacteria that reside in the colon in order to break down indigestible components in complex fiber. In conditions like IBS, indigestible fiber can become difficult to break down, because these patients lack specific types of bacterial species needed to process this prebiotic in the colon (El-Salhy & Gundersen, 2015; Shepherd, Lomer, & Gibson, 2013). Another benefit of prebiotics is the release of postbiotics (short-chain fatty acids), and examples include acetates, isobutyric, propionic, and succinic acids (Atarashi et al., 2013; Furusawa et al., 2013; Grenier, 1992; Grenier, 1995; Mayhew, Onderdonk, & Gorbach, 1975; Narushima et al., 2014). These short-chain fatty acids are important for biofilm homeostasis. Prebiotics therefore play a role in maintaining a balanced gut microbiome. Gut colonizing commensal bacteria appear to play a key role in the production of the common neurotransmitters in the human brain, such as gamma-aminobutyric acid (GABA) and serotonin (de Weerth, 2017; Dinan & Cryan, 2016). Their loss can influence the functioning of the hypothalamic–pituitary–adrenal (HPA) axis, which is a key mechanism in the coordination of stress-related responses (O'Mahony et al., 2009) via the gut–brain axis. Literature suggests that changes in the biodiversity of human gut biofilm consortia could be the result of several host and environmental factors, including gender, age, genetics, lifestyles, medication (particularly the use of antibiotics), geography, diet, pet ownership, and exercise (Kussmann & Fay, 2008; Maleki et al., 2018; Mayer, 2018; Tun et al., 2017). The question as to why nature has provided so much flexibility, allowing shifts in the microbes in the human GI tract to take place quickly, remains intriguing.

It is only recently that we have started to understand the health consequences of microbial biofilm dysbiosis (Hajishengallis & Lamont, 2012; Lamont & Hajishengallis, 2015). Dysbiosis is the homeostatic breakdown of the natural symbiotic biofilm, resulting in a microbial imbalance with reduced microbial biodiversity, and leads to a greater number of specific pathogens in the biofilm. For example, research has revealed the subtle effects of dysbiosis on the humoral immune responses. Increases in virulent forms of bacteria resulting from dysbiosis can lead the host to secrete defective IgA that enables pathogenic bacteria to adhere to the gut mucosa (Peterson, McNulty, Guruge, & Gordon, 2007). This can have serious health consequences, because by adhering to otherwise refractive mucosal surfaces pathogenic bacteria can erode the protective epithelial barriers. Erosion of the epithelial cell barrier can then allow leakage of pathogenic bacteria, with an inflammatory phenotype, into the blood circulation (Hajishengallis et al., 2012; Olsen, 2008; Singhrao et al., 2016; Tomas, Diz, Tobias, Scully, & Donos, 2012). The leakage of pathogens into the bloodstream means that the bacteria can potentially cause damage to disparate organs (see reviews by Olsen, Chen, & Tribble, 2018; Olsen, Singhrao, & Potempa, 2018). One such disparate organ of importance here is the brain (Singhrao et al., 2014; Zhao, Jaber, & Lukiw, 2017). As more studies, including those by the Human Microbiome Project consortium (2012), give greater prominence to the idea that microbial dysbiosis can be a contributing factor in some chronic and complex diseases, their management by dietary adjustments (such as the use of probiotics) may become popular. However, more research is needed, especially focusing on which specific diet adjustments are useful. In addition, we need more research-based evidence to understand how we can reestablish healthy bacterial biofilms in the oral cavity and the gut. We also need to understand the interaction between bacteria and host genes, in order to support good gut health and physical health and mental well-being throughout life (Fig. 4.1).

The human gut microbiome is a delicately balanced community of mixed microbes from different kingdoms and phyla that are prone to undergoing swift population shifts under a variety of environmental fluctuations. One of these fluctuations is diet, as demonstrated in one short-term study conducted by David et al. (2014). These researchers found that eating an entirely animal-based or entirely plant-based diet, led to rapid changes in microbial communities. People who ate the herbivorous diet showed proliferation in the members of the phylum Firmicutes. An increase in the level of Firmicutes represents greater biodiversity of microbes, which in turn equates to a healthy digestive system. However, people in the carnivorous diet group experienced an increase in bacteria of the Bacteroidetes phylum, which are potentially pathogenic (David et al., 2014). The bacteria of the *Bacteroides* genus are opportunistic, meaning they will take advantage of their host's health status. If the host is vulnerable to, for example, infection, these bacteria will

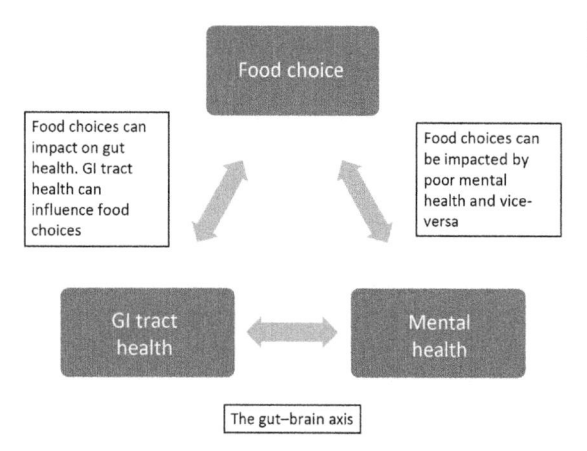

FIGURE 4.1 The relationship between gut health, food choices, and mental health.

overcome protective host barriers and gain greater virulence by exchanging genetic material amongst different bacterial strains. This results in the bacteria of the *Bacteroides* genus losing their commensal (harmless) status to pathogenic/disease causing forms (Olsen, Chen, et al., 2018; Olsen & Singhrao, 2018; Olsen, Singhrao, et al., 2018; Prindiville et al., 2000; Vogt et al., 2017). Therefore the GI tract microbiota appears to be very sensitive to changes in the hosts' diet and these dietary changes may allow shifts at interphylum level on a daily basis.

How Do Bacteria Adapt so Quickly?

Bacteria have a form of communication system of their own known as Quorum Sensing (Bassler, 1999). This system relies on the release of actively transportable chemicals across bacterial cell membranes or via passive diffusion within the biofilm matrix. The chemicals then either switch off or turn on the transcription of certain genes, which may be advantageous for bacterial survival (Reuter, Steinbach, & Helms, 2016). Such bacterial cell-to-cell communication has a role, for example, in forming biofilms, expressing virulence factors, and producing antibiotics to suppress the growth of some species over others, and even resisting the host's immune responses that are directed to kill bacteria. Furthermore, bacterial cell-to-cell communication can support the transfer of genetic material for appropriate bacterial phyla to outcompete those that may be less adaptable to the host's environment (Papenfort & Bassler, 2016; Reuter et al., 2016). Another example of microbial population shifts is the creation of an inflammophilic environment as the host's immune responses try to combat infection. Although the inflammophilic environment can help us to fight an infection, it is also hostile to the survival of most nonpathogenic bacteria found in the host, and in particular within subgingival biofilm communities dispersing elsewhere in the body (Hajishengallis et al., 2012; Singhrao, Harding, Poole, Kesavalu, & Crean, 2015).

What Are Probiotics?

Probiotics are living microorganisms that when administered in appropriate quantities give health benefits to the host (Hill et al., 2014). Examples of probiotics include "bio live yogurts" from various manufacturers stacked on shelves in the dairy section of supermarkets, which can increase levels of bacteria such as *Bifidobacterium* species in the gut (Kumar et al., 2015). In addition, traditional fermented foods can also be considered as probiotic foods. Fermented foods not only have a better shelf life at room temperature than probiotic yogurts, but also have unique flavors, hues, and tastes, which are enjoyable. For example, in Africa the traditional diet includes fermented foods prepared from cereals, such as maize, rice, millet, or sorghum (Achi & Asamudo, 2017). Other traditional fermented foods from around the world include pickled vegetables (sauerkraut, carrots, and gherkins), dairy (yogurts, cheese, kefir, paneer, tofu, and tempeh), and cured fish (Chilton, Burton, & Reid, 2015).

Some foods are fermented using the lacto fermentation process in which *Lactobacillus, Streptococcus, Enterococcus, Lactococcus,* and *Bifidobacterium* species of bacteria belonging to the Firmicute phylum are utilised (Masood, Qadir, Shirazi, & Khan, 2011). These genera of bacteria belong to probiotic bacteria suited to living in an anaerobic fermenting environment. These bacteria convert lactose sugars to lactic acid in natural food products. For patients who suffer from lactose intolerance, the natural "milk-based sugar" conversion into lactic acid prior to eating makes the subsequent digestibility easier. We know little about the health benefits of probiotic yeasts but research is underway to examine the benefits of adding probiotic yeasts to craft beer production to increase the health benefits of drinking beer (Capece et al., 2018). Quorn is a mycoprotein commercially manufactured from a specific fungus (*Fusarium venenatum*). It is a prebiotic and it is popular with vegetarians as a substitute for animal protein. Although many tolerate it, a small number of individuals with no underlying gastrointestinal pathology have reported intolerance to Quorn after eating it (https://www.quorn.co.uk/intolerance). Caution and personalized nutrition therefore are key to going forward.

The inclusion of probiotics as part of the diet in theory, at least, implies that dysbiosis is correctable. However, it is difficult for an individual to know whether they are harboring a dysbiotic gut microbiome prior to disease symptom development or even if there is underlying intolerance. Tests are underway for early indications of disease initiation and it is now possible to have feces analyzed for the predominant types of bacteria in order to monitor the health of a person's gut. The results will indicate the absence of specific genera of bacteria from a person's feces. Research is now focused on building libraries of bacteria, taken from healthy human donor's feces, which support certain desired traits (lean versus obese). The bacteria can then be included in probiotics for human consumption.

Global uptake of probiotic consumption, because it appears to promote health, has an enormous potential in dairy probiotic-based food industries. At the consumer level, the introduction of missing bacteria via probiotics is a highly desirable approach but the understanding of its efficacy is lacking. There may be several reasons as to why such information is missing. For instance, has the correct species of the universal health-mediating bacteria been isolated? Should probiotic use be personalized to achieve the desired outcome because the GI tract microbiome varies from person to person, and some people may show intolerance to certain prebiotics? In addition, the "adequate" probiotic dose for each person (dose of bacteria to gain sufficient colony forming units of commensals/person), and over what time span probiotics should be taken is unknown. We do not know if there will be a lifelong dependency on consuming beneficial probiotics to keep topping up desired bacteria, or whether they will be lost through feces over time. For example, whilst *Akkermansia* species are associated with lean and healthy people, the understanding of the specific mechanisms that could lead to discovering the "obesity bacterium" is more challenging. Perry et al. (2016) have shown that obesity is the result of harboring certain bacteria that signal to the brain, via the vagus nerve, that the host should eat high calorie foods. The consumption of high calorie foods causes an increased insulin secretion, which in turn leads to a negative cycle of excessive eating, which the body stores as fat. However, currently it is not clear what imbalances in the bacteria can cause the host to overeat, and what probiotic treatments would help to rectify the imbalance for a healthy gut in an obese person.

Importance of a GI Tract Symbiotic Microbiome for Micronutrients

Humans rely on essential vitamins from external sources (chemically synthesized supplements, dietary sources, and from the sun, e.g., vitamin D). Surprisingly, some species of bacteria from the GI tract healthy microbiome provide the host with vitamin K and the majority of B class vitamins (biotin, cobalamin, folates, nicotinic acid, pantothenic acid, pyridoxine, riboflavin, and thiamine) (Hill, 1997; LeBlanc et al., 2011, 2013). The site of absorption within the GI tract for microbial derived vitamins is the colon, whereas chemically synthesized supplements are absorbed in the small intestine (Said & Mohammed, 2006).

People developing the late-onset form of AD, have been found to also have nutritional deficiencies, specifically in the class of B-vitamins, folic acid, and vitamin D (Engelborghs, Gilles, Ivanoiu, & Vandewoude, 2014; Landel, Annweiler, Millet, Morello, & Feron, 2016; Mooijaart et al., 2005). Previous explanations have suggested that the observed micronutrient deficiencies were due to inadequate nutritional intake, such as low levels of vitamin D due to a diet low in foods such as oily fish. However, another potential cause is that elderly people may have lost specific genera of commensal bacteria that normally live in the gut, and which synthesize essential vitamins for the host (LeBlanc et al., 2011, 2013). Further research, which looked at vitamin D production in germ-free mice, found lower levels of this vitamin compared to mice that were reexposed to commensals. Currently the administration of synthesized vitamins is the only way to address human deficiencies. However, this may do little to restore the commensal bacteria in the colon, which could naturally produce vitamins for the host. In the future, as our knowledge of vitamin production by bacteria increases, we may be able to support the production of certain vitamins through probiotics use. Specifically, some researchers suggest that by consuming probiotics containing *Bifidobacterium*, *Lactobacillus*, *Streptococcus*, and *Lactococcus* species, we may promote the growth of other beneficial bacteria, which may result in a heterogeneous microbial biodiversity capable of providing essential vitamins for the host (Hill, 1997; LeBlanc et al., 2011, 2013; Vulevic, Rastall, & Gibson, 2004).

Environmental factors can also influence the health of the GI tract. For example, when physical exercise is undertaken alongside probiotics this produces dual benefits for the host and their biofilm consortia (de Oliveira & Burini, 2009; O'Sullivan et al., 2015). Regular physical exercise appears to have an antiinflammatory and antioxidant effect (Rosado-Perez, Santiago-Osorio, Oritiz, & Mendoza-Núñez, 2012). These antiinflammatory and antioxidant effects are opposite to the inflammophilic environments created by pathogenic bacteria undergoing phylotype shifts, which then create dysbiosis. Therefore exercise that lowers the levels of proinflammatory cytokines and reactive oxidative stress (Mendoza-Núñez, Hernández-Monjaraz, Santiago-Osorio, Betancourt-Rule, & Ruiz-Ramos, 2014; Rosado-Perez et al., 2012; Taafe, Harris, Ferrucci, Rowe, & Seeman, 2000) is important for helping commensal populations to flourish in the host's GI tract.

Importance of a GI Tract Symbiotic Microbiome for the Immune System

Firmicutes are largely Gram-positive cocci; examples include the genera *Prevotela*, *Clostridium*, *Veillonella*, *Selenomonas*, *Listeria*, *Staphylococcus*, *Streptococcus*, and *Enterococcus*. With the exception of *Staphylococcus aureus*, these bacteria are largely obligate anaerobic, endospore forming, rod-shaped bacteria residing mainly in the small intestine. Following the work of Schaedler et al. (1965), some coliform bacteria and *Clostridium* species that they investigated were termed as the "Schaedler flora" (Wells, Sugiyama, & Bland, 1982). These bacteria demonstrate a positive impact on cellular and adaptive immune responses via a subpopulation of T helper 17 lymphocytes, known as regulatory (T_{reg}) cells, and are found in the colon (Atarashi et al., 2013). Forkhead box P3 (Foxp3) is a host derived transcription factor that induces the host gene activation for the development and differentiation of T cells into T_{regs} in lymphoid organs (Sawant & Vignali, 2014). T_{regs} are regulatory cells providing immunological tolerance to the individual and actively restrain the immune system from damaging self-tissues (Anderson et al., 2014). T_{regs} control and suppress the activities of myeloid lineage cells, such as dendritic cells, macrophages, and microglia that contribute to innate immunity (Anderson et al., 2014). The balance between Th17 and T_{reg} cells controls inflammation and depends on several proteins, which together regulate the immune response through the secretion of pro- or antiinflammatory cytokines. The presence of T_{reg} with inflammatory phenotype (Foxp3+ derived T helper lymphocytes) in oral mucosa and in periodontal pockets is documented (Hajishengallis, 2014), and these are the major source of IL-17 cytokine. Some pathogenic bacteria can suppress the secretion of certain cytokines that are essential for T cell differentiation, and thereby subvert the proliferation of T_{regs} (Olsen, Taubman, & Singhrao, 2016).

It is now clear that short-chain fatty acids induce differentiation of T_{reg} cells (Atarashi et al., 2011; Honda & Littman, 2016; Smith et al., 2013) and suppress the expression of proinflammatory cytokines in dendritic cells (Singh et al., 2014). In this way, commensal bacteria can find a safe, short-term sanctuary in dendritic cells, whilst the GI tract undergoes cleansing of some biofilm shifts by the host's immune system (Macpherson & Uhr, 2004). This enables local commensals to stay within their original niche in the gut. Short-chain fatty acids therefore appear beneficial to the host, and in turn support the biodiversity of microbes (Atarashi et al., 2013; Furusawa et al., 2013; Narushima et al., 2014). Similarly *Lactobacillus* and *Bacteroides* genera also regulate T_{reg} cells in the small intestine to benefit the bidirectional homeostasis between host and bacteria.

Why is Dysbiosis of the Gut Microbiota Detrimental to General Health?

Many factors can cause changes in the microbial populations found in the GI tract. For example, the use of antibiotics can disturb the diversity of the microbes within microbiomes by their inability to distinguish populations of commensals from pathogens, thus destroying both the health promoting and pathogenic bacteria (David et al., 2014; Francino, 2016; Maleki et al., 2018; Tun et al., 2017). These adverse changes in the gut microbiota can lead to negative changes in the regulation of metabolic pathways. Further changes in the gut microbiota can induce epigenetic modifications involved in cell processes and can cause the breakdown of the gut barrier, allowing microbes to access disparate organs in the body. It is therefore plausible that dysbiosis may initiate or exacerbate developing pathologies such as cardiovascular, metabolic (diabetes, obesity) disorders, or mental health conditions such as AD (Singhrao et al., 2016).

Dysbiosis in IBS

Dysbiosis of the GI tract microbiome can cause problems within the GI tract itself, with conditions other than IBS. However, studies highlight that dysbiosis may only be the cause of subtypes of IBS. For example, IBS patients who experienced severe pain were likely to have an altered gut microbiome, whereas those who suffered from mild pain symptoms did not (Kassinen et al., 2007; Kerckhoffs et al., 2009; Malinen et al., 2005; Mättö et al., 2005). Furthermore, the gut microbiome organisms in patients with mild IBS were similar to those without IBS (Mayer, 2018). This research suggests that some subsets of IBS are due to altered gut composition (Mayer, 2018). It should, however, be remembered that other host and environmental factors may influence IBS onset and progression. For example, advancing age can cause shifts in the ecology of the human GI tract, with Bacteroidetes phylum members increasing over those of Firmicutes (Pistollato et al., 2016). This ecological shift can cause progressive inflammatory degeneration of the human nervous system (DuPont & DuPont, 2011) and affect metabolic syndromes through the production of acetic short-chain fatty acid metabolites (Perry et al., 2016). Hence, any intervention proposed to reduce pathogenic bacteria, and encourage the growth of commensals to improve health, would need to consider the influence of other factors, such as age and overlapping comorbidities.

Oral Biofilm Dysbiosis and Brain Health

The oral cavity, at the start of the GI tract, has its own microbiome (Aas et al., 2005). Caries and periodontitis are diseases typical of microbial dysbiosis within the mouth (Lamont & Hajishengallis, 2015). The keystone pathogen, *Porphyromonas gingivalis*, of the phylum Bacteroidetes is negatively associated with cardiovascular disorders, metabolic conditions, and autoimmune and mental health diseases (Bale, Doneen, & Vigerust, 2016; Ding, Ren, Yu, Yu, & Zhou, 2018; Ilievski et al., 2018; Ishida et al., 2017; Olsen, Chen, et al., 2018; Olsen, Singhrao, et al., 2018; Poole, Singhrao, Kesavalu, Cutis, & Crean, 2013; Singhrao et al., 2014, 2016). Pathogens are detected in AD brains (Maheshwari & Eslick, 2017; Miklossy, 2011;) but their contributions to dementia are not considered environmental as they are not classically part of the host's dysbiotic microbiomes. A "planktonic" bacterial contribution from the host's dysbiotic subgingival microbiome in AD development (Ding et al., 2018; Ilievski et al., 2018; Poole et al., 2013; Riviere, Riviere, & Smith, 2002) is implicated. The planktonic forms of bacteria are those that disseminate from mature host biofilms, and may reach the brain via the hematogenous route, although other pathways for microbial translocation are also possible (Singhrao et al., 2014). Supporting data show periodontal disease initiation in vivo, with *P. gingivalis* monoinfection seeding this bacterium in the brain from its oral niche (Ilievski et al., 2018; Poole et al., 2015; Singhrao et al., 2017).

On arrival in the brain, the bacterium recapitulates plaques and neurofibrillary tangles composed of amyloid beta (Aβ) and hyperphosphorylated tau protein, respectively (Ilievski et al., 2018). These key neuropathological hallmarks define AD (Alzheimer, 1907). Ilievski et al. (2018) have unequivocally demonstrated the presence of both intra- and extracellular Aβ$_{42}$ and ser396 residue phosphorylation of tau protein on neurofibrillary tangles in their experimental mouse model, with established periodontitis following chronic infection with *P. gingivalis*. Ishida et al. (2017) and Ding et al. (2018) performed functional tests and demonstrated statistically significant outcomes for impaired learning and memory in the middle aged *P. gingivalis* infected mice compared to the younger and middle aged uninfected mice (wild type and transgenic mice). These results are significant and contribute to our growing knowledge of the grave dangers arising from a dysbiotic subgingival biofilm. Wu et al. (2017) recently showed that chronic exposure to lipopolysaccharide (LPS) from *P. gingivalis* elicited AD-like phenotypes in middle aged, cathepsin B sufficient mice. The phenotypes included learning and memory deficits and intraneuronal Aβ accumulation. This research provides evidence to support a causal relationship between chronic exposure to a keystone periodontal pathogen and emerging hallmark proteins of AD depositing in areas of pathology together with functional correlates.

However, recent research suggests imbalanced microbiomes can be a causal factor in the development of dementia in later life (Ding et al., 2018; Ilievski et al., 2018; Ishida et al., 2017; Wu et al., 2017). Prospective and retrospective epidemiological studies suggest a 10-year period, following chronic periodontitis, for this risk factor to impact on AD development (Chen, Wu, & Chang, 2017; Sparks Stein et al., 2012), with the risk of developing late-onset AD increasing twofold (Gatz et al., 2006; Noble et al., 2009).

Importance of Symbiotic Oral/Gut Biofilms for Normal Brain Function

Literature suggests bacteria within our gut influence the normal functioning of the brain in several ways. For example, brain development and behavior are dependent on a bidirectional communication through the gut–brain axis (Cryan & Dinan, 2012). The communication between the gut and the brain involves multiple neural, immune, endocrine, and humoral pathways via the vagus nerve, as well as increasing levels of neurotransmitter precursors, such as the amino acid tryptophan (Bested, Logan, & Selhub, 2013). As bacteria contribute to the production of GABA and serotonin (de Weerth, 2017) their retention in the gut is essential in order to improve the functioning of the HPA axis, and alleviate stress. Therefore dysbiosis may cause a paucity of neurotransmitters, or affect HPA axis regulation, which can affect cognition and mental health conditions such as anxiety and depression (Dinan & Cryan, 2016) (see Fig. 4.2).

Dysbiosis in Depressive Mental Health Disorders

Depressive illnesses collectively affect the brain (elicited by dysthymia, bipolar, postpartum depression, seasonal affective disorders, and posttraumatic stress), which can have a significant impact on an individual's quality of life. People with depressive disorders experience a wide range of symptoms including sadness, feelings of guilt, loss of interest,

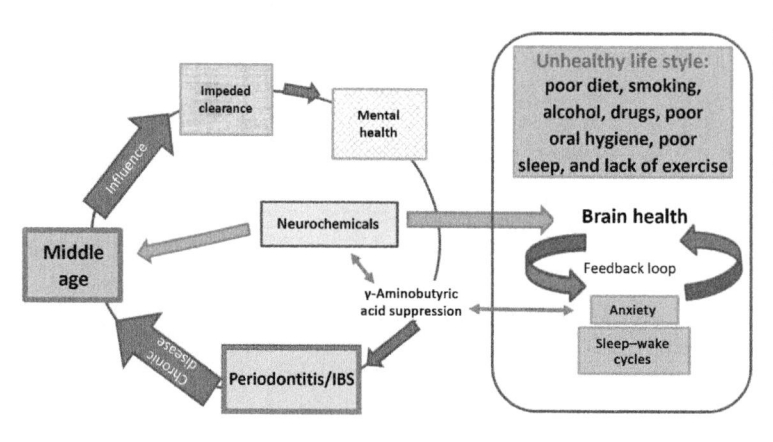

FIGURE 4.2 Cycle of events from a dysbiotic GI tract microbiome on the disruption of mental health well-being and poor quality of life as a result. *IBS*, irritable bowel syndrome.

low self-worth, poor sleep, reduced appetite, fatigue, and difficulty concentrating (World Health Organization, 2017). Depression can often be difficult to treat, with the underlying cause frequently attributed to psychological issues, such as relationship problems or work strain. However, growing evidence suggests that there is a marked difference in the microbiome of people with mental health conditions. For example, reduced bacterial biodiversity has been found to be present in depressed people (Zheng et al., 2016). This suggests that changes in gut bacteria are associated with depression and if this is the case research in this area might offer a new therapeutic approach. For example, IBS patients treated with *Bifidobacterium longum* NCC3001 showed a reduction in depression compared to a control group.

The mechanism by which the gut and the brain communicate is complex. For example, we know that levels of neurotransmitter precursors, such as the amino acid tryptophan, are regulated by the gut microbiota. The brain has a limited store of tryptophan and depends on the intestines to top it up on a regular basis. If the gut is colonized with bacteria, which directly absorb tryptophan, then there is a reduced supply of this amino acid available to the host (Dinan & Cryan, 2017). As tryptophan is a precursor for the neurotransmitter serotonin, which is related to a positive mood state, it is possible that tryptophan-absorbing bacteria within the gut could lead to mental health problems, such as depression.

Higher levels of stress hormones (cortisol and corticotrophin releasing factor) are indicators of depression (Dinan & Cryan, 2016). However, research is starting to explore how certain microbes may be involved in the development of depressive mood states. To this end, Jiang et al. (2015) examined the fecal samples taken from acutely depressed patients. Following their molecular analysis, they discovered that depressed patients had lower representation of Firmicutes, but higher levels of Bacteroidetes, Proteobacteria, and Actinobacteria phyla members of bacteria compared to nondepressed controls. Furthermore, dysregulation of the HPA axis, due to dysbiosis, can cause elevations in levels of cortisol and corticotrophin releasing factor (Dinan & Cryan, 2016). Dinan and Cryan (2016) therefore suggest that microbial shifts within our gut can make us more susceptible to poor mental health. In order to treat depressive conditions by consuming probiotics, molecular identification of bacteria at the species level would be an advantage, because broad identification of bacteria at the phylum level is not helpful in selecting the right species of bacteria for their inclusion in probiotics. Therefore methodological refinements in order to identify the specific types of bacteria that can support mental health are vital alongside the development of probiotic therapies for conditions such as depression (Fig. 4.1).

Dysbiosis in Other Mental Health Disorders

In vivo animal models and the limited human studies point to specific changes in gut bacteria that collectively influence mental illnesses related to anxiety, autism, and post-traumatic stress disorder. These are bacteria belonging to Actinobacteria, Lentisphaerae, and Verrucomicrobia phyla (Hemmings et al., 2017). Furthermore, data from animal model studies support the idea that bacterial population shifts occurring within the gut microbiome can induce mental health conditions. For example, Bercik et al. (2011) found that mice belonging to a low anxiety strain started to show behaviors associated with anxiety when given a fecal transplant from mice belonging to a high anxiety mouse strain. Furthermore, some negative mental health symptoms have shown a reduction when certain bacteria are administered. For example, cancer patients given *Clostridium butyricum* prior to surgery showed a reduction in self-reported anxiety (Yang et al., 2016).

The relationship between gut bacteria and mental health status is complex. For example, exercise can affect the relationship between gut bacteria and mood status. As skeletal muscle increases so does the production of kynurenine acid, which in turn reduces the level of kynurenine in the central nervous system. As kynurenine is involved in inflammation, immune response, and excitatory transmission, which have been linked to mental health disorders, a reduction in kynurenine can have a positive impact on mental health and reduce stress levels (Cervenka, Agudelo, & Ruas, 2017). In addition, the gut microbiota is sensitive to increases of stress and emotion, as the release of stress hormones or sympathetic neurotransmitters can alter the gut microbiome (Montiel-Castro, González-Cervantes, Bravo-Ruiseco, & Pacheco-López, 2013). Therefore interventions that promote exercise and relaxation can also help to stabilize the gut microbiota and so improve mental health.

Microbial Intervention

If the carefully balanced collaboration between humans and microbials is what makes us healthy, then our diet is an important part in maintaining a healthy biofilm. The two major *Bacteroides* species, namely *P. gingivalis* and *B. fragilis*, can break down the indigestible fiber to produce short-chain fatty acids (Grenier, 1992, 1995; Mayhew et al., 1975). So why is it that an imbalance from Firmicutes to Bacteroidetes becomes pathogenic (Hajishengallis et al., 2012; Prindiville et al., 2000; Vogt et al., 2017)? One plausible explanation is that Bacteroidetes members produce different types of short-chain fatty acids to those produced by Firmicutes. One short-chain fatty acid (acetate) released by the former phylum (Bacteroidetes) has been shown to be detrimental to people who are prone to obesity (Perry et al., 2016). However, other factors, such as diet, lifestyle, and genetic factors, can contribute to greater virulence from the dominant pathogenic bacteria, encouraging a shift from homeostasis to dysbiosis (Harding, Robinson, Crean, & Singhrao, 2017a) in opportunistic microbial populations in any person (Olsen, Chen, et al., 2018). Although several other factors may be involved in maintaining a healthy biofilm, the focus here will remain on dietary interventions.

What are Prebiotics?

Prebiotics are essentially fiber-containing components of foods, which are broken down in the GI tract by bacteria present in the colon. Eating fiber can selectively stimulate the growth of commensals that improve the host's gut health (Foster, 2017). Dietary fiber can be broken down into short-chain and long-chain carbohydrates and can be fermentable or nonfermentable (Biesiekierski et al., 2011; Bijkerk, Muris, Knottnerus, Hoes, & de Wit, 2004; Chouinard, 2011; Heizer, Southern, & McGovern, 2009; Muir et al., 2009). Prebiotic rich foods include sweet potatoes, carrots, onions, asparagus, and squash. When eaten regularly prebiotics, such as galactooligosaccharides and fructooligosaccharides, encourage the growth of beneficial gut bacteria (Sohn & Underwood, 2017; Wilson & Whelan, 2017). Recently research has undertaken the task of creating prebiotics which can be used to manufacture functional foods. For example, Costabile et al. (2015) evaluated a prebiotic bread made using Bimuno (galactooligosaccharide mixture) and found that participants who ate the bread had significantly higher levels of *Bifidobacteria* and *Lactobacillus* species (Firmicutes) compared to controls.

However, in some conditions, such as IBS, insoluble fiber can have an adverse effect (Bijkerk et al., 2004; Moayyedi, Marshall, Yuan, & Hunt, 2014). Instead, those suffering from IBS are encouraged to supplement their diet with psyllium and avoid eating bran-based foods. This is because psyllium is a long-chain, intermediate viscosity, moderately soluble, and fermentable dietary fiber, that results in lower gas production and helps to alleviate painful symptoms related to gas production (Anderson et al., 2009; Chutkan, Fahey, Wright, & McRorie, 2012; Dikeman & Fahey, 2006; Ford et al., 2014), whilst bran has the opposite effect.

Management of Subgingival Microbiome via Diet to Protect the Brain

Earlier in this chapter it was noted that a dysbiotic subgingival microbiome can negatively affect brain health in later life. The oral cavity represents the start of the GI tract, and the maintenance of a healthy symbiotic biofilm can help us to avoid oral diseases, such as dental caries and periodontal disease. Periodontitis is an inflammatory condition that occurs because of an interaction between pathogenic (dysbiotic) microorganisms and the host's immune responses (Haffajee et al., 1988). This can result in bleeding gums, inflammation, and pocket formation around teeth (for more details see Singhrao et al., 2014). As mentioned above and supported by research, periodontal pathogens disseminate from their primary subgingival niche and have the potential to affect the functioning of the brain later in life, with particular emphasis on late-onset AD. Therefore those individuals who suffer from periodontal disease should attempt to keep the numbers of the pathogens low through better management of their oral health, and so maintain their brain health (Harding et al., 2017a; Harding, Gonder, Robinson, Crean, & Singhrao, 2017b; Singhrao et al., 2014).

Certain dietary factors influence the health of the oral cavity and influence the homeostasis of the commensals. For example, a diet rich in fruits which provide the host with antioxidants, a natural product found in vitamins and minerals, appears beneficial to periodontal health. Antioxidants appear to be able to reduce oxidative damage from immune cells, fighting infection within periodontal tissues. As antioxidants are constituents of vitamins and minerals, deficiencies in vitamin C and calcium can promote periodontal disease (Nishida et al., 2000). Magnesium supplements, on the other hand, have been found to improve periodontal health (Meisel et al., 2005), whilst vitamin E reduces inflammation in periodontal tissues (Asman, Wijkander, & Hjerpe, 1994). Malnutrition can have a detrimental effect on innate and adaptive immune responses, and so elicits adverse alterations in the oral microbiome (Ewanwu, 1995).

Other dietary interventions that are beneficial for the digestive system are probiotics, as they encourage symbiosis of the gut bacteria through reducing the numbers of pathogens. As periodontal disease is a polymicrobial dysbiosis, it would seem reasonable that the use of probiotics may encourage a balance of the normal flora into a more symbiotic state. When assessing the potential benefit of probiotics in the reduction of periodontal disease most studies have used the *Lactobacillus* species, with results showing a limited and temporary improvement in periodontal parameters (Jayaram, Chatterjee, & Raghunathan, 2016). *L. brevis* lozenges have also been shown to improve both clinical and microbiological aspects of periodontal disease for up to 60 days (Shah, Gujjari, & Chandrasekhar, 2013) and delay onset of gingival inflammation (Lee, Kim, Ko, Ouwehand, & Ma, 2015). Other studies using *L. reuteri* have had mixed results. Some studies showed a reduction in bleeding scores, inflammation, and pocket depth (Teughels et al., 2013; Twetman et al., 2009; Vivekananda, Vandana, & Bhat, 2010), whereas others demonstrated no improvement (Iniesta et al., 2012; Tekce et al., 2015). The consensus is that currently there is insufficient evidence to support the use of probiotics in the prevention of periodontal disease, however, probiotics may have a short-term beneficial effect in treating periodontal disease.

Management of IBS via Diet

A suggested trigger for IBS is the consumption of diets enriched in poorly absorbable and fermentable oligo-, di-, monosaccharides, and polyols (FODMAPs) (El-Salhy, Ystad, Mazzawi, & Gundersen, 2017; Francis & Whorwell, 1994; Shepard & Gibson, 2006). Examples of FODMAPs are fructans, lactose, fructose, glucose, mannitol, sorbitol, maltitol, and xylitols. These foods consist of α-linked galactose and α-linked glucose and a terminal β-linked fructose, and are malabsorbed in IBS patients. A diet low in FODMAPs is effective in 75% of patients suffering from IBS (Halmos, 2017). However, a low FODMAP diet restricts the intake of fermentable carbohydrates, and this in turn has a negative impact on some key gut microbes (Wilson & Whelan, 2017). Therefore in the future a better treatment for IBS may be to reestablish the bacteria that have the enzymes capable of breaking down FODMAPs back into the gut.

Management of Mental Health via Diet

Animal models suggest that probiotics may positively affect mental health by increasing serotonin synthesis, reducing serotonin metabolism, and increasing the levels of available tryptophan (Desbonnet, Garrett, Clarke, Bienenstock, & Dinan, 2008; Luo et al., 2014). Human interventional studies in which probiotics were consumed show mixed results (Wallace & Milev, 2017). For example, petrochemical workers demonstrated general health benefits and improvements in levels of depression after taking multispecies probiotic capsules for 6 weeks (Mohammadi et al., 2015). Furthermore, consumption of probiotics appears to alter brain activity, as monitored by functional magnetic resonance imaging of individuals (Dinan & Cryan, 2017). Probiotics and prebiotics that are used to promote mental health benefits are referred to as "psychobiotics" (Dinan & Cryan, 2012; Wall et al., 2014). If inflammation is central to symptoms of dementing brain diseases such as AD, then the long awaited magic bullet of psychobiotics with the potential to mop up inflammatory mediators, such as proinflammatory cytokines (from the bloodstream and the brain parenchyma), would be of great interest. However, in order for this to take place, double-blind randomized control trials on appropriate patients need to be completed to assess the efficacy of the psychobiotics.

Some bacteria appear to be important suppliers of neurotransmitters to their host. For example, *Candida*, *Streptococcus*, *Escherichia*, and *Enterococcus* genera can produce serotonin (Lyte, 2013). However, our understanding is still limited as to which specific prebiotics and probiotics have positive effects on mental health. For example, the neurodevelopmental condition autism may be a relevant example of a reduction in the hormone known as oxytocin. In addition, we know that 70% of children presenting with autism have abdominal symptoms, which in turn suggests poor gut health. Probiotics can elevate oxytocin levels (Borre et al., 2014), which could alleviate some of the symptoms of autism. However, we currently do not have the knowledge of which bacterial species would allow us to reestablish a healthy gut microbiome in those individuals who suffer from autism. Most studies which have attempted to improve mental health via bacterial interventions to date have taken a cocktail approach, administrating a broad range of different prebiotics and probiotics. Additional studies are now necessary to examine whether a cocktail or a single probiotic/prebiotic approach is best (Foster, 2017).

Future Perspectives

In the oral cavity, periodontitis is a disease of a known cause, namely polymicrobial dysbiosis of the biofilm beneath the gum line. From their original oral niche these disease-causing bacteria can reach surprising places in the body. If they are the culprits of disparate organ microbiome dysbiosis they could affect other related diseases. Research suggests that some subsets of IBS are directly related to altered gut microflora as they cannot digest certain food components and this leads to severe pain symptoms. Advancing age may also be responsible for the loss of specific types of bacteria that normally provide essential vitamins (B and D class vitamins), which in turn help to lower inflammation. Other anxiety and depressive mental illnesses directly point to the loss of bacteria that supplement the brain with common neurotransmitters. Dietary intervention with effective probiotics and prebiotics, where bacteria have the role of nutritional aids, appears to offer a timely solution to manage the aforementioned conditions that are currently lacking adequate medical treatments.

However, the understanding of the human microbiome superimposed with dybiosis is in its infancy. It is, however, clear that the host is dependent on the microbial diversity of the Firmicutes wthin its microbiome to enable and optimise overall health. This is a paradigm shift. Scientists now need to further explore the impact of microbial−host interactions in different health conditions, and explain how dysbiosis may contribute to disease processes. Once we have established the role of specific bacteria in certain health conditions, we may be able to reestablish beneficial bacteria in the GI tract in order to treat these health conditions. Additional research is needed to ascertain their efficacy and which methodological approach is most appropriate when reestablishing beneficial bacteria in the gut. We know diet choices are important and specific dietary advice is needed in order to help people to maintain a healthy GI tract, and so prevent certain disease conditions. Further, if specific interventions are needed to support gut functioning we need to know which prebiotic and probiotic supplements are the most effective, and what dosage/length of treatment. Finally, it should be noted that the GI tract microbiome is not only affected by diet but can also be impacted by different factors, such as genetics, stress, pet ownership, and exercise, and a holistic approach is likely to be needed in order to support gut health.

Conclusions on the Role of Bacteria in Personalized Nutrition

Humans and microbiomes have a codependency for a healthy existence. A shift towards Bacteroidetes members can cause dysbiosis and the development of an inflammatory milieu. Dysbiosis can either lead to health problems at a local level, such as periodontal disease and IBS, or if the microbes leak from their primary niche into the bloodstream, and access secondary niches, they can cause problems elsewhere in the body, including cardiovascular diseases, mental health conditions, type 2 diabetes, and AD, primarily through inflammation. Periodontitis is a typical example whereby dominance of the keystone pathogen *P. gingivalis*, belonging to the phylum Bacteroidetes, can cause so much damage to the host. Furthermore, we know that the GI tract microbiome directly communicates with the brain, and consequently can influence human behavior. Therefore to keep our GI tract healthy we should consume a balanced diet that contains sufficient amounts of fiber in order to maintain the biodiversity of Firmicutes over other phyla, especially Bacteroidetes, within the GI tract. In time, research may find commensal bacterial strains that will be part of probiotics with the potential to mop up inflammatory mediators, and so help to manage a wide range of related diseases.

Now that we are beginning to understand how an unhealthy microbiome can lead to ill health, we can start to use this knowledge to produce interventions to improve health conditions. In the future, dietary advice in order to maintain a healthy GI tract microbiome is needed. Once we have a good understanding of how dysbiosis, or the absence of certain gut bacteria, can impact on disease processes, dieticians can offer dietary interventions to correct these deficits and potentially "cure" certain health conditions.

References

Aas, J. A., Paster, B. J., Stokes, L. N., Olsen, I., & Dewhirst, F. E. (2005). Defining the normal bacterial flora of the oral cavity. *Journal of Clinical Microbiology*, 43(11), 572–5732.

Achi, O. K., & Asamudo, N. U. (2017). Cereal-based fermented foods of Africa as functional foods. In *Bioactive molecules in food* (pp. 1–32). Springer.

Asman, B., Wijkander, P., & Hjerpe, A. (1994). Reduction of collagen degradation in experimental granulation tissue by vitamin E and selenium. *Journal of Clinical Periodontology*, 21(1), 45–47.

Alzheimer, A. (1907). Uber eine eigenartige Erkankung der Hirnrinde. *Allgemeine Zeitschrift fur Psychiatre*, 64, 146–148.

Anderson, J. W., Baird, P., Davis, R. H., Jr., Ferreri, S., Knudtson, M., Koraym, A., ... Williams, C. L. (2009). Health benefits of dietary fiber. *Nutrition Reviews*, 67, 188–205. Available from https://doi.org/10.1111/j.1753-4887.2009.00189.x.

Anderson, K. M., Olson, K. E., Estes, K. A., Flanagan, K., Gendelman, H. E., & Mosley, R. L. (2014). Dual destructive and protective roles of adaptive immunity in neurodegenerative disorders. *Translational Neurodegeneration*, 3, 25. Available from https://doi.org/10.1186/2047-9158-3-25.

Atarashi, K., Tanoue, T., Oshima, K., Suda, W., Nagano, Y., Nishikawa, H., ... Honda, K. (2013). Treg induction by a rationally selected mixture of *Clostridia* strains from the human microbiota. *Nature*, 500, 232–236. Available from https://doi.org/10.1038/nature12331.

Atarashi, K., Tanoue, T., Shima, T., Imaoka, A., Kuwahara, T., Momose, Y., ... Honda, K. (2011). Induction of colonic regulatory T cells by indigenous *Clostridium* species. *Science*, 331, 337–341. Available from https://doi.org/10.1126/science.1198469.

Bale, B. F., Doneen, A. L., & Vigerust, D. J. (2016). High-risk periodontal pathogens contribute to the 477 pathogenesis of atherosclerosis. *Postgraduate Medical Journal*, 93, 215–220. Available from https://doi.org/10.1136/postgradmedj-2016-134279.

REFERENCES

Bassler, B. L. (1999). How bacteria talk to each other: Regulation of gene expression by quorum sensing. *Current Opinion in Microbiology, 2*, 582–587.

Bercik, P., Denou, E., Collins, J., Jackson, W., Lu, J., Jury, J., … Collins, S. M. (2011). The intestinal microbiota affect central levels of brain-derived neurotropic factor and behavior in mice. *Gastroenterology, 141*(2), 599–609. Available from https://doi.org/10.1053/j.gastro.2011.04.052, 609.e1–3.

Bested, A. C., Logan, A. C., & Selhub, E. M. (2013). Intestinal microbiota, probiotics and mental health: From Metchnikoff to modern advances: Part II—Contemporary contextual research. *Gut Pathogens, 5*(1), 3. Available from https://doi.org/10.1186/1757-4749-5-3.

Bhattacharjee, S., & Lukiw, W. J. (2013). Alzheimer's disease and the microbiome. *Frontiers in Cellular Neuroscience, 7*, 153. Available from https://doi.org/10.3389/fncel.2013.00153.

Biesiekierski, J. R., Rosella, O., Rose, R., Liels, K., Barrett, J. S., Shepherd, S. J., … Muir, J. G. (2011). Quantification of fructans, galacto-oligosacharides and other short-chain carbohydrates in processed grains and cereals. *Journal of Human Nutrition and Dietetics, 24*, 154–176. Available from https://doi.org/10.1111/j.1365-277X.2010.01139.x.

Bijkerk, C. J., Muris, J. W., Knottnerus, J. A., Hoes, A. W., & de Wit, N. J. (2004). Systematic review: The role of different types of fibre in the treatment of irritable bowel syndrome. *Alimentary Pharmacology & Therapeutics, 19*, 245–251. Available from https://doi.org/10.1111/j.0269-2813.2004.01862.x.

Bokulich, N. A., Chung, J., Battaglia, T., Henderson, N., Jay, M., Li, H. D., … Blaser, M. J. (2016). Antibiotics, birth mode, and diet shape microbiome maturation during early life. *Science Translational Medicine, 8*(343), 343–382.

Borre, Y. ,E., O'Keeffe, G. W., Clarke, G., Stanton, C., Dinan, T. G., & Cryan, J. F. (2014). Microbiota and neurodevelopmental windows: Implications for brain disorders. *Trends in Molecular Medicine, 20*(9), 509–518. Available from https://doi.org/10.1016/j.molmed.2014.05.002.

Capece, A., Romaniello, R., Pietrafesa, A., Siesto, G., Pietrafesa, R., Zambuto, M., & Romano, P. (2018). Use of *Saccharomyces cerevisiae* var. *boulardii* in co-fermentations with *S. cerevisiae* for the production of craft beers with potential healthy value-added. *International Journal of Food Microbiology, 284*, 22–30. Available from https://doi.org/10.1016/j.ijfoodmicro.2018.06.028.

Cervenka, I., Agudelo, L. Z., & Ruas, J. L. (2017). Kynurenines: Tryptophan's metabolites in exercise, inflammation, and mental health. *Science, 357*(6349), eaaf9794. Available from https://doi.org/10.1126/science.aaf9794.

Chen, C. K., Wu, Y. T., & Chang, Y. C. (2017). Association between chronic periodontitis and the risk of Alzheimer's disease: A retrospective, population-based, matched-cohort study. *Alzheimers Research & Therapy, 9*(1), 56. Available from https://doi.org/10.1186/s13195-017-0282-6.

Chilton, S. N., Burton, J. P., & Reid, G. (2015). Inclusion of fermented foods in food quides around the world. *Nutrients, 7*(1), 390–404. Available from https://doi.org/10.3390/nu7010390.

Chouinard, L. E. (2011). The role of psyllium fibre supplementation in treating irritable bowel syndrome. *Canadian Journal of Dietetic Practice and Research, 72*, e107–e114. Available from https://doi.org/10.3148/72.1.2011.48.

Chutkan, R., Fahey, G., Wright, W. L., & McRorie, J. (2012). Viscous versus nonviscous soluble fiber supplements: Mechanisms and evidence for fiber-specific health benefits. *The Journal of the American Association of Nurse Practitioners, 24*, 476–487. Available from https://doi.org/10.1111/j.1745-7599.2012.00758.x.

Costabile, A., Walton, G. E., Tzortzis, G., Vulevic, J., Charalampopoulos, D., & Gibson, G. R. (2015). Development of a bread delivery vehicle for dietary prebiotics to enhance food Functionality targeted at those with metabolic syndrome. *Gut Microbes, 6*(5), 300–309. Available from https://doi.org/10.1080/19490976.2015.1064577.

Cryan, J. F., & Dinan, T. G. (2012). Mind-altering microorganisms: The impact of the gut microbiota on brain and behaviour. *Nature Reviews Neuroscience, 13*, 701–712. Available from https://doi.org/10.1038/nrn3346.

David, L. A., Maurice, C. F., Carmody, R. N., Gootenberg, D. B., Button, J. E., Wolfe, B. E., … Turnbaugh, P. J. (2014). Diet rapidly and reproducibly alters the human gut microbiome. *Nature, 505*(7484), 559–563. Available from https://doi.org/10.1038/nature12820.

de Oliveira, E. P., & Burini, R. C. (2009). The impact of physical exercise on the gastrointestinal tract. *Current Opinion in Clinical Nutrition & Metabolic Care, 12*(5), 533–538. Available from https://doi.org/10.1097/MCO.0b013e32832e6776.

de Weerth, C. (2017). Do bacteria shape our development? Crosstalk between intestinal microbiota and HPA axis. *Neuroscience & Biobehavioral Reviews, 83*, 458–471. Available from https://doi.org/10.1016/j.neubiorev.2017.09.016.

Desbonnet, L., Garrett, L., Clarke, G., Bienenstock, J., & Dinan, T. G. (2008). The probiotic Bifidobacteria infantis: An assessment of potential antidepressant properties in the rat. *Journal of Psychiatric Research, 43*(2), 164−174. Available from https://doi.org/10.1016/j.jpsychires.2008.03.009.

Dikeman, C. L., & Fahey, G. C., Jr. (2006). Viscosity as related to dietary fiber: A review. *Critical Reviews in Food Science and Nutrition, 46*, 649−663. Available from https://doi.org/10.1080/10408390500511862.

Dinan, T. G., & Cryan, J. F. (2012). Regulation of the stress response by the gut microbiota: Implications for psychoneuroendocrinology. *Psychoneuroendocrinology, 37*, 1369−1378.

Dinan, T. G., & Cryan, J. F. (2016). Mood by microbe: Towards clinical translation. *Genome Medicine, 8*(1), 36. Available from https://doi.org/10.1186/s13073-016-0292-1.

Dinan, T. G., & Cryan, J. F. (2017). Gut instincts: Microbiota as a key regulator of brain development, ageing and neurodegeneration. *Journal of Physiology, 595*(2), 489−503. Available from https://doi.org/10.1113/JP273106.

Ding, Y., Ren, J., Yu, H., Yu, W., & Zhou, Y. (2018). *Porphyromonas gingivalis*, a periodontitis causing bacterium, induces memory impairment and age-dependent neuroinflammation in mice. *Immunity & Ageing, 15*, 6. Available from https://doi.org/10.1186/s12979-017-0110-7.

Dominguez-Bello, M. G., De Jesus-Laboy, K. M., Shen, N., Cox, L. M., Amir, A., Gonzalez, A., ... Clemente, J. C. (2016). Partial restoration of the microbiota of cesarean-born infants via vaginal microbial transfer. *Nature Medicine, 22*(3), 250−253. Available from https://doi.org/10.1038/nm.4039.

DuPont, A. W., & DuPont, H. L. (2011). The intestinal microbiota and chronic disorders of the gut. *Nature Reviews Gastroenterology & Hepatology, 8*, 523−531. Available from https://doi.org/10.1038/nrgastro.2011.133.

Ebersole, J. L., Holt, S. C., & Delaney, J. E. (2014). Acquisition of oral microbes and associated systemic responses of newborn nonhuman primates. *Clinical and Vaccine Immunology, 21*(1), 21−28. Available from https://doi.org/10.1128/CVI.00291-13.

El-Salhy, M., & Gundersen, D. (2015). Diet in irritable bowel syndrome. *Nutrition Journal, 14*, 36. Available from https://doi.org/10.1186/s12937-015-0022-3.

El-Salhy, M., Ystad, S. O., Mazzawi, T., & Gundersen, D. (2017). Dietary fiber in irritable bowel syndrome (review). *International Journal of Molecular Medicine, 40*(3), 607−613. Available from https://doi.org/10.3892/ijmm.2017.3072.

Engelborghs, S., Gilles, C., Ivanoiu, A., & Vandewoude, M. (2014). Rationale and clinical data supporting nutritional intervention in Alzheimer's disease. *Acta Clinica Belgica, 69*, 17−24, 1310.

Ewanwu, C. O. (1995). Interface of malnutrition and periodontal disease. *American Journal of Clinical Nutrition, 61*(2), 430S−436S.

Francino, M. P. (2016). Antibiotics and the human gut microbiome: Dysbioses and accumulation of resistances. *Frontiers in Microbiology, 6*, 1543. Available from https://doi.org/10.3389/fmicb.2015.01543.

Francis, C. Y., & Whorwell, P. J. (1994). Bran and irritable bowel syndrome: Time for reappraisal. *The Lancet, 344*, 39−40. Available from https://doi.org/10.1016/S0140-6736(94)91055-3.

Ford, A. C., Moayyedi, P., Lacy, B. E., Lembo, A. J., Saito, Y. A., Schiller, L. R., ... Quigley, E. M. (2014). American College of Gastroenterology monograph on the management of irritable bowel syndrome and chronic idiopathic constipation. *The American Journal of Gastroenterology, 109*(Suppl 1), S2−S26. Available from https://doi.org/10.1038/ajg.2014.187.

Foster, J. A. (2017). Targeting the microbiome for mental health: Hype or hope? *Biological Psychiatry, 82*(7), 456−457. Available from https://doi.org/10.1016/j.biopsych.2017.08.002.

Furusawa, Y., Obata, Y., Fukuda, S., Endo, T. A., Nakato, G., Takahashi, D., ... Ohno, H. (2013). Commensal microbe-derived butyrate induces the differentiation of colonic regulatory T cells. *Nature, 504*, 446−450. Available from https://doi.org/10.1038/nature12721.

Gatz, M., Mortimer, J. A., Fratiglioni, L., Johansson, B., Berg, S., Reynolds, C. A., ... Pedersen, N. L. (2006). Potentially modifiable risk factors for dementia in identical twins. *Alzheimers & Dementia, 2*, 110−117. Available from https://doi.org/10.1016/j.jalz.2006.01.002.

Grenier, D. (1992). Nutritional interactions between two suspected periodontopathogens, *Treponema denticola* and *Porphyromonas gingivalis*. *Infection and Immunity, 60*(12), 5298−5301.

Grenier, D. (1995). Characterization of the trypsin-like activity of *Bacteroides forsythus*. *Microbiology, 141*, 921−926.

Haffajee, A. D., Socransky, S. S., Dzink, J. L., Taubman, M. A., Ebersole, J. L., & Smith, D. J. (1988). Clinical, microbiological and immunological features of subjects with destructive periodontal diseases. *Journal of Clinical Periodontology, 15*, 240−246.

Hajishengallis, G. (2014). Immunomicrobial pathogenesis of periodontitis: Keystones, pathobionts, and host response. *Trends in Immunology, 35*(1), 3–11. Available from https://doi.org/10.1016/j.it.2013.09.001.

Hajishengallis, G., Darveau, R. P., & Curtis, M. A. (2012). The keystone pathogen hypothesis. *Nature Reviews Microbiology, 10*, 717–725. Available from https://doi.org/10.1038/nrmicro2873.

Hajishengallis, G., & Lamont, R. J. (2012). Beyond the red complex and into more complexity: The polymicrobial synergy and dysbiosis (PSD) model of periodontal disease etiology. *Molecular Oral Microbiology, 27*(6), 409–419. Available from https://doi.org/10.1111/j.2041-1014.2012.00663.x.

Halmos, E. P. (2017). When the low FODMAP diet does not work. *Journal of Gastroenterology and Hepatology, 32* (Suppl 1), 69–72. Available from https://doi.org/10.1111/jgh.13701.

Harding, A., Gonder, U., Robinson, S. J., Crean, S., & Singhrao, S. K. (2017b). Exploring the association between Alzheimer's disease, oral health, microbial endocrinology and nutrition. *Frontiers in Aging Neuroscience, 9*, 398. Available from https://doi.org/10.3389/fnagi.2017.00398.

Harding, A., Robinson, S., Crean, S., & Singhrao, S. K. (2017a). Can better management of periodontal disease delay the onset and progression of Alzheimer's disease? *Journal of Alzheimer's Disease, 58*, 337–348. Available from https://doi.org/10.3233/JAD-170046.

Heizer, W. D., Southern, S., & McGovern, S. (2009). The role of diet in symptoms of irritable bowel syndrome in adults: A narrative review. *Journal of American Dietetic Association, 109*, 1204–1214. Available from https://doi.org/10.1016/j.jada.2009.04.012.

Hemmings, S. M. J., Malan-Müller, S., van den Heuvel, L. L., Demmitt, B. A., Stanislawski, M. A., Smith, D. G., ... Lowry, C. A. (2017). The microbiome in posttraumatic stress disorder and trauma-exposed controls: An exploratory study. *Psychosomatic Medicine, 79*(8), 936–946. Available from https://doi.org/10.1097/PSY.0000000000000512.

Hill, C., Guarner, F., Reid, G., Gibson, G. R., Merenstein, D. J., Pot, B., ... Sanders, M. E. (2014). Expert consensus document: The International Scientific Association for Probiotics and Prebiotics consensus statement on the scope and appropriate use of the term probiotic. *Nature Reviews Gastroenterology & Hepatology, 11*(8), 506–514. Available from https://doi.org/10.1038/nrgastro.2014.66.

Hill, M. J. (1997). Intestinal flora and endogenous vitamin synthesis. *European Journal of Cancer Prevention, 6*(1), S43–S45.

Honda, K., & Littman, D. R. (2016). The microbiota in adaptive immune homeostasis and disease. *Nature, 535* (7610), 75–84. Available from https://doi.org/10.1038/nature18848.

Ilievski, V., Zuchowska, P. K., Green, S. J., Toth, P. T., Ragozzino, M. E., Le, K., ... Watanabe, K. (2018). Chronic oral application of a periodontal pathogen results in brain inflammation, neurodegeneration and amyloid beta production in wild type mice. *PLoS One, 13*(10), e0204941.

Iniesta, M., Herrera, D., Montero, E., Zurbriggen, M., Matos, A. R., Marín, M. J., ... Sanz, M. (2012). Probiotic effects of orally administered *Lactobacillus reuteri*-containing tablets on the subgingival and salivary microbiota in patients with gingivitis. A randomized clinical trial. *Journal of Clinical Periodontology, 39*, 736–744.

Ishida, N., Ishihara, Y., Ishida, K., Tada, H., Funaki-Kato, Y., Hagiwara, M., ... Matsushita, K. (2017). Periodontitis induced by bacterial infection exacerbates features of Alzheimer's disease in transgenic mice. *Aging and Mechanisms of Disease, 3*, 15. Available from https://doi.org/10.1038/s41514-017-0015-x.

Jayaram, P., Chatterjee, A., & Raghunathan, V. (2016). Probiotics in the treatment of periodontal disease: A systematic review. *Journal of Indian Society of Periodontology, 20*(5), 488–495. Available from https://doi.org/10.4103/0972-124X.207053.

Jiang, H., Ling, Z., Zhang, Y., Mao, H., Ma, Z., Yin, Y., ... Ruan, B. (2015). Altered fecal microbiota composition in patients with major depressive disorder. *Brain, Behavior, and Immunity, 48*, 186–194. Available from https://doi.org/10.1016/j.bbi.2015.03.016.

Kassinen, A., Krogius-Kurikka, L., Mäkivuokko, H., Rinttilä, T., Paulin, L., Corander, J., ... Palva, A. (2007). The fecal microbiota of irritable bowel syndrome patients differs significantly from that of healthy subjects. *Gastroenterology, 133*, 24–33.

Kennedy, P. J., Cryan, J. F., Dinan, T. G., & Clarke, G. (2014). Irritable bowel syndrome: A microbiome–gut–brain axis disorder? *World Journal of Gastroenterology, 20*(39), 14105–14125. Available from https://doi.org/10.3748/wjg.v20.i39.14105.

Kerckhoffs, A. P., Samsom, M., van der Rest, M. E., de Vogel, J., Knol, J., Ben-Amor, K., & Akkermans, L. M. (2009). Lower Bifidobacteria counts in both duodenal mucosa-associated and fecal microbiota in irritable bowel syndrome patients. *World Journal of Gastroenterology, 15*, 2887–2892.

Kumar, H., Salminen, S., Verhagen, H., Rowland, I., Heimbach, J., Bañares, S., ... Lalonde, M. (2015). Novel probiotics and prebiotics: Road to the market. *Current Opinion in Biotechnology, 32*, 99–103. Available from https://doi.org/10.1016/j.copbio.2014.11.021.

Kussmann, M., & Fay, L. B. (2008). Nutrigenomics and personalized nutrition: Science and concept. *Personalized Medicine, 5*(5), 447–455.

Lamont, R. J., & Hajishengallis, G. (2015). Polymicrobial synergy and dysbiosis in inflammatory disease. *Trends in Molecular Medicine, 21*(3), 172–183. Available from https://doi.org/10.1016/j.molmed.2014.11.004.

Landel, V., Annweiler, C., Millet, P., Morello, M., & Feron, F. (2016). Vitamin D, cognition and Alzheimer's disease: The therapeutic benefit is in the D-tails. *Journal of Alzheimer's Disease, 53*(2), 419–444. Available from https://doi.org/10.3233/JAD-150943.

LeBlanc, J. G., Laino, J. E., del Valle, M. J., Vannini, V., van Sinderen, D., Taranto, M. P., ... Sesma, F. (2011). B-group vitamin production by lactic acid bacteria—Current knowledge and potential applications. *Journal of Applied Microbiology, 111*, 1297–1309.

LeBlanc, J. G., Milani, C., de Giori, G. S., Sesma, F., van Sinderen, D., & Ventura, M. (2013). Bacteria as vitamin suppliers to their host: A gut microbiota perspective. *Current Opinion in Biotechnology, 24*(2), 160–168. Available from https://doi.org/10.1016/j.copbio.2012.08.005.

Lee, J. K., Kim, S. J., Ko, S. H., Ouwehand, A. C., & Ma, D. S. (2015). Modulation of the host response by probiotic *Lactobacillus brevis* CD2 in experimental gingivitis. *Oral Disease, 21*, 705–712.

Lukiw, W. J. (2016). The microbiome, microbial-generated proinflammatory neurotoxins, and Alzheimer's disease. *Journal of Sport and Health Science, 5*, 393–396. Available from https://doi.org/10.1016/j.jshs.2016.08.008.

Luo, J., Wang, T., Liang, S., Hu, X., Li, W., & Jin, F. (2014). Ingestion of *Lactobacillus* strain reduces anxiety and improves cognitive function in the hyperammonemia rat. *Science China Life Sciences, 57*(3), 327–335. Available from https://doi.org/10.1007/s11427-014-4615-4.

Lyte, M. (2013). Microbial endocrinology in the microbiome–gut–brain axis: How bacterial production and utilization of neurochemicals influence behavior. *PLoS Pathogens, 9*(11), e1003726.

Macpherson, A. J., & Uhr, T. (2004). Induction of protective IgA by intestinal dendritic cells carrying commensal bacteria. *Science, 303*, 1662–1665.

Maheshwari, P., & Eslick, G. D. (2017). Bacterial infection increases the risk of Alzheimer's disease: An evidence-based assessment. *Journal of Alzheimer's Disease.* Available from https://doi.org/10.3233/JAD-160362.

Maleki, B. H., Tartibian, B., Mooren, F. C., FitzGerald, L. Z., Krüger, K., Chehrazi, M., & Malandish, A. (2018). Low-to-moderate intensity aerobic exercise training modulates irritable bowel syndrome through antioxidative and inflammatory mechanisms in women: Results of a randomized controlled trial. *Cytokine, 102*, 18–25.

Malinen, E., Rinttilä, T., Kajander, K., Mättö, J., Kassinen, A., Krogius, L., ... Palva, A. (2005). Analysis of the fecal microbiota of irritable bowel syndrome patients and healthy controls with real-time PCR. *The American Journal of Gastroenterology, 100*, 373–382.

Masood, M. I., Qadir, M. I., Shirazi, J. H., & Khan, I. U. (2011). Beneficial effects of lactic acid bacteria on human beings. *Critical Reviews in Microbiology, 37*, 91–98. Available from https://doi.org/10.3109/1040841X.2010.536522.

Mättö, J., Maunuksela, L., Kajander, K., Palva, A., Korpela, R., Kassinen, A., & Saarela, M. (2005). Composition and temporal stability of gastrointestinal microbiota in irritable bowel syndrome—A longitudinal study in IBS and control subjects. *FEMS Immunology and Medical Microbiology, 43*, 213–222.

Mayer, E. A. (2018). The role of gut–brain interactions in influencing symptoms of irritable bowel syndrome. *Gastroenterology & Hepatology (New York), 14*(1), 44–46.

Mayhew, J. W., Onderdonk, A. B., & Gorbach, S. L. (1975). Effects of time and growth media on short-chain fatty acid production by *Bacteroides fragilis*. *Applied Microbiology, 29*(4), 472–475.

Meisel, P., Schwahn, C., Luedemann, J., John, U., Kroemer, H. K., & Kocher, T. (2005). Magnesium deficiency is associated with periodontal disease. *Journal of Dental Research, 84*(10), 937–941.

Mendoza-Núñez, V. M., Hernández-Monjaraz, B., Santiago-Osorio, E., Betancourt-Rule, J. M., & Ruiz-Ramos, M. (2014). Tai chi exercise increases SOD activity and total antioxidant status in saliva and is linked to an improvement of periodontal disease in the elderly. *Oxidative Medicine and Cellular Longevity, 2014*, 603853. Available from https://doi.org/10.1155/2014/603853.

Miklossy, J. (2011). Alzheimer's disease—A neurospirochetosis. Analysis of the evidence following Koch's and Hill's criteria. *Journal of Neuroinflammation, 8*, 90.

Moayyedi, P., Marshall, J. K., Yuan, Y., & Hunt, R. (2014). Canadian Association of Gastroenterology Position statement: Fecal microbiota transplant therapy. *Canadian Journal of Gastroenterology and Hepatology*, 28(2), 66−68.

Mohammadi, A. A., Jazayeri, S., Khosravi-Darani, K., Solati, Z., Mohammadpour, N., Asemi, Z., ... Eghtesadi, S. (2015). Effects of probiotics on biomarkers of oxidative stress and inflammatory factors in petrochemical workers: A randomized, double-blind, placebo-controlled trial. *International Journal of Preventive Medicine*, 6, 82. Available from https://doi.org/10.4103/2008-7802.164146.

Montiel-Castro, A. J., González-Cervantes, R. M., Bravo-Ruiseco, G., & Pacheco-López, G. (2013). The microbiota−gut−brain axis: Neurobehavioral correlates, health and sociality. *Frontiers in Integrative Neuroscience*, 7, 70. Available from https://doi.org/10.3389/fnint.2013.00070.

Mooijaart, S. P., Gussekloo, J., Frolich, M., Jolles, J., Stott, D. J., Westendorp, R. G. J., & de Craen, A. J. M. (2005). Homocysteine, vitamin B-12, and folic acid and the risk of cognitive decline in old age: The Leiden 85-plus study. *American Journal of Clinical Nutrition*, 82, 866−871.

Muir, J. G., Rose, R., Rosella, O., Liels, K., Barrett, J. S., Shepherd, S. J., & Gibson, P. R. (2009). Measurement of short-chain carbohydrates in common Australian vegetables and fruits by high-performance liquid chromatography (HPLC). *Journal of Agricultural and Food Chemistry*, 57, 554−565. Available from https://doi.org/10.1021/jf802700e.

Narushima, S., Sugiura, Y., Oshima, K., Atarashi, K., Hattori, M., Suematsu, M., & Honda, K. (2014). Characterization of the 17 strains of regulatory T cell inducing human-derived *Clostridia*. *Gut Microbes*, 5, 333−339. Available from https://doi.org/10.4161/gmic.28572.

Nishida, M., Grossi, S. G., Dunford, R. G., Ho, A. W., Trevisan, M., & Genco, R. G. (2000). Dietary vitamin C and the risk for periodontal disease. *Journal of Periodontology*, 71(8), 1215−1223.

Noble, J. M., Borrell, L. N., Papapnou, P. N., Elkind, M. S. V., Scarmeas, N., & Wright, C. B. (2009). Periodontitis is associated with cognitive impairment among older adults: Analysis of NHANES-III. *Journal of Neurology, Neurosurgery, and Psychiatry*, 80, 1206−1211.

Olsen, I. (2008). Update on bacteraemia related to dental procedures. *Transfusion and Apheresis Science*, 39, 173−178. Available from https://doi.org/10.1016/j.transci.2008.06.008.

Olsen, I., Chen, T., & Tribble, G. D. (2018). Genetic exchange and reassignment in *Porphyromonas gingivalis*. *Journal of Oral Microbiology*, 10(1), 1457373. Available from https://doi.org/10.1080/20002297.2018.1457373.

Olsen, I., & Singhrao, S. K. (2018). Importance of heterogeneity in *Porphyromonas gingivalis* lipopolysaccharide lipid A in tissue specific inflammatory signaling. *Journal of Oral Microbiology*, 10(1), 1440128. Available from https://doi.org/10.1080/20002297.2018.1440128.

Olsen, I., Singhrao, S. K., & Potempa, J. (2018). Citrullination as a plausible link to periodontitis, rheumatoid arthritis, atherosclerosis and Alzheimer's disease. *Journal of Oral Microbiology*, 10(1), 1487742.

Olsen, I., Taubman, M. A., & Singhrao, S. K. (2016). *Porphyromonas gingivalis* suppresses adaptive immunity in periodontitis, atherosclerosis and Alzheimer's disease. *Journal of Oral Microbiology*, 8, 33029. Available from https://doi.org/10.3402/jom.v8.33029.

O'Mahony, S. M., Marchesi, J. R., Scully, P., Codling, C., Ceolho, A. M., Quigley, E. M., ... Dinan, T. G. (2009). Early life stress alters behavior, immunity, and microbiota in rats: Implications for irritable bowel syndrome and psychiatric illnesses. *Biological Psychiatry*, 65(3), 263−267. Available from https://doi.org/10.1016/j.biopsych.2008.06.026.

O'Sullivan, O., Cronin, O., Clarke, S. F., Murphy, E. F., Molloy, M. G., Shanahan, F., & Cotter, P. D. (2015). Exercise and the microbiota. *Gut Microbes*, 6(2), 131−136. Available from https://doi.org/10.1080/19490976.2015.1011875.

Papaioannou, W., Gizani, S., Haffajee, A. D., Quirynen, M., Mamai-Homata, E., & Papagiannoulis, L. (2009). The microbiota on different oral surfaces in healthy children. *Oral Microbiology and Immunology*, 24(3), 183−189. Available from https://doi.org/10.1111/j.1399-302X.2008.00493.x.

Papenfort, K., & Bassler, B. L. (2016). Quorum sensing signal-response systems in Gram-negative bacteria. *Nature Reviews Microbiology*, 14(9), 576−588. Available from https://doi.org/10.1038/nrmicro.2016.89.

Perry, R. J., Peng, L., Barry, N. A., Cline, G. W., Zhang, D., Cardone, R. L., ... Shulman, G. I. (2016). Acetate mediates a microbiome-brain-β-cell axis to promote metabolic syndrome. *Nature*, 534(7606), 213−217. Available from https://doi.org/10.1038/nature18309.

Peterson, D. A., McNulty, N. P., Guruge, J. L., & Gordon, J. I. (2007). IgA response to symbiotic bacteria as a mediator of gut homeostasis. *Cell Host & Microbe*, 2, 328–339.

Pistollato, F., Sumalla Cano, S., Elio, I., Masias Vergara, M., Giampieri, F., & Battino, M. (2016). Role of gut microbiota and nutrients in amyloid formation and pathogenesis of Alzheimer disease. *Nutrition Reviews*, 74, 624–634. Available from https://doi.org/10.1093/nutrit/nuw023.

Poole, S., Singhrao, S. K., Chukkapalli, S., Rivera, M., Velsko, I., Kesavalu, L., & Crean, S. (2015). Active invasion of *Porphyromonas gingivalis* and infection-induced complement activation in ApoE−/− mice brains. *Journal of Alzheimer's Disease*, 43, 67–80. Available from https://doi.org/10.3233/JAD-140315.

Poole, S., Singhrao, S. K., Kesavalu, L., Cutis, M. A., & Crean, S. (2013). Determining the presence of perodontopathic virulence factors in short-term postmortem Alzheimer's disease brain tissue. *Journal of Alzheimer's Disease*, 36(4), 655–677.

Prindiville, T. P., Sheikh, R. A., Cohen, S. H., Tang, Y. J., Cantrell, M. C., & Silva, J., Jr. (2000). *Bacteroides fragilis* enterotoxin gene sequences in patients with inflammatory bowel disease. *Emerging Infectious Disease*, 6, 171–174. Available from https://doi.org/10.3201/eid0602.000210.

Reid, G. (2004). When microbe meets human. *Clinical Infectious Disease*, 39, 827–830.

Reuter, K., Steinbach, A., & Helms, V. (2016). Interfering with bacterial quorum sensing. *Perspectives in Medicinal Chemistry*, 8, 1–15.

Riviere, G. R., Riviere, K. H., & Smith, K. S. (2002). Molecular and immunological evidence of oral 767 Treponema in the human brain and their association with Alzheimer's disease. *Oral Micriobiology and Immunology*, 17(2), 113–118, pmid:11929559 769 770 22.

Rosado-Perez, J., Santiago-Osorio, E., Oritiz, R., & Mendoza-Núñez, V. M. (2012). Tai chi diminishes oxidative stress in maxican older adults. *The Journal of Nutrition, Health & Aging*, 16(7), 642–646.

Rosier, B. T., Marsh, P. D., & Mira, A. (2018). Resilience of the oral microbiota in health: Mechanisms that prevent dysbiosis. *Journal of Dental Research*, 97(4), 371–380. Available from https://doi.org/10.1177/0022034517742139.

Said, H. M., & Mohammed, Z. M. (2006). Intestinal absorption of water-soluble vitamins: An update. *Current Opinion in Gastroenterology*, 22(2), 140–146.

Sawant, D. V., & Vignali, D. A. (2014). Once a Treg, always a Treg? *Immunological Reviews*, 259(1), 173–191. Available from https://doi.org/10.1111/imr.12173.

Schaedler, R. W., Dubos, R., & Costello, R. (1965). Association of germfree mice with bacteria isolated from normal mice. *The Journal of Experimental Medicine*, 122, 77–83.

Shah, M. P., Gujjari, S. K., & Chandrasekhar, V. S. (2013). Evaluation of the effect of probiotic (inersan) alone, combination of probiotic with doxycycline and doxycycline alone on aggressive periodontitis—A clinical and microbiological study. *Journal of Clinical Diagnostic Research*, 7, 595–600.

Shepard, S. J., & Gibson, P. R. (2006). Fructose malabsorption and symptoms of irritable bowel syndrome: Guidelines for effective dietary management. *Journal of the American Dietetic Association*, 106, 1631–1639.

Shepherd, S. J., Lomer, M. C., & Gibson, P. R. (2013). Short-chain carbohydrates and functional gastrointestinal disorders. *American Journal of Gastroenterology*, 108, 707–717.

Singh, N., Gaurav, A., Sivaprakasam, S., Brady, E., Padia, R., Shi, H., ... Ganapathy, V. (2014). Activation of Gpr109a, receptor for niacin and the commensal metabolite butyrate, suppresses colonic inflammation and carcinogenesis. *Immunity*, 40, 128–139. Available from https://doi.org/10.1016/j.immuni.2013.12.007.

Singhrao, S. K., Chukkapalli, S., Poole, S., Velsko, I., Crean, S., & Kesavalu, L. (2017). Chronic *Porphyromonas gingivalis* infection accelerates the occurrence of age-related granules in ApoE−/− mice. *Journal of Oral Microbiology*, 9. Available from https://doi.org/10.1080/20002297.2016.1270602.

Singhrao, S. K., Harding, A., Chukkapalli, S., Olsen, I., Kesavalu, L., & Crean, S. (2016). Apoliporpotein E related co-morbidities and Alzheimer's disease. *Journal of Alzheimer's Disease*, 51(4), 935–948. Available from https://doi.org/10.3233/JAD150690.

Singhrao, S. K., Harding, A., Poole, S., Kesavalu, L., & Crean, S. (2015). *Porphyromonas gingivalis* periodontal infection and its putative links with Alzheimer's disease. *Mediators of Inflammation*, 137357. Available from https://doi.org/10.1155/2015/137357, 2015.

Singhrao, S. K., Harding, A., Simmons, T., Robinson, S., Kesavalu, L., & Crean, S. (2014). Oral inflammation, tooth loss, risk factors and association with progression of Alzheimer's disease. *Journal of Alzheimer's Disease*, 42(3), 723–737. Available from https://doi.org/10.3233/JAD-140387.

REFERENCES

Smith, P. M., Howitt, M. R., Panikov, N., Michaud, M., Gallini, C. A., Bohlooly-Y, M., ... Garrett, W. S. (2013). The microbial metabolites, short-chain fatty acids, regulate colonic Treg cell homeostasis. *Science*, *341*, 569–573. Available from https://doi.org/10.1126/science.1241165.

Sohn, K., & Underwood, M. A. (2017). Prenatal and postnatal administration of prebiotics and probiotics. *Seminars in Fetal Neonatal Medicine*, *22*(5), 284–289. Available from https://doi.org/10.1016/j.siny.2017.07.002.

Sparks Stein, P., Steffen, M. J., Smith, C., Jicha, G., Ebersole, J. L., Abner, E., & Dawson, D. (2012). Serum antibodies to periodontal pathogens are a risk factor for Alzheimer's disease. *Alzheimer's & Dementia*, *8*, 196–203.

Taafe, D. R., Harris, T. B., Ferrucci, L., Rowe, J., & Seeman, T. E. (2000). Cross-sectional and prospective relationships of interleukin-6 and C-reactive protein with physical performance in elderly persons: MacArthur studies of successful aging. *The Journal of Gerontology Series A: Biological Sciences and Medical Sciences*, *5*, M709–M715.

Tekce, M., Ince, G., Gursoy, H., Dirikan Ipci, S., Cakar, G., Kadir, T., & Yilmaz, S. (2015). Clinical and microbiological effects of probiotic lozenges in the treatment of chronic periodontitis: A 1-year follow-up study. *Journal of Clinical Periodontology*, *42*, 363–372. Available from https://doi.org/10.1111/jcpe.12387.

Teughels, W., Durukan, A., Ozcelik, O., Pauwels, M., Quirynen, M., & Haytac, M. C. (2013). Clinical and microbiological effects of *Lactobacillus reuteri* probiotics in the treatment of chronic periodontitis: A randomized placebo-controlled study. *Journal of Clinical Periodontology*, *40*, 1025–1035.

Thaiss, C. A., Zmora, N., Levy, M., & Elinav, E. (2016). The microbiome and innate immunity. *Nature*, *535*(7610), 65–74. Available from https://doi.org/10.1038/nature18847.

Tomas, I., Diz, P., Tobias, A., Scully, C., & Donos, N. (2012). Periodontal health status and bacteraemia from daily oral activities: Systematic review/meta-analysis. *Journal of Clinical Periodontology*, *39*, 213–228.

Tun, H. M., Konya, T., Takaro, T. K., Brook, J. R., Chari, R., Field, C. J., ... CHILD Study Investigators. (2017). Exposure to household furry pets influences the gut microbiota of infant at 3–4 months following various birth scenarios. *Microbiome*, *5*(1), 40. Available from https://doi.org/10.1186/s40168-017-0254-x.

Twetman, S., Derawi, B., Keller, M., Ekstrand, K., Yucel-Lindberg, T., & Stecksen-Blicks, C. (2009). Short-term effect of chewing gums containing probiotic *Lactobacillus reuteri* on the levels of inflammatory 318 mediators in gingival crevicular fluid. *Acta Odontologica Scandinavica*, *67*, 19–24.

Vivekananda, M. R., Vandana, K. L., & Bhat, K. G. (2010). Effect of the probiotic *Lactobacilli reuteri* (Prodentis) in the management of periodontal disease: A preliminary randomized clinical trial. *Journal of Oral Microbiology*, *2*, 5344. Available from https://doi.org/10.3402/jom.v2i0.5344.

Vogt, N. M., Kerby, R. L., Dill-McFarland, K. A., Harding, S. J., Merluzzi, A. P., Johnson, S. C., ... Rey, F. E. (2017). Gut microbiome alterations in Alzheimer's disease. *Scientific Reports*, *7*, 13537. Available from https://doi.org/10.1038/s41598-017-13601-y.

Vulevic, J., Rastall, R. A., & Gibson, G. R. (2004). Developing a quantitative approach for determining the in vitro prebiotic potential of dietary oligosaccharides. *FEMS Microbiology Letters*, *236*, 153–159.

Wall, R., Cryan, J. F., Ross, R. P., Fitzgerald, G. F., Dinan, T. G., & Stanton, C. (2014). Bacterial neuroactive compounds produced by psychobiotics. *Advances in Experimental Medicine and Biology*, *817*, 221–239. Available from https://doi.org/10.1007/978-1-4939-0897-4_10.

Wallace, C. J. K., & Milev, R. (2017). The effects of probiotics on depressive symptoms in humans: A systematic review. *Annals of General Psychiatry*, *16*, 14. Available from https://doi.org/10.1186/s12991-017-0138-2.

Wells, C. L., Sugiyama, H., & Bland, S. E. (1982). Resistance of mice with limited intestinal flora to enteric colonization by *Clostridium botulinum*. *The Journal of Infectious Diseases*, *146*(6), 67–76.

Wilson, B., & Whelan, K. (2017). Prebiotic inulin-type fructans and galacto-oligosaccharides: Definition, specificity, function and application in gastrointestinal disorders. *Journal of Gastroenterology and Hepatology*, *32*(Suppl 1), 64–68. Available from https://doi.org/10.1111/jgh.13700.

World Health Organization. (2017). *Depression and other common mental disorders: Global health estimates*. Geneva: WHO.

Wu, Z., Ni, J., Liu, Y., Teeling, J. L., Takayama, F., Collcutt, A., ... Nakanishi, H. (2017). Cathepsin B plays a critical role in inducing Alzheimer's disease like phenotypes following chronic systemic exposure to lipopolysaccharide from *Porphyromonas gingivalis* in mice. *Brain, Behavior and Immunity*, *65*, 350–361. Available from https://doi.org/10.1016/j.bbi.2017.06.002.

Yang, H., Zhao, X., Tang, S., Huang, H., Zhao, X., Ning, Z., ... Zhang, C. (2016). Probiotics reduce psychological stress in patients before laryngeal cancer surgery. *Asia-Pacific Journal of Clinical Oncology*, *12*(1), e92–e96. Available from https://doi.org/10.1111/ajco.12120.

Yoo, B. B., & Mazmanian, S. K. (2017). The enteric network: Interactions between the immune and nervous systems of the gut. *Immunity, 46*(6), 910–926. Available from https://doi.org/10.1016/j.immuni.2017.05.011.

Zhao, Y., Jaber, V., & Lukiw, W. J. (2017). Secretory products of the human GI tract microbiome and their potential impact on Alzheimer's disease (AD): Detection of lipopolysaccharide (LPS) in AD hippocampus. *Frontiers in Cellular and Infection Microbiology, 7*, 318. Available from https://doi.org/10.3389/fcimb.2017.00318.

Zheng, P., Zeng, B., Zhou, C., Liu, M., Fang, Z., Xu, X., ... Xie, P. (2016). Gut microbiome remodeling induces depressive-like behaviors through a pathway mediated by the host's metabolism. *Molecular Psychiatry, 21*(6), 786–796. Available from https://doi.org/10.1038/mp.2016.44.

Further Reading

Bijkerk, C. J., de Wit, N. J., Muris, J. W., Whorwell, P. J., Knottnerus, J. A., & Hoes, A. W. (2009). Soluble or insoluble fibre in irritable bowel syndrome in primary care? Randomised placebo controlled trial. *BMJ, 339*, b3154. Available from https://doi.org/10.1136/bmj.b3154.

Dewhirst, F. E., Chen, T., Izard, J., Paster, B. J., Tanner, A. C., Yu, W. H., ... Wade, W. G. (2010). The human oral microbiome. *Journal of Bacteriology, 192*, 5002–5017. Available from https://doi.org/10.1128/JB.00542-10.

Emery, D. C., Shoemark, D. K., Batstone, T. E., Waterfall, C. M., Coghill, J. A., Cerajewska, T. L., ... Allen, S. J. (2017). 16S rRNA next generation sequencing analysis shows bacteria in Alzheimer's post-mortem brain. *Frontiers in Aging Neuroscience, 9*. Available from https://doi.org/10.3389/fnagi.2017.00195.

Ford, A. C., Talley, N. J., Spiegel, B. M., Foxx-Orenstein, A. E., Schiller, L., Quigley, E. M., & Moayyedi, P. (2008). Effect of fibre, antispasmodics, and peppermint oil in the treatment of irritable bowel syndrome: Systematic review and meta-analysis. *BMJ, 337*, a2313. Available from https://doi.org/10.1136/bmj.a2313.

Kawamoto, S., Maruya, M., Kato, L. M., Suda, W., Atarashi, K., Doi, Y., ... Fagarasan, S. (2014). Foxp3 + T cells regulate immunoglobulin a selection and facilitate diversification of bacterial species responsible for immune homeostasis. *Immunity, 41*, 152–165. Available from https://doi.org/10.1016/j.immuni.2014.05.016.

Kulkami, V., Bhatavadekar, N. B., & Uttamani, J. R. (2014). The effect of nutrition on periodontal disease: A systematic review. *Journal of the California Dental Association, 42*(5), 302–311.

Roberfroid, M., Gibson, G. R., Hoyles, L., McCartney, A. L., Rastall, R., Rowland, I., ... Meheust, A. (2010). Prebiotic effects: Metabolic and health benefits. *British Journal of Nutrition, 104*, S1–S63. Available from https://doi.org/10.1017/S0007114510003363.

Tzortzis, G., & Vulevic, J. (2009). *Galacto-oligosaccharide prebiotics. Prebiotics and probiotics science and technology* (pp. 207–244). New York: Springer.

CHAPTER 5

Cognitive Dissonance in Food and Nutrition

Andy S.J. Ong

School of Health & Social Sciences, Nanyang Polytechnic, Singapore, Singapore

OUTLINE

Introduction	105	Using the FCD Conceptual Framework in Research—Construct Instrumentation	120
Dietary Choices and the Attitude–Behavior Link	106	Using the FCD Conceptual Framework in Public Health and Nutrition Research—Illustration(s)	121
Cognitive Dissonance Theory in Food and Nutrition	107	Locating Cognitive Dissonance (and Its Role) in the Overall Scheme of Food and Nutrition Research	124
CDT and Health/Nutrition Messages About Food	108		
CDT and Changing Food Attitudes/Behaviors	110	Conclusion	127
Need for Unified Cognitive Dissonance Theorization in Food and Nutrition	115	References	128
The Food Cognition Dissonance (FCD) Conceptual Framework	116	Further Reading	133

INTRODUCTION

Food consumption plays a vital role in health, as evidenced by research showing that poor nutrition is a causal factor for many diseases that predominate in developed countries like cancer, heart disease, and diabetes (Dibsdall, Lambert, & Frewer, 2002; World Health Organisation & Food & Agriculture Organisation of the United Nations, 2003). "Historically, the public health approach to dietary change has been based on the premise that consumers will abandon those dietary behaviours that are demonstrably unhealthy in order to prevent future illness" (Nestle et al., 1998, p. S50). Correspondingly, many intra- and international health bodies have increased their efforts over the years in defining and promoting healthy diets (Dibsdall et al., 2002), in the hope that the impact of numerous later-life diseases, such as osteoporosis, obesity, hypertension, diabetes, heart disease, and certain cancers, may be reduced with greater compliance to such healthy diets (Miller & Cassady, 2012). Given that nutrition is inextricably linked to health and illness (Ross, Caballero, Cousins, Tucker, & Ziegler, 2012), the process of food choice becomes a critical issue in prevention and treatment; understanding this process is pivotal to promoting health (Devine, Connors, Bisogni, & Sobal, 1998) as knowing how and why individuals choose their foods is essential to motivating them to modify their eating and food habits toward dietary recommendations (Zandstra, de Graaf, & van Staveren, 2001).

Dietary Choices and the Attitude—Behavior Link

The study of attitudes is a means by which understanding food choice and behavior may be achieved (Ajzen & Fishbein, 1980; Roininen & Tuorila, 1999; Dahm, Samonte, & Shows, 2009). Attitude has been found to influence, guide, or be related to eating and food behavioral outcomes, whether independently (e.g., Harvey et al., 2001; Zandstra et al., 2001) or as part of a larger theoretical framework like the health belief model (HBM; Becker & Rosenstock, 1984; Deshpande, Basil, & Basil, 2009), the protection motivation theory (PMT; Cox, Anderson, Lean, & Mela, 1998; Rogers, 1975), the theory of reasoned action (TRA; Fishbein & Ajzen, 1975; Shepherd & Stockley, 1985), the theory of planned behavior (TPB; Ajzen, 1985; Povey, Conner, Sparks, James, & Shepherd, 2000), and the health action process approach (HAPA; Garcia & Mann, 2003; Schwarzer, 1992). The general notion of a positive relationship between attitude and behavior in such studies is exemplified by Lechner and Brug's (1997) study in which a positive attitude toward fruit and vegetable consumption was found to predict higher self-ratings of the consumption of fruits and vegetables. Given the link between eating/food attitudes and eating/food behavior, it is generally acknowledged by researchers concerned with optimizing food choices in the direction of health that a change in dietary behavior might occur through changing food-related attitudes (Aikman, Crites, & Fabrigar, 2006; Contento, 2012; Nestle et al., 1998; Worsley, 2002).

Despite the best attempts made by public health practitioners and attitude researchers, however, getting individuals to eat right has not been an easy task (Ronteltap, Sijtsema, Dagevos, & de Winter, 2012). For example, even as efforts have been expended on trying to get individuals to at least balance red meat consumption with increased fiber—namely fruits and vegetables—intake (Hall, Moore, Harper, & Lynch, 2009; Talukder, 2015), actual fruit and vegetable consumption still falls short of public health recommendations (e.g., Moore & Thompson, 2015). Indeed, although health has been found to be "among the most important motives for food choice" (Steptoe, Pollard, & Wardle, 1995; Verbeke, 2008, cited in Ronteltap et al., 2012, p. 333), there is ironically a critical rise in the prevalence rates of obesity and other dietary-linked ailments, such as diabetes and coronary heart disease, globally (Delpeuch, Maire, Monnier, & Holdsworth, 2009; Popkin, 2009; WHO, 2003, cited in Ronteltap et al., 2012). Ronteltap et al. (2012) pointed out that "it is striking that, despite all efforts in public health interventions and product development, and despite the importance consumers claim to attach to health, the health status of many people is decreasing" (p. 333). This sentiment is corroborated by Hornick et al. (2013) who, in a 5-year retrospective look at American's attitudes toward food, nutrition, and health, noted that "although food and health communications may have fostered general awareness, a disconnect remains among Americans' perceptions, attitudes, and actual behaviours when it comes to achieving a healthful lifestyle" (p. 14). Specifically, the authors found that even when food and nutrition information/knowledge is widely and instantaneously accessible to Americans, "they are not acting on this knowledge when it comes to making decisions about food and health" (Hornick et al., 2013, p. 14). This finding is apparently not a recent phenomenon as Girois, Kumanyika, Morabia, and Mauger (2001) had earlier and similarly found that although "many professionals and policy makers advocate changes in food practices among Americans for health, safety or environmental reasons, yet success in achieving these planned changes is often elusive" (cited in Bisogni, Connors, Devine, & Sobal, 2002, p. 128).

In light of the less than optimal outcomes produced by the existing strategies that underlie current health promotion efforts in getting individuals to change their dietary nutritional habits for better health, the time seems right to explore new and/or alternative ways through which positive change(s) in dietary behavior might be achieved. Accordingly, the current chapter examines and discusses the potential utility of cognitive dissonance as a tool in this regard.

COGNITIVE DISSONANCE THEORY IN FOOD AND NUTRITION

Festinger (1957, as cited in Harmon-Jones & Harmon-Jones, 2007), in his original basic conception of the cognitive dissonance theory (denoted CDT henceforth), postulated that individuals would experience an aversive, psychological state of discomfort, that is, dissonance, when faced with two or more inconsistent cognitions, which might include "attitudes and beliefs or awareness of one's own behavior" (Alfnes, Yue, & Jensen, 2010, p. 147). They would then attempt to remove/reduce this unpleasant psychological tension experienced by restoring cognitive consistency. Festinger (1957) further elaborated that the degree of dissonance experienced by an individual with regard to a specific cognition is denoted by the ratio $D/D + C$, where D is the sum of dissonant cognitions and C is the sum of consonant cognitions, the cognitions each weighted by its importance. In other words, the magnitude of dissonance pertaining to a certain cognition depends on the number as well as the psychological significance of cognitions dissonant (inconsistent) and consonant (consistent) with that cognition such that "dissonance will increase as the number and importance of dissonant cognitions relative to consonant cognitions increase" (Harmon-Jones, 2002, p. 100). Given thus dissonance might be reduced by (1) removing dissonant cognitions, (2) inserting consonant cognitions, and/or (3) reducing the importance of dissonant cognitions and augmenting the importance of consonant cognitions (Harmon-Jones, 2002; Harmon-Jones & Harmon-Jones, 2007). The actual manifestation of these might be in the form of "attitude, belief, value, or behavior maintenance or change," typically affecting "the cognition least resistant to change" (Harmon-Jones, 2002, p. 100).

CDT and Health/Nutrition Messages About Food

CDT provides an avenue through which the apparent ineffectiveness of current dietary health promotion efforts may be potentially examined and explained. Specifically, the premise of a need for cognitive consistency that underlies CDT makes it a potentially relevant and appropriate theory to be used in the study of food attitudes and the food choice process given that "today's consumers are at the centre of a perplexing and changing nutrition environment, particularly when it comes to eating healthfully" (Hornick et al., 2013, p. 14). The latter phenomenon is due, in part, to the complication arising from the ongoing search for a clear scientific definition of what constitutes healthy eating (Lobstein & Davies, 2009). Numerous nutritional studies with contradictory findings on the health effects of certain foods like red meat or dairy products continue to be published (Givens, 2010) and widely disseminated to meet and sustain public interest in health and nutrition but "leaving consumers puzzled on what healthy food is and is not" (Ronteltap et al., 2012, p. 333). Thus faced with a great and extensive variety of foods, from which daily food choices need to be made, it is not surprising that, contemporary consumers in modern societies "have fears and conflicts involving food and health" (Mennell, Murcott, & van Otterloo, 1992; Rozin, Fischler, Imada, Sarubin, & Wrzesniewski, 1999; Senauer, Asp, & Kinsey, 1991; cited in Connors, Bisogni, Sobal, & Devine, 2001, p. 189).

Indeed, Patterson, Satia, Kristal, Neuhouser, and Drewnowski (2001) who conducted a survey research to study the potential negative impact of nutrition messages on dietary behavior, agreed that "giving the public comprehensible and useful information on the relationships between diet and health is a major component of public health efforts to promote healthful dietary patterns" (p. 37). However, the same researchers noted that whilst consumer interest in nutrition was high (Byers & Lyle, 1999), several factors worked against consumer confidence in nutrition communication. Firstly, due to continued advances in scientific research and knowledge in food and human nutrition, messages regarding diet and health had often changed over time—for instance, after years of being told to choose margarine instead of butter, consumers were livid, confused, and skeptical (Goldberg, 1992) when subsequently told that the trans fatty acids in margarine had negative effects on serum cholesterol concentrations and therefore were bad for the heart (Mensink & Katan, 1990). Secondly, new scientific knowledge created through research had necessarily led to increasing complexity in diet and health messages, often resulting in disharmonized information, depending on the sources of the message and their markedly different agendas (Goldberg, 1992). Patterson et al. (2001) used the term "nutrition backlash" to refer to "a broad gamut of negative feelings about dietary recommendations, which could include scepticism, anger, guilt, worry, fear, and helplessness" (p. 38) and found it to be associated with less healthful dietary patterns, implying that individuals who were more skeptical and had more negative feelings toward diet and health messages also ate more fat-related diets and less fruit-and-vegetables diets. While Patterson et al.'s (2001) research generated some interesting findings, a limitation in their study was that they only focused on nutrition backlash as *"one consequence of inconsistent and confusing diet and health messages"* (p. 38), and had neglected to consider the possible role played by cognitive dissonance in such a situation of incongruity. This in turn could be attributed to the failure of the researchers to explicitly manipulate the inconsistency in health messages (to create dissonance) before examining its effects against the backdrop of participants' preexisting attitudes toward diet and health (which were not measured either).

Against this, Albarracín, Cohen, and Kumkale (2003) conducted a study to investigate the hypothesis of increased resistance to persuasion when message recommendations conflict with a postmessage behavior. Here, Albarracín et al. (2003) exposed experimental subjects to preventive, consumer education messages that either opposed or recommended the moderate consumption of an alcohol-like product (i.e., simulated alcohol) before letting half of the participants try the product and half of the participants perform a filler task. Primary results showed that (1) in the absence of trial condition, there was no significant difference in terms of participants' intentions to use the product in the future between recipients of the two different messages but (2) in the trial condition, recipients of the abstinence-promoting preventive message who did try the product expressed stronger intentions to use the product in the future than recipients of the moderation message. The researchers related the exact experimental conditions to a different sample of study participants who were then asked to estimate, amongst other things, the intentions of those participants involved in the experiment to use the alcohol-like product in the future and found the same pattern of results as that of the actual initial experiment. Vis-à-vis the findings the researchers explained that "recipients who act in ways that conflict with an earlier message are likely to resist that message to a greater extent than recipients who experience no post-message conflict" (p. 7); and "accordingly, forceful abstinence presentations to people who will nevertheless perform the behavior may 'backfire', inducing greater resistance than more moderate appeals" (p. 8). Although Albarracín et al. (2003) considered cognitive dissonance to be a possible factor in producing the results obtained, they eventually contended that self-perception (i.e., individuals inferring their attitudes or intentions from the implications of a salient behavior of theirs; Bem, 1965, 1967) was the "primary causal factor" (p. 10). Dismissing cognitive dissonance in favor of self-perception as causality could be traced to the authors' failure to account for subjects' initial attitudes toward alcohol (or like products), a point that the authors had implicitly acknowledged when they asserted that the application of "direct attributional reasoning" due to self-perception "is even more likely whenever pre-existing attitudes are uncertain" (p. 11). This is a limitation reminiscent of Patterson et al.'s (2001) study. Additionally, the dismissal of cognitive dissonance as an explanatory factor was somewhat premature, given the authors' failure to formally and explicitly measure the construct itself.

Nonetheless, Albarracín et al.'s (2003) study shows the potential applicability of cognitive dissonance in an incongruous situation, in which a discrepancy exists between eating/food cognition and behavior. This in turn suggests that cognitive dissonance might also therefore be applicable in the aforementioned incongruous situation found in developed countries where "there is still a discrepancy between the dietary recommendations and actual food consumption" (Zandstra et al., 2001, p. 75) despite "an increased awareness of the consequences of dietary choices and actions, and the risks associated with bad dietary habits" (Schönfeldt & Hall, 2012, p. 152). This situation of incongruity is exacerbated by the "surge in contradictory messages related to health and nutrition" in recent times (Schönfeldt & Hall, 2012, p. 152), which raises the odds of cognitive dissonance being pertinent to the investigation of eating/food cognition and behavior in a food and human nutrition context. However, a formal study of this nature has yet to materialize, which underscores the fact that cognitive dissonance has generally been a poorly studied construct in food and human nutrition research.

CDT and Changing Food Attitudes/Behaviors

Given that cognitive dissonance resolution could potentially occur in terms of attitudinal and/or behavioral change(s) (Harmon-Jones, 2002), CDT additionally provides a basis for purposeful formulation of strategies to influence positive changes to food and food-related attitudes/behaviors toward health. Such potential utility of CDT was recognized by Worsley (2002) more than a decade ago when he noted then that very little, if anything at all, had been done with CDT in this manner within the public health domain "during the past 20 years" (p. S580). In fact, up to 2016, no study may be found that has purposefully engaged cognitive dissonance to influence food attitudes/behaviors (Ong, Frewer, & Chan, 2017a; Ong, Frewer, & Chan, 2017b).

To be sure, cognitive dissonance has been employed in food-related studies in *other ways* in the domains of food risk/safety, food-related consumer behavior, health/nutrition communication, and meat consumption dietary health behavior (Ong et al., 2017b). Taking only research that has explicitly used cognitive dissonance as a focal point of investigation, in which a priori theorization and hypothesis formulation, and subsequently, experimental manipulation, relate directly to the construct, 17 studies to date[1] may be identified to have been conducted as such. Fourteen of these were covered by Ong et al. (2017b), and shall not be repeated here. A summary of the other three new study additions are presented in Table 5.1.

The objective of Choi et al.'s (2017) study was to examine how the effectiveness of interactive advertising varied depending on product and endorser types. In a 2 × 2

---

[1] Ong et al. (2017b) found 14 studies to come under such a classification in their review that was carried out from March 1, 2014 to October 1, 2014. Ong et al. (2017a) reported that four new publications were found in a literature-database search from October 1, 2014 to August 18, 2016, using the terms "cognitive dissonance," "food" and "nutrition." In retrospect, of these, one (i.e., Cao, Just, Turvey, & Wansink, 2015) was actually a same study that had already been included in Ong et al.'s (2017b) review (i.e., Cao, Just, & Wansink, 2014), one (i.e., Onwezen & van der Weele, 2016) was a qualitative study that had used cognitive dissonance as a nonfocal part of a larger framework in *a priori* theorization without hypothesis formulation, leaving just two (i.e., Gaspar et al., 2016; Tian, Hilton, & Becker, 2016) that could be added to this category. Picking up from where Ong et al.'s (2017a) search ended, a new literature-database search (from August 18, 2016 to June 1, 2018) conducted for this chapter article revealed three new potential publications. On closer scrutiny, one of the three (i.e., Westerwick, Johnson, & Knobloch-Westerwick, 2017) reported the exact study by Knobloch-Westerwick, Johnson, and Westerwick (2013) that had been covered in the review by Ong et al. (2017b) but with additional secondary data analyses based exclusively on the Selective Exposure Self- and Affect-Management (SESAM) model by Knobloch-Westerwick (2015) and was thus excluded. Similarly, another study by Wilson, Knobloch-Westerwick, and Robinson (2018) had focused on the SESAM model, bypassing basic cognitive dissonance foundations—just as how assimilation theory had superseded cognitive dissonance theory in consumer research (Ong et al., 2017b)—and was thus also excluded. Only one study by Choi, Kim, Sung, and Yu (2017) in the domain of food-related consumer behavior met Ong et al.'s (2017b) inclusion criteria, and was added to the list.

TABLE 5.1 Summary of New Food-Related Studies That had Explicitly/Directly Used Cognitive Dissonance in a priori Theorization and Hypothesis-Testing (October 1, 2014–June 1, 2018).

Topic Area	Authors	Brief Description of Study	Sample Characteristics	Main Result(s)	Cognitive Dissonance Measurement	Implications for Use of Cognitive Dissonance Theory in Research into Dietary Choice and Public Health
Food-related consumer behavior	Choi et al. (2017)	Experimentally investigated how the advertising factor in terms of type of endorser would impact on attitudes toward virtue/healthy (mixed fruit-vegetable juice) vs. vice/unhealthy (carbonated soft drink) products.	Undergraduate and graduate students in the South Korea (N = 186).	Participants exposed to self-endorsed advertisements for unhealthy food had a more positive attitude toward carbonated soft drinks compared to those exposed to friend-endorsed advertisements for the product. The relationship between self-endorsement and attitude toward the unhealthy food was mediated by self-justification.	Cognitive dissonance arousal was not directly measured but somewhat experimentally manipulated and inferred from the outcome variables instead.	To reduce cognitive dissonance due to conflict arising from self-endorsement of unhealthy food, self-justification emerges to promote a positive attitude toward the unhealthy food.
Food risk/safety	Gaspar et al. (2016)	Investigated how the provision of risk and benefit information to red meat consumers, who were assumed to possess a natural propensity to avoid such information, would relate to their attitudes toward red meat and knowledge regarding red meat risks.	International participants from the United Kingdom (n = 80), Belgium (n = 80), and Portugal (n = 84).	Using a longitudinal design, when exposed to both health-nutritional or nonhealth risk and benefit information on red meat, individuals who had a higher tendency to avoid such information showed more positive attitude toward red meat and greater experienced cognitive dissonance, lower risk information seeking behavior, and lower systematic processing of information.	Cognitive dissonance arousal was manipulated (indirectly at best) but not controlled. Cognitive dissonance was assessed through a proxy measure that is study discontentment.	Cognitive dissonance is positively related to risk information avoidance and negatively related to information seeking, therein posing a potential barrier to effective health risk communication.

(Continued)

TABLE 5.1 (Continued)

Topic Area	Authors	Brief Description of Study	Sample Characteristics	Main Result(s)	Cognitive Dissonance Measurement	Implications for Use of Cognitive Dissonance Theory in Research into Dietary Choice and Public Health
Meat consumption	Tian et al. (2016)	Examined experimentally how the connection between meat and its animal origin would affect individuals' willingness to consume meat and their mind perceptions of the concerned animal.	Young adults from France ($n = 243$; $n = 301$) and China ($n = 277$; $n = 217$).	Via two experiments, in which one focused on the stage of meat production and the other on meat consumption, participants were exposed to stimuli that depicted varying levels of dissociation between meat and its animal origin. Only in the first study was a clear, statistically significant result obtained that showed French participants indicating less willingness to eat beef when this was measured first before mind perception of cows than when it was measured following the assessment of mind perception of cows.	Cognitive dissonance arousal was experimentally manipulated, although actual cognitive dissonance onset was not directly measured but implicitly inferred from the outcome variables in the two studies.	Cognitive dissonance elicited by the association between meat and its animal origin might increase willingness to consume the meat for individuals from certain cultures, particularly if these individuals are not asked about animal mind perception beforehand.

between-subjects experimental design, participants, who could only take part in the study if they came in pairs with a friend, were randomly assigned to one of four conditions: (1) self-endorsed advertisement of carbonated soft drinks—participants were shown three advertisements for carbonated soft drinks with their pictures included within; (2) friend-endorsed advertisement of carbonated soft drinks—participants were shown three advertisements for carbonated soft drinks with their friend's pictures included within; (3) self-endorsed advertisement of mixed fruit and vegetable juice—participants were shown three advertisements for mixed fruit and vegetable juice with their pictures included within; and (4) friend-endorsed advertisement of mixed fruit and vegetable juice—participants were shown three advertisements for mixed fruit and vegetable juice with their friend's pictures included within. Manipulation checks showed that participants made a differentiation between the carbonated soft drinks as unhealthy and the mixed fruit and vegetable juice as healthy. With attitudes toward the two products as outcome measures, the researchers found that participants exposed to the self-endorsement condition for the vice product of carbonated soft drink evaluated the product more favorably than those exposed to the friend-endorsement condition. No significant difference, however, was found between endorser types with respect to the virtue product of mixed fruit and vegetable juice. Using a self-justification measure that was adapted from studies of Franke, Keinz, and Steger (2009) and Inman and Zeelenberg (2002), the researchers additionally reported that self-justification mediated the relationship between product and endorser types in terms of product attitude such that it predicted more positive attitude toward the carbonated soft drink when the vice product had been advertised via self-endorsement. While Choi et al.'s (2017) study represented a novel study of the effectiveness of interactive advertising, it was inadequate from the perspective of cognitive dissonance scholarship. Specifically, although cognitive dissonance theory was used to guide hypothesis formulation, cognitive dissonance was not focused upon sufficiently for the construct to be precisely manipulated nor explicitly measured. If it was, then measures of product attitudes would have been additionally taken prior to experimental manipulation so as to ascertain if self-endorsement of the products constituted a situation of cognitive conflict or not.

Gaspar et al. (2016) examined the effects of presenting red meat risks information to red meat consumers, who were assumed to possess a natural propensity to avoid such information, on their attitudes toward red meat and knowledge regarding red meat risks. The researchers hypothesized that avoidance of risk information would be positively related to attitudes toward red meat and cognitive dissonance, and negatively related to additional risk information seeking and both systematic and heuristic processing. It was further anticipated that individuals who avoided risk information would show less change in attitudes toward red meat and perceived risk knowledge than those who did not avoid risk information. Using a longitudinal design, measures of red meat risks information avoidance, attitudes toward red meat, and perceived knowledge about red meat risks were taken from study participants at time 1. Immediately after, the participants were presented with information regarding both health-nutritional (e.g., chronic disease) as well as nonhealth (e.g., environmental, socioeconomic, etc.) risks and benefits of red meat consumption. After information exposure, measures of attitudes toward red meat, perceived knowledge of red meat risks, and systematic and heuristic processing were taken (time 2). Two weeks following the information exposure (time 3), participants were asked to complete a final questionnaire set measuring attitudes toward red meat, perceived knowledge of red meat risks and overall satisfaction with the study. The hypothesized correlations between avoidance of risk information and red meat attitude, cognitive dissonance, risk information seeking, and systematic processing were confirmed but the remaining hypotheses were not confirmed. Whilst Gaspar et al.'s (2016) use of a longitudinal study design and the conscious assessment of cognitive dissonance were a credit to the research, a major flaw rested in the authors' use of overall satisfaction with study (i.e., study discontentment) as an operationalization of the cognitive dissonance construct. Such operational definition misalignment aside, the assessment of cognitive dissonance would also have been more appropriately carried out immediately following (at time 2) rather than two weeks after (at time 3) risk information exposure.

The awareness of the "meat paradox" (i.e., "liking to eat meat but not wanting to kill animals," p. 186) and the strategies used to reduce the resultant cognitive dissonance amongst individuals from different cultural backgrounds were examined by Tian et al. (2016) in two survey-based experimental studies. Adapting Bastian, Loughnan, Haslam, and Radke's (2012) methodological procedure, the first study focused on cognitive dissonance arousal at the meat production stage, whereby Chinese and French participants were exposed to one of four conditions that varied in "the transparency of the connection between meat and its animal origin" (p. 188). Specifically, with the exception of the control condition, in increasing level of dissociation between meat and its animal origin, a picture of a cow was shown in two of the experimental conditions accompanied either by the statement that it would be sent to the abattoir (abattoir condition) or another pasture (pasture condition) the next day, whilst in the remaining experimental condition, the same picture was diagrammatically dissected into the different kinds of beef that derived from the various parts of the cow (meat condition). In all conditions, participants had to subsequently indicate their willingness to eat meat and their mind perception of cows as dependent measures, for which the presentation order was varied and factored as a second independent variable. The researchers reported that participants in the abattoir condition were less willing to eat beef than those in the meat condition, even though the difference in terms of study conditions was not statistically significant. A significant interaction, however, was found between participant nationality and order of dependent measures presentation, in which French participants indicated less willingness to eat beef when this was measured first before mind perception of cows than when it was measured following the assessment of mind perception of cows; no such difference was found for the Chinese participants. In terms of mind perceptions of cows, whilst a significant interaction between participant nationality and study condition was indicated, the reported simple main effects analyses, showing that French participants in the pasture and meat conditions attributed less mind to cows than those in the control condition, were not statistically significant. The same dependent variables were used in the second study that focused on cognitive dissonance arousal at the meat consumption stage, where the connection between meat and its animal origin was now represented descriptively as a dish recipe (in which beef was the main ingredient) instead. Apart from the control condition in which no stimulus was presented, in increasing level of dissociation between meat and animal origin, one condition presented the meat recipe together with an animal image, another presented the recipe with a dish image—much like that depicted in restaurants' menus—and the last experimental condition presented the recipe alone. Although the researchers specifically reported that participants in the recipe alone condition were more willing to eat beef compared to those in the control condition, this was not statistically significant. Likewise, whilst it was reported that less mind was attributed to cows by (1) French participants compared to Chinese participants, and (2) those in the recipe with animal and dish image conditions compared to the recipe alone condition, these were not statistically significant. Using and reporting results that, by and large, did not meet the minimum $p \leq .05$ level of statistical significance but were merely "marginally significant" (p. 189) constituted a major flaw of the study. In addition, Tian et al.'s (2016) failure to explicitly measure cognitive dissonance is problematic in a "meat paradox" study such as this as it fails to separate cognitive dissonance from guilt, a potential affect experienced by meat eaters due to moral conscience (Bastian et al., 2012; Graca, Calheiros, & Oliveira, 2016; Šedová, Slovák, & Ježková, 2016), which is distinct from (albeit related to) cognitive dissonance (Breslavs, 2013). In a situation like this, any effects on outcome variables might then be erroneously attributed to cognitive dissonance when they could in reality be due to feelings of guilt instead.

Need for Unified Cognitive Dissonance Theorization in Food and Nutrition

From all the 17 studies reviewed—14 by Ong et al. (2017b) and three in the current chapter—current cognitive dissonance scholarship in food and nutrition appears to be dogged by the following issues:

1. *Disparities in how cognitive dissonance was used in research conceptualization*—across the different topical areas within the food and nutrition domain, cognitive dissonance was conceptualized and operationalized differently, with some studies explicitly ensuring the existence of cognitive conflict prior to dissonance arousal (e.g., Albarracín et al., 2003; Tian et al., 2016) and some other studies failing to do so (e.g., Knobloch-Westerwick et al., 2013; Nordvall, 2014), resulting in disparate research findings.
2. *Variations in how cognitive dissonance arousal was experimentally evoked without clear adherence to established cognitive dissonance paradigms*—although the basic cognitive dissonance process comprises the stages of dissonance arousal and dissonance resolution, the latter has been studied relatively more extensively than the former, which has been largely and substantially neglected; the major paradigms associated with dissonance arousal, which include *free choice, induced compliance, belief disconfirmation, hypocrisy,* and *effort justification* (see Harmon-Jones, 2002; and/or Harmon-Jones, & Harmon-Jones, 2007; for paradigm descriptions), have therefore almost always been overlooked in the manipulation of cognitive dissonance arousal in food and/or food-related studies.
3. *General lack of explicit measurement of cognitive dissonance itself (subsequent to its arousal)*—following experimental manipulation, actual cognitive dissonance arousal was rarely explicitly assessed or measured but instead inferred from "observable manifestations of attempts to reduce it" (Carlsmith & Aronson, 1963, p. 151), which Rothgerber (2014) noted, "While important, these demonstrations only offer indirect support for a dissonance-based explanation" (p. 38).

Apart from the identified issues, a main takeaway from the research review is that all 17 studies reviewed rarely examined the utility of cognitive dissonance in influencing and/or altering food/food-related attitudes, reflecting the fact that whilst the potential of cognitive dissonance to influence attitudes and behaviors in food and nutrition has been recognized and acknowledged (e.g., Worsley, 2002), it has yet to be fully explored and exploited. It is thus in the interest of food science and nutrition scholars to become more engaged in cognitive dissonance research applied in the area of food choice and dietary practice, with the ultimate goal of optimizing the utility of cognitive dissonance in the design of effective policies and promotional strategies in public health.

As the unsystematic and disconnected approach taken in the examination of cognitive dissonance in food-related studies could have contributed to the disparate findings vis-à-vis the effects of cognitive dissonance across those studies, Ong et al. (2017b) opined that going forward a conceptual framework integrating the basic principles of cognitive dissonance theory with the relevant attitude and context-specific theorizations associated with food and nutrition was required to facilitate systematic research in this area as a precursor to application.

THE FOOD COGNITION DISSONANCE (FCD) CONCEPTUAL FRAMEWORK

The FCD conceptual framework was proposed by Ong et al. (2017a) as an integrated theoretical framework that could serve to guide systematic cognitive dissonance research in the food and nutrition domain, particularly with regards to investigating cognitive dissonance effects on food-related attitudes. The proposed framework is derived from amalgamating the fundamental principles underlying Festinger's (1957) cognitive dissonance theory with those of a contemporary view of the tripartite model of attitude (Breckler, 1984), supported by relevant food and/or food-related studies.

In defining the framework's core cognitive dissonance construct and its conceptualization, Ong et al. (2017a) noted that although "Festinger's early explanation of dissonance did not clearly identify whether dissonance is cognitive or emotional" (Sweeney, Hausknecht, & Soutar, 2000, p. 373), the construct has been, and still is, typically described in emotional terms despite its cognitive label, being frequently referred to as an aversive motivational state (Harmon-Jones, 2002) and/or a psychological state of tension or discomfort (Carlsmith & Aronson, 1963; Elliot & Devine, 1994). An emotional dimension of cognitive dissonance is thus suggested, which has been associated with, albeit seen to be separate from and not necessarily synonymous with, anxiety and (dis)satisfaction (Hawkins, 1972; Oshikawa, 1972; Sweeney et al., 2000). However, a cognitive dimension to cognitive dissonance is also implied, given Festinger's postulation that "dissonance... is the existence of nonfitting relations among cognitions," with the latter specified to "mean any knowledge, opinion, or belief about the environment, about oneself, or about one's behavior" (Festinger, 1957, p. 3). Taking these into consideration, Ong et al (2017a) stipulated that a conceptualization of cognitive dissonance (arousal) must therefore include both cognitive and emotional aspects (Sweeney et al., 2000) and, using Harmon-Jones' (2002) typology taken against a food and nutrition context, respectively referred to these as *food-related cognitive discrepancy* (i.e., inconsistency between two or more food-related cognitions) and *food-related dissonance* (i.e., psychological tension or discomfort experienced as a result of food-related cognitive inconsistency).

Food-related cognition is equated to food-related attitude (Alfnes et al., 2010) in the FCD framework, in which attitude is seen as a response to an antecedent stimulus or attitude object alongside affective (emotional response), behavioral (overt actions and behavioral intentions), and cognitive (beliefs, knowledge structures, perceptual responses, and thoughts) tendencies toward the attitude object (Breckler, 1984). The definition of attitude premised on a contemporary view of the tripartite model, in which all three components are seen as bases of an attitude (Fabrigar, MacDonald, & Wegener, 2005), essentially captures what has been termed as the internal structure of attitude, that is, *intraattitudinal structure*, which comprises attitude, with its tricomponential cognitive, affective, and behavioral dimensions, toward an attitude object (Fabrigar & Wegener, 2010). Whilst all three components, varying on a common evaluative continuum, might be sufficiently distinct from each other to preclude high intercomponential correlation (Breckler, 1984, citing Greenwald, 1982 and Zajonc, 1980), there is normally some degree of positive correlation amongst the three components that establishes a situation of triadic consistency. This is particularly so when attitude measurement may be derived from cognitive representations of each component, a provision allowed for in the tripartite model. Furthermore, as attitude objects may be delineated in terms of relative concreteness or abstraction (Eagly & Chaiken, 1998), in which a less concrete (and thus more abstract) object may be termed a *superordinate* attitude object, and a more concrete (and thus less abstract) object termed a *subordinate* attitude object, it is possible for attitudes toward superordinate attitude objects to subsume attitudes toward subordinate attitude objects in a way that is generally consistent with each other. For example, an individual who holds a positive attitude toward environmentalism is also likely to possess a positive attitude toward organic food (e.g., Nordvall, 2014) and a negative attitude toward meat consumption (e.g., Hjelmar, 2011). Such linkages or associations between attitudes constitute what has been termed as the external structure of attitude, that is, *interattitudinal structure* (Dreezens, Martijn, Tenbult, Kok, & de Vries, 2005a; Dreezens, Martijn, Tenbult, Kok, & de Vries, 2005b; Eagly & Chaiken, 1998; Fabrigar & Wegener, 2010), which may also include attitudinal links between subordinate—subordinate and superordinate—superordinate attitude object pairings.

Based on (1) the tripartite model's allowance for an assumption of tendency toward triadic consistency amongst the intraattitudinal components, as well as potential consistency in the interattitudinal links amongst attitude objects, and (2) core cognitive dissonance theory principles, the proposed FCD framework stipulates that food-related cognitive dissonance arousal may occur within and/or across food-related attitudinal structures. Any cognitive inconsistency amongst the evaluative tricomponents within the internal structure of a food-related attitude is termed *intraattitudinal, food-related cognitive discrepancy* (*Intra-FCDp*), with the aversive state of tension or psychological discomfort resulting from it correspondingly termed *intraattitudinal, food-related dissonance* (Intra-FD). These two terms collectively define intraattitudinal, food-related cognitive dissonance arousal.[2] Any cognitive inconsistency that occurs in the external linkages between food-related attitudes of different attitude objects is termed *interattitudinal, food-related cognitive discrepancy* (Inter-FCDp), with the resulting aversive state of tension or psychological discomfort correspondingly termed *interattitudinal, food-related dissonance* (Inter-FD). These two terms collectively define interattitudinal, food-related cognitive dissonance arousal[2]. Both intra- and interattitudinal dimensions of food-related cognitive dissonance may be aroused via the use of appropriate cognitive dissonance paradigms. A slightly modified graphical representation of the FCD framework from that published by Ong et al. (2017a) is shown in Fig. 5.1.[2]

In the framework, value, which refers to abstract ideals/principles that provide general orientation and organization for life (Austin & Vancouver, 1996; Maio, Olson, Bernard, & Luke, 2003; Rohan, 2000), is included as part of an extended attitude structure, in which it places hierarchically above attitude. This is because attitudes are seen to derive from values (Dreezens et al., 2005a, b; Eagly & Chaiken, 1995; Verplanken & Holland, 2002) such that "causality flows from values through attitudes to behavior" (Dreezens et al., 2005a, p. 116, citing Bernard, Maio, & Olson, 2003; Homer & Kahle, 1988; Luzar & Cosse, 1998; Maio & Olson, 1994; Stienstra, Ruelle, & Bartels, 2002; Thøgersen & Ölander, 2002). By serving as standards or archetypes for attitude development (Homer & Kahle, 1988; Luzar & Cosse, 1998; Rokeach, 1973), values have implications for attitudinal consistency insofar as qualitative similarities and differences amongst the values exist. The latter is particularly well illustrated in the domain of food and nutrition where individuals are often caught in a conundrum in terms of having to negotiate opposing values within a personal food system when making food choice decisions (Falk, Bisognit, & Sobal, 1996; Furst, Connors, Bisogni, Sobal, & Falk, 1996), such as cost versus quality, or taste versus health considerations (Connors et al., 2001; Hauser, Jonas, & Riemann, 2011; Shepherd, 1999).

Based on the illustration of the FCD framework presented in Fig. 5.1, some hypotheses may be drawn about the framework mechanism concerning the direction and mobility of cognitive dissonance effects within and across attitude structures. Within an extended intraattitudinal structure, a change in attitude toward an attitude object may occur due to dissonance-based alterations in (1) the tricomponential bases of the attitude (bottom-up) or (2) the value from which the attitude derives (top-down). The overall disruption and change in the intraattitudinal structure of that attitude could likely then cause interattitudinal cognitive dissonance to emerge in terms of its external attitudinal link with another (related) attitude object (assuming consistency between the attitudinal structures of both attitude objects prior to the former's intraattitudinal structure disruption/change). If these

---

[2] In Ong et al.'s (2017a) original writing, intraattitudinal food-related cognitive discrepancy and dissonance were reflected as defining intraattitudinal food-related cognitive dissonance, and likewise, interattitudinal cognitive discrepancy and dissonance were reflected as defining interattitudinal food-related cognitive dissonance. In retrospect, cognitive discrepancy and dissonance should be more precisely referred to as constituents of cognitive dissonance *arousal* rather than cognitive dissonance per se. This was actually acknowledged and depicted in Fig. 1 of Ong et al.'s (2017a) same work but missed out on in the articulation of FCD framework. The errata are thus addressed herewith.

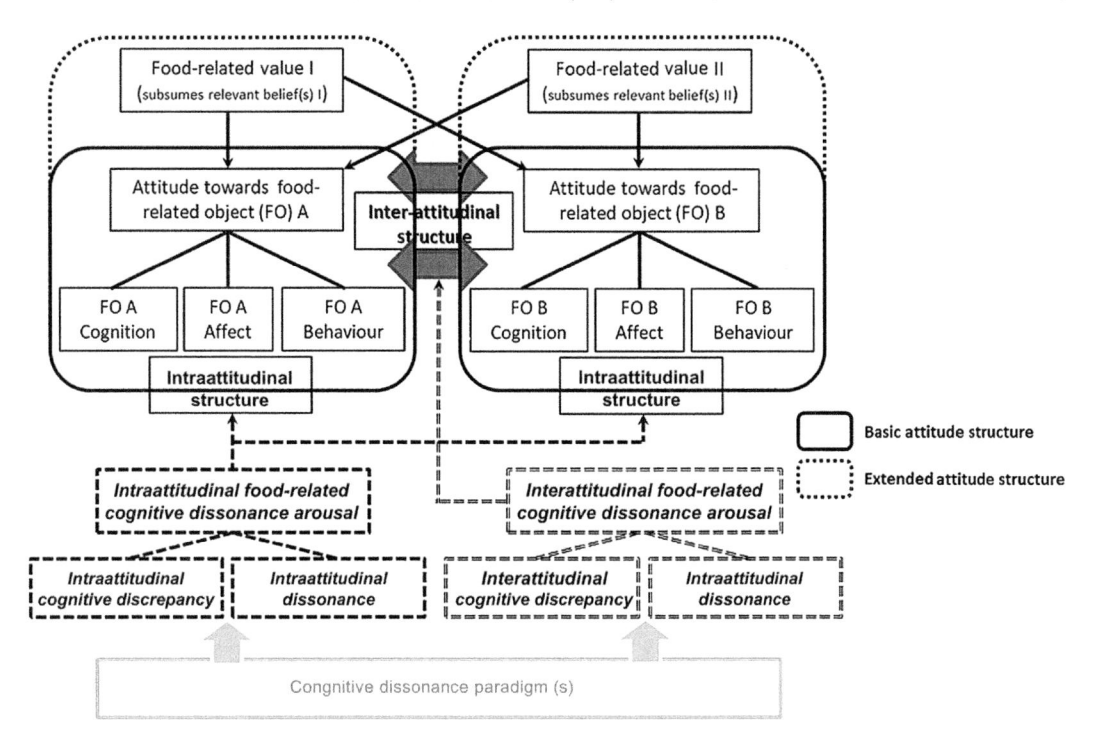

FIGURE 5.1 The food cognition dissonance (FCD) conceptual framework. *Source: Minor modification from Ong, A. S. J., Frewer, L. J., & Chan, M. Y. (2017a). Cognitive dissonance in food and nutrition—A conceptual framework. Trends in Food Science and Technology, 59(1), 60–69.*

are strong enough, corresponding cognitive dissonance effects will bear on the intraattitudinal structure of the second related attitude object to ultimately change it and bring it in line with the altered intraattitudinal structure of the first attitude object, *ceteris paribus*. The hypothesis that a change in attitude toward an attitude object would correspondingly influence a change in attitude toward another related attitude object has been (1) supported by research on interattitudinal structure and attitude change, which showed the spreading activation effect to apply across various attitude object level pairings (i.e., superordinate–superordinate, superordinate–subordinate, subordinate–superordinate, subordinate–subordinate), regardless of the initial attitude object level from which the attitude change began (Dinauer & Fink, 2005); and (2) suggested by specific food research examining associations between food-related attitudes such as Bergmann, von der Heidt, and Maller's (2010) study, which advocated influencing meat consumption via leveraging on consumers' ethical concerns about the impact of factory farming on the environment, including animal welfare. However, the hypothesized cognitive dissonance mechanism underlying such attitude alterations amongst linked attitude objects, as postulated in the FCD framework, are yet to be empirically tested. Additionally, whilst the basis of the ongoing discussion is predicated on intra- and interattitudinal cognitive dissonance occurring sequentially in that order, it is theoretically possible for the sequence to occur in the reverse order, or for the interaction to occur simultaneously. The actual effects of these latter two theoretical possibilities would likewise require empirical testing. It is, however, suspected that the effects might be lesser if the sequence is reversed but strongest when both types of attitudinal cognitive dissonance are activated simultaneously (particularly if both of these complement each other and work in unison to drive linked attitudes in the same direction).

Using the FCD Conceptual Framework in Research—Construct Instrumentation

The proposed FCD conceptual framework provides a theoretical basis for developing formal measures of food-related cognitive dissonance, plugging a major gap in cognitive dissonance research in food and nutrition. In this instance, the nature of the FCD framework in terms of its conceptual makeup dictates that any research conceptualization using the framework necessarily ought to take into consideration both (1) the intra- and interattitudinal dimensions of food-related cognitive dissonance (arousal), as well as (2) the affective-motivational state (i.e., dissonance) and the cognitive inconsistency that produces it (i.e., cognitive discrepancy) separately. Additionally, both (1) and (2) need to be taken in the context of all relevant food-related attitudes and/or behavior that are being examined. Explicit measurements of the relevant cognitive dissonance and attitude/behavior constructs must correspondingly take place. Some considerations related to construct instrumentation, particularly with regard to the novel attitudinal dimensions of cognitive dissonance arousal, are:

- *Attitude object-centered research conceptualization*—in the process of research conceptualization, it is important for researchers to be particularly mindful of the specific attitude object(s), including the number of these and the relationships between them, that a study is examining. Such mindfulness is crucial in determining (1) the exact attitudinal dimensions of cognitive dissonance arousal to be measured and (2) the precise nature in which cognitive dissonance arousal should be experimentally manipulated.
- *Measurement of attitudinal dimensions of food-related cognitive dissonance*—a general principle regarding measurement of the attitudinal dimensions of food-related cognitive dissonance is that it should be carried on a *per attitude object* basis. To elaborate and illustrate, in the context of two attitude objects A and B, there should be assessments of intraattitudinal cognitive dissonance arousal related to A and B separately and an assessment of interattitudinal cognitive dissonance arousal related to the external attitudinal link between them. Furthermore, within each assessment, there should be measurements of cognitive discrepancy and dissonance, that is, intraattitudinal cognitive discrepancy and dissonance related to attitude object A, intraattitudinal cognitive discrepancy and dissonance related to attitude object B, and interattitudinal cognitive discrepancy and dissonance related to attitude objects A and B. Thus for two attitude objects, there would be a total of six assessments in terms of the attitudinal dimensions of food-related cognitive dissonance arousal.

- *Experimental manipulation of cognitive dissonance arousal*—based on the notion of spreading activation effect that any (dissonance-based) change in attitude toward an attitude object would potentially cause a corresponding change in attitude toward another related attitude object (Dinauer & Fink, 2005), it may be extrapolated that a single manipulation (through the use of one cognitive dissonance paradigm) would be sufficient to arouse food-related cognitive dissonance within and across attitudinal dimensions. Specifically, in the ongoing illustration of attitude objects A and B, for example, the *belief disconfirmation* paradigm may be used to arouse intraattitudinal cognitive discrepancy and dissonance in A, which would then cause corresponding cognitive discrepancies and dissonances in the intraattitudinal structure of B, as well as in the interattitudinal structure linking A and B.[3]

For clarity, especially for an initial empirical test of the FCD framework, it is proposed that the number of attitude objects examined be capped at two. The two attitude objects selected should be conceptually driven such that a logical, theoretical relationship may be established between the two for an interattitudinal dimension of cognitive dissonance to be conceivably and soundly derived. Extrapolating from the tripartite model's allowance for attitude measurement to be derived from cognitive representations of each attitude component that may be assessed via self-reports, the mode of measurement for the attitudinal dimensions of food-related cognitive dissonance is also via self-reports. This aligns well with the focus of cognitive dissonance theory on cognitive consistency, and its propositional thoughts-based analysis.

Using the FCD Conceptual Framework in Public Health and Nutrition Research—Illustration(s)

In providing a unified theoretical framework for the study of cognitive dissonance in food and nutrition, apart from potentially providing the avenue to reconcile disparate findings regarding cognitive dissonance effects across diverse topical food and nutrition research, in the context of promoting public health, the proposed FCD framework further paves the way for potentially discovering (1) the reasons that might explain the relative ineffectiveness of health and nutrition communication in increasing/decreasing healthy/unhealthy eating, and (2) new methods to influence positive food attitude and behaviors. An illustration of each, with details regarding measurement of the various attitudinal dimensions of cognitive dissonance, is given herewith.

1. *Public health and nutrition communication*

    Patterson et al.'s (2001) research that warned against nutrition backlash vis-à-vis health and nutrition communication provides a suitable platform from which the FCD framework's theorization(s) might be tested. The study indicated that when people's health beliefs and expectations of a food were violated, they were more likely to go the opposite way to engage in less healthful dietary behaviors. This is in contrast to food

---

[3] A single manipulation to arouse cognitive discrepancy and dissonance in the external attitudinal structure linking A and B may also be possible, with corresponding reverberations then occurring within the internal attitude structures of A and B separately.

risk/safety studies that found food risk/safety information violations to actually sustain current dietary behaviors (e.g., Cao et al., 2015). Patterson et al.'s (2001) finding is significant as it suggests a rejection of the authenticity of health and nutrition communication messages as a whole as a consequence of consumer reactance to contradictory health and nutrition communication regarding specific foods. The FCD framework may be used to assess and verify if and to what extent such a scenario plays out.

To illustrate, it should first be noted that the above represents a subordinate–superordinate attitude object pairing situation, in which changes in the internal attitude structure of a specific food (subordinate attitude object) affect changes to the internal attitude structure of health in food considerations (superordinate attitude object). Using the FCD framework, we can choose to study a specific food (e.g., yogurt[4]) and health considerations in food choice as two attitude objects. The *belief disconfirmation* paradigm might then be used to arouse intraattitudinal cognitive discrepancy and dissonance with respect to the food, following which measurements of (1) intraattitudinal cognitive discrepancy (e.g., "I am consuming more yogurt than I should") and dissonance (e.g., "I feel bothered that I am consuming more yogurt than I should") related to the food; (2) intraattitudinal cognitive discrepancy (e.g., "I am not eating as healthily as I should") and dissonance (e.g., "I feel bothered that I am not eating as healthily as I should") related to attitude toward health in food; and (3) interattitudinal cognitive discrepancy (e.g., "I am consuming more yogurt than I should to be considered healthy eating") and dissonance (e.g., "I feel bothered that I am consuming more yogurt than I should to be considered healthy eating") related to the food and attitude toward health in food, are taken. Measurements of attitudes toward the food and health considerations in food choice ought to be collected before and after the experimental manipulation of arousal. Apart from allowing for any attitudinal and/or behavioral change(s) to be tracked and measured, these, particularly the initial attitude measurements before experimental arousal, could be used to assist in the differentiation, if any, of actual dissonance aroused between belief violation of a positive versus negative attitude.

A study such as this would allow public health practitioners to determine the existence of Patterson et al.'s (2001) notion of nutrition backlash and, if it does exist, obtain potential insights into its underlying mechanics, which are very likely to be linked to the processes of cognitive dissonance arousal and resolution (Ong et al., 2017a). The ultimate aim is to then use the insights gained to tweak public health and nutrition communication in ways that would optimize its intended health promotional effects and minimize nutrition backlash.

2. *Influencing positive food (and food-related) attitude(s) and/or behavior(s)*

The phenomenon of individuals being frequently caught in a dilemma when making food choices based on contrasting values in a personal food system (Connors et al., 2001) provides a suitable context for the study of how the FCD framework might be

---

[4] Yogurt is used in the illustration as it is a food that could potentially trigger nutrition backlash since it is perceived as a health food but, scientifically, may not necessarily have the same health benefits for everyone (German, 2014).

used to influence positive attitudes and/or behaviors linked to an immunogenic food value (e.g., health, quality) over those linked to a pathogenic food value (e.g., taste, convenience).

As an illustration, consider public health efforts to promote the value of health over convenience in making food choices. In this instance, the conflict between food choice considerations of health versus convenience (e.g., Hanks, Just, Smith, & Wansink, 2012; Hauser et al., 2011; Remnant & Adams, 2015) may be manipulated to trigger the arousal of various attitudinal dissonances in such a way as to drive positive attitude and/or behavior toward the former over the latter as a means of dissonance resolution. The key to such a regulated arousal of cognitive dissonance lies in the use of appropriate cognitive dissonance paradigm(s) to trigger the arousal. Of the five major cognitive dissonance paradigms (as mentioned earlier), *hypocrisy* and *induced compliance* are the two paradigms that have been most frequently adopted in the context of effecting health-related changes (Freijy & Kothe, 2013). Between these two paradigms, although *induced compliance*—which assumes that dissonance is aroused when an individual does or says something that contradicts a prior held belief or attitude—has been successfully applied to the prevention of disordered eating (e.g., Stice, Marti, & Cheng, 2014), *hypocrisy*—which assumes that dissonance is aroused whenever individuals are induced to publicly make statements consistent with some normative standards and thereafter reminded of times when they did not act in accordance with these standards—"appears most effective in inciting change across a range of non-clinical health behavior" (Freijy & Kothe, 2013, p. 311). Indeed, with respect to *nonclinical* health behavior, "studies based on the induced compliance paradigm produced mixed findings at best" whilst the *hypocrisy* paradigm "appears to most reliably lead to changes in attitude, intention or behavior" (Freijy & Kothe, 2013, p. 330). This could be attributed to the fact that the latter involves a relatively standardized protocol governing the arousal of cognitive dissonance (Aronson, Fried & Stone, 1991), whereas studies adopting the former "reported a variety of dissonance-arousing techniques" (Freijy & Kothe, 2013, p. 326).

Correspondingly, the *hypocrisy* paradigm may be applied to arouse cognitive dissonance in attitude toward convenience in food, with measurements of (1) intraattitudinal cognitive discrepancy (e.g., "I am choosing food based on convenience more than I should") and dissonance (e.g., "I feel bothered that I am choosing food based on convenience more than I should") taken of it, along with (2) intraattitudinal cognitive discrepancy (e.g., "I am not choosing food based on health as much as I should") and dissonance (e.g., "I feel bothered that I am not choosing food based on health as much as I should") related to attitude toward health in food, and (3) interattitudinal cognitive discrepancy (e.g., "I am choosing food based on convenience more than choosing food based on health") and dissonance (e.g., "I feel bothered that I am choosing food based on convenience more than choosing food based on health") based on the spreading activation effect (Dinauer & Fink, 2005). Measurements of attitude toward convenience in food and attitude toward health in food, along with corresponding behavioral assessments, are taken before and after experimental manipulation to gauge attitudinal and/or behavioral changes.

A study such as the above represents an efficacy test of the utility of the FCD framework in guiding health promotional efforts, particularly in terms of influencing positive food attitudes and/or behaviors. This is a research focus that food/nutrition academics and practitioners alike, particularly those with a specific interest in public health promotion, are encouraged to adopt going forward. Efforts in this area will not only verify the validity of the framework's principles, but also help fine-tune them, if or when necessary. In this way, the potential utility of the framework in deriving strategies that would effectively facilitate the modification of food attitudes and/or behaviors in a positive direction might then be actualized.

LOCATING COGNITIVE DISSONANCE (AND ITS ROLE) IN THE OVERALL SCHEME OF FOOD AND NUTRITION RESEARCH

In summary, cognitive dissonance is a construct that hitherto has been relatively understudied in the food and nutrition domain. This is despite an existing awareness of its potential application to the domain, particularly in terms of modifying food-related attitudes/behaviors (Worsley, 2002), amongst food/nutrition researchers. For example, Hjelmar (2011) reported that reflexive shopping practices (i.e., deliberated shopping behavior based on careful consideration of issues such as health, nutrition, environmental welfare, etc.) "can be sparked by...news capable of creating a "cognitive dissonance" among consumers" (p. 336). Šedová et al. (2016) reported that environmental students dealing with attitude—behavior incongruity regarding meat consumption sought to resolve their "feelings of guilt" (p. 416) by using specific coping strategies like "perceived behavioural change and promises for improved future behavior" (p. 421) due to their specialized knowledge and awareness. Thus reiterating the call made by Ong et al. (2017b), it is strongly recommended that food and nutrition researchers begin work to realize the potential of cognitive dissonance in influencing food-related attitudes and/or behaviors in earnest. Furthermore, it is recommended that such work be approached systematically via the use of the FCD framework, which focuses on the cognitive dissonance arousal process based on the logic that its understanding would facilitate a better gauge of the cognitive dissonance resolution process that follows, which includes attitude change.

Ultimately, instead of being subsumed into a marginalized role within broader frameworks examining food/nutrition-related phenomena and given cursory attention (e.g., Quick & Heiss, 2009; Schifferstein, Kole, & Mojet, 1999;), it is hoped that cognitive dissonance (and its study via the FCD framework) might be integrated as an important (and independent) portion of these larger frameworks that incorporate other crucial processes working both separately as well as together to drive and support strategic public health promotion efforts. This chapter concludes with an exemplar of such an integrative approach, which is based on a recent study conducted by Stoll-Kleemann and Schmidt (2017) who formalized cognitive dissonance into their model of factors influencing meat-eating behavior (see Fig. 5.2).

In the model, cognitive dissonance was presented both as a barrier and an opportunity to reducing meat consumption. It was contended that although "people tend to avoid or resist information about the negative consequences of meat-eating because they contradict or threaten basic perspectives on fairness and ethical behavior" (p. 1267), the cognitive

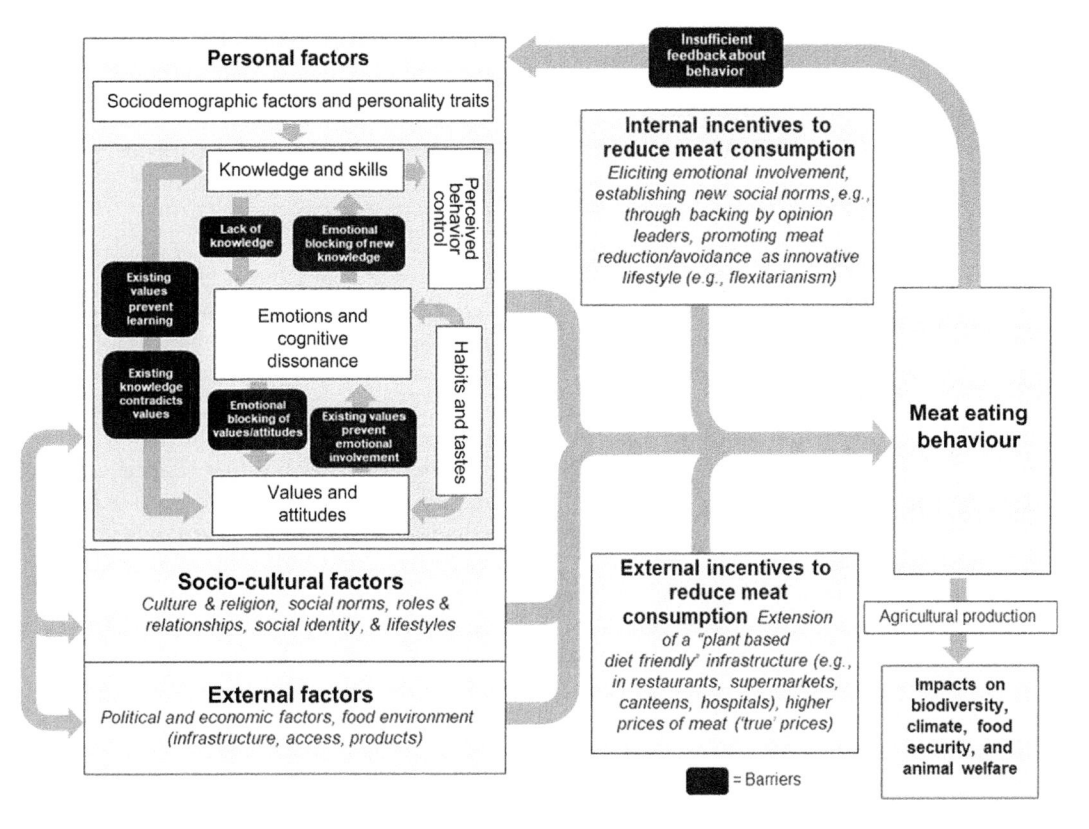

FIGURE 5.2 Model of factors influencing meat-eating behavior. *Source: From Stoll-Kleemann, S., & Schmidt, U. J. (2017). Reducing meat consumption in developed and transition countries to counter climate change and biodiversity loss: A review of influence factors. Regional Environmental Change, 17(5), 1261–1277.*

dissonance aroused as a result of such encounters with contradictory information, nonetheless, could lead to the use of *denial* and *delegation* (i.e., refusal to accept personal responsibility and to blame others) as strategies to remove the negative feelings experienced, thereby sustaining the meat-eating behavior. The solution, according to the authors, was to activate appropriate social norms, established through associating with individuals of the right attitude toward food and personal integrity, to pressure the enactment of the correct response to cognitive dissonance instead, which was to reduce meat consumption.

How cognitive dissonance might be turned from being a barrier to reducing meat-eating behavior into an opportunity to do precisely the opposite might be supplemented through the FCD framework. The FCD framework provides a suitable theoretical basis for studying how food-related cognitive discrepancy in food-related attitude(s) might be strategically manipulated to arouse food-related dissonance, which would serve as an aversive motivational state to prompt positive attitudinal and/or behavioral change(s) as a means of reducing the food-related cognitive discrepancy to restore cognitive consistency. This entails future research work in this area verifying/testing both the structural and mechanical aspects of the FCD framework, which would include, but not necessarily be limited to, the following general notions:

- *Interplay between intra- and interattitudinal cognitive discrepancy sources of food-related cognitive dissonance*—as alluded to, great potential benefits might be gained from investigating possible interaction effects between the intra- and interattitudinal discrepancy sources of food-related cognitive dissonance deriving from different values that simultaneously impinge on same-level attitude objects (i.e., superordinate–superordinate or subordinate–subordinate object pairings). In influencing food-related attitudes, ideally dissonance should be simultaneously created using both intra- and interattitudinal cognitive discrepancies in a congruent manner such that they complement each other to drive positive dietary attitudinal and behavioral change in a single, consistent direction—for example, as mentioned earlier, encouraging healthy eating by reminding an individual that he/she has not been eating healthily despite his/her belief in doing so and additionally highlighting that he/she has compromised health for something less consequential such as convenience (e.g., Connors et al., 2001; Dave, An, Jeffery, & Ahluwalia, 2009; Sijtsema, Jesionkowska, Symoneaux, Konopacka, & Snoek, 2012). The potential of cumulative benefits would be tested in this instance. However, as also noted, intra- and interattitudinal cognitive discrepancies can also realistically occur in opposite directions simultaneously. For example, opting for a less tasty food choice based on its health benefits, only to be told subsequently that the food is not as healthy as it was originally thought to be (Goldberg & Sliwa, 2011; Patterson et al., 2001). Determining which cognition is least resistant to change under such circumstances, and hence the net result(s) of such opposing attitudinal sources of food-related cognitive dissonance, have important implications, particularly for the design and execution of effective dietary attitude change interventions (e.g., food health/nutrition communication). This warrants verification through empirical testing.
- *Relating cognitive dissonance paradigms to the arousal of intra- versus interattitudinal food-related cognitive dissonance*—careful analysis of the use of the different cognitive dissonance paradigms in terms of how each might be appropriate or inappropriate for the arousal of intra- versus interattitudinal food-related cognitive dissonance, including the outcome(s) of such pairings on dietary attitude and/or behavior, is required. This would be particularly useful for identifying and matching appropriate cognitive dissonance paradigms to the differential arousal of attitudinal dimensions of food-related cognitive dissonance *simultaneously* in order to achieve optimal attitudinal/behavioral change outcomes (i.e., toward health and nutrition). Whilst somewhat discernible (albeit largely still ambiguous), cognitive dissonance paradigms could be identified for some of the studies reviewed by Ong et al. (2017b) as the source of intra- versus interattitudinal cognitive dissonance arousal—for example, the latter could be seen in meat consumption studies where it resulted in meat-consumption sustenance through selective cognitive modification (e.g., Bastian et al., 2012; Rothgerber, 2014). Current cognitive dissonance research in food and nutrition has generally been lackadaisical in the requisite use of cognitive dissonance paradigms to elicit dissonance arousal. A systematic study into both intra- and interattitudinal discrepancy sources of

food-related dissonance in relation to the various cognitive dissonance paradigms is thus needed.
- *Domain-specific versus global values, and food-related cognitive dissonance*—although both domain-specific and global values have been examined in food and nutrition studies (e.g., Dreezens et al., 2005b; Furst et al., 1996; Worsley, 2003), these have not been done so utilizing the cognitive dissonance perspective. Specifically, whilst studies have looked at how food-related values could be in conflict with one another such that "satisfying one value would prevent meeting another" (Connors et al., 2001, p. 194), these were largely qualitative in nature. As such, no definitive conclusion, in terms of actual cognitive dissonance effects on dietary attitudes and/or behaviors, could be drawn from such studies. Moreover, most food and nutrition studies have been conducted looking at domain-specific, food-related values, with few examining global values like Worsley (2003), who investigated the association between global, personal values and use of, as well as trust in, nutrition information sources. The lack in relating values conflict to cognitive dissonance and the inequitable focus on food-related versus global values, particularly in food choice research, are issues that need to be reviewed and rectified in food and nutrition research. Although the FCD conceptual framework relates specifically to domain-specific, food-related values, it may be easily adapted to include global values as the focus of investigation, especially since it has been suggested that global values are hierarchically located one level atop domain-specific values (Hauser et al., 2011). An empirical investigation into which type of values—domain-specific, food-related values such as health, quality/indulgence, price/cost, etc. (Connors et al., 2001; Hauser et al., 2011) or global values such as stimulation, hedonism, universalism, etc. (Schwartz, 1992, 2012)—to target in dissonance-based interventions, in order to achieve maximal or optimal effectiveness in terms of attitudinal and/or behavioral change(s), would be useful at some point in the future.

Ensuring that explicit measurements of food-related cognitive dissonance accompany all manner of hypothesis-testing utilizing the FCD framework, the examination of these aforementioned ideas, within the context of Stoll-Kleemann and Schmidt's (2017) broader model of factors influencing meat-eating behavior, could potentially lead to new discoveries regarding dissonance-based management of such behavior, similar to that developed by Stice and colleagues for disordered eating (Stice, Chase, Stormer, & Appel, 2001; Stice, Mazotti, Weibel, & Agras, 2000).

CONCLUSION

This chapter has shown how current cognitive dissonance research in the food and nutrition domain continues to be limited and is yet to be fully explored since Ong et al.'s (2017b) published review. Research in this area needs to begin in earnest in order to advance cognitive dissonance scholarship in food and nutrition, particularly with respect to how the construct might be utilized to optimize food-related attitudes and/or behaviors to achieve favorable health and nutrition outcomes. The proposed FCD conceptual framework by Ong et al. (2017a) represents a step toward facilitating a systematic approach to the study of cognitive dissonance in food and nutrition, with this ultimate goal in mind. It specifically focuses on understanding the dissonance arousal process, which has hitherto been inadequately studied, to attain an understanding of the dissonance resolution process that includes attitude change. The proposed FCD framework not only opens up prospective new directions in food science and nutrition research but also potentially brings a logical, consistent explanatory structure to the varied findings that plague current cognitive dissonance scholarship in food and nutrition. With more work done using the FCD framework, a relatively precise explanation of food-related cognitive dissonance effects could be established that would in turn aid the development of effective dissonance-based strategies within nutrition programs to influence positive dietary attitudes (and thus behaviors) and to facilitate public health promotion.

References

Aikman, S. N., Crites, S. L., Jr., & Fabrigar, L. R. (2006). Beyond affect and cognition: Identification of the informational bases of food attitudes. *Journal of Applied Social Psychology, 36*(2), 340–382.

Ajzen, I. (1985). From intentions to actions: A theory of planned behaviour. In J. Kuhl, & J. Beckman (Eds.), *Action control: From cognition to behaviour* (pp. 11–39). Heidelberg: Springer.

Ajzen, I., & Fishbein, M. (1980). *Understanding attitudes and predicting social behaviour*. Englewood Cliffs, NJ: Prentice-Hall.

Albarracín, D., Cohen, J. B., & Kumkale, G. T. (2003). When communications collide with recipients' actions: Effects of post-message behaviour on intentions to follow the message recommendation. *Personality and Social Psychology Bulletin, 29*(7), 1–12.

Alfnes, F., Yue, C. Y., & Jensen, H. H. (2010). Cognitive dissonance as a means of reducing hypothetical bias. *European Review of Agricultural Economics, 37*(2), 147–163.

Aronson, E., Fried, C., & Stone, J. (1991). Overcoming denial and increasing the intention to use condoms through the induction of hypocrisy. *American Journal of Public Health, 81*(12), 1636–1638.

Austin, J. T., & Vancouver, J. B. (1996). Goal constructs in psychology: Structure, process, and content. *Psychological Bulletin, 120*(3), 338–375.

Bastian, B., Loughnan, S., Haslam, N., & Radke, H. R. (2012). Don't mind meat? The denial of mind to animals used for human consumption. *Personality and Social Psychology Bulletin, 38*(2), 247–256.

Becker, M. H., & Rosenstock, L. M. (1984). Compliance with medical advice. In A. Steptoe, & A. Mathes (Eds.), *Health care and human bBehaviour* (pp. 135–152). London: Academic Press Inc.

Bem, D. J. (1965). An experimental analysis of self-persuasion. *Journal of Personality and Social Psychology, 1*, 199–218.

Bem, D. J. (1967). Self-perception: An alternative interpretation of cognitive dissonance phenomena. *Psychological Review, 74*, 183–200.

Bergmann, I., von der Heidt, T., & Maller, C. (2010). Cognitive dissonance and individuals' response strategies as a basis for audience segmentation to reduce factory farmed meat consumption. In R. Russell-Bennett & and S. Rundle-Thiele (Eds.), *Connecting Thought and Action: Proceedings of the 2010 International Nonprofit & Social Marketing (INSM) Conference, Brisbane, Australia* (pp. 32–35). Lismore, NSW: ePublications@SCU.

Bernard, M. M., Maio, G. R., & Olson, J. M. (2003). The vulnerability of values to attack: Inoculation of values and value-relevant attitudes. *Personality and Social Psychology Bulletin, 29*(1), 63–75.

Bisogni, C. A., Connors, M., Devine, C. M., & Sobal, J. (2002). Who we are and how we eat: A qualitative study of identities in food choice. *Journal of Nutrition Education and Behaviour, 34*(3), 128–139.

Breckler, S. J. (1984). Empirical validation of affect, behaviour and cognition as distinct components of attitude. *Journal of Personality and Social Psychology, 47*(6), 1191–1205.

Breslavs, G. M. (2013). Moral emotions, conscience, and cognitive dissonance. *Psychology in Russia: State of the Art, 6*(4), 65–72.

Byers, T., & Lyle, B. (1999). The role of epidemiology in determining when evidence is sufficient to support nutrition recommendations: Summary statement. *American Journal of Clinical Nutrition, 69*(suppl), 1365S–1367S.

REFERENCES

Cao, Y., Just, D. R., Turvey, C., & Wansink, B. (2015). Existing food habits and recent choices lead to disregard of food safety announcements. *Canadian Journal of Agricultural Economics, 63*(4), 491–511.

Cao, Y., Just, D. R., & Wansink, B. (2014). *Cognitive dissonance, confirmatory bias and inadequate information processing: Evidence from experimental auctions.* Paper presented at the Agricultural & Applied Economic Association's AAEA/EAAE/CAES Joint Symposium: Social Networks, Social Media and the Economics of Food 2014, Montreal, Canada.

Carlsmith, J. M., & Aronson, E. (1963). Some hedonic consequences of the confirmation and disconfirmation of expectations. *Journal of Abnormal and Social Psychology, 66*(2), 151–156.

Choi, J., Kim, Y., Sung, J., & Yu, H. (2017). Are self-endorsed advertisements for unhealthy food more effective than friend-endorsed advertisements?. *Social Behaviour and Personality: An International Journal, 45*, 1069–1084.

Connors, M., Bisogni, C. A., Sobal, J., & Devine, C. M. (2001). Managing values in personal food systems. *Appetite, 36*(3), 189–200.

Contento, I. R. (2012). *Nutrition education: Linking research, theory, and practice* (2nd ed.). Sudbury, MA: Jones & Bartlett Publishers.

Cox, D. N., Anderson, A. S., Lean, M. E. J., & Mela, D. J. (1998). UK consumer attitudes, beliefs and barriers to increasing fruit and vegetable consumption. *Public Health Nutrition, 1*(1), 61–68.

Dahm, M. J., Samonte, A. V., & Shows, A. R. (2009). Organics foods: Do eco-friendly attitudes predict eco-friendly behaviours?. *Journal of American College Health, 58*(3), 195–202.

Dave, J. M., An, L. C., Jeffery, R. W., & Ahluwalia, J. S. (2009). Relationship of attitudes toward fast food and frequency of fast-food intake in adults. *Obesity, 17*(6), 1164–1170.

Delpeuch, F., Maire, B., Monnier, E., & Holdsworth, M. (2009). *Globesity: A planet out of control?* London: Earthscan Publications Ltd.

Deshpande, S., Basil, M. D., & Basil, D. Z. (2009). Factors influencing healthy eating habits among college students: An application of the health belief model. *Health Marketing Quarterly, 26*(2), 145–164.

Devine, C. M., Connors, M., Bisogni, C. A., & Sobal, J. (1998). Life-course influences on fruit and vegetable trajectories: Qualitative analysis of food choices. *Journal of Nutrition and Behaviour, 30*(6), 361–370.

Dibsdall, L. A., Lambert, N., & Frewer, L. J. (2002). Using interpretative phenomenology to understand the food-related experiences and beliefs of a select group of low-income UK women. *Journal of Nutrition Education and Behaviour, 34*(6), 298–309.

Dinauer, L. D., & Fink, E. L. (2005). Interattitude structure and attitude dynamics: A comparison of the hierarchical and Galileo spatial-linkage models. *Human Communication Research, 31*(1), 1–32.

Dreezens, E., Martijn, C., Tenbult, P., Kok, G., & de Vries, N. K. (2005a). Food and values: An examination of values underlying attitudes toward genetically modified- and organically grown food products. *Appetite, 44*(1), 115–122.

Dreezens, E., Martijn, C., Tenbult, P., Kok, G., & de Vries, N. K. (2005b). Food and the relation between values and attitude characteristics. *Appetite, 45*(1), 40–46.

Eagly, A. H., & Chaiken, S. (1995). Attitude strength, attitude structure and resistance to change. In R. E. Petty, & J. A. Krosnick (Eds.), *Attitude strength: Antecedents and consequences. Ohio State University series on attitudes and persuasion* (Vol. 4, pp. 413–432). Hillsdale, NJ: Lawrence Erlbaum Associates, Inc.

Eagly, A. H., & Chaiken, S. (1998). Attitude structure and function. In D. T. Gilbert, S. T. Fiske, & G. Lindzey (Eds.), *The handbook of social psychology* (4th ed., pp. 269–322). New York: McGraw-Hill.

Elliot, A. J., & Devine, P. G. (1994). On the motivational nature of cognitive dissonance: Dissonance as psychological discomfort. *Journal of Personality and Social Psychology, 67*(3), 382–394.

Fabrigar, L. R., MacDonald, T. K., & Wegener, D. T. (2005). The structure of attitudes. In D. Albarracín, B. T. Johnson, & M. P. Zanna (Eds.), *The handbook of attitudes* (pp. 79–124). Abingdon: Routledge.

Fabrigar, L. R., & Wegener, D. T. (2010). Attitude structure. In R. F. Baumeister, & E. J. Finkel (Eds.), *Advanced social psychology: The state of the science* (pp. 177–216). New York: Oxford University Press.

Falk, L., Bisognit, C., & Sobal, J. (1996). Food choice processes of older adults: A qualitative investigation. *Journal of Nutrition Education, 28*(5), 257–265.

Festinger, L. (1957). *A theory of cognitive dissonance.* Stanford, CA: Stanford University Press.

Fishbein, M., & Ajzen, I. (1975). *Belief, attitude, intention and behaviour: An introduction to theory and research.* Reading, MA: Addison Wesley.

Franke, N., Keinz, P., & Steger, C. J. (2009). Testing the value of customization: When do customers really prefer products tailored to their preferences? *Journal of Marketing, 73*, 103–121.

Freijy, T., & Kothe, E. J. (2013). Dissonance-based interventions for health behaviour change: A systematic review. *British Journal of Health Psychology, 18*(2), 310–337.

Furst, T., Connors, M., Bisogni, C., Sobal, J., & Falk, L. (1996). Food choice: A conceptual model of the process. *Appetite, 26*(3), 247–265.

Garcia, K., & Mann, T. (2003). From "I wish" to "I will": Social-cognitive predictors of behavioural intentions. *Journal of Health Psychology, 8*, 347–360.

Gaspar, R., Luís, S., Seibt, B., Lima, M. L., Marcu, A., Rutsaert, P., ... Barnett, J. (2016). Consumers' avoidance of information on red meat risks: Information exposure effects on attitudes and perceived knowledge. *Journal of Risk Research, 19*(4), 533–549.

German, J. B. (2014). The future of yogurt: Scientific and regulatory needs. *American Journal of Clinical Nutrition, 99* (5), 1271S–1278S.

Girois, S. B., Kumanyika, S. K., Morabia, A., & Mauger, E. (2001). A comparison of knowledge and attitudes about diet and health among 35- to 75-yearold adults in the United States and Geneva, Switzerland. *American Journal of Public Health, 91*(3), 418–424.

Givens, D. I. (2010). Milk and meat in our diet. Good or bad for health? *Animal, 4*(12), 1941–1952.

Goldberg, J. P. (1992). Nutrition and health communication: The message and the media over half a century. *Nutrition Reviews, 50*(3), 71–77.

Goldberg, J. P., & Sliwa, S. A. (2011). Getting balanced nutrition messages across communicating actionable nutrition messages: Challenges and opportunities. Symposium on Nutrition: Getting the balance right in 2010. In *Proceedings of the Nutrition Society, 70, 26–37.* A meeting of the Nutrition Society hosted by the Irish Section was held at the University of Ulster, Coleraine, 16–18 June 2010.

Graca, J., Calheiros, M. M., & Oliveira, A. (2016). Situating moral disengagement: Motivated reasoning in meat consumption and substitution. *Personality and Individual Differences, 90*, 353–364.

Greenwald, A. G. (1982). Is anyone in charge? Personalysis versus the principle of personal unity. In J. Suls (Ed.), *Psychological perspectives on the self* (1, pp. 151–181). Hillsdale, NJ: Erlbaum.

Hall, J. N., Moore, S., Harper, S. B., & Lynch, J. W. (2009). Global variability in fruit and vegetable consumption. *American Journal of Preventive Medicine, 36*(5), 402–409, e5.

Hanks, A. S., Just, D. R., Smith, L. E., & Wansink, B. (2012). Healthy convenience: Nudging students toward healthier choices in the lunchroom. *Journal of Public Health, 34*(3), 370–376.

Harmon-Jones, E. (2002). A cognitive dissonance theory perspective on persuasion. In J. P. Dillard, & M. W. Pfau (Eds.), *The persuasion handbook: Developments in theory and practice* (pp. 99–116). Thousand Oaks, CA: Sage Publications Inc.

Harmon-Jones, E., & Harmon-Jones, C. (2007). Cognitive dissonance theory after 50 years of development. *Zeitschrift für Sozialpsychologie, 38*(1), 7–16.

Harvey, J., Erdos, G., Challinor, S., Drew, S., Taylor, S., Ash, R., ... Moffat, C. (2001). The relationship between attitudes, demographic factors and perceived consumption of meats and other proteins in relation to the BSE crisis: a regional study in the United Kingdom. *Health, Risk and Society, 3*(2), 181–197.

Hauser, M., Jonas, K., & Riemann, R. (2011). Measuring salient food attitudes and food-related values. An elaborated, conflicting and interdependent system. *Appetite, 57*(2), 329–338.

Hawkins, D. I. (1972). Reported cognitive dissonance and anxiety: Some additional findings. *Journal of Marketing, 36*(3), 63–66.

Hjelmar, U. (2011). Consumers' purchase of organic food products. A matter of convenience and reflexive practices. *Appetite, 56*(2), 336–344.

Homer, P. M., & Kahle, L. R. (1988). A structural equation test of the value-attitude-behaviour hierarchy. *Journal of Personality and Social Psychology, 54*(4), 638–646.

Hornick, B. A., Childs, N. M., Edge, M. S., Kapsak, W. R., Dooher, C., & White, C. (2013). Is it time to rethink nutrition communications? A 5-year retrospective of Americans' attitudes toward food, nutrition, and health. *Journal of the Academy of Nutrition and Dietetics, 113*(1), 14–23.

Inman, J. J., & Zeelenberg, M. (2002). Regret in repeat purchase versus switching decisions: The attenuating role of decision justifiability. *Journal of Consumer Research, 29*, 116–128.

Knobloch-Westerwick, S. (2015). The selective exposure self- and affect management (SESAM) model: Applications in the realms of race, politics, and health. *Communication Research, 42*(7), 959–985.

REFERENCES

Knobloch-Westerwick, S., Johnson, B. K., & Westerwick, A. (2013). To your health: Self-regulation of health behaviour through selective exposure to online health messages. *Journal of Communication, 63*(5), 807–829.

Lechner, L., & Brug, J. (1997). Consumption of fruit and vegetables: How to motivate the population to change their behaviour. *Cancer Letters, 114*(1–2), 335–336.

Lobstein, T., & Davies, S. (2009). Defining and labelling 'healthy' and 'unhealthy' food. *Public Health Nutrition, 12*(3), 331–340.

Luzar, E. J., & Cosse, K. J. (1998). Willingness to pay or intention to pay: The attitude-behaviour relationship in contingent valuation. *Journal of Socio-Economics, 27*(3), 427–444.

Maio, G. R., & Olson, J. M. (1994). Value-attitude-behaviour relations: The moderation role of attitude functions. *British Journal of Social Psychology, 33*(3), 301–312.

Maio, G. R., Olson, J. M., Bernard, M. M., & Luke, M. A. (2003). Ideologies, values, attitudes, and behaviour. In J. Delamater (Ed.), *Handbook of social psychology* (pp. 283–308). New York: Kluwer Academic/Plenum Publishers.

Mennell, S., Murcott, A., & van Otterloo, A. H. (1992). *The sociology of food: Eating, diet and culture*. Newbury Park: Sage.

Mensink, R. P., & Katan, M. B. (1990). Effect of dietary trans fatty acids on high-density and low-density lipoprotein cholesterol levels in healthy subjects. *The New England Journal of Medicine, 323*(7), 439–445.

Miller, L. M., & Cassady, D. L. (2012). Making healthy food choices using nutrition facts panels. The roles of knowledge, motivation, dietary modifications goals, and age. *Appetite, 59*(1), 129–239.

Moore, L. V., & Thompson, F. E. (2015). Adults meeting fruit and vegetable intake recommendations—United States, 2013. *Morbidity & Mortality Weekly Report (Centers for Disease Control & Prevention), 65*(26), 709–713.

Nestle, M., Wing, R., Birch, L., DiSogra, L., Drewnowski, A., Middleton, S., ... Economos, C. (1998). Behavioural and social influences on food choice. *Nutrition Reviews, 56*, S50–S74.

Nordvall, A. C. (2014). Consumer cognitive dissonance behaviour in grocery shopping. *International Journal of Psychology and Behavioural Sciences, 4*(4), 128–135.

Ong, A. S. J., Frewer, L. J., & Chan, M. Y. (2017a). Cognitive dissonance in food and nutrition—A conceptual framework. *Trends in Food Science and Technology, 59*(1), 60–69.

Ong, A. S. J., Frewer, L. J., & Chan, M. Y. (2017b). Cognitive dissonance in food and nutrition: A review. *Critical Reviews in Food Science and Nutrition, 57*(11), 2330–2342.

Onwezen, M. C., & van der Weele, C. N. (2016). When indifference is ambivalence: Strategic ignorance about meat consumption. *Food Quality and Preference, 52*, 96–105.

Oshikawa, S. (1972). The measurement of cognitive dissonance: Some experimental findings. *Journal of Marketing, 36*(1), 64–67.

Patterson, R. E., Satia, J. A., Kristal, A. R., Neuhouser, M. L., & Drewnowski, A. (2001). Is there a consumer backlash against the diet and health message? *Journal of the American Dietetic Association, 101*(1), 37–41.

Popkin, B. (2009). *The world is fat. The fads, trends, policies, and products that are fattening the human race*. New York: Avery.

Povey, R., Conner, M., Sparks, P., James, R., & Shepherd, R. (2000). Application of the theory of planned behaviour to two dietary behaviours: Roles of perceived control and self-efficacy. *British Journal of Health Psychology, 5*, 121–139.

Quick, B. L., & Heiss, S. N. (2009). An investigation of value-, impression-, and outcome-relevant involvement on attitudes, purchase intentions, and information seeking. *Communication Studies, 60*(3), 253–267.

Remnant, J., & Adams, J. (2015). The nutritional content and cost of supermarket ready-meals. Cross-sectional analysis. *Appetite, 92*, 36–42.

Rogers, R. W. (1975). A protection motivation theory of fear appeals and attitude change. *The Journal of Psychology: Interdisciplinary and Applied, 91*(1), 93–114.

Rohan, M. J. (2000). A rose by any name? The value construct. *Personality and Social Psychology Review, 4*(3), 255–277.

Roininen, K., & Tuorila, H. (1999). Health and taste attitudes in the prediction of use frequency and choice between less healthy and more healthy snacks. *Food Quality and Preference, 10*(4–5), 357–365.

Rokeach, M. (1973). *The nature of human values*. New York: Free Press.

Ronteltap, A., Sijtsema, S. J., Dagevos, H., & de Winter, M. A. (2012). Construal levels of healthy eating. Exploring consumers' interpretation of health in the food context. *Appetite, 59*(2), 333–340.

Ross, A. C., Caballero, B., Cousins, R. J., Tucker, K. L., & Ziegler, T. R. (2012). *Modern nutrition in health and disease* (11th ed.). Philadelphia, PA: Lippincott Williams & Wilkins.

Rothgerber, H. (2014). Efforts to overcome vegetarian-induced dissonance among meat eaters. *Appetite, 79*(1), 32–41.

Rozin, P., Fischler, C., Imada, S., Sarubin, A., & Wrzesniewski, A. (1999). Attitudes to food and the role of food in life in the U.S.A., Japan, Flemish Belgium and France: Possible implication for the diet-health debate. *Appetite, 33*(2), 163–180.

Schifferstein, H. N. J., Kole, A. P. W., & Mojet, J. (1999). Asymmetry in the disconfirmation of expectations for natural yogurt. *Appetite, 32*(3), 307-239.

Schönfeldt, H. C., & Hall, N. G. (2012). Consumer education on the health benefits of red meat: A multidisciplinary approach. *Food Research International, 47*(2), 152–155.

Schwartz, S. H. (1992). Universals in the content and structure of values: Theoretical advances and empirical tests in 20 countries. In M. P. Zanna (Ed.), *Advances in experimental social psychology* (Vol. 25, pp. 1–65). Waterloo: Academic Press, Inc.

Schwartz, S. H. (2012). An overview of the Schwartz theory of basic values. *Online Readings in Psychology and Culture, 2*(1). Available from https://doi.org/10.9707/2307-0919.1116.

Schwarzer, R. (1992). Self-efficacy in the adoption and maintenance of health behaviours: Theoretical approaches and a new model. In R. Schwarzer (Ed.), *Self-efficacy: Thought control of action* (pp. 217–243). Washington, DC: Hemisphere.

Šedová, I., Slovák, L., & Ježková, I. (2016). Coping with unpleasant knowledge: Meat eating among students of environmental studies. *Appetite, 107*, 415–424.

Senauer, B., Asp, E., & Kinsey, J. (1991). *Food trends and the changing consumer*. St. Paul, MN: Eagan Press.

Shepherd, R. (1999). Social determinants of food choice. *Proceedings of the Nutrition Society, 58*(4), 807–812.

Shepherd, R., & Stockley, L. (1985). Fat consumption and attitudes towards food with a high fat content. *Human Nutrition: Applied Nutrition, 39A*, 431–442.

Sijtsema, S. J., Jesionkowska, K., Symoneaux, R., Konopacka, D., & Snoek, H. (2012). Perceptions of the health and convenience characteristics of fresh and dried fruits. *LWT—Food Science & Technology, 49*(2), 275–281.

Steptoe, A., Pollard, T. M., & Wardle, J. (1995). Development of a measure of the motives underlying the selection of food: The Food Choice Questionnaire. *Appetite, 25*, 267–284.

Stice, E., Chase, A., Stormer, S., & Appel, A. (2001). A randomized trial of a dissonance-based eating disorder prevention program. *International Journal of Eating Disorders, 29*(3), 247–262.

Stice, E., Marti, C. N., & Cheng, H. Z. (2014). Effectiveness of a dissonance-based eating disorder prevention program for ethnic groups in two randomised controlled trials. *Behaviour Research and Therapy, 55*, 54–64.

Stice, E., Mazotti, L., Weibel, D., & Agras, W. S. (2000). Dissonance prevention program decreases thin-ideal internalization, body dissatisfaction, dieting, negative affect, and bulimic symptoms: A preliminary experiment. *Journal of Eating Disorders, 27*(2), 206–217.

Stienstra, J., Ruelle, H., & Bartels, G. (2002). A closer look at eleven years of environment perception through laddering. In G. Bartels, & W. Nelissen (Eds.), *Marketing for sustainability: Towards transactional policy-making*. Amsterdam: IOS Press.

Stoll-Kleemann, S., & Schmidt, U. J. (2017). Reducing meat consumption in developed and transition countries to counter climate change and biodiversity loss: A review of influence factors. *Regional Environmental Change, 17*(5), 1261–1277.

Sweeney, J. C., Hausknecht, D., & Soutar, G. N. (2000). Cognitive dissonance after purchase: A multidimensional scale. *Psychology and Marketing, 17*(5), 369–385.

Talukder, S. (2015). Effect of dietary fiber on properties and acceptance of meat products: A review. *Critical Review in Food Science and Nutrition, 55*(7), 1005–1011.

Thøgersen, J., & Ölander, F. (2002). Human values and the emergence of a sustainable consumption pattern: A panel study. *Journal of Economic Psychology, 23*(5), 605–630.

Tian, Q., Hilton, D., & Becker, M. (2016). Confronting the meat paradox in different cultural contexts: Reactions among Chinese and French participants. *Appetite, 96*, 187–194.

Verbeke, W. (2008). Impact of communication on consumers' food choices. *The Proceedings of the Nutrition Society, 67*(3), 281–288.

Verplanken, B., & Holland, R. W. (2002). Motivated decision making: Effects of activation and self-centrality of values on choices and behaviour. *Journal of Personality and Social Psychology, 82*(3), 434–447.

Westerwick, A., Johnson, B. K., & Knobloch-Westerwick, S. (2017). Change your ways: Fostering health attitudes toward change through selective exposure to online health messages. *Health Communication, 32*(5), 639–649.

Wilson, B., Knobloch-Westerwick, S., & Robinson, M. J. (2018). Picture yourself healthy—How users select mediated images to shape health intentions and behaviors. *Health Communication*. Available from https://doi.org/10.1080/10410236.2018.1437527.

World Health Organisation, & Food and Agriculture Organisation of the United Nations. (2003). Diet, nutrition and the prevention of chronic diseases: Report of a joint WHO/FAO expert consultation, 28 January–1 February 2002, Geneva, Switzerland. WHO Technical Report Series, Technical report 916, World Health Organization, Geneva.

Worsley, A. (2002). Nutrition knowledge and food consumption: Can nutrition knowledge change food behaviour? *Asia Pacific Journal of Clinical Nutrition, 11*(Suppl 3), S579–S585.

Worsley, A. (2003). Consumers' personal values and sources of nutrition information. *Ecology of Food and Nutrition, 42*(2), 129–151.

Zajonc, R. B. (1980). Feeling and thinking: Preferences need no inferences. *American Psychologist, 35*(2), 151–175.

Zandstra, E. H., de Graaf, C., & van Staveren, W. A. (2001). Influence of health and taste attitudes on consumption of low- and high-fat foods. *Food Quality and Preference, 12*(1), 75–82.

Further Reading

Bratanova, B., Loughnan, S., & Bastian, B. (2011). The effect of categorization as food on the perceived moral standing of animals. *Appetite, 57*(1), 193–196.

SECTION B

APPLICATIONS OF PERSONALIZED NUTRITION

CHAPTER 6

Trends, Insights, and Approaches to Diet and Obesity

I. Iglesia[1,2,3,*], P. De Miguel-Etayo[1,2,4,*], T. Battelino[5,6] and L.A. Moreno[1,2,4]

[1]Growth, Exercise, NUtrition and Development (GENUD) Research Group, Faculty of Health Sciences, Agri-food Institute of Aragón (IA2), University of Zaragoza, Zaragoza, Spain [2]Health Research Institute of Aragón (IIS Aragón), Zaragoza, Spain [3]Maternal and child health and development network (SAMID), Carlos III Health Institute, Madrid, Spain [4]Biomedical Research Center in the Physiopathology of Obesity and Nutrition network (CIBERObn), Carlos III Health Institute, Madrid, Spain [5]Department of Pediatric Endocrinology, Diabetes and Metabolism, University Children's Hospital (UMC), Ljubljana, Slovenia [6]Faculty of Medicine, University of Ljubljana, Ljubljana, Slovenia

OUTLINE

General Concepts	138	Factors Associated With Obesity: Sociodemographic Factors	144
Diagnosis Criteria	138	Associated Comorbidities	145
Epidemiology	139	Prevention Obesity Strategies	146
Causes	141	Environmental Factors	147
Genetic Factors	142	Behavioral Strategies	149
Psychological Factors	142	Support of Health Services and Clinical Interventions	150
Dietary Factors	142		
Sedentarism and Physical Activity	144		
Sleep Habits	144	Future Approaches	151

[*] These authors contributed equally to the writing of this Chapter.

Obesity Treatment	151	Conclusion	158
Obesity Treatment Objectives	151	References	159
Specific Treatment Components	153		

GENERAL CONCEPTS

Obesity is a multifactorial disease resulting from a combination of genetic, physiological, and environmental factors. Overweight and obesity are defined as abnormal or excessive fat accumulation that may impair health (World Health Organization, 2016). Apart from genetic factors, obesity is the result of the disequilibrium between energy intake and expenditure associated with alterations of different metabolic pathways. Excessive fat accumulation is linked with disturbances in some organs and human systems (Milagro, Mansego, De Miguel, & Martinez, 2013). Obesity is responsible for an increase in cardiovascular diseases, type 2 diabetes, some types of cancers, many other diseases, and low quality of life in the short and long terms (Guh et al., 2009).

DIAGNOSIS CRITERIA

BMI is a simple index of weight-for-height that is commonly used to identify overweight and obesity in adults. This index is defined as a person's weight (kilograms) divided by the square of their height (meters) (kg/m^2). In adults the body mass index (BMI) provides a useful population-level measure of overweight and obesity as the cutoffs are the same for both sexes and for all age groups. However, it should be considered as a rough guide because it may not correspond to the same degree of fatness in different individuals (WHO, 2016). BMI is considered internationally a good index of cardiometabolic risk, but it may not be a good index of adiposity at the individual level since it cannot distinguish between fat and lean mass.

For adults, the WHO and Organisation for Economic Co-operation and Development (OECD) define overweight as a BMI greater than or equal to $25 \, kg/m^2$, and obesity as a BMI greater than or equal to $30 \, kg/m^2$ (Organisation for Economic Co-operation and Development (OECD), 2018; WHO, 2016). However, lower BMI cutoff points apply for some ethnic populations, such as Southeast Asians. For children the age needs to be considered when defining overweight and obesity (WHO, 2016). Moreover, this index should be used with caution in elderly populations (Gill, Bartels, & Batsis).

Taking into consideration the technological advances, the development of devices, and the equipment to measure body fat, such as air-displacement plethysmography (BodPod), dual X-ray absorptiometry (DEXA), and bioelectrical impedance analysis (BIA), makes it easier to classify individuals according to their body fat stores, independently of BMI. Using skinfold thickness measurements, total body fat from body density can be estimated using available equations for men and women (Siri, 1993). However, the main limitations of this method are the reproducibility, the inter- and intraindividual variations, and the difficulty to obtain accurate measures in subjects with severe obesity (Mei et al., 2002).

Other anthropometric indices are more accurate indicators of total adiposity, such as the fat mass index [FMI = fat mass (kg) divided by height (m^2)] (Ortega, Sui, Lavie, & Blair, 2016; Vanltallie, Yang, Heymsfield, Funk, & Boileau, 1990). The BMI takes into account body weight and height, while the FMI requires information on body weight, height, and fat mass content (Peltz, Aguirre, Sanderson, & Fadden, 2010). The FMI has high sensitivity to slight changes in body fat stores compared to the use of BMI or percentage body fat in adolescence (Schutz, Kyle, & Pichard, 2002) making it an interesting index for assessing nutritional status. However, the FMI has not had wide application because appropriate reference standards are not yet available.

Intraabdominal fat is associated with elevated metabolic and cardiovascular risk (WHO, 2016; Zhu et al., 2002). Waist circumference (WC) is an accurate predictor of diseases and has been shown to be a better marker of mortality than BMI (Zhang et al., 2007) and can be used as a proxy for abdominal fat (Zhu et al., 2002). WC is measured at the level of the narrowest point between the lower costal (10th rib) border and the iliac crest. The subject should breathe normally, and the measurement is taken at the end of a normal expiration (end tidal). If there is no obvious narrowing, the measurement is taken at the mid-point between the lower costal (10th rib) border and the iliac crest. The subject assumes a relaxed standing position with the arms folded across the thorax (International Society for the Advancement of Kinanthropometry (ISAK)). The International Diabetes Federation (IDF) defined central obesity as a WC $\geq$ 94 cm in men and $\geq$ 80 cm in nonpregnant women, however, lower cutoff points apply for some ethnic groups (Alberti, Zimmet, & Shaw, 2005).

EPIDEMIOLOGY

The worldwide prevalence of obesity nearly tripled between 1975 and 2016 (WHO, 2016). The public health relevance of obesity worldwide is unquestionable, with it being considered a global epidemic (NCD Risk Factor Collaboration NCD-RisC, 2016; WHO, 2016, 2018b, 2018c). Over the past decade the prevalence of overweight and obesity has increased in Canada, France, Mexico, Switzerland, and the United States, while it has been stabilized in England, Italy, Korea, and Spain (OECD).

Obesity is a common disease in developed countries and also in most of the developing countries. In 2015 across the OECD 19.5% of the adult population had obesity (Fig. 6.1). The lowest prevalences were observed in Korea and Japan (6%) while the highest adult obesity prevalences are in the United States, Mexico, New Zealand, and Hungary (30%).

In 2016 more than 1.9 billion adults were overweight. Among them over 650 million adults had obesity. Overall about 13% of the world's adult population (11% of men and 15% of women) had obesity in 2016 (WHO, 2016). In addition, the prevalence of obesity is projected to increase further by 2030. If the recent trends continue 60% of the world's population could have obesity in the future (Kelly, Yang, Chen, Reynolds, & He, 2008). In 2017 the WHO reported that in the European region the overall obesity prevalence among adults is 20% and 29.9% in males and females, respectively (WHO, 2018). However, the prevalence of obesity in Sweden, Denmark, Switzerland, Austria, Slovakia, and Italy was lower than 19.9% in females (WHO, 2018).

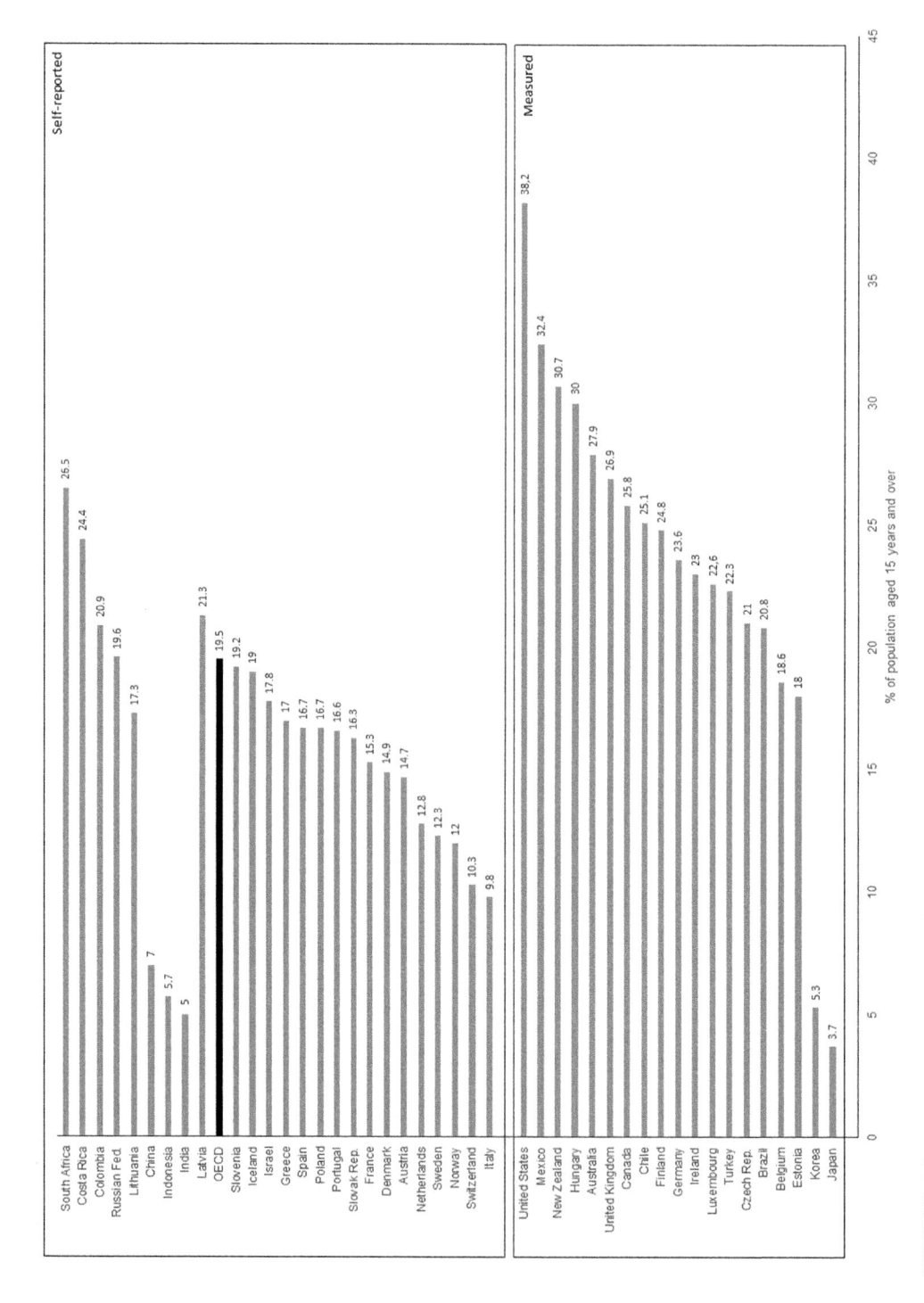

FIGURE 6.1 Worldwide obesity prevalence among adults, per country, in 2015 or nearest year (OECD).

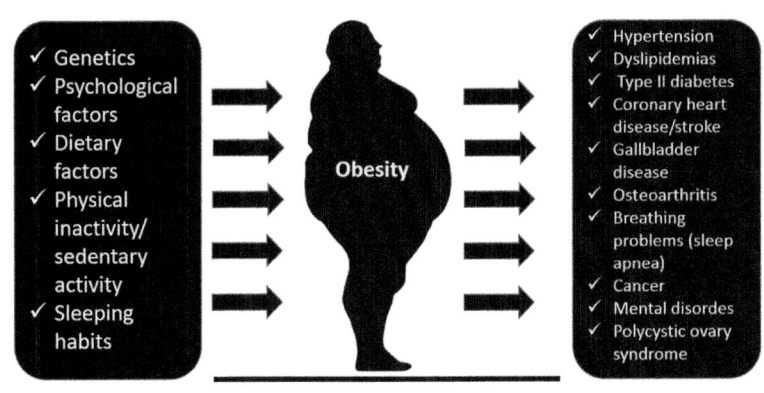

FIGURE 6.2 Obesity. Causes and consequences.

The overweight (including obesity) rate in adults aged 15–74 years has been rising in most countries. The highest increase is observed in the United States (Fig. 6.2).

Obesity rates are expected to be particularly high in the United States, Mexico, and England, where 47%, 39%, and 35% of the population, respectively, could be obese in 2030. In contrast, the increase is expected to be weaker in Italy and Korea, with obesity rates projected to be 13% and 9% in 2030, respectively. The level of obesity in France is projected to nearly match that of Spain at 21% in 2030.

Social inequalities and overweight and obesity are highly related, especially among women. In about half of the eight countries in the OECD organization, less educated women are two to three times more likely to be overweight than those with a higher level of education (OECD).

Inequalities have grown in Italy, Spain, Korea, and England between 2010 and 2014 for both men and women. However, in the United States the prevalence has been increasing most rapidly among the highly educated population.

Currently more than one in two adults and nearly one in six children have overweight or obesity from North and South America to Europe and Asia Pacific (OECD). The obesity epidemic has spread further in the past 5 years, but prevalences have been increasing at a slower pace than before.

CAUSES

Obesity's primary cause is an imbalance between calories consumed and calories expended (Hruby & Hu, 2016). However, this energetic imbalance is multifactorial. An important component is due to individual factors, such as genetics or psychology, which combine with the so-called energy balance–related behaviors, which include food intake, physical activity practice, sleep quality, sedentary behaviors, and stress levels (Fishbein, 2001).

Fig. 6.2 shows a summary of the causes and comorbidities associated with obesity in adults.

Genetic Factors

In the last decade research has focused on identifying lifestyle factors linked with genetic predisposition to obesity, together with the description of hundreds of novel common genetic variants associated with body composition parameters, such as weight and height, BMI, WC, or waist to hip circumference ratio (Hruby et al., 2016). Genome-wide studies have identified several common genetic variants associated with obesity (Bradfield et al., 2012; Hosseini-Esfahani et al., 2017). Among the most studied associations, the fat mass and obesity-associated gene (FTO) locus and obesity represent a big burden with consistent results (Peng et al., 2011), increasing BMI by 0.22–0.66 per risk allele. However, the interactions between lifestyle factors with genetic variants and obesity could better provide insights into the roles of diet/environmental factors in the pathogenesis of obesity.

For instance, based on three US cohorts, it was shown that B vitamins intake (Huang et al., 2015), sugared-sweetened beverages (SSB) intake (Qi, Chu, et al., 2012), fried foods (Qi et al., 2014), television viewing, or physical activity practicing interacted with the genetic risk of obesity (Qi, Li, et al., 2012).

Psychological Factors

There is a significant body of literature available in relation to obesity and psychiatric illness, especially for depression. However, most of the studies were cross-sectional and therefore establishment of cause–effect is not possible. Nevertheless, a recent systematic review (Rajan & Menon, 2017), based on longitudinal studies, tried to answer this question. A large heterogeneity was found among the studies included: effect sizes, differences in the cutoffs used for measuring BMI, differences in methods used to measure psychiatric outcomes such as depression, varying lengths of follow-ups, the nature of the effect estimate used, or the effect of some characteristics such as age or gender in these associations. The conclusion was that the evidence is strong and reciprocal for depression; modest and inconsistent for anxiety disorders; and inadequate for other psychiatric conditions (Rajan & Menon, 2017), since it was only for depression that causal relationships could be established. Depression may cause shifts in hormone levels and immune system function, which might lead to weight gain. Besides, depression can also downregulate the motivation for movement while increasing overeating and binge eating (National Center for Eating Disorders, 2012).

Dietary Factors

Nutrients, Foods, and Beverages

Traditionally dietary fat was considered the main cause of obesity. However, in an 8-year follow-up from the Nurses' Health Study (NHS) in the United States, total fat intake was only weakly related to weight gain, whereas increasing energy intakes from animal, saturated, and, remarkably, trans fatty acids were positively associated with weight gain, particularly in women who were already overweight

(Field, Willett, Lissner, & Colditz, 2007). In a 12-year follow-up from the NHS, higher whole grain intake was negatively associated with gained weight in women, in contrast with what occurred with higher refined grain intake (Liu et al., 2003). Additionally, women who increased the intake of whole grains or total dietary fiber throughout the follow-up decreased their risk of having obesity by 19% and 34%, respectively, while the intake of refined grains had the opposite effect (Liu et al., 2003). Nuts have also been shown to reduce the risk of obesity, central obesity, diabetes, and metabolic syndrome (MetS) in Spanish adults (Ibarrola-Jurado et al., 2013). However, the effect of the consumption of nuts remains unclear because some other studies did not show the same effect (Jiang et al., 2002).

Beverages also have gained attention over recent years in relation to their association with weight gain. In this respect SSB or fruit juices intake have been shown to be associated with weight gain (Brunkwall et al., 2016; Schulze et al., 2004). A nonlinear relationship was drawn with alcohol intake in NHS II, showing that women who drank up to 30 g/day were less likely to gain weight than nondrinkers or heavy drinkers (Wannamethee, Field, Colditz, & Rimm, 2004), while in another study the daily intake of water, coffee (without added sugar), or one serving of a diet beverage in women showed a protective effect for weight loss over a period of 4 years (Pan et al., 2013).

Dietary Patterns

Foods are not consumed in isolation and for this reason it seems important to explore dietary patterns in relation to health outcomes (Iglesia et al., 2018). Besides, by analyzing individual nutrients and foods, problems of collinearity might be found (Cespedes et al., 2015). Consequently, in order to strengthen the evidence for public health recommendations and to prevent obesity, recent nutrition research has been focused on dietary patterns. For instance, a dietary pattern described as Western (characterized by higher levels of consumption of red and processed meats, refined grains, sweets or desserts, SSBs, and potatoes) was associated with an increase in weight of women during a 8-year follow-up study, while those showing adherence to a named prudent pattern (consisting of high intakes of fruits, vegetables, whole grains, fish, poultry, and salad dressing) gained the least weight in the cited follow-up (Schulze, Fung, Manson, Willett, & Hu, 2006).

However, apart from these "a posteriori" methods, there are also other "a priori" methods based on the scientific evidence and dietary recommendations, which consist of several diet quality scores. From those it is possible to highlight the Alternate Healthy Eating Index 2010 (AHEI-2010), which has been shown to be consistently associated with a lower risk of chronic diseases in clinical and epidemiological investigations, the Dietary Approach to Stop Hypertension (DASH), or the Alternate Mediterranean Diet (AMED), which focuses on a Mediterranean dietary pattern. In previous studies it has been shown that the higher the adherence to these three diet quality scores, the lower the weight gain (Wang et al., 2018). These results were similar to those also shown in seven European countries where adults demonstrating greater adherence to the Mediterranean diet (MedDiet) pattern presented better anthropometric and biochemical markers, even in the presence of an elevated genetic risk (San-Cristobal et al., 2017).

Sedentarism and Physical Activity

The industrial revolution, modern technology, and the development of motor-based transport systems for commuting, have diminished dramatically the former high-energy demanding daily living activities (Church et al., 2011). The direct consequence is a sedentary lifestyle, which might result in an imbalance of energy, which in turn might produce overweight or obesity and/or a progressive atrophy or physical weakness in the whole organism, and even an increased morbidity (Gonzalez-Gross & Melendez, 2013).

On the other side of the energy balance equation, the lack of physical activity is an important determinant of overweight or obesity. It has been shown in a number of longitudinal studies that exercise is the most important component of total daily energy expenditure, and thus it has the potential to affect energy balance (Wiklund, 2016).

Ideally, in order to prevent overweight or obesity an increase in the time spent on physical activity and a reduction in sedentary time should be recommended. However, few studies have analyzed the combined influence of sedentary behaviors and physical activity on obesity and the results we have are still contradictory, so further research in this respect is highly needed (Gonzalez-Gross & Melendez, 2013).

Sleep Habits

Habitual sleep duration was first assessed in the Nurses' Health Study in 1986. It was shown that throughout 16 years of follow-up, women sleeping 5 or fewer hours per night presented 32% more risk to gain 15 or more kilograms and women who slept 6 hours had 12% more risk, compared to those sleeping 7–8 hours (Patel & Hu, 2008). In addition, a recent systematic review focusing on the effect of sleep time and health outcomes revealed that those who can be considered as short sleepers have 38% higher risk of obesity than normal sleepers (Itani, Jike, Watanabe, & Kaneita, 2017). In a recent systematic review with meta-analyses (Wu, Zhai, & Zhang, 2014), which for the first time included prospective studies involving 197,906 participants for short sleep duration and 164,016 participants for long sleep duration, a strong association between short sleep duration and increased risk of obesity was identified, while long sleep duration had no contribution to future obesity in adults. However, the subsequent mechanisms are still not fully elucidated. Some evidence indicates that levels of appetite-regulating hormones such as leptin and ghrelin may be deranged in conditions of chronic sleep restriction, which lead to increased appetite and subsequently increased food intake (Brondel, Romer, Nougues, Touyarou, & Davenne, 2010; Taheri, Lin, Austin, Young, & Mignot, 2004). Another possibility is that individuals with longer awake time also have more time to eat (Knutson, 2012). Finally, there is also the theory that short sleep duration produces fatigue and significantly reduces physical activity affecting the energy balance–related behaviors (Patel, Malhotra, White, Gottlieb, & Hu, 2006).

Factors Associated With Obesity: Sociodemographic Factors

Excess of body weight is a crucial topic when considering both genders worldwide. Obesity is much more prevalent among women than men because women's bodies store more fat to adapt them for reproduction (Power & Schulkin, 2008). Nevertheless, the causes of obesity are biological and social and both of them vary considerably by sex or gender. Gender mediates differences in food consumption (women often report consuming healthier foods, apart from sweets, than men). In some countries a larger body size is favored by women and men as a sign of fertility, healthfulness, or prosperity (Kanter & Caballero, 2012). After considering all these gender- and sex-related factors, in the end it is males who are presenting higher obesity rates in Europe (European Comission, 2017), while it is females in the United States (Flegal, Kruszon-Moran, Carroll, Fryar, & Ogden, 2016).

It is well known that disadvantaged socioeconomic circumstances are associated with increased health risks throughout the life span. A number of socioeconomic factors such as family income, education, or occupational status have been associated with a wide range of health, cognitive, and socioemotional outcomes (Salonen et al., 2009). These concepts refer to the position of individuals or groups within the societal structure (Lynch & Kaplan, 2000).

An individual's own occupation can be considered as a reflection of his/her own societal position. Education can be seen as a useful indicator of socioeconomic status from early adult life on, since it is usually completed in early adulthood and normally remains stable through the life course (Beebe-Dimmer et al., 2004). Income, which affects health through a direct effect on the resources available, is the most commonly used indicator of socioeconomic status when measuring economic resources, but it must be taken into account that is not very stable and might change longitudinally (Galobardes, Shaw, Lawlor, Lynch, & Davey Smith, 2006). Marital status has also been shown to be associated with the risk of being overweight or obese, in the sense that being married is positively associated with overweight and obesity (Teachman, 2016).

In many epidemiological studies, the educational level is used as a proxy of sociodemographic characteristics. When investigating the association between educational level and obesity there is a consistent inverse relationship, so that at lower educational levels the prevalence of obesity is more elevated (Serra-Majem & Bautista-Castano, 2013). Obesity prevalence is high in the socioeconomically disadvantaged groups in developed countries, whereas in the less developed countries the high socioeconomic groups present a higher risk, probably due to the incorporation of Western lifestyles (Serra-Majem & Bautista-Castano, 2013). Also it has been shown that, while in the United States (Befort, Nazir, & Perri, 2012) and developing countries obesity prevalence is higher in rural areas than in urban ones, it is the opposite for developing or emerging countries (Carrillo-Larco et al., 2015; Obirikorang, Osakunor, Anto, Amponsah, & Adarkwa, 2015). Nevertheless, there is no difference in prevalence of obesity between rural and urban areas in Europe (Peytremann-Bridevaux, Faeh, & Santos-Eggimann, 2007).

ASSOCIATED COMORBIDITIES

Obesity is characterized by an increase in body fat deposits leading to a greater risk of comorbidities and affecting both quality of life and life expectancy (NHLBI Obesity Education Initiative Expert Panel on the Identification, Evaluation, and Treatment of Obesity in Adults). This is because adipose tissue interferes in energy homeostasis. Adipocytes synthesize and release a variety of substances including tumor necrosis factor α, C-reactive protein, intercellular adhesion molecule, angiotensinogen, plasminogen activator inhibitor, adiponectin, and resistin, among others (Guerre-Millo, 2002). All of them are involved in the pathogenesis of chronic diseases.

Evidence obtained through prospective studies with prolonged follow-ups indicates that both overweight and obesity are associated with increased all-cause mortality in specific parts of the world. A recent systematic review including 239 prospective studies determined that this association was consistent in four continents for both overweight and obesity (BMIMC et al., 2016). It has been shown that people who have obesity, compared to normal weight people, are at increased risk for many serious diseases and health conditions, including high blood pressure (hypertension), hypercholesterolemia or dyslipidemia, type 2 diabetes, coronary heart disease, stroke, gallbladder disease, osteoarthritis, sleep apnea and breathing problems, some types of cancers, mental disorders and physical functioning impairment (Centers for Disease, Control and Prevention, 2018), or polycystic ovary syndrome (PCOS) in the case of women (Barber, Dimitriadis, & Franks, 2016).

PREVENTION OBESITY STRATEGIES

Major attention has been focused in recent years on the development and implementation of obesity prevention strategies. Preventive interventions are implemented in unselected populations that may be normal weight or with obesity, with the aim to avoid weight gain (Sharma, 2007). These interventions have been based on factors contributing to obesity, such as those related to lifestyle, or environments, or have actively involved different stakeholders (Chan & Woo, 2010). Population-based strategies for the prevention of excess weight gain are of great importance based on the calls for action on public health in recent years (Aranceta, Moreno, Moya, & Anadon, 2009).

Sacks, Swinburn, & Lawrence (2009) proposed a number of items that should be covered in the development and implementation of effective public health strategies for obesity prevention (Fig. 6.3):

1. food, physical activity, and socioeconomic environments;
2. behavior modifications to improve eating and physical activity behaviors; and
3. support of health services and clinical interventions.

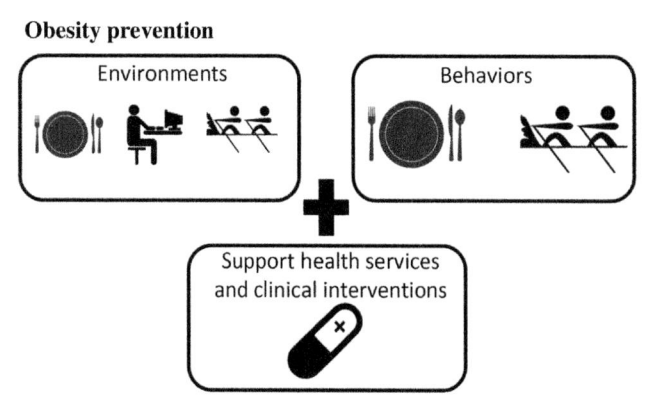

FIGURE 6.3 Proposed items to be covered by effective public health strategies for obesity prevention (Sacks, Swinburn, & Lawrence, 2009).

In this chapter, there is special attention paid to food and diet-related factors in association with obesity, so focusing on these three aspects, diet is going to be examined as a prevention factor for obesity development.

Environmental Factors

Policies targeting *food environments* have included fiscal food policies, such as the taxes applied on sugared beverages (Powell & Maciejewski, 2018), the mandatory nutrition panels about the formulation of manufactured foods or nutrition labeling, and restricting advertising on unhealthy foods (Sacks et al., 2009).

Some studies have showed that food prices are determinants in the purchase of foods (Chan & Woo, 2010), mainly in low socioeconomic status groups (Nicholls, Gwozdz, Reisch, & Voigt, 2011). In this sense, taxes on food groups are considered one of the best alternatives. However, these taxes can discriminate between foods either in positive or in negative ways. There are two different strategies that can be used: either increasing taxes on the energy-dense and low-nutrient foods (i.e., fizzy drinks, chips, sweets, or salty savory snacks, etc.), or decreasing taxes applied to the low-energy high-nutrient food groups (i.e., fruits and vegetables, grains, and cereals etc.). For instance, in the United Kingdom, as well as in France, the first strategy of the abovementioned taxes is already working. Food bought in restaurants and takeaways, together with confectionery, attracts a sales tax (VAT) of 20% in the United Kingdom, while in France sweets, chocolates, margarine, and vegetable fat are subject to VAT of 20.6%, compared to the standard 5.5% VAT for other food (Leicester & Windmeijer, 2004). In other countries, such as Romania or Denmark, preparations are underway to enact these taxes in the coming years. In Denmark it was planned that food products such as meat, dairy products, animal fats, and vegetable oils will be "punished" with €2.15 per kg of saturated fat if the content of saturated fat exceeds 2.3%. This would increase food prices by up to 35% depending on the food category. Besides, a 25% increase in taxation on ice cream, chocolate, and sweets was also proposed. However, these strategies failed to be implemented, in large extent due to strong public resistance (Nicholls et al., 2011). Furthermore, in the name of equity and social justice, taxation of unhealthy foods, without subsidization of healthier options, might be considered as counterproductive, because it will imply that lower-income groups, who are precisely those who consume higher amounts of unhealthy foods, would spend a greater percentage of their income on food (Robertson, Lobstein, & Knai, 2007). Theoretically, increasing taxes over unhealthy products can be compensated by subsidy systems on healthy foods and thus allow low-income groups to keep their food budgets constant. In fact apart from the effect on relative expenditure, tax-subsidy systems might have differential effects in terms of health outcomes, for instance in terms of consumption patterns in low-income groups, relative to affluent groups (Powell & Chaloupka, 2009). Consequently, tax-subsidy schemes could be a possible instrument in tackling health inequalities (Nicholls et al., 2011). However, even if the available literature is consistent in terms of reducing mortality or morbidity throughout tax-subsidy policies (Mytton, Gray, Rayner, & Rutter, 2007), the corresponding studies refer to simulations based on assumptions that may not hold in the real world and empirical data is urgently required (Nicholls et al., 2011).

When translating policies into real changes, it has been shown that apart from changes in prices, the major determinant for the consumer is really the availability of food products. A study performed in a cafeteria in the 1990s (Jeffery, French, Raether, & Baxter, 1994) showed that increasing the variety of fruits and vegetables in a cafeteria and reducing their price by half roughly tripled the consumption of these food items in one case. More recently in another study performed in community stores (Rushakoff et al., 2017), an increase of 40% in stocks of fresh products and of 20% in the variety of products produced a statistically significant increase in the frequency of healthy food consumption by the consumers. This was also corroborated by a review (Harvard, 2018) of experts from the Centers for Disease Control and Prevention, the Institute of Medicine, and the WHO, among others, in relation to worksite environments in relation with foods. This review recommended:

1. "Create a worksite environment that promotes healthy eating."
2. "Implement formal worksite policies to promote healthy food."
3. "Use marketing strategies to encourage healthier food and beverage choices or discourage unhealthy choices at the workplace."
4. "Promote breastfeeding or pumping, such as by setting up lactation rooms and giving female employees time to breastfeed or pump."

However, there is another agent participating in all these strategies. Obviously the food industry supports the hypothesis that obesity is mainly caused by the low levels of physical activity of the population and is in favor of providing more places where people can undertake physical activity and more healthy alternatives in food stores (James & Gill, 2008; Kumanyika & Daniels, 2006). Nonetheless, it remains unclear if price-sensitive consumers may benefit from these strategies since "healthy" food items are usually more expensive than their unhealthy counterparts and since new technologies have to be effectively implemented (Bray).

The home environment is also an important setting in preventing overweight and obesity because 68% of calories come from home food sources for US adults and considerable leisure time is spent at home (Lin & Guthrie, 2012). It has been shown that the availability of high-fat foods at home has been associated with fat intake (Rosenkranz & Dzewaltowski, 2008) and fruit and vegetable availability relates to fruit and vegetable consumption (Larson, Laska, Story, & Neumark-Sztainer, 2012) and lower fat intake (Gattshall, Shoup, Marshall, Crane, & Estabrooks, 2008). Besides, overweight adults had more high-fat snacks and less low-fat snacks and fruits and vegetables at home than normal weight adults. This availability of healthy and nonhealthy foods is determined by grocery shopping behavior, use of nonhome sources, and food preparation methods (Kegler et al., 2014). Unsurprisingly, studies have shown that overweight individuals purchased foods higher in fat and calories than those with normal weight (Ransley et al., 2003) and that more frequent shopping is related to better diets (Bhargava, Jolliffe, & Howard, 2008). However, aspects such as the frequency of occasions eating outside has demonstrated to have implications for eating control (Fulkerson et al., 2011).

Finally, family rules about eating behaviors while watching television are another dimension of the home food environment. In fact, television viewing is consider as an independent risk factor for obesity (World Cancer Research Fund and American Institute for Cancer Research, 2007), not only because of its connection with nibbling behavior but also because of the influence that advertising messages may have on people.

As social inequality is associated with the increase in risk of developing obesity (Drewnowski, 2009), it is crucial that any kind of intervention is done for well-defined population groups in terms of socioeconomic levels to suit them. For this reason, policies focused in reducing obesity prevalence, must cover financial, educational, social and employ-related aspects to have a real impact on population health (Sacks et al., 2009).

Behavioral Strategies

As it has been already described, obesity occurs due to the levels of exposure to causative agents in different vulnerable populations and involves energy intake and/or expenditure-related factors. Decreasing levels of energy expenditure usually derive from decreased physical activity in leisure time, increased television viewing, the usage of electronic devices, unsafe neighborhoods, and the increased use of automobiles rather than active commuting (Office of the Surgeon General, 2001), while the increasing energy intakes usually derive from high intakes of energy-dense and low-nutrient foods (i.e., not eating enough fruits and vegetables, elevated consumption of SSB, etc.). This situation might be reversed through changes in lifestyle behaviors, which have been shown to be more successful when interventions target both physical activity and nutrition behaviors (Sharma, 2007).

Lifestyle interventions for obesity typically target changes in diet and physical activity through strategies focusing on enhancing the subjects' motivation and providing guidance in the use of a variety of self-monitoring skills to influence and maintain behavior change (Teixeira et al., 2015).

To achieve a behavior modification through "comprehensive lifestyle interventions" (Jensen et al., 2013) must be the target in obesity prevention and treatment interventions. However, so far results of randomized controlled trials evaluating the effectiveness of programs in changing behaviors have shown mixed effects or very discrete ones for positive cases (Teixeira et al., 2015). Only a few studies have analyzed the reasons why interventions are successful for some individuals but not for others. There is still a knowledge gap for identifying causal predictors of these differences in the literature (Rossner, Hammarstrand, Hemmingsson, Neovius, & Johansson, 2008).

Individual behavior changes by intervention approaches are an important topic of interest in obesity research because these interventions typically focus on diet and physical activity, which are directly related with consequences for health, even if not necessarily with weight loss. The effects of the intervention should be sustainable to promote an impact on health, mainly because the change in one behavior usually supports the change in other health behaviors (Mata et al., 2009). In this sense, although some individual interventions may be ineffective by themselves, they can contribute to the effectiveness of strategies that integrate multiple levels (i.e., strategies combining both individual and environmental-level approaches) (Lakerveld et al., 2012). Besides, the dissemination of the intervention activities has an impact by itself if at least, those having either overweight or obesity, ask for health advice to professionals at any point in their lives (Teixeira et al., 2015).

Success or failure in the self-regulation of health behaviors involves several psychological and behavioral aspects that should be taken into account (Teixeira et al., 2015). For instance, in a recent European-based systematic review (Panter, Tanggaard Andersen, Aro, & Samara, 2018) the final conclusion was that there was not a clear relationship between BMI changes and some intervention settings, while some of the inconclusive results might have been due to poorly fulfilled representativeness and randomization, or due to having no available information on the attributability of the intervention, even if the comparability of baseline data and attrition rates or evaluation was appropriate. These inconclusive results were also observed some years before (Peirson et al., 2014).

Some examples of strategies that have been found to be effective in changing behaviors:

- Formal and informal education sessions, regular educational sessions (reducing intake of refined carbohydrates, and increasing consumption of fruits and vegetables), physical activity groups, cooking classes, and store tours (Rowley et al., 2000).
- Computer-tailored interventions targeting increasing physical activity and improving eating habits (Vandelanotte, De Bourdeaudhuij, Sallis, Spittaels, & Brug, 2005).
- Multicomponent interventions: worksite wellness for adults and community-based health promotion based on healthy cooking demonstrations, classes on exercise techniques, supermarket tours, social marketing using TV documentary series, and TV advertisements (Bachar et al., 2006).

Support of Health Services and Clinical Interventions

There is not much information or many results available in relation to clinical interventions focused on obesity prevention in adulthood. This is for sure a consequence of the number of limitations that the clinicians may deal with. In their daily routine clinicians normally do not have enough time to address these kinds of issues, while in parallel there is also a lack of incentives and a lack of training to do it (Villagra, 2009). However, the limitations are present also at patient level, such as the feeling of weight stigmatization (MacLean et al., 2009), lack of incentives (Villagra, 2004), or difficulties they might find to access any weight management service (Jones, Furlanetto, Jackson, & Kinn, 2007). To deal with all these circumstances the inclusion or the increase in the number of dietitians and nutritionists in primary care health services and hospitals (Sacks et al., 2009) probably could be one of the most cost-effective strategies to prevent overweight or obesity in the population. For instance, in the United States it has been calculated that the total associated costs with diabetes (obesity comorbidity) are nearly US$132 billion each year (American Heart Association Heart Disease and Stroke Statistics, 2006). In total, obesity costs the United States around US$117 billion per year (US Department of Health and Human Services, 2013). It has been proved that lifestyle interventions would cost about US$8800 per quality-adjusted life year while metformin intervention would cost US$29,900 for diabetes. This shows the cost-effectiveness of lifestyle interventions compared to the use of medicines. This also shows how dietitians may have a positive impact not only on health but also on an economic level.

Besides, a systematic review, whose aim was to determine the existence and effectiveness of interventions to improve health professionals' management of obesity or the organization of care for overweight and obese people (Harvey, Glenny, Kirk, & Summerbell, 2001), showed inconclusive results due to the heterogeneity of the studies. However, reminder systems, brief training interventions, shared care, inpatient care, and dietitian-led treatments might represent an opportunity for further research (Stitzel, 2006).

FUTURE APPROACHES

The current knowledge supports the need to create guidelines for setting-based interventions as they already exist for clinical trials. When creating guidelines, issues such as the minimum period of follow-up required to see BMI changes or using adequate representative and randomized samples should be considered. Based also on another systematic review, there is a need for all interventions to be based on behavioral theories, to target worksite and community settings, and to ensure that interventions are at least longer than 6 months. In that systematic review it was also identified that wherever possible one-on-one counseling should be used as an educational approach (Sharma, 2007).

OBESITY TREATMENT

Obesity treatment is challenging and often ineffective. Results are also compromised by the high attrition rate during the necessarily long follow-up. A comprehensive medical history, physical examination, and laboratory assessment in adults with obesity should be performed (Kushner, 2012; National Institutes of Health, 2018; National Institute for Health and Care Excellence, 2014). The aims for the management and treatment of obesity should include weight loss, risk reduction, and health improvement.

Obesity Treatment Objectives

Appropriate individualized SMART (Specific, Measurable, Attainable, Relevant, and Timely) goals for weight loss should be established to achieve and improve health (Kushner, 2012; National Institute for Health and Care Excellence, 2014). Weight loss promotion, maintenance, and weight regain prevention should be also included in the obesity treatment algorithm (Fig. 6.4). A 5%–15% weight loss over a period of 6 months is a realistic goal and a health benefit should be observed (Brunkwall et al., 2016; Jensen et al., 2013). An initial weight loss of 20% or more might be considered for those patients with severe obesity (BMI ≥ 35 kg/m^2). Modest weight losses (5%–10% of initial weight) and lifestyle modifications may be associated with significant clinical benefits (Knowler et al., 2002; Pietrobelli & Heymsfield, 2002; Slentz et al., 2004; Yumuk, Fruhbeck, Oppert, Woodward, & Toplak, 2014). Obesity is considered as a chronic disease, therefore follow-up supervision is necessary to prevent weight regain and to monitor comorbidities (Anderson, Konz, Frederich, & Wood, 2001). In overweight patients without comorbidities, prevention is an appropriate goal.

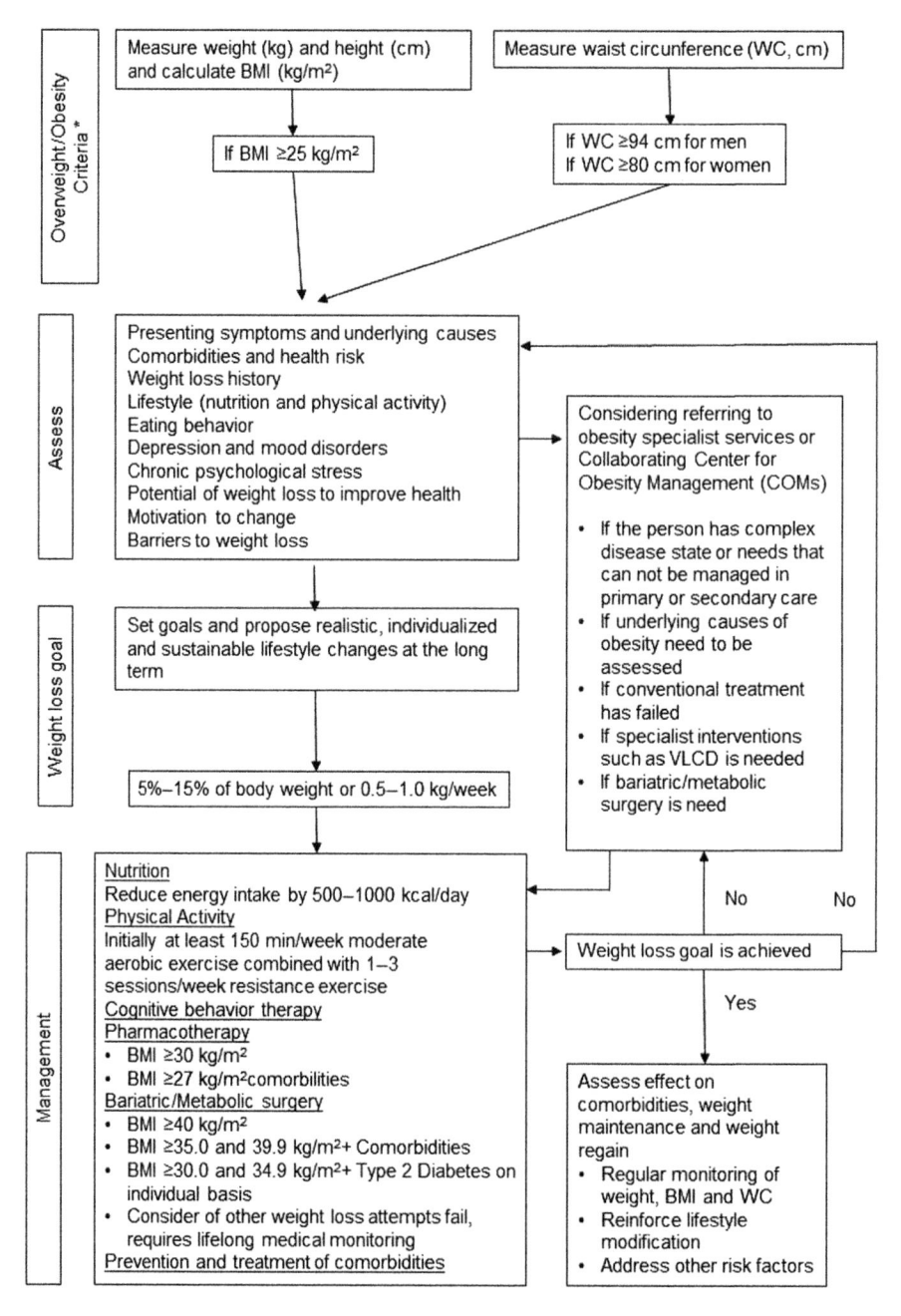

FIGURE 6.4 Algorithm for the assessment and stepwise management of overweight and obese adults (Yumuk et al., 2014). *BMI and WC cutoff points are different for some ethnic groups (see text).

Specific Treatment Components

Dietary Advice

Prior to providing dietary advice, it could be useful to address the motivation for change (Armstrong et al., 2011; Christie & Channon, 2014). The advice should be individualized and take into account the nutritional habits, physical activity, comorbidities, and previous dietary treatment attempts. Prescribing an energy restriction and encouraging healthy eating habits should require the professional intervention of a registered nutritionist (Yumuk et al., 2014). There is great variation in energy requirements between individuals depending on gender, age, BMI, and physical activity level. However, misreporting, mainly underreporting, of energy intake by patients with obesity is common (Mendez et al., 2011).

Diets focused in a concrete distribution of macronutrients have not proved better effects than a balanced hypocaloric diet, except for low-glycemic load diets in the short term (Larsen et al., 2010; Sacks et al., 2009; Shai et al., 2008). Diets providing fewer than 1200 kcal/day may be associated with some micronutrients deficiencies, which could show untoward nutritional and weight management outcome effects.

A balanced diet should be tailored to individual patients on the basis of their personal and cultural preferences in order to obtain the best chance for long-term success (Dernini & Berry, 2015; Estruch et al., 2013). As the genetic contribution to the variance in human adiposity is estimated to be around 40%–70%, the prescription of future individualized treatments may need the knowledge of the subject's genotype.

Individuals respond differently to dietary and lifestyle interventions because of genetic variants that influence how dietary components are absorbed, metabolized, and utilized (Hesketh, 2013; Simopoulos, 2010). Personalized nutrition is a new and important part of medicine and may help in establishing guidelines for specific subgroups based on phenotype and genotype.

The conceptual idea for personalized nutrition is that individual nutritional advice will be more effective than any other more generic approach. The main bases are the biological evidence of differential responses to nutrients depending on genotype and phenotypic characteristics and the knowledge of the current behavior, preferences, barriers, objectives, and interventions, which can be motivatation to perform the appropriate changes in the eating pattern.

The suffix "omics," meaning "global," is used as a modifier for a wide range of activities, such as the comprehensive analysis of genes (genomics), DNA modifications (epigenomics), messenger RNA or transcripts (transcriptomics), proteins (proteomics), metabolites (metabolomics), lipids (lipidomics), food (foodomics), and microbiota (microbiomics, metagenomics). The "omic" technologies are growing and allow the development of new knowledge aimed at providing a better understanding of nutrient–gene interactions, depending on the genotype, with the main goal of developing personalized nutrition strategies for optimal health and disease prevention (Corella & Ordovas, 2009; Ferguson, 2009; Kaput, 2008; Ordovas & Corella, 2004; Simopoulos, 2010; Trujillo, Davis, & Milner, 2006). All of these techniques can be applied individually or together for a better understanding of health metabolism and disease development (Ordovas, 2007). The information regarding genes and molecular pathways related to the use and metabolism of nutrients is a key approach for personalized nutrition (Scalbert et al., 2009).

Nutrigenomics and nutrigenetics are defined as the science of the effect of genetic variation on dietary response and the role of nutrients and bioactive food compounds in gene expression, respectively (Corella & Ordovas, 2009; Ferguson, 2009; Kaput, 2008; Ordovas & Corella, 2004; Simopoulos, 2010; Trujillo, Davis, Milner, & 2006).

Nutrigenomics and nutrigenetics are related terms, however, they are not interchangeable. Therefore it is important to note the difference. The field of nutrigenomics includes multiple disciplines and dietary effects on genome stability (DNA damage at the molecular and chromosome level), epigenome alterations (DNA methylation), RNA and microRNA expression (transcriptomics), protein expression (proteomics), and metabolite changes (metabolomics). However, nutrigenetics specifically investigates the modifying effects of inheritance (or acquired mutations) in nutrition-related genes on micronutrient uptake and metabolism as well as dietary effects on health.

This new arm of dietary advice shows the great diversity of the genomes between ethnic groups and individuals which affects nutrient bioavailability and metabolism. Moreover, people differ greatly in their food/nutrient availability and choices depending on cultural, economic, and geographical factors and taste perception. On the other hand, malnutrition (deficiency or excess) can affect gene expression and genome stability; the latter leading to mutations at the gene sequence or chromosomal level which may cause abnormal gene dosage and gene expression leading to adverse phenotypes during the various life stages (Fenech et al., 2011). These advances in genetic science will help us answering how personalized nutrition provides solutions from the perspective of public health and constituting a sizable tool for reducing the risk and prevalence of nutrition related diseases (Ferguson et al., 2016).

As we mentioned before, nutrigenomics is a growing science that studies the response of individuals to a dietary component or components depending on their genotype (Gillies, 2003; Subbiah, 2007). The field of nutrigenomics offers novel tools to study the roles of obesity-related genes and to understand how we may modulate them through personalized nutrition. Advances in nutrigenomics are based on the understanding that the genetic makeup determines unique nutritional requirements, and these advances rely on the sequencing of the human genome and the subsequent analysis of human genetic variation, as well as studies that associate gene variants with diseases (Fenech et al., 2011). Nutritional outcomes can also be determined by gene-mediated biochemical pathways that regulate nutrient absorption, distribution, metabolism, and excretions, as well as other cellular processes (Jenab, Slimani, Bictash, Ferrari, & Bingham, 2009). The prevention and treatment of obesity should be independently considered in each case by considering the individual's potential response to lifestyle modifications or drug treatment depending on the genotype.

The "omics" techniques and the use of a genetic profile in nutritional advice are linked with ethical, legal, and social issues (Kohlmeier, 2013), including the use of genetic tests, nutrigenetics research and clinical practice (Camp & Trujillo, 2014), the collection and storage of samples, children's involvement, and information passed on to the family (Castle & Ries, 2007).

There is increasing evidence that nutrigenetics and nutrigenomics are taking a central role in the investigation of the effect of nutrition on health outcomes, and that the impacts of nutrients can be evaluated comprehensively by a multitude of "omic" technologies and biomarkers. Some of these technologies are still in their early stages while others are much more mature and therefore differ significantly in their validation status with respect to health outcomes. Therefore there is an emerging need to carefully evaluate published papers on nutrient−genotype interactions with respect to whether the results are of sufficiently strong clinical relevance that they could be used to guide dietetic practice and recommendations to consumers (Fenech et al., 2011).

The main implementation challenge for scientists in this area are concerns about overpromising (Joost et al., 2007; Stenne, Hurlimann, & Godard, 2012), individually (Hurlimann et al., 2014; Stenne, Hurlimann, & Godard, 2013) as well as through institutional guidelines and statements (Camp & Trujillo, 2014; Ferguson, Allayee, et al., 2016; Ferguson, De Caterina, et al., 2016; Grimaldi et al., 2016; Kohlmeier et al., 2016; Ramos-Lopez et al., 2017). However, the most evidence on the effectiveness of personalized nutrition has come from observational studies with risk factor as the main outcomes, rather than from randomized controlled trials using clinical outcomes. Therefore we have limited information to assess if personalized nutrition can produce greater and more appropriate changes in behaviors than traditional approaches and if these changes result in a better health. There are no studies with an appropriate population group, on a large scale, and with a sufficient follow-up period (Ordovas, Ferguson, Tai, & Mathers, 2018).

A recent systematic review (Horne, Madill, O'Connor, Shelley, & Gilliland, 2018) concluded that behavior change can be facilitated using genetic tests, because to promote the change the behavioral plan should be established at the same time as communicating the genetic results.

Moreover, logistical and practical challenges and the financial costs of nutrition intervention studies with disease risk are large and will be increased in a personalized nutrition intervention design.

The development of personalized nutrition needs a strong development of the theoretical framework, taking into consideration the identification of the individual characteristics on which to base personalization. Moreover, the evidence for efficacy and cost-effectiveness from well designed intervention studies will be required as well. There must also be a regulatory framework designed to give confidence to the public, health professionals, and policy markers (Ordovas, Ferguson, Tai, & Mathers, 2018).

The practical application of nutritional genomics for complex chronic diseases is a new science and the use of nutrigenetic testing to provide dietary advice is not ready for routine practice. However, future nutrigenomic studies to examine how diet and dietary patterns affect gene expression might help to guide clinicians in classifying obese patients to accurately design a weight loss process from a long term point of view (Rudkowska & Perusse, 2012).

The application of nutritional genomics to the practice of dietetics requires the knowledge of an individual's susceptibility to disease. Although this information may be obtained from several tools, including family history, biochemical parameters, and the presence of risk factors, the results from genetic testing may provide useful information relating to an individual's risk of developing disease or maintaining health.

The availability of genetic testing has increased in recent years. There are about 2000 genetic tests available for use in a clinical setting (Khoury, Gwinn, Bowen, & Dotson, 2012). However, there is a need to establish the validity and usefulness of the genetic tests offered in medical settings and directly to consumers in predicting disease and to determine whether identifying mutations will improve patient outcomes. Nowadays, public health messages provide important nutrition guidance for the general population. Nutritional genomics may help registered dieticians in their individualization of dietary guidance. Although nutritional genomics promise a diet tailored to a personal genotype to influence the prevention of the development of chronic diseases, the science is still developing (Camp & Trujillo, 2014).

Nutritional genomics requires an evidence-based approach to validate that the personalized recommendations result in health benefits to individuals (Fenech et al., 2011) and do not cause harm (Camp & Rohr, 2009).

In summary the main goal of personalized nutrition is to preserve or increase health by using genetic, phenotypic, medical, and nutritional information from individuals to deliver specific healthy eating guidance and services (Ordovas et al., 2018).

The management of obesity requires an understanding of the genetic and environmental contributions to an individual's health status including the identification of polymorphisms and the interpretation of responses to nutritional interventions that may be affected by genetic determinants. Therefore the efforts of international consortia are aimed at describing genetic variants that contribute to obesity in order to characterize nutrient—gene interactions and to implement dietary counseling for obesity prevention and management via a tailored route (Marti, Goyenechea, & Martinez, 2010).

Monogenic obesity disorders have confirmed that the hypothalamic leptin—melanocortin system is critical for energy balance in humans, because disruption of these pathways causes the most severe obesity phenotypes (Farooqi & O'Rahilly, 2005). Around 20 different genes have been implicated in monogenic causes of obesity. However, they account for less than 5% of all severe obesity cases. At least 50 genes have been implicated in obesity phenotypes and adiposity in animal and human studies (Fenech et al., 2011). In most cases obesity has a polygenic background, with each causative gene variation having a small relevance to the disease but a considerable importance in the development of a personalized treatment (Martinez et al., 2008). Individuals susceptible to excessive fat gain may carry gene variants that influence appetite control [neuropeptide Y; proopiomelanocortin; melanocortin 4 receptor (MC4R), nuclear and cytoplasm regulatory machinery (FTO), adipogenesis and lipid metabolism (adrenoceptor beta 3); peroxisome proliferator-activated receptor (PPAR); apolipoproteins (APOs), etc.], energy expenditure (uncoupling proteins), insulin signaling (insulin receptors; ISR/2), and inflammation (interleuquine-6); adiponectin (ADIPOQ; Resistin) (Walley, Asher, & Froguel, 2009). Most obesity cases are attributed to the interaction of multiple factors including polymorphisms on several genes.

Taking into consideration the effects on energy intake and expenditure, although their primary effect appears to be on the regulation of appetite and satiety (Lee, 2009), MC4R is a strong obesity candidate gene.

This receptor is a 332-amino acid protein encoded by a single exon on chromosome 18q22 (Dernini & Berry, 2015; Estruch et al., 2013) and is widely expressed in the brain. The endogenous ligand for MC4R is the α-melanocyte stimulating hormone (α-MSH).

MC4R mutations have been associated with inherited severe obesity in humans (Hesketh, 2013; Simopoulos, 2010). Although defects in MC4R seem to constitute the most common form of monogenic obesity, prevalence rates ranging from 0.5% to 5.8%, (Corella & Ordovas, 2009; Ferguson, 2009), and different expressivity of the mutations and potential environment interactions configure a variety of obesity phenotypes. The features concerning MC4R deficiency are characterized by several disorders such as hyperphagia, hyperinsulinemia, or increased fat mass (Mendez et al., 2011).

On the other hand, FTO polymorphisms appear to have the most important effects on obesity susceptibility (Ordovas & Corella, 2004). The FTO gene is composed of nine exons on chromosome 16. The effect in humans remains to be fully established (Trujillo, Davis, & Milner, 2006), although there is increasing evidence for associations between the FTO genotype and differences in eating behavior, satiety, and dietary intake, but not in energy expenditure, at least in children (Ordovas, 2007).

Moreover, PPARγ2 encodes a transcription factor (PPARγ2) that controls the expression of genes involved in adipocyte differentiation, lipid storage, and insulin sensitization (Scalbert et al., 2009). This gene is one of those most studied as being potentially linked to the development of obesity, and especially related to the interactions with lifestyle factors (Fenech et al., 2011; Ferguson, De Caterina, et al., 2016). The Pro12Ala polymorphism of the PPARγ2 protein is the most frequently found genetic variant of PPARγ2, whose frequency has been reported to vary from 2% to 25%, depending on ethnicity. The 12Ala carriers would be expected to be protected against excessive adiposity due to the reduced functionality of the receptor. However, there are studies in human subjects showing that the 12Ala allele was associated with increased adiposity (Gillies, 2003; Jenab, Slimani, Bictash, Ferrari, & Bingham, 2009; Subbiah, 2007).

Physical Activity

Exercise is considered an important component of weight management in addition to energy restriction. Several studies report some extra benefits of combining exercise with energy restriction on the reduction on body weight and body fat and the maintenance of the fat-free mass as compared with dietary advice alone. In obesity management the physical activity objectives should be to reduce sedentary behaviors and increase daily life activities. An increase in physical activity reduces intraabdominal fat, increases lean (muscle and bone) mass, reduces blood pressure, and improves glucose tolerance, insulin sensitivity, lipid profile, and physical fitness (Kay & Fiatarone Singh, 2006; Lee et al., 2005; Ross et al., 2004).

All scientific guidelines recommend at least 150 min/week of moderate aerobic exercise that should be combined with three weekly sessions of resistance training in order to increase muscle strength (Geliebter, Ochner, Dambkowski, & Hashim, 2014; Poirier & Despres, 2001; Willis et al., 2012). According to the literature, aerobic training is the optimal exercise to reduce fat mass while resistance training is needed for the increase in lean mass in the middle-aged and individuals with overweight/obesity (Geliebter et al., 2014; Willis et al., 2012). Exercise advice must be tailored to the patient's skills and health, and focus on a gradual increase to levels that are safe (Yumuk et al., 2015).

Given the fact that the FTO gene might participate in the control of energy expenditure, variations of this gene are receiving attention in the study of gene variation–lifestyle interactions on body weight (Razquin, Marti, & Martinez, 2011). In European adults no evidence of interaction between physical activity and this FTO gene variant on body weight was found (Centers for Disease 2018; Powell & Maciejewski, 2018; Sacks et al., 2009), although Andreasen et al. (2008) suggest that low physical activity may accentuate the effect of FTO rs9939609 on body fat accumulation.

Cognitive Behavioral Therapy

Cognitive behavioral therapy (CBT) is a blend of cognitive therapy and behavioral therapy aiming to support patients to modify their insight and understanding of thoughts and beliefs concerning weight management, obesity, and its consequences. Also it is necessary to address behaviors requiring change for successful weight loss and maintenance. CBT elements are self-monitoring techniques to control the eating process, with stimulus control and reenforcement as well as cognitive and relaxation techniques. These elements should be considered as a part of routine weight management. CBT can be provided by registered psychologists or other trained health professionals such as physicians, registered nutritionists, or exercise physiologists (Yumuk et al., 2015).

Pharmacological Support

Pharmacological support should be considered as a part of a comprehensive strategy for disease management (Hainer, Toplak, & Mitrakou, 2008; Toplak et al., 2015). Drugs should be used according to their license indications and restrictions. Their efficacy should be evaluated after the first 3 months. Drug therapy may contribute to maintaining compliance, improving obesity-related risks, decreasing comorbidities, and improving quality of life.

Pharmacological support is only recommended in adult patients with a BMI $\geq 30 \text{ kg/m}^2$ or BMI $\geq 27 \text{ kg/m}^2$ with obesity-related diseases (Yumuk et al., 2015).

Bariatric and Metabolic Surgery

Surgery is a treatment option in morbid patients and is considered as the most effective treatment in terms of long-term weight loss and improvements in co/morbidities, quality of life, and decreased overall mortality (Berrington de Gonzalez et al., 2010; Flegal, Kit, Orpana, & Graubard, 2013; Neovius et al., 2012; Pories, 2008; Sjostrom, 2013). Surgery is considered for adult patients (18–60 years) with a BMI $\geq 40 \text{ kg/m}^2$ or with a BMI between 35 and 39.90 kg/m² and comorbidities (Buchwald et al., 2009; Fried et al., 2013).

Multidisciplinary skills are needed to support surgical interventions. The decision to offer surgery should follow a comprehensive interdisciplinary assessment from physicians, surgeons, anesthesiologists, psychologists or psychiatrists, nutritionists, nurse practitioners, and social workers (DeMaria, 2007; Sauerland et al., 2005).

CONCLUSION

Obesity has dramatically increased worldwide in the last decades and this trend is projected to continue in the coming years. BMI has been widely used to define both overweight and obesity and has been identified as a good marker of cardiovascular risk.

However, this index misses the real amount of fat in the body as it only takes into account height and weight, so it must be interpreted with caution and, whenever possible, with other markers, such as the FMI, or in combination with body composition assessed with high accuracy methods (DXA, BODPOD).

Obesity, which is a multifactorial disease, is defined by an excess of fat deposits, which may lead to alterations in the functioning of the body. Genetic, psychological, and lifestyle factors can be considered as the main reasons to develop the disease, which later may be linked with other comorbidities such as hypertension, dyslipidemia, type 2 diabetes, or cardiovascular disease. In recent years the science has been focused on discerning what are the influences of the lifestyle factors, such as dietary factors, physical activity, or sleeping habits, on the main preventable related causes. That is why obesity prevention strategies should be one of the major focuses for health policies, mainly by targeting the food environment, food-related behaviors, or by performing clinical interventions supported by health services. Whenever established, multifactorial treatment approaches are recommended, including psychological and lifestyle modifications. However, when these strategies do not succeed, pharmacological support or bariatric surgery might be the option to consider.

References

Alberti, K. G., Zimmet, P., & Shaw, J. (2005). The metabolic syndrome—a new worldwide definition. *Lancet*, *366* (9491), 1059–1062.

American Heart Association Heart Disease and Stroke Statistics. (2006). *2006 Update*. Dallas, TX: American Heart Association.

Anderson, J. W., Konz, E. C., Frederich, R. C., & Wood, C. L. (2001). Long-term weight-loss maintenance: A meta-analysis of US studies. *American Journal of Clinical Nutrition*, *74*(5), 579–584.

Andreasen, C. H., Stender-Petersen, K. L., Mogensen, M. S., Torekov, S. S., Wegner, L., Andersen, G., et al. (2008). Low physical activity accentuates the effect of the FTO rs9939609 polymorphism on body fat accumulation. *Diabetes*, *57*(1), 95–101.

Aranceta, J., Moreno, B., Moya, M., & Anadon, A. (2009). Prevention of overweight and obesity from a public health perspective. *Nutrition Reviews*, *67*(Suppl 1), S83–S88.

Armstrong, M. J., Mottershead, T. A., Ronksley, P. E., Sigal, R. J., Campbell, T. S., & Hemmelgarn, B. R. (2011). Motivational interviewing to improve weight loss in overweight and/or obese patients: A systematic review and meta-analysis of randomized controlled trials. *Obesity Reviews*, *12*(9), 709–723.

Bachar, J. J., Lefler, L. J., Reed, L., McCoy, T., Bailey, R., & Bell, R. (2006). Cherokee Choices: A diabetes prevention program for American Indians. *Preventing Chronic Disease*, *3*(3), A103.

Barber, T. M., Dimitriadis, G. K., & Franks, S. (2016). In S. Ahmad, & S. Imam (Eds.), *Polycystic ovary syndrome and obesity* (pp. 199–210). Cham: Obesity Springer.

Beebe-Dimmer, J., Lynch, J. W., Turrell, G., Lustgarten, S., Raghunathan, T., & Kaplan, G. A. (2004). Childhood and adult socioeconomic conditions and 31-year mortality risk in women. *American Journal of Epidemiology*, *159* (5), 481–490.

Befort, C. A., Nazir, N., & Perri, M. G. (2012). Prevalence of obesity among adults from rural and urban areas of the United States: Findings from NHANES (2005-2008). *Journal of Rural Health*, *28*(4), 392–397.

Berrington de Gonzalez, A., Hartge, P., Cerhan, J. R., Flint, A. J., Hannan, L., MacInnis, R. J., et al. (2010). Body-mass index and mortality among 1.46 million white adults. *New England Journal of Medicine*, *363*(23), 2211–2219.

Bhargava, A., Jolliffe, D., & Howard, L. L. (2008). Socio-economic, behavioural and environmental factors predicted body weights and household food insecurity scores in the Early Childhood Longitudinal Study-Kindergarten. *British Journal of Nutrition*, *100*(2), 438–444.

Bradfield, J. P., Taal, H. R., Timpson, N. J., Scherag, A., Lecoeur, C., Warrington, N. M., et al. (2012). A genome-wide association meta-analysis identifies new childhood obesity loci. *Nature Genetics, 44*(5), 526−531.

Bray, G. A. (2000). Prevention of obesity. In L. J. De Groot, G. Chrousos, K. Dungan, et al. (Eds.) *Endotext [Internet].* South Dartmouth (MA): MDText.com, Inc. Available from https://www.ncbi.nlm.nih.gov/books/NBK279120/.

Brondel, L., Romer, M. A., Nougues, P. M., Touyarou, P., & Davenne, D. (2010). Acute partial sleep deprivation increases food intake in healthy men. *American Journal of Clinical Nutrition, 91*(6), 1550−1559.

Brunkwall, L., Chen, Y., Hindy, G., Rukh, G., Ericson, U., Barroso, I., et al. (2016). Sugar-sweetened beverage consumption and genetic predisposition to obesity in 2 Swedish cohorts. *American Journal of Clinical Nutrition, 104*(3), 809−815.

Buchwald, H., Estok, R., Fahrbach, K., Banel, D., Jensen, M. D., Pories, W. J., et al. (2009). Weight and type 2 diabetes after bariatric surgery: Systematic review and meta-analysis. *American Journal of Medicine, 122*(3), 248−256.e5.

Camp, K., & Rohr, F. J. (2009). Advanced practitioners and what they do that is different, roles in genetics. *Topics in Clinical Nutrition, 23*(3), 2019−2230.

Camp, K. M., & Trujillo, E. (2014). Position of the Academy of Nutrition and Dietetics: Nutritional genomics. *Journal of the Academy of Nutrition and Dietetics, 114*(2), 299−312.

Carrillo-Larco, R. M., Bernabe-Ortiz, A., Pillay, T. D., Gilman, R. H., Sanchez, J. F., Poterico, J. A., et al. (2015). Obesity risk in rural, urban and rural-to-urban migrants: Prospective results of the PERU MIGRANT study. *International Journal of Obesity (London), 40*(1), 181−185.

Castle, D., & Ries, N. M. (2007). Ethical, legal and social issues in nutrigenomics: The challenges of regulating service delivery and building health professional capacity. *Mutation Research, 622*(1-2), 138−143.

Centers for Disease, Control and Prevention. Adult obesity. Causes and consequences. [updated 29/08/2017 21/06/2018]. Available from https://www.cdc.gov/obesity/adult/causes.html.

Cespedes, E. M., Hu, F. B., Redline, S., Rosner, B., Gillman, M. W., Rifas-Shiman, S. L., et al. (2015). Chronic insufficient sleep and diet quality: Contributors to childhood obesity. *Obesity (Silver Spring), 24*(1), 184−190.

Chan, R. S., & Woo, J. (2010). Prevention of overweight and obesity: How effective is the current public health approach. *International Journal of Environmental Research and Public Health, 7*(3), 765−783.

Christie, D., & Channon, S. (2014). The potential for motivational interviewing to improve outcomes in the management of diabetes and obesity in paediatric and adult populations: A clinical review. *Diabetes, Obesity and Metabolism, 16*(5), 381−387.

Church, T. S., Thomas, D. M., Tudor-Locke, C., Katzmarzyk, P. T., Earnest, C. P., Rodarte, R. Q., et al. (2011). Trends over 5 decades in U.S. occupation-related physical activity and their associations with obesity. *PLoS One, 6*(5), e19657.

Corella, D., & Ordovas, J. M. (2009). Nutrigenomics in cardiovascular medicine. *Circulation: Cardiovascular Genetics, 2*(6), 637−651.

DeMaria, E. J. (2007). Bariatric surgery for morbid obesity. *New England Journal of Medicine, 356*(21), 2176−2183.

Dernini, S., & Berry, E. M. (2015). Mediterranean diet: From a healthy diet to a sustainable dietary pattern. *Frontiers in Nutrition, 2,* 15.

Drewnowski, A. (2009). Obesity, diets, and social inequalities. *Nutrition Reviews, 67*(Suppl 1), S36−S39.

Estruch, R., Ros, E., Salas-Salvado, J., Covas, M. I., Corella, D., Aros, F., et al. (2013). Primary prevention of cardiovascular disease with a Mediterranean diet. *New England Journal of Medicine, 368*(14), 1279−1290.

European Comission. EUROSTAT Statistics explained. Overweight and obesity-BMI Statistics. [updated 28 April 2017, at 17:02 18/06/2018]. Available from http://ec.europa.eu/eurostat/statistics-explained/index.php/Overweight_and_obesity_-_BMI_statistics.

Farooqi, I. S., & O'Rahilly, S. (2005). Monogenic obesity in humans. *Annual Review of Medicine, 56,* 443−458.

Fenech, M., El-Sohemy, A., Cahill, L., Ferguson, L. R., French, T. A., Tai, E. S., et al. (2011). Nutrigenetics and nutrigenomics: Viewpoints on the current status and applications in nutrition research and practice. *Journal of Nutrigenetics and Nutrigenomics, 4*(2), 69−89.

Ferguson, J. F., Allayee, H., Gerszten, R. E., Ideraabdullah, F., Kris-Etherton, P. M., Ordovas, J. M., et al. (2016). Nutrigenomics, the microbiome, and gene-environment interactions: New directions in cardiovascular disease research, prevention, and treatment: A scientific statement from the American Heart Association. *Circulation: Cardiovascular Genetics, 9*(3), 291−313.

Ferguson, L. R., De Caterina, R., Gorman, U., Allayee, H., Kohlmeier, M., Prasad, C., et al. (2016). Guide and position of the international society of nutrigenetics/nutrigenomics on personalised nutrition: Part 1—Fields of precision nutrition. *Journal of Nutrigenetics and Nutrigenomics*, 9(1), 12−27.

Ferguson, L. R. (2009). Nutrigenomics approaches to functional foods. *Journal of the American Dietetic Association*, 109(3), 452−458.

Fishbein, L. (2001). Causes of obesity. *Lancet*, 357(9272), 8−9, 1977; author reply.

Field, A. E., Willett, W. C., Lissner, L., & Colditz, G. A. (2007). Dietary fat and weight gain among women in the Nurses' Health Study. *Obesity (Silver Spring)*, 15(4), 967−976.

Flegal, K. M., Kit, B. K., Orpana, H., & Graubard, B. I. (2013). Association of all-cause mortality with overweight and obesity using standard body mass index categories: A systematic review and meta-analysis. *JAMA*, 309(1), 71−82.

Flegal, K. M., Kruszon-Moran, D., Carroll, M. D., Fryar, C. D., & Ogden, C. L. (2016). Trends in obesity among adults in the United States, 2005 to 2014. *JAMA*, 315(21), 2284−2291.

Fried, M., Yumuk, V., Oppert, J. M., Scopinaro, N., Torres, A. J., Weiner, R., et al. (2013). Interdisciplinary European Guidelines on metabolic and bariatric surgery. *Obesity Facts*, 6(5), 449−468.

Fulkerson, J. A., Farbakhsh, K., Lytle, L., Hearst, M. O., Dengel, D. R., Pasch, K. E., et al. (2011). Away-from-home family dinner sources and associations with weight status, body composition, and related biomarkers of chronic disease among adolescents and their parents. *Journal of the American Dietetic Association*, 111(12), 1892−1897.

Galobardes, B., Shaw, M., Lawlor, D. A., Lynch, J. W., & Davey Smith, G. (2006). Indicators of socioeconomic position (part 1). *Journal of Epidemiology and Community Health*, 60(1), 7−12.

Gattshall, M. L., Shoup, J. A., Marshall, J. A., Crane, L. A., & Estabrooks, P. A. (2008). Validation of a survey instrument to assess home environments for physical activity and healthy eating in overweight children. *International Journal of Behavioral Nutrition and Physical Activity*, 5, 3.

Geliebter, A., Ochner, C. N., Dambkowski, C. L., & Hashim, S. A. (2014). Obesity-related hormones and metabolic risk factors: A randomized trial of diet plus either strength or aerobic training versus diet alone in overweight participants. *Journal of Diabetes and Obesity*, 1(1), 1−7.

Gill, L. E., Bartels, S. J., & Batsis, J. A. (2015). Weight management in older adults. *Current Obesity Reports*, 4(3), 379−388.

Gillies, P. J. (2003). Nutrigenomics: The Rubicon of molecular nutrition. *Journal of the American Dietetic Association*, 103(12Suppl 2), S50−S55.

Global BMIMC., Di Angelantonio, E., Bhupathiraju Sh, N., Wormser, D., Gao, P., Kaptoge, S., et al. (2016). Body-mass index and all-cause mortality: Individual-participant-data meta-analysis of 239 prospective studies in four continents. *Lancet*, 388(10046), 776−786.

Gonzalez-Gross, M., & Melendez, A. (2013). Sedentarism, active lifestyle and sport: Impact on health and obesity prevention. *Nutricion Hospitalaria* (Suppl 5), 89−98.

Grimaldi, K. A., van Ommen, B., Ordovas, J. M., Parnell, L. D., Mathers, J. C., Bendik, I., et al. (2016). Proposed guidelines to evaluate scientific validity and evidence for genotype-based dietary advice. *Genes & Nutrition*, 12, 35.

Guerre-Millo, M. (2002). Adipose tissue hormones. *Journal of Endocrinological Investigation*, 25(10), 855−861.

Guh, D. P., Zhang, W., Bansback, N., Amarsi, Z., Birmingham, C. L., & Anis, A. H. (2009). The incidence of co-morbidities related to obesity and overweight: A systematic review and meta-analysis. *BMC Public Health*, 25(9), 88.

Hainer, V., Toplak, H., & Mitrakou, A. (2008). Treatment modalities of obesity: What fits whom? *Diabetes Care*, 31 (Suppl 2), S269−S277.

Harvard, T. H. (2018). *Creating a Healthy Worksite Food Environment*. Chan. School of Public Health.

Harvey, E. L., Glenny, A., Kirk, S. F., & Summerbell, C. D. (2001). Improving health professionals' management and the organisation of care for overweight and obese people. *Cochrane Database Syst Rev* (2), CD000984.

Hesketh, J. (2013). Personalised nutrition: How far has nutrigenomics progressed? *European Journal of Clinical Nutrition*, 67(5), 430−435.

Horne, J., Madill, J., O'Connor, C., Shelley, J., & Gilliland, J. (2018). A systematic review of genetic testing and lifestyle behaviour change: Are we using high-quality genetic interventions and considering behaviour change theory?. *Lifestyle Genome*, 11(1), 49−63.

Hosseini-Esfahani, F., Koochakpoor, G., Daneshpour, M. S., Sedaghati-Khayat, B., Mirmiran, P., & Azizi, F. (2017). Mediterranean dietary pattern adherence modify the association between FTO genetic variations and obesity phenotypes. *Nutrients*, *9*(10).

Hruby, A., & Hu, F. B. (2016). The epidemiology of obesity: A big picture. *Pharmacoeconomics*, *33*(7), 673−689.

Hruby, A., Manson, J. E., Qi, L., Malik, V. S., Rimm, E. B., Sun, Q., et al. (2016). Determinants and consequences of obesity. *American Journal of Public Health*, *106*(9), 1656−1662.

Huang, T., Zheng, Y., Qi, Q., Xu, M., Ley, S. H., Li, Y., et al. (2015). DNA methylation variants at HIF3A locus, B-vitamin intake, and long-term weight change: Gene-diet interactions in two U.S. cohorts. *Diabetes*, *64*(9), 3146−3154.

Hurlimann, T., Menuz, V., Graham, J., Robitaille, J., Vohl, M. C., & Godard, B. (2014). Risks of nutrigenomics and nutrigenetics? What the scientists say. *Genes & Nutrition*, *9*(1), 370.

Ibarrola-Jurado, N., Bullo, M., Guasch-Ferre, M., Ros, E., Martinez-Gonzalez, M. A., Corella, D., et al. (2013). Cross-sectional assessment of nut consumption and obesity, metabolic syndrome and other cardiometabolic risk factors: The PREDIMED study. *PLoS One*, *8*(2), e57367.

Iglesia, I., Huybrechts, I., Mouratidou, T., Santabarbara, J., Fernandez-Alvira, J. M., Santaliestra-Pasias, A. M., et al. (2018). Do dietary patterns determine levels of vitamin B6, folate, and vitamin B12 intake and corresponding biomarkers in European adolescents? *The Healthy Lifestyle in Europe by Nutrition in Adolescence (HELENA) study. Nutrition*, *50*, 8−17.

International Society for the Advancement of Kinanthropometry (ISAK). International Standards for Anthropometric Assessment. ISBN 0868037125.2001.

Itani, O., Jike, M., Watanabe, N., & Kaneita, Y. (2017). Short sleep duration and health outcomes: A systematic review, meta-analysis, and meta-regression. *Sleep Med*, *32*, 246−256.

James, W. P. T., & Gill, T. P. (2008). Prevention of obesity. In G. A. Bray, & C. Bouchard (Eds.), *Handbook of Obesity: Clinical Applications* (pp. 157−175). New York: Informa Healthcare.

Jeffery, R. W., French, S. A., Raether, C., & Baxter, J. E. (1994). An environmental intervention to increase fruit and salad purchases in a cafeteria. *Preventive Medicine*, *23*(6), 788−792.

Jenab, M., Slimani, N., Bictash, M., Ferrari, P., & Bingham, S. A. (2009). Biomarkers in nutritional epidemiology: Applications, needs and new horizons. *Human Genetics*, *125*(5−6), 507−525.

Jensen, M. D., Ryan, D. H., Apovian, C. M., Ard, J. D., Comuzzie, A. G., Donato, K. A., et al. (2013). AHA/ACC/TOS guideline for the management of overweight and obesity in adults: A report of the American College of Cardiology/American Heart Association Task Force on Practice Guidelines and The Obesity Society. *Circulation*, *129*(25Suppl 2), S102−S138.

Jiang, R., Manson, J. E., Stampfer, M. J., Liu, S., Willett, W. C., & Hu, F. B. (2002). Nut and peanut butter consumption and risk of type 2 diabetes in women. *JAMA*, *288*(20), 2554−2560.

Jones, N., Furlanetto, D. L., Jackson, J. A., & Kinn, S. (2007). An investigation of obese adults' views of the outcomes of dietary treatment. *Journal of Human Nutrition and Dietetics*, *20*(5), 486−494.

Joost, H. G., Gibney, M. J., Cashman, K. D., Gorman, U., Hesketh, J. E., Mueller, M., et al. (2007). Personalised nutrition: Status and perspectives. *British Journal of Nutrition*, *98*(1), 26−31.

Kanter, R., & Caballero, B. (2012). Global gender disparities in obesity: A review. *Advances in Nutrition*, *3*(4), 491−498.

Kaput, J. (2008). Nutrigenomics research for personalized nutrition and medicine. *Current Opinion in Biotechnology*, *19*(2), 110−120.

Kay, S. J., & Fiatarone Singh, M. A. (2006). The influence of physical activity on abdominal fat: A systematic review of the literature. *Obesity Reviews*, *7*(2), 183−200.

Kegler, M. C., Alcantara, I., Haardorfer, R., Gazmararian, J. A., Ballard, D., & Sabbs, D. (2014). The influence of home food environments on eating behaviors of overweight and obese women. *Journal of Nutrition Education and Behavior*, *46*(3), 188−196.

Kelly, T., Yang, W., Chen, C. S., Reynolds, K., & He, J. (2008). Global burden of obesity in 2005 and projections to 2030. *International Journal of Obesity (London)*, *32*(9), 1431−1437.

Khoury, M. J., Gwinn, M., Bowen, M. S., & Dotson, W. D. (2012). Beyond base pairs to bedside: A population perspective on how genomics can improve health. *American Journal of Public Health*, *102*(1), 34−37.

Knowler, W. C., Barrett-Connor, E., Fowler, S. E., Hamman, R. F., Lachin, J. M., Walker, E. A., et al. (2002). Reduction in the incidence of type 2 diabetes with lifestyle intervention or metformin. *New England Journal of Medicine*, *346*(6), 393−403.

Knutson, K. L. (2012). Does inadequate sleep play a role in vulnerability to obesity? *American Journal of Human Biology, 24*(3), 361–371.

Kohlmeier, M., De Caterina, R., Ferguson, L. R., Gorman, U., Allayee, H., Prasad, C., et al. (2016). Guide and position of the international society of nutrigenetics/nutrigenomics on personalized nutrition: Part 2—Ethics, challenges and endeavors of precision nutrition. *Journal of Nutrigenetics and Nutrigenomics, 9*(1), 28–46.

Kohlmeier, M. (2013). Pratical uses of nutrigenetics. *Nutrigenetics: Applying the Science of Personalized Nutrition*. (pp. 307–333) Amsterdam, Elsevier.

Kumanyika, S. K., & Daniels, S. R. (2006). Obesity Prevention. In G. A. Bray & D.H. Ryan (Eds.), *Overweight and the Metabolic Syndrome: From Bench to Bedside* (Endocrine Updates) (pp. 233–254), New York: Springer Verlay.

Kushner, R. F. (2012). Clinical assessment and management of adult obesity. *Circulation, 126*(24), 2870–2877.

Lakerveld, J., Brug, J., Bot, S., Teixeira, P. J., Rutter, H., Woodward, E., et al. (2012). Sustainable prevention of obesity through integrated strategies: The SPOTLIGHT project's conceptual framework and design. *BMC Public Health, 12*, 793.

Larsen, T. M., Dalskov, S., van Baak, M., Jebb, S., Kafatos, A., Pfeiffer, A., et al. (2010). The Diet, Obesity and Genes (Diogenes) Dietary Study in eight European countries—A comprehensive design for long-term intervention. *Obesity Reviews, 11*(1), 76–91.

Larson, N., Laska, M. N., Story, M., & Neumark-Sztainer, D. (2012). Predictors of fruit and vegetable intake in young adulthood. *Journal of the Academy of Nutrition and Dietetics, 112*(8), 1216–1222.

Lee, S., Kuk, J. L., Davidson, L. E., Hudson, R., Kilpatrick, K., Graham, T. E., et al. (2005). Exercise without weight loss is an effective strategy for obesity reduction in obese individuals with and without Type 2 diabetes. *Journal of Applied Physiology, 99*(3), 1220–1225.

Lee, Y. S. (2009). The role of leptin-melanocortin system and human weight regulation: Lessons from experiments of nature. *Annals, Academy of Medicine, Singapore, 38*(1), 34-11.

Leicester, A., & Windmeijer, F. (2004). *The 'Fat Tax': Economic Incentives to Reduce Obesity*. London: Institute for Fiscal Studies.

Lin, B.-H., & Guthrie, J. (2012). *Nutritional Quality of Food Prepared at Home and Away From Home, 1977–2008*. Washington, DC: United States Department ofAgriculture, Economic Research Service. <http://www.ers.usda.gov/publications/eib-economic-information-bulletin/eib105.aspx#.UvKS0PldXE0> Accessed 05.02.14.

Liu, S., Willett, W. C., Manson, J. E., Hu, F. B., Rosner, B., & Colditz, G. (2003). Relation between changes in intakes of dietary fiber and grain products and changes in weight and development of obesity among middle-aged women. *American Journal of Clinical Nutrition, 78*(5), 920–927.

Lynch, J., & Kaplan, G. (2000). Socioeconomic position. In L. F. Berkman, & I. Kawachi (Eds.), *Social Epidemiology* (1st ed., pp. 13–35). Oxford, UK: Oxford University Press.

MacLean, L., Edwards, N., Garrard, M., Sims-Jones, N., Clinton, K., & Ashley, L. (2009). Obesity, stigma and public health planning. *Health Promotion International, 24*(1), 88–93.

Marti, A., Goyenechea, E., & Martinez, J. A. (2010). Nutrigenetics: A tool to provide personalized nutritional therapy to the obese. *Journal of Nutrigenetics and Nutrigenomics, 3*(4-6), 157–169.

Martinez, J. A., Parra, M. D., Santos, J. L., Moreno-Aliaga, M. J., Marti, A., & Martinez-Gonzalez, M. A. (2008). Genotype-dependent response to energy-restricted diets in obese subjects: Towards personalized nutrition. *Asia Pacific Journal of Clinical Nutrition, 17*(Suppl 1), 119–122.

Mata, J., Silva, M. N., Vieira, P. N., Carraca, E. V., Andrade, A. M., Coutinho, S. R., et al. (2009). Motivational "spill-over" during weight control: Increased self-determination and exercise intrinsic motivation predict eating self-regulation. *Health Psychology, 28*(6), 709–716.

Mei, Z., Grummer-Strawn, L. M., Pietrobelli, A., Goulding, A., Goran, M. I., & Dietz, W. H. (2002). Validity of body mass index compared with other body-composition screening indexes for the assessment of body fatness in children and adolescents. *American Journal of Clinical Nutrition, 75*(6), 978–985.

Mendez, M. A., Popkin, B. M., Buckland, G., Schroder, H., Amiano, P., Barricarte, A., et al. (2011). Alternative methods of accounting for underreporting and overreporting when measuring dietary intake-obesity relations. *American Journal of Epidemiology, 173*(4), 448–458.

Milagro, F. I., Mansego, M. L., De Miguel, C., & Martinez, J. A. (2013). Dietary factors, epigenetic modifications and obesity outcomes: Progresses and perspectives. *Molecular Aspects of Medicine, 34*(4), 782–812.

Mytton, O., Gray, A., Rayner, M., & Rutter, H. (2007). Could targeted food taxes improve health? *Journal of Epidemiology and Community Health, 61*, 689–694.

National Center for Eating Disorders. *Compulsive eating & binge eating disorder.* (2012) [19/06/2018]. Available from https://eating-disorders.org.uk/information/compulsive-overeating-binge-eating-disorder/.

National Institute for Health and Care Excellence. *Obesity: Identification, assessment and management clinical guideline* [CG189] Published date: November 2014 Accessed: 16 July 2018.

National Institutes of Health: The practical guide Identification. *Evaluation, and treatment of overweight and obesity in adults.* NHLBI Obesity Education Initiative Expert Panel on the Identification, Evaluation, and Treatment of Overweight and Obesity in Adults. <https://www.nhlbi.nih.gov/files/docs/guidelines/prctgd_c.pdf>. Accessed 16.07.18.

NCD Risk Factor Collaboration (NCD-RisC). (2016). Trends in adult body-mass index in 200 countries from 1975 to 2014: A pooled analysis of 1698 population-based measurement studies with 19.2 million participants. *Lancet, 387*(10026), 1377−1396.

Neovius, M., Narbro, K., Keating, C., Peltonen, M., Sjoholm, K., Agren, G., et al. (2012). Health care use during 20 years following bariatric surgery. *JAMA, 308*(11), 1132−1141.

NHLBI Obesity Education Initiative Expert Panel on the Identification, Evaluation, and Treatment of Obesity in Adults. *Clinical guidelines on the identification, evaluation, and treatment of overweight and obesity in adults.* Report No. 98-4083. Bethesda, MD: National Heart, Lung, and Blood Institute; 1998. <http://www.ncbi.nlm.nih.gov/books/NBK2003/>. Accessed 21.06.18.

Nicholls, S. G., Gwozdz, W., Reisch, L. A., & Voigt, K. (2011). Fiscal food policy: Equity and practice. *Perspectives in Public Health, 131*(4), 157−158.

Obirikorang, C., Osakunor, D. N., Anto, E. O., Amponsah, S. O., & Adarkwa, O. K. (2015). Obesity and cardiometabolic risk factors in an urban and rural population in the ashanti region-ghana: A comparative cross-sectional study. *PLoS One, 10*(6), e0129494.

Office of the Surgeon General. (2001). *The Surgeon General's call to action to prevent and decrease overweight and obesity.* Rockville, MD: Office of the Surgeon General.

Ordovas, J. M., & Corella, D. (2004). Nutritional genomics. *Annual Review of Genomics and Human Genetics, 5*, 71−118.

Ordovas, J. M., Ferguson, L. R., Tai, E. S., & Mathers, J. C. (2018). Personalised nutrition and health. *BMJ, 361*, bmjk2173.

Ordovas, J. M. (2007). Gender, a significant factor in the cross talk between genes, environment, and health. *Gender Medicine, 4*(Suppl B), S111−S122.

Organisation for Economic Co-operation and Development (OECD). *Obesity Update 2017.* <http://www.oecd.org/health/obesity-update.htm>. Accessed 16.07.18.

Ortega, F. B., Sui, X., Lavie, C. J., & Blair, S. N. (2016). Body mass index, the most widely used but also widely criticized index: Would a criterion standard measure of total body fat be a better predictor of cardiovascular disease mortality? *Mayo Clin Proc, 91*(4), 443−455.

Pan, A., Malik, V. S., Hao, T., Willett, W. C., Mozaffarian, D., & Hu, F. B. (2013). Changes in water and beverage intake and long-term weight changes: Results from three prospective cohort studies. *International Journal of Obesity (London), 37*(10), 1378−1385.

Panter, J., Tanggaard Andersen, P., Aro, A. R., & Samara, A. (2018). Obesity Prevention: A systematic review of setting-based interventions from Nordic Countries and the Netherlands. *Journal of Obesity 2018*, 7093260.

Patel, S. R., & Hu, F. B. (2008). Short sleep duration and weight gain: A systematic review. *Obesity (Silver Spring), 16*(3), 643−653.

Patel, S. R., Malhotra, A., White, D. P., Gottlieb, D. J., & Hu, F. B. (2006). Association between reduced sleep and weight gain in women. *American Journal of Epidemiology, 164*(10), 947−954.

Peirson, L., Douketis, J., Ciliska, D., Fitzpatrick-Lewis, D., Ali, M. U., & Raina, P. (2014). Prevention of overweight and obesity in adult populations: A systematic review. *CMAJ Open, 2*(4), E268−E272.

Peltz, G., Aguirre, M. T., Sanderson, M., & Fadden, M. K. (2010). The role of fat mass index in determining obesity. *Am J Hum Biol, 22*(5), 639−647.

Peng, S., Zhu, Y., Xu, F., Ren, X., Li, X., & Lai, M. (2011). FTO gene polymorphisms and obesity risk: A meta-analysis. *BMC Medicine, 9*, 71.

Peytremann-Bridevaux, I., Faeh, D., & Santos-Eggimann, B. (2007). Prevalence of overweight and obesity in rural and urban settings of 10 European countries. *Preventive Medicine, 44*(5), 442−446.

Pietrobelli, A., & Heymsfield, S. B. (2002). Establishing body composition in obesity. *Journal of Endocrinological Investigation, 25*(10), 884–892.
Poirier, P., & Despres, J. P. (2001). Exercise in weight management of obesity. *Cardiology Clinics, 19*(3), 459–470.
Pories, W. J. (2008). Bariatric surgery: Risks and rewards. *Journal of Clinical Endocrinology and Metabolism, 93* (11Suppl 1), S89–S96.
Powell, L. M., & Chaloupka, F. J. (2009). Food prices and obesity: Evidence and policy implications for taxes and subsidies. *Milbank Quarterly, 87*, 229–257.
Powell, L. M., & Maciejewski, M. L. (2018). Taxes and sugar-sweetened beverages. *JAMA, 319*(3), 229–230.
Power, M. L., & Schulkin, J. (2008). Sex differences in fat storage, fat metabolism, and the health risks from obesity: Possible evolutionary origins. *British Journal of Nutrition, 99*(5), 931–940.
Qi, Q., Chu, A. Y., Kang, J. H., Huang, J., Rose, L. M., Jensen, M. K., et al. (2014). Fried food consumption, genetic risk, and body mass index: Gene-diet interaction analysis in three US cohort studies. *BMJ, 348*, g1610.
Qi, Q., Chu, A. Y., Kang, J. H., Jensen, M. K., Curhan, G. C., Pasquale, L. R., et al. (2012). Sugar-sweetened beverages and genetic risk of obesity. *New England Journal of Medicine, 367*(15), 1387–1396.
Qi, Q., Li, Y., Chomistek, A. K., Kang, J. H., Curhan, G. C., Pasquale, L. R., et al. (2012). Television watching, leisure time physical activity, and the genetic predisposition in relation to body mass index in women and men. *Circulation, 126*(15), 1821–1827.
Rajan, T. M., & Menon, V. (2017). Psychiatric disorders and obesity: A review of association studies. *Journal of Postgraduate Medicine, 63*(3), 182–190.
Ramos-Lopez, O., Milagro, F. I., Allayee, H., Chmurzynska, A., Choi, M. S., Curi, R., et al. (2017). Guide for current nutrigenetic, nutrigenomic, and nutriepigenetic approaches for precision nutrition involving the prevention and management of chronic diseases associated with obesity. *Journal of Nutrigenetics and Nutrigenomics, 10* (1-2), 43–62.
Ransley, J. K., Donnelly, J. K., Botham, H., Khara, T. N., Greenwood, D. C., & Cade, J. E. (2003). Use of supermarket receipts to estimate energy and fat content of food purchased by lean and overweight families. *Appetite, 41* (2), 141–148.
Razquin, C., Marti, A., & Martinez, J. A. (2011). Evidences on three relevant obesogenes: MC4R, FTO and PPARgamma. Approaches for personalized nutrition. *Molecular Nutrition & Food Research, 55*(1), 136–149.
Robertson, A., Lobstein, T., & Knai, C. (2007). *Obesity and socioeconomic groups in Europe: Evidence review and implications for action*. Brussels: European Union.
Rosenkranz, R. R., & Dzewaltowski, D. A. (2008). Model of the home food environment pertaining to childhood obesity. *Nutrition Reviews, 66*(3), 123–140.
Ross, R., Janssen, I., Dawson, J., Kungl, A. M., Kuk, J. L., Wong, S. L., et al. (2004). Exercise-induced reduction in obesity and insulin resistance in women: A randomized controlled trial. *Obesity Research, 12*(5), 789–798.
Rossner, S., Hammarstrand, M., Hemmingsson, E., Neovius, M., & Johansson, K. (2008). Long-term weight loss and weight-loss maintenance strategies. *Obesity Reviews, 9*(6), 624–630.
Rowley, K. G., Daniel, M., Skinner, K., Skinner, M., White, G. A., & O'Dea, K. (2000). Effectiveness of a community-directed 'healthy lifestyle' program in a remote Australian aboriginal community. *Australian and New Zealand Journal of Public Health, 24*(2), 136–144.
Rudkowska, I., & Perusse, L. (2012). Individualized weight management: What can be learned from nutrigenomics and nutrigenetics? *Progress in Molecular Biology and Translational Science, 108*, 347–382.
Rushakoff, J. A., Zoughbie, D. E., Bui, N., DeVito, K., Makarechi, L., & Kubo, H. (2017). Evaluation of Healthy2Go: A country store transformation project to improve the food environment and consumer choices in Appalachian Kentucky. *Preventive Medicine Reports, 7*, 187–192.
Sacks, F. M., Bray, G. A., Carey, V. J., Smith, S. R., Ryan, D. H., Anton, S. D., et al. (2009). Comparison of weight-loss diets with different compositions of fat, protein, and carbohydrates. *New England Journal of Medicine, 360* (9), 859–873.
Sacks, G., Swinburn, B., & Lawrence, M. (2009). Obesity Policy Action framework and analysis grids for a comprehensive policy approach to reducing obesity. *Obesity Reviews, 10*(1), 76–86.
Salonen, M. K., Kajantie, E., Osmond, C., Forsen, T., Yliharsila, H., Paile-Hyvarinen, M., et al. (2009). Role of socioeconomic indicators on development of obesity from a life course perspective. *Journal of Environmental and Public Health, 2009*, 625168.

San-Cristobal, R., Navas-Carretero, S., Livingstone, K. M., Celis-Morales, C., Macready, A. L., Fallaize, R., et al. (2017). Mediterranean diet adherence and genetic background roles within a web-based nutritional intervention: The Food4Me Study. *Nutrients, 9*(10).

Sauerland, S., Angrisani, L., Belachew, M., Chevallier, J. M., Favretti, F., Finer, N., et al. (2005). Obesity surgery: Evidence-based guidelines of the European Association for Endoscopic Surgery (EAES). *Surgical Endoscopy, 19*(2), 200−221.

Scalbert, A., Brennan, L., Fiehn, O., Hankemeier, T., Kristal, B. S., van Ommen, B., et al. (2009). Mass-spectrometry-based metabolomics: Limitations and recommendations for future progress with particular focus on nutrition research. *Metabolomics, 5*(4), 435−458.

Schulze, M. B., Fung, T. T., Manson, J. E., Willett, W. C., & Hu, F. B. (2006). Dietary patterns and changes in body weight in women. *Obesity (Silver Spring), 14*(8), 1444−1453.

Schulze, M. B., Manson, J. E., Ludwig, D. S., Colditz, G. A., Stampfer, M. J., Willett, W. C., et al. (2004). Sugar-sweetened beverages, weight gain, and incidence of type 2 diabetes in young and middle-aged women. *JAMA, 292*(8), 927−934.

Schutz, Y., Kyle, U. U., & Pichard, C. (2002). Fat-free mass index and fat mass index percentiles in Caucasians aged 18-98 y. *International Journal of Obesity and Related Metabolic Disorders, 26*(7), 953−960.

Serra-Majem, L., & Bautista-Castano, I. (2013). Etiology of obesity: Two "key issues" and other emerging factors. *Nutricion Hospitalaria, 28*(Suppl 5), 32−43.

Shai, I., Schwarzfuchs, D., Henkin, Y., Shahar, D. R., Witkow, S., Greenberg, I., et al. (2008). Weight loss with a low-carbohydrate, Mediterranean, or low-fat diet. *New England Journal of Medicine, 359*(3), 229−241.

Sharma, M. (2007). Behavioural interventions for preventing and treating obesity in adults. *Obesity Reviews, 8*(5), 441−449.

Simopoulos, A. P. (2010). Nutrigenetics/nutrigenomics. *Annual Review of Public Health, 31*, 53−68.

Siri, W. E. (1993). Body composition from fluid spaces and density: Analysis of methods. 1961. *Nutrition, 9*(5), 480−491, discussion, 92.

Sjostrom, L. (2013). Review of the key results from the Swedish Obese Subjects (SOS) trial—prospective controlled intervention study of bariatric surgery. *Journal of Internal Medicine, 273*(3), 219−234.

Slentz, C. A., Duscha, B. D., Johnson, J. L., Ketchum, K., Aiken, L. B., Samsa, G. P., et al. (2004). Effects of the amount of exercise on body weight, body composition, and measures of central obesity: STRRIDE—a randomized controlled study. *Archives of Internal Medicine, 164*(1), 31−39.

Stenne, R., Hurlimann, T., & Godard, B. (2012). Are research papers reporting results from nutrigenetics clinical research a potential source of biohype? *Account Research, 19*(5), 285−307.

Stenne, R., Hurlimann, T., & Godard, B. (2013). Benefits associated with nutrigenomics research and their reporting in the scientific literature: Researchers' perspectives. *Account Research, 20*(3), 167−183.

Stitzel, K. F. (2006). Position of the American Dietetic Association: The roles of registered dietitians and dietetic technicians, registered in health promotion and disease prevention. *Journal of the American Dietetic Association, 106*(11), 1875−1884.

Subbiah, M. T. (2007). Nutrigenetics and nutraceuticals: The next wave riding on personalized medicine. *Translational Research, 149*(2), 55−61.

Taheri, S., Lin, L., Austin, D., Young, T., & Mignot, E. (2004). Short sleep duration is associated with reduced leptin, elevated ghrelin, and increased body mass index. *PLoS Medicine, 1*(3), e62.

Teachman, J. (2016). Body weight, marital status, and changes in marital status. *Journal of Family Issues, 37*(1), 74−96.

Teixeira, P. J., Carraca, E. V., Marques, M. M., Rutter, H., Oppert, J. M., De Bourdeaudhuij, I., et al. (2015). Successful behavior change in obesity interventions in adults: A systematic review of self-regulation mediators. *BMC Medicine, 13*, 84.

Toplak, H., Woodward, E., Yumuk, V., Oppert, J. M., Halford, J. C., & Fruhbeck, G. (2015). 2014 EASO position statement on the use of anti-obesity drugs. *Obesity Facts, 8*(3), 166−174.

Trujillo, E., Davis, C., & Milner, J. (2006). Nutrigenomics, proteomics, metabolomics, and the practice of dietetics. *Journal of the American Dietetic Association, 106*(3), 403−413.

US Department of Health and Human Services, National Institute of Diabetes and Digestive and Kidney Diseases. *Statistics related to overweight and obesity.* NIH. Publication No. 03-4158. July 2003. <http://win.niddk.nih.gov/statistics/index.htm>. Accessed 11.05.06.

Vandelanotte, C., De Bourdeaudhuij, I., Sallis, J. F., Spittaels, H., & Brug, J. (2005). Efficacy of sequential or simultaneous interactive computer-tailored interventions for increasing physical activity and decreasing fat intake. *Annals of Behavioral Medicine, 29*(2), 138−146.

Vanltallie, T. B., Yang, M. U., Heymsfield, S. B., Funk, R. C., & Boileau, R. A. (1990). Height-normalized indices of the body's fat frere mass and fat mass: Potentially useful indicators of nutritional status. *American Journal of Clinical Nutrition, 52*(6), 953−959.

Villagra, V. (2004). Strategies to control costs and quality: A focus on outcomes research for disease management. *Medical Care, 42*(4 Suppl), III24−III30.

Villagra, V. G. (2009). An obesity/cardiometabolic risk reduction disease management program: A population-based approach. *American Journal of Medicine, 122*(4Suppl 1), S33−S36.

Walley, A. J., Asher, J. E., & Froguel, P. (2009). The genetic contribution to non-syndromic human obesity. *Nature Reviews Genetics, 10*(7), 431−442.

Wang, T., Heianza, Y., Sun, D., Huang, T., Ma, W., Rimm, E. B., et al. (2018). Improving adherence to healthy dietary patterns, genetic risk, and long term weight gain: Gene-diet interaction analysis in two prospective cohort studies. *BMJ, 360*, j5644.

Wannamethee, S. G., Field, A. E., Colditz, G. A., & Rimm, E. B. (2004). Alcohol intake and 8-year weight gain in women: A prospective study. *Obesity Research, 12*(9), 1386−1396.

Wiklund, P. (2016). The role of physical activity and exercise in obesity and weight management: Time for critical appraisal. *Journal of Sport and Health Science, 5*, 151−154.

Willis, L. H., Slentz, C. A., Bateman, L. A., Shields, A. T., Piner, L. W., Bales, C. W., et al. (2012). Effects of aerobic and/or resistance training on body mass and fat mass in overweight or obese adults. *Journal of Applied Physiology, 113*(12), 1831−1837.

World Cancer Research Fund and American Institute for Cancer Research. Food, nutrition, physical activity, and the prevention of cancer: A global perspective; American Institute for Cancer Research: Washington, DC, 2007

World Health Organization (WHO). *Global Health Observatory (GHO) data. Topic: Noncommunicable diseases.* (2018a). <http://gamapserver.who.int/mapLibrary/app/searchResults.aspx>. Accessed 13.09.18.

World Health Organization (WHO). *Obesity: Preventing and managing the global epidemic Report of a WHO Consultation (WHO Technical Report Series 894).* (2018b). <http://www.who.int/nutrition/publications/obesity/WHO_TRS_894/en/>. Accessed 16.07.18.

World Health Organization (WHO). *Physical status: The use and interpretation of anthropometry.* Report of a WHO Expert Committee. (2018c) <http://www.who.int/childgrowth/publications/physical_status/en/>. Accessed 16.07.18.

World Health Organization. *Obesity and overweight.* Factsheet. Updated June 2016. <http://www.who.int/mediacentre/factsheets/fs311/en/>. Accessed 26.09.18.

Wu, Y., Zhai, L., & Zhang, D. (2014). Sleep duration and obesity among adults: A meta-analysis of prospective studies. *Sleep Medicine, 15*(12), 1456−1462.

Yumuk, V., Fruhbeck, G., Oppert, J. M., Woodward, E., & Toplak, H. (2014). An EASO position statement on multidisciplinary obesity management in adults. *Obesity Facts, 7*(2), 96−101.

Yumuk, V., Tsigos, C., Fried, M., Schindler, K., Busetto, L., Micic, D., et al. (2015). European guidelines for obesity management in adults. *Obesity Facts, 8*(6), 402−424.

Zhang, X., Shu, X. O., Yang, G., Li, H., Cai, H., Gao, Y. T., et al. (2007). Abdominal adiposity and mortality in Chinese women. *Archives of Internal Medicine, 167*(9), 886−892.

Zhu, S., Wang, Z., Heshka, S., Heo, M., Faith, M. S., & Heymsfield, S. B. (2002). Waist circumference and obesity-associated risk factors among whites in the third National Health and Nutrition Examination Survey: Clinical action thresholds. *American Journal of Clinical Nutrition, 76*(4), 743−749.

CHAPTER 7

Personalized Nutrition for Women, Infants, and Children

Elizabeth Wambui Kimani-Murage[1,2], Carolyn K. Nyamasege[3], Sandrine Mutoni[4], Teresia Macharia[1], Milka Wanjohi[1], Eva W. Kamande[1], Elizabeth Mwaniki[1], Peter G. Muriuki[1,5], Frederick Murunga Wekesah[1,6], Caroline Wainaina[1], Maurice Mutisya[1] and Taddese Alemu Zerfu[1]

[1]Maternal and Child Wellbeing Unit, African Population and Health Research Center, Nairobi, Kenya [2]Wellcome Trust, London, United Kingdom [3]Graduate School of Comprehensive Human Sciences, University of Tsukuba, Tsukuba, Japan [4]School of Human Nutrition, McGill University, Montreal, Canada [5]University of Global Health Equity, Kigali, Rwanda [6]Julius Global Health, Julius Center for Health Sciences and Primary Care, University Medical Center Utrecht, Utrecht, The Netherlands

OUTLINE

Introduction	170	Complications of Inadequate Nutrient Intake During Pregnancy and Preconception	173
Personalized Nutrition for Women: Maternal and Adolescent Nutrition	172	Personalized Interventions to Promote Maternal Nutrition During Pregnancy	173
Introduction	172		
Global and Regional Epidemiology of Maternal Malnutrition	172	Personalized Nutrition for Infants and Children	174
Nutritional Requirements During Pregnancy and Preconception	172	Introduction	174

Child Nutritional Status (Undernutrition and Overweight)	175	Interventions for Women, Infants, and Children	186
Factors Affecting the Nutrition Status of Children	176	Impending Implementation Research of Personalized Nutrition Programs for Women, Infants, and Children in LMICs	187
Factors Influencing Child Feeding Practices in Urban Poor Settings (Breastfeeding and Complementary Feeding)	179	Human Milk Banking	187
Personalized Nutrition Interventions to Address Child Undernutrition	182	Workplace Support for Breastfeeding	188
Economic and Social Returns on Investments of Personalized Nutrition		Conclusion	189
		References	189

INTRODUCTION

Globally malnutrition is linked, either directly or indirectly, to the major causes of death and disability. It is a significant global public health concern, affecting one in three people globally, and a major risk factor for the global burden of disease (International Food Policy Research Institute, 2016). Worldwide, about 101 million and 165 million of children under 5 years of age are underweight and stunted, respectively. The majority of these cases are reported from low-income countries. For example, in sub-Saharan Africa (SSA), approximately 40% of all children under 5 years (56 million) are estimated to be stunted (Ahmed, Hossain, & Sanin, 2012). Wasting, including severe wasting with implications on child survival, is also prevalent in low-income countries (Kerac, Blencowe, Grijalva-Eternod, McGrath, Shoham, Cole, & Seal, 2011). The greatest burden of undernutrition is often among the poorest households who are more likely to experience food and nutritional insecurity as a result of lack of resources, inadequate food, low levels of education and nutritional health information, and poor access to and utilization of health care (Goudet, Kimani-Murage, Wekesah, Wanjohi, Griffiths, Bogin, & Madise, 2017). Additionally, the burden of unhealthy diets, for example, obesity, is now shifting from those of higher socioeconomic status to those of lower socioeconomic status. There are reports that a total of 43 million children are overweight or obese in developing countries (Popkin, Adair, & Ng, 2012).

Undernutrition in children is associated with adverse short-term and long-term effects on their health, development, and survival. Moreover, it is associated with increased morbidity and mortality, that is, increased burden of disease, mental and motor development, and increased risk of obesity and metabolic diseases later in the life course (Grantham-McGregor, Cheung, Cueto, Glewwe, Richter, & Strupp, 2007; Lanigan & Singhal, 2009; Oddy, Kendall, Blair, De Klerk, Stanley, Landau, & Zubrick, 2003; Victora et al., 2008; World Health Organization (WHO), 2009). On the other hand, overweight and obesity in children are also associated with adverse effects including risk for noncommunicable diseases (Guo, Wu, Chumlea, & Roche, 2002), that is, cardiovascular diseases diabetes, musculoskeletal diseases, and cancers, which are a leading cause of death in adults. Overweight and obesity in childhood are also the cause of breathing difficulties, increased risk of fractures and psychological effects in childhood, and a higher risk of obesity, disability, and premature death in adulthood (Whitaker, Wright, Pepe, Seidel, & Dietz, 1997). The double burden of malnutrition, with the coexistence of both undernutrition and overnutrition within the same community, or households with overnutrition result in increased health care cost and low productivity, thereby perpetuating the poverty cycle (Victora et al., 2008). The economic consequences of malnutrition are enormous, representing losses of 11% of gross domestic product every year in Africa and Asia (Bain, Awah, Geraldine, Kindong, Sigal, Bernard, & Tanjeko, 2013). Thereby both malnutrition and overnutrition are confirmed as a major public health challenges worldwide (Lanigan & Singhal, 2009).

Research into personalized nutrition is gaining traction, and this approach will be crucial for preventing complicated and highly individualized conditions such as metabolic diseases. The emerging nutrition research continues to provide convincing evidence on the benefits for the implementation of personalized nutrition in health care. For example, as a result of the evidence in the United States, the Food and Drug Administration established a Division of Personalized Nutrition within its National Center for Toxicological Research. On the other hand, personalized nutrition interventions for women, infants, and children are becoming the next big thing in addressing the global public health challenge of malnutrition (Walsh & Kuhn, 2012). Personalized nutrition in this context refers to developing unique nutrition guidelines for women, infants, and children that are appropriate to maintain optimal health, by taking into account individual dietary and lifestyle patterns and preferences, phenotypic status, and genetic makeup (Kaput, Kussmann, Mendoza, Le Coutre, Cooper, & Roulin, 2015).

This book chapter explores different personalized nutrition interventions and their ultimate impact in improving the nutrition and well-being of women, infants, and children. The chapter is structured into four different parts: in the first part empirical findings from personalized nutrition status and intervention studies including maternal, adolescent, and child nutrition are presented. Maternal nutrition is presented at the levels of preconception, pregnancy, and during lactation. In addition, the maternal and adolescents' anthropometric dynamics of this group are examined to provide the linkages with personalized nutrition. Infant and child nutrition is presented in the second part. Part two covers breastfeeding and interventions put in place to promote breastfeeding and complementary feeding as a key element in infant and child nutrition. This part also evaluates anthropometric dynamics of infant nutrition and evidence from intervention studies in respect to implementing infant and child nutrition programs. The third part demonstrates the social returns on investments on personalized nutrition for women, infants, and young children, in this case the costs and cost-effectiveness, as well as the social returns accruing from the implementation of personalized nutrition interventions, and the methods of determination therein. Part four presents the impending implementation research of personalized nutrition programs for women, infants, and children population in low- and middle-income countries (LMICs) and the research gaps.

PERSONALIZED NUTRITION FOR WOMEN: MATERNAL AND ADOLESCENT NUTRITION

Introduction

Maternal nutritional status is a strong predictor of growth and development in the first 1000 days of life and may influence susceptibility to noncommunicable diseases in adulthood. Nowadays, new initiatives are targeting maternal nutrition. For example, the established mission of the US Department of Agriculture, Food and Nutrition Service Special Supplemental Nutrition Program for Women, Infants, and Children is to safeguard the health of low-income women who are at risk for poor nutrition.

Global and Regional Epidemiology of Maternal Malnutrition

Maternal malnutrition is a serious developmental challenge contributing to a considerable (7%) share of the global burden of disease (Kassebaum et al., 2014). Evidence shows that at least one-fifth of maternal deaths are attributed to malnutrition, along with the increased probability of poor pregnancy outcomes. SSA is home to some of the most nutritionally insecure people in the world, as some countries in the region have maternal undernutrition prevalence as high as 35% (Fanzo, 2012).

Poor infrastructure and limited resources compounded with conflict, HIV, and poor access to health services are factors that have contributed to the staggering levels of malnutrition and food insecurity on the continent. Despite these enormous challenges, some countries in SSA are making progress toward food and nutrition security and there has never been a better time to work toward improved human development that has nutrition as a goal.

Nutritional Requirements During Pregnancy and Preconception

In a woman's life cycle there is no time where nutrition is more important than before and/or during pregnancy (Marangoni et al., 2016). Likewise, nutritional needs during this critical anabolic phase of life change significantly and drastically (King, 2000; Marangoni et al., 2016). Requirements for almost all nutrients are increased during pregnancy compared to other adults. Generally, during pregnancy requirements for both macro- and micronutrients increase sharply to accommodate the high demands of the growing fetus and maternal tissue deposition.

For example, during the third trimester of pregnancy, the need for macronutrients (energy and protein) and several micronutrients, including iron, iodine, zinc, magnesium, selenium, folate, vitamin B6, niacin, riboflavin, thiamine, pantothenic acid, vitamin C, vitamin A, vitamin B-12, and choline, is increased by between 6% and 50%, although the requirements for biotin, vitamin D, vitamin E, vitamin K, calcium, phosphorus, and fluoride remain the same (Ladipo, 2000). As such, pregnant women need to consume extra vitamins and minerals, increase their calorie intake (Blumfield, Hure, Macdonald-Wicks, Smith, & Collins, 2012), and avoid certain foods to optimize the growth and development of their baby and to support the alterations in maternal tissues and metabolism.

Complications of Inadequate Nutrient Intake During Pregnancy and Preconception

Nutrition during pregnancy is among the leading environmental factors strongly associated with pregnancy and perinatal outcomes (Abu-Saad & Fraser, 2010). Poor maternal diet during the periods of pregnancy and lactation poses a potential threat to maternal and child health. Short maternal stature, which occurs due to chronic malnutrition in childhood, may lead to obstructed labor and maternal and/or fetal or neonatal death. Inadequate maternal dietary intake during pregnancy is among the leading causes of adverse pregnancy outcomes including low birth weight, stillbirth, preterm birth, and early infant death in LMICs (Abu-Saad & Fraser, 2010).

Personalized Interventions to Promote Maternal Nutrition During Pregnancy

A lifetime and a continuum of care/interventions are needed to end the high burden of maternal malnutrition, particularly in the poor settings of SSA. According to WHO's essential interventions guidelines for reproductive, maternal, newborn, and child health, interventions should start as early as during adolescence (Lassi., Salam, Das, & Bhutta, 2014). Folic acid fortification/supplementation and family planning (to avoid or delay adolescent pregnancies) are critical nutrition interventions during adolescence (Cox & Phelan, 2008). Similarly, during preconception and pregnancy, iron, folic acid, and calcium supplementation, as well as smoking cessation, have been found to be most effective (Cox & Phelan, 2008). Nutrition counseling and treating maternal anemia or supplementation with iron, folic acid, and calcium are recommended during the postpartum period as effective nutrition interventions.

The African Population and Health Research Center (APHRC) in 2015 designed a study to identify effective interventions to address the poor antenatal practices and the issue of poor access to professional nutritional support for mothers in urban slum settings (Kimani-Murage et al., 2013). The study primarily tested the effectiveness of personalized, home-based nutritional counseling by community health volunteers on maternal nutrition and breastfeeding practices among women in the slums. Following the 3-year intervention study, personalized home-based nutrition counseling may have influenced the pregnant women's knowledge gaps, which translated to the adoption of good nutrition and antenatal care practices. This was evidenced by positive changes in some of the maternal outcomes, such as more antenatal care visits and better nutrition status among women in the intervention group when compared to those in the control group. The prevalence of undernutrition and overnutrition in the intervention group was reduced, as revealed by the comparison of the baseline and follow-up mid-upper arm circumference measurements. Moreover, women in the intervention group had a reduction in such practices as the consumption of soil and mineral stones, which is a form of pica caused by micronutrient deficiency, mostly iron deficiency (Nyamasege, Kimani, Wanjohi, Kaindi, Ma, Fukushige,& Wagatsuma, 2018). Soil consumption (pica) may increase the transmission of soil helminths such as hookworms, which may lead to anemia and later low birth weight (Luoba et al., 2005). Hence there is a need for new product developers to design micronutrient supplements which mimic the mineral stones in terms of scent and appearance to enable these women with pica to have an alternative which is hygienically safe and of nutritional importance.

Extant reviews and findings from previous studies show that training health care providers to deliver a personalized nutritional educational intervention in the form of advice during usual antenatal care and primary health care services was associated with an improvement in pregnant women's diet by increasing their protein intake, improved infant and young child feeding practices (IYCF), increased fetal growth, and increased child birth weight and head circumference (Nikièma, Huybregts, Martin-Prevel, Donnen, Lanou, Grosemans, Kolsteren, 2017). In the intervention by APHRC, there was a relative reduction in preterm birth for nutritional advice in energy and protein compared with no nutritional counseling (Kimani-Murage et al., 2015c; Nyamasege et al., 2018). From the foregoing, it can be seen that personalized nutritional counseling based on individual needs may be beneficial to pregnant women. This finding demonstrates the potential effectiveness of a community health strategy in promoting optimal antenatal care, especially in underserved settings such as among the urban poor (Kimani-Murage et al., 2015c). However, there is inadequate literature on personalized nutrition for adolescents and women in the reproductive age group, as well as not enough evidence on other interventions such as isocaloric protein supplements, which currently appear to be unhelpful, and high protein supplements, which may be harmful.

PERSONALIZED NUTRITION FOR INFANTS AND CHILDREN

Introduction

Child nutrition is a major global public health agenda. The sustainable development goal 3 underscores its importance by calling for an end to preventable deaths of infants and children under 5 (United Nations, 2015). Poverty for children has a negative long-term effect on physical, social, and mental development (Casey et al., 2006; Martorell, 1999). Indeed, childhood malnutrition contributes to nearly one-third of under-5 deaths globally and to up to 11% of disability-adjusted life years; 80% of the deaths occur in LMICS (Black, Allen, Bhutta, Caulfied, de Onis, & Ezzati, 2008).

One key contributor to malnutrition is poor nutritional practices. In the last decade, progress has been made in generating the evidence on the link between poor nutritional practices and poor health outcomes, particularly in maternal and child health in SSA. It is becoming highly evident that countries are going through nutrition transitions resulting in a double burden of nutrition-related diseases—undernutrition and obesity. Many authors describe the nutrition transition as a shift from healthier diets including mainly fiber-rich starchy carbohydrates, fruits, and vegetables to unhealthy diets high in animal food sources and sweetened foods, and thus higher in lipid (mainly cholesterol) and added salt and/or sugar. This nutrition transition thus constitutes an important window for nutrition-sensitive and nutrition-specific programs to achieve great returns, both in the short and long term. On the one hand, the region still faces undernutrition and its negative health effects, mainly in relation to infectious diseases, while on the other hand, obesity and other noncommunicable diseases such as diabetes and cardiovascular diseases, which have long been thought to be a concern primarily for high-income countries, are now rising at faster pace. The most vulnerable populations remain mainly infants and young children—doubly exposed to undernutrition with limited access to healthy diets on one side; and on the other side exposed to obesogenic disease-prone foods. Multiple studies support the importance of targeted and scalable interventions to improve more efficiently the nutritional status of infants and children, and ultimately nutrition-related health issues.

Child Nutritional Status (Undernutrition and Overweight)

Despite improvements in child nutrition globally, the progress is low and off target for most of the maternal and child nutrition indicators (wasting, stunting, overweight, and anemia) (Akombi, Agho, Merom, Renzaho, & Hall, 2017). Globally many health and nutrition indicators, such as life expectancy, child undernutrition and micronutrient deficiencies, maternal nutrition and mortality, and under-5 mortality rates have all improved. Despite the gains, the progress is not uniform, with the SSA region among the regions showing the slowest progress, with a reduction of stunting by only 18% between 2000 and 2016 compared to a 37% and 40% decline in Asia and Latin America, respectively, during the same period. The reduction in the proportion of stunted children tells a different story, given that the absolute numbers of stunted children in SSA increased by 17%. In fact, more than one-third of stunted children under the age of 5 years lived in Africa in 2014. Comparing numbers of stunted children under the age of 5 years from 2000 to 2016, Africa is the only region where stunting has increased. Moreover, three out of the five subregions with the highest stunted children under the age of 5 years are in Africa, namely Eastern, Western, and Central Africa. Furthermore, subregional differences exist with a higher proportion of stunted children living in East Africa (37%), compared to 32.5% in Central Africa, 31% Western Africa, and 28% in Southern Africa in 2016 on one hand, and West Africa experiencing the highest increase in wasting between 2000 and 2016 on the other hand. Moreover, West Africa experienced the highest increase in wasting between 2000 and 2016 (UNICEF, WHO, & World Bank, 2017).

Within countries there are also differences between the urban and rural settings and between regions. For instance, the 2014 Kenya demographic and health surveys showed stunting prevalence of 26% among rural and 20% among urban children aged below 5 years, respectively (KNBS, 2015). Moreover, with rapid urbanization there is a growing urban poor population experiencing worse health outcomes compared to the rural and better urban settings (Fotso, 2006, 2007). For instance, about two in every three in children living in Nairobis slums' experience stunting before the age of 2 years. Indeed, recent evidence has shown that urban poor settings in SSA are particularly experiencing the problem of a double burden of malnutrition. For instance, Kimani-Murage et al. (2015a) reported a stunting prevalence close to 50% among children aged less than 5 years, along with close to 10% of overweight/obesity among children of this age group and 32% of overweight/obesity among mothers of children of the same age group in Nairobi slums (Kimani-Murage et al., 2015a). A large proportion of overweight and obese mothers (43% and 37%, respectively) had stunted children. The prevalence of overweight/obesity among mothers of children aged under 5 years is slightly higher than the 25% of all women of reproductive age at the national level in Kenya but relatively lower than the 40% recorded among women of reproductive age in urban areas (Kenya National Bureau of Statistics, Ministry of Health, National AIDS Control Council, Kenya Medical Research Institute, & National Council for Population and Development, 2015). This research may reflect the implication of urbanization in SSA, which has resulted in overcrowded informal settlements and shanty towns with poorer health and nutritional conditions than in rural areas (African Population & Health Research Center (APHRC), 2014; APHRC, 2002; Kimani-Murage et al., 2014a). This research, reflecting the implications of urbanization on health and nutritional outcomes, is in agreement with a study by Fotso et al. conducted in 15 SSA countries which reported a shift in urban–rural health and nutritional gaps (Fotso, 2007). Fotso et al. demonstrated that urban–rural differentials have narrowed in most countries in SSA due primarily to an increase in urban malnutrition, while in a few other countries they have widened due to a sharp decline in urban malnutrition. However, when socioeconomic status is controlled for, these urban–rural differentials are eliminated, suggesting a need to pay particular attention to the urban poor.

Factors Affecting the Nutrition Status of Children

UNICEF has grouped the causes of malnutrition into three main categories: immediate, underlying, and basic (Engle, Menon, & Haddad, 1999; UNICEF, 1990). The immediate causes include inadequate dietary intake and health status of the child. The underlying causes include food insecurity, childcare practices, health service delivery, and environment. The basic causes include economic, political, and ideological structures. Later frameworks include intrauterine growth restrictions as an immediate cause (Fenske, Burns, Hothorn, & Rehfuess, 2013). Fenske et al.'s (2013) framework also expanded the underlying (intermediate) causes to include water and sanitation, breastfeeding practices, health care, and household food security among others. Irrespective of the framework the factors are intertwined and in most cases do not occur in isolation.

Research in the urban poor settings by APHRC indicated how these factors identified in the UNICEF model influence nutritional status for children in low-income settings. Key factors associated with child nutritional status include overall social and structural factors, including poor knowledge and perceptions of child feeding and hence poor feeding practices, poor professional and social support, socioeconomic status including poverty, poor livelihoods/living conditions, inadequate education of the mothers, and food insecurity (Abuya, Ciera, & Kimani-Murage, 2012; Goudet et al., 2017; Kimani-Murage et al., 2015a).

The major issues affecting the nutrition integrity of women, infants, and children are directly related to inadequate or excessive dietary intakes as well as the presence of illnesses. In LMICs a smaller proportion of children benefit from the required meal frequency and food diversity (Lutter et al., 2011). In the informal settlements of Nairobi most households are food insecure and cope by consuming the same type of food and reduced frequency, hence predisposing children to foods that lack the key nutrients required for optimal growth (Kimani-Murage et al., 2014b). Moreover, in these settings diarrhea and pneumonia are the most common diseases among children (Kyobutungi, Ziraba, Ezeh, & Yé, 2008). While there are still debates as to whether diarrheal disease is associated with stunting, a multicountry analysis of the effects of diarrhea on childhood stunting showed that the risk of stunting increased with increased episodes of the disease (Checkley et al., 2008). Urban poor settings are characterized by the lack of water and sanitation facilities and a poor environment, which is likely to predispose children into several episodes of diarrhea, especially during the cold and wet seasons (Mutisya, Orindi, Emina, Zulu, & Ye, 2010). Besides, many other factors may indirectly influence the nutrition of the children including household food security, maternal and childcare practices, breastfeeding practices, health services, genetic factors, and the environment.

At child level, nutritional status varies with gender, age, and birth weight. For instance, boys have a higher prevalence of stunting, underweight, and wasting (51%, 13%, and 3%, respectively) than girls (40%, 9%, and 2%, respectively). However, there is no variation in the prevalence of overweight/obese, reported at 9% for each gender group. Mutisya et al. (2015) also show boys have a higher chance of being stunted than girls, at 54% and 44%, respectively (Mutisya, Kandala, Ngware, & Kabiru, et al., 2015). In terms of age groups, statistics indicate stunting to be lower in children aged 23 months or younger (about 43%) than children aged 24 months and older (about 48%), while wasting and overweight/obesity show the opposite results (3.6% and 10.6% in the former and 1.0% and 6.6% in the latter, respectively) (Kimani-Murage et al., 2015a). With regards to child growth trajectories, data collected from 2007 to 2010 show an overall increase in stunting from the first 3 months of life (10% in early infancy) to an alarming 60% at the age of 15–17 months (Fotso, Madise, Baschieri, Cleland, Zulu, Mutua, & Essendi, 2012). On the basis of birth weight, Abuya et al. (2012) report that children born with low birth weight (less than 2500 g) have a higher chance of stunting (62%) compared to those born with optimal birth weight (36%). In a qualitative study among the residents of the slums of Nairobi, community members perceived suboptimal child feeding practices including early introduction and poor quality of complementary feeding as among the causes of poor child nutrition in their community (Goudet et al., 2017).

Similarly, using qualitative data from the same settings, Goudet et al. (2017) demonstrated how the factors affecting child nutrition in urban poor settings align with the factors identified in the UNICEF model. The most important themes that emerge include: (1) maternal health and nutrition; (2) infant and young children feeding practices; (3) working mothers; (4) family planning; (5) water, sanitation, and hygiene and related diseases; (6) alcohol; and (7) inadequate food and street food, as shown in Fig. 7.1.

At maternal level education plays a major role in the burden of malnutrition among women and children in the slums along with other factors such as marital age and employment status, parity, pregnancy intentions, and place of delivery (Abuya et al., 2012; Mutisya et al., 2015). Evidence indicates a higher prevalence of stunted children born to mothers with at most a primary education level (43%) compared to those born to mothers with at least a secondary level of education (37%). The results further show a lesser burden of stunting among women whose pregnancy is wanted/planned at the time of conception (35%) than later (44%). Children born in health facilities have a lower prevalence of stunting (37%) than those born at home or with the assistance of traditional birth attendants (45%). Parity is also an important maternal factor in child nutrition in urban poor settings, as mothers with one birth are less likely to have stunted children (35%), than those with two (41%) or three (43%) (Abuya et al., 2012). Maternal work, alcoholism, and family planning were also perceived as important influencers of child nutrition status by communities living in urban slums.

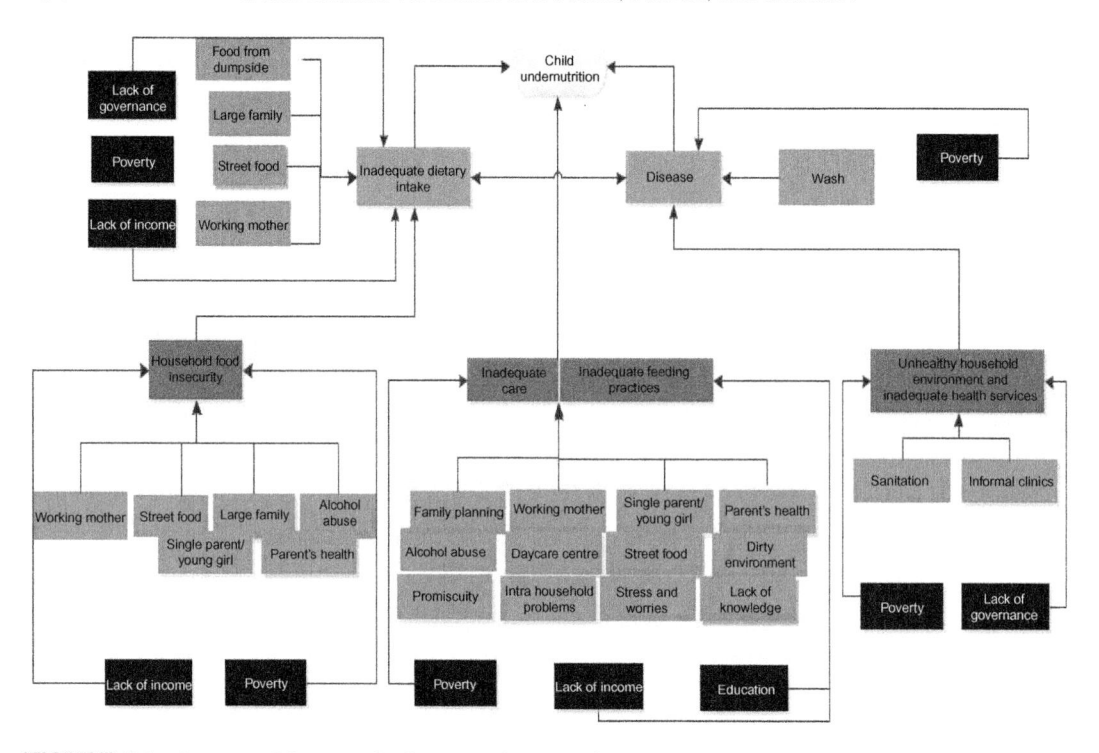

FIGURE 7.1 Conceptual framework of perceived causes of undernutrition mapped to the UNICEF conceptual framework (Goudet et al., 2017).

Working mothers were said to have inadequate time to feed and care for their children while alcoholic mothers were said to often neglect their children and provide inadequate food, resulting in poor growth and child nutrition. Lack of family planning due to poor access to health services was perceived as a cause for large family sizes leading to less time and resources for the mothers to sufficiently feed and care for their children (Goudet et al., 2017).

At the household level evidence indicates the important role household level factors, including socioeconomic status and food security play in nutritional status (Fotso et al., 2012). Existing evidence shows that slum residents greatly experience chronic poverty (Mutisya et al., 2015) and food insecurity (Faye, Baschieri, Falkingham, & Muindi, 2011; Mutisya, Ngware, Kabiru, & Kandala, 2016), which is significantly associated with nutritional status. Fotso et al. (2012) showed the role of various dimensions of poverty, namely food poverty, assets poverty, expenditure poverty, and subjective poverty, at the household level on malnutrition, with children from poorer households being more likely to be stunted or underweight. Malnutrition was shown to be significantly associated with food poverty among children aged 6–11 months, while the association only exists with the subjective and assets dimensions among older children (children aged 12 months or older and those aged 24 months or older, respectively) (Fotso et al., 2012). Household head characteristics such as gender, age, and education were also positively associated with child's nutrition status in an urban poor neighborhood (Dominguez-Salas et al., 2016).

Poverty is closely associated with food insecurity, and studies have documented high levels of food insecurity in the urban poor settings (Kimani-Murage et al., 2011a). For instance, Kimani-Murage et al. (2014b) showed very high prevalence of food insecurity (85%) among households in these settings, with 50% of them being severely food insecure (Kimani-Murage et al., 2014b). Poor livelihoods make it hard to purchase food with adequate quantity, quality, and variety, and instead make people rely on cheap street foods with questionable nutrition and safety values. Some (close to one in five) residents barely survive on one meal a day, which is monotonous and solely consists of maize meal (ugali), collard greens (sukuma wiki), and occasionally tea (in the morning), and food of very insufficient nutritive value (e.g., potato chips) is considered a good meal for children. In these settings, meat is not only consumed rarely, but is also of low quality (mostly offal).

The situation of food insecurity worsens during periods of crisis, such as postelection violence as experienced after the 2007 election in Kenya, when scarcity increases, reportedly leading to severe malnutrition and even death (Kimani-Murage et al., 2011a). Mutisya et al. (2015) showed an increased risk of stunting (by 12%) among children aged 6–23 months living in urban poor households with food insecurity (Mutisya et al., 2015). Poor hygiene and sanitation, a common problem in urban poor settings, has also been highlighted as a probable cause of frequent child infections and worm infestations, which are linked to poor child nutrition (Goudet et al., 2017).

Factors Influencing Child Feeding Practices in Urban Poor Settings (Breastfeeding and Complementary Feeding)

The WHO recommends exclusive breastfeeding in the first 6 months, beginning from the first hour of life, to meet the infant's nutritional requirements and achieve optimal growth, development, and health. The mother is advised to continue breastfeeding up to 2 years of age or more and begin nutritionally adequate, safe, and appropriately-fed complementary foods at the age of 6 months in order to meet the evolving needs of the growing infant (WHO, 2002).

Child feeding practices observed in urban poor settings, however, fail to achieve these WHO infant and young child feeding recommendations (Goudet et al., 2017; Kimani-Murage et al., 2011b; Kimani-Murage et al., 2015b). For example, Kimani-Murage et al. (2011b) showed that less than 2% of children were exclusively breastfed cumulatively for the first 6 months. The study goes further to show that close to two in five infants were not started on breast milk within the first hour of life, and about the same proportion were given prelacteal feeds, for example, plain water and sweetened/flavored water within the first 3 days of life, mainly due to perceptions of inadequate milk (42%) or infants having stomach upsets (32%). Plain water and sweetened/flavored water were introduced in the first month of life for the majority of the infants (approximately 70% and 40%, respectively), while other liquids/semisolid foods including porridge and milk were mainly introduced between the second and third months of life. Further, the studies conducted in urban poor settings in Nairobi, Kenya show that 15% of children are not breastfed beyond 1 year, even though nearly all (99%) have ever been breastfed (Kimani-Murage et al., 2011b). Knowledge and agreement do exist regarding the benefits of breastfeeding to children. For example, the majority (two-thirds) of mothers in urban poor settings in Nairobi know that children should be exclusively breastfed for 6 months. Findings from a qualitative research carried out among mothers and other key informants in the urban poor settings reveal good knowledge and agreement about breastfeeding, including breastfeeding within the first hour, the benefits of feeding on colostrum, and about exclusive breastfeeding for the first 6 months of life, but seemingly this knowledge does not translate to optimal practices due to various social, cultural, and structural barriers (Kimani-Murage et al., 2015b; Wanjohi et al., 2017).

The research done in the urban slums demonstrates various factors that influence IYCF practices, In a conceptual framework on factors affecting breastfeeding in these settings, adapted from Hector et al.'s conceptual framework (Hector, King, Webb, & Heywood, 2005), Kimani-Murage et al. demonstrated that various social and structural barriers affect IYCF practices, hence making it impractical to actualize WHO recommendations (Fig. 7.2). The conceptual framework proposes three levels of factors that influence breastfeeding practices in the urban poor settings: individual level factors, relating directly to the mother, child, and the "mother–child dyad"; group level factors, constituting the attributes of the environments where the mother and the child live which enable the mother to

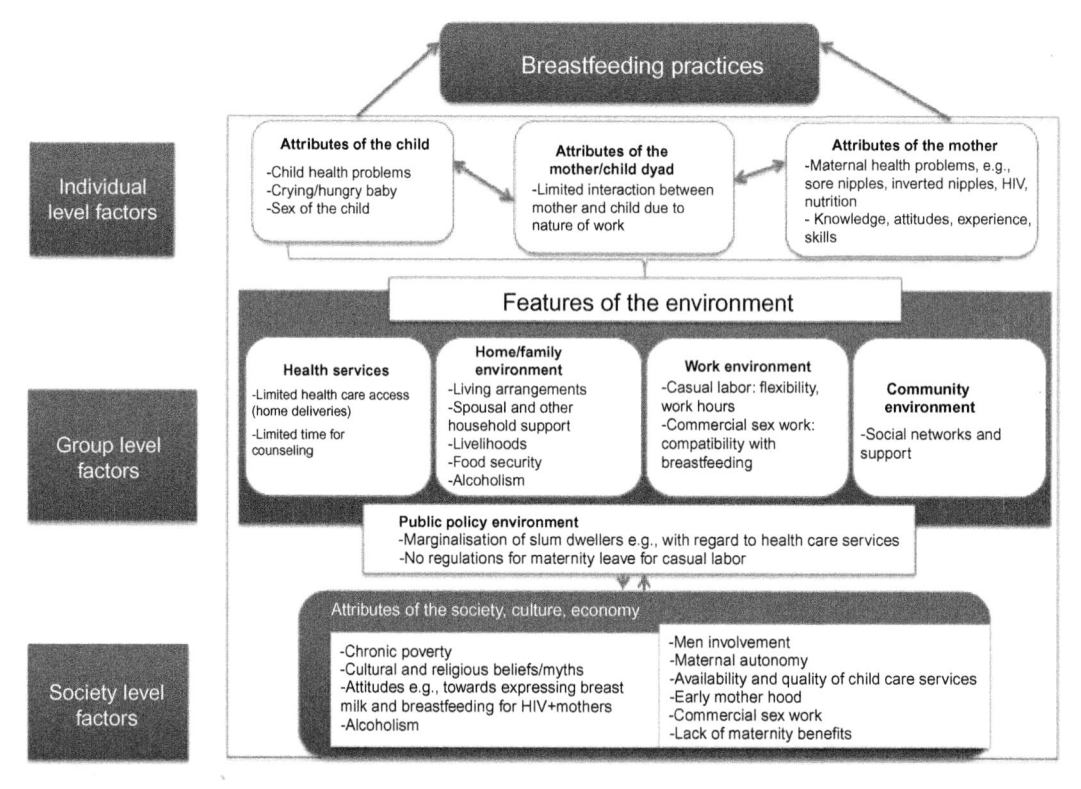

FIGURE 7.2 Conceptual framework of factors affecting breastfeeding practices in urban poor settings (Kimani-Murage et al., 2015b).

breastfeed; and the society level factors, which influence the acceptability and expectations regarding breastfeeding and provide the context for breastfeeding (Kimani-Murage et al., 2015b). These factors include:

1. poverty, livelihoods, and living conditions;
2. early and single motherhood;
3. poor social and professional support;
4. poor knowledge, myths, and misconceptions;
5. HIV; and
6. unintended pregnancies.

Household and societal level factors including poverty, livelihoods, and living conditions are perceived as major barriers to optimal IYCF (Fenske et al., 2013). Indeed, the lack of maternity leave and insufficient income force mothers to seek employment quickly after giving birth, and work for long hours such that it becomes challenging to breastfeed and work. The lack of workplace support for breastfeeding parallels a lack of social support for breastfeeding mothers, mainly from their husbands/partners—the major decision-makers in the household. Since childcare and nutrition are socially and culturally the responsibility of women, male involvement is suboptimal. Evidence also indicates that some men go as far as complaining about the reduced attention they get from their spouses who take time to breastfeed. Moreover, women in urban poor settings do most of the domestic chores in their households, even after delivery, unlike in urban wealthier groups who engage house helps or those in rural areas who are normally supported by relatives. This affects optimal child feeding, thereby impacting the duration of exclusive breastfeeding or any breastfeeding (Kimani-Murage et al., 2015b). Poor feeding practices have been reported to be dire even for young mothers who are not yet mature or self-confident enough to handle early motherhood on their own (Kimani-Murage et al., 2015b).

Adolescent and young mothers lack the knowledge and confidence in infant feeding practices, and are more worried about younger generations' concerns like body image, whereby breastfeeding is said to result in sagging breasts. Further, many younger mothers are still in school and breastfeeding a baby may be a disruption to their studies—often those who continue schooling abandon breastfeeding. Other important factors include commercial sex work and substance and alcohol use (Kimani-Murage et al., 2015b).

Inappropriate/inadequate feeding practices are also influenced by maternal level factors including health status and nutritional status. Results from a qualitative study in urban poor settings in Kenya revealed stress, poor nutrition, and health status of the mother as causes of insufficient breast milk production and hence a barrier to exclusive breastfeeding and a reason for early introduction of complementary feeding and cessation of breastfeeding (Goudet et al., 2017). Poor maternal nutritional status, heightened by the high prevalence of food insecurity in the urban poor settings, and the perceived associations are major barriers to optimal breastfeeding (Kimani-Murage et al., 2014b, 2015b). Women, often living in food insecure households, are said to have inadequate food, and this is perceived to affect breast milk production and flow, leading to the early introduction of complementary foods or the cessation of breastfeeding all together (Kramer & Kakuma, 2012). HIV status and misperceptions regarding breastfeeding while living with HIV are also considered an important barrier to optimal breastfeeding practices. This is important given the high prevalence of HIV in the urban poor settings, at 12% (Madise et al., 2012). There is also reportedly constantly changing advice regarding breastfeeding for HIV positive women which makes the matter worse (Kimani-Murage et al., 2015b).

Feeding practices are also influenced by child level characteristics, including the child's sex and birth weight, according to perceptions by residents of the urban slums. Boys and small-sized babies are perceived to have higher nutritional needs/requirements, which breast milk alone cannot solely satisfy, and are thus more likely to be given other foods at earlier ages (Kimani-Murage et al., 2015b). Cultural beliefs and practices are also highlighted as important factors influencing breastfeeding and complementary feeding practices (Wanjohi et al., 2017). Findings from a recent study documents both positive and negative cultural beliefs in urban poor settings that promote and hinder optimal breastfeeding practices, respectively (Wanjohi et al., 2017).

Personalized Nutrition Interventions to Address Child Undernutrition

Globally there has been an interest in designing and evaluating interventions and programs whose aim is to increase parental efforts toward improving infant and young child nutrition and health (Engle et al., 2007). Besides, multiple studies conducted in SSA, where child malnutrition is still high, have for close to a decade now supported the importance of targeted and scalable interventions to improve the nutritional status and ultimately the nutrition-related health issues of children (Akombi et al., 2017). These interventions are through the partnerships of national governments with nongovernmental organizations with the aim of improving parental behavior toward appropriate child feeding through nutrition-specific interventions and also through nutrition-sensitive interventions.

Optimal nutrition-targeted interventions are imperative in early childhood to alleviate the persistent growth and development issues related to poor nutritional status in SSA (Prentice, Ward, Goldberg, Jarjou, Moore, Fulford, & Prentice, 2013). To be precise, these interventions help to prevent the loss of human capital due to short-term negative health consequences, such as childhood illnesses due to infectious diseases and mortality, and long-term effects, such as noncommunicable diseases and disabilities in adulthood.

Interestingly numerous authors report considerable actions that have been taken across the globe to address these developmental issues by improving nutritional status in infants and young children (Bhutta et al., 2008; Gillespie, Haddad, Mannar, Menon, & Nisbett, 2013). Overall, LMICs, which include nearly all SSA subregions, show the least improvements as the prevalence of stunting, underweight, and wasting remain high. Moreover, SSA is the second region after Asia with the greatest numbers of children who are stunted, wasted, and also with a rapid increase in overweight. Hence identifying nutrition interventions which have been utilized to improve developmental issues could help in scaling up the successes while decreasing the shortcomings.

To date, nutrition-specific interventions targeting immediate determinants of poor infant and child nutrition include maternal dietary or micronutrient supplementation during pregnancy, promotion of exclusive and continued breastfeeding, interventions on proper complementary feeding, dietary supplementation for undernourished children, micronutrient supplementation or food fortification, treatment of severe acute malnutrition, disease prevention and management, and nutrition in emergencies. On the other hand, nutrition-sensitive interventions which target the underlying determinants of child nutrition include food security, access to health services, a safe and hygienic environment, and adequate caregiving resources at the maternal, household, and community levels (Bhutta et al., 2008). Most of these interventions have been actualized in different SSA countries.

Promotion of Optimal Breastfeeding

Generally, optimal nutrition/feeding in infants and young children comprises exclusive breastfeeding in the first 6 months of life, and breastfeeding in combination with adequate complementary feeding from 6 months to 2 years of age. The WHO recommends initiation of breastfeeding within 1 hour of birth, exclusive breastfeeding of infants until 6 months of age, and safe and nutritionally adequate complementary feeding while breastfeeding until 2 years of age or older (Kramer & Kakuma, 2012). Hence to increase exclusive breastfeeding, the WHO launched the Baby Friendly Hospital Initiative, a tool containing 10 steps for successful initiation of breastfeeding in the hospital immediately after delivery (Yotebieng & Behets, 2016). A study by Imdad, Yakoob, & Bhutta (2011) on education or counseling on breastfeeding promotion interventions reported increases in exclusive breastfeeding by 43% on day 1, by 30% until 1 month, and by 90% from 1 to 5 months. Hence interventions toward promoting optimal breastfeeding, such as the Baby Friendly Hospital Initiative, professional provider-led interventions, and optimal complementary feeding interventions, are estimated to be able to prevent almost one-fifth of under-5 mortality in developing countries (Jones, Steketee, Black, Bhutta, & Morris, 2003). However, in SSA, the progress on exclusive and continued breastfeeding is still suboptimal and uneven. Given the difficulty of reaching the majority of poor women through the Baby Friendly Hospital Initiative due to limited health care access and utilization around the time of delivery, some sub-Saharan countries such as Kenya, Gambia, Nigeria, and others have explored the adoption of another strategy recommended by the WHO, the Baby Friendly Community Initiative. This is a community-based intervention strategy delivered through community health volunteers to promote optimal breastfeeding and IYCF and hence to enhance health coverage.

In Kenya the community health strategy (a government strategy that uses community health volunteers to promote health at the community level) is the main avenue for the implementation of the Baby Friendly Community Initiative. In contrast to the Baby Friendly Hospital Initiative, the Baby Friendly Community Initiative promotes breastfeeding and optimal infant feeding in the community with the help of community health volunteers through personalized community or personalized home-based nutrition education interventions. Through a cluster-randomized controlled trial of the key components of the Baby Friendly Community Initiative, Kimani-Murage et al. followed slightly over 1000 mother–child pairs during pregnancy and for 1 year after birth regarding their breastfeeding and infant feeding practices in urban poor settings in Kenya. The study primarily tested the effectiveness of personalized, home-based nutritional counseling by community health volunteers on breastfeeding practices among women in Nairobi's urban informal settlements. The study indicated an increase in exclusive breastfeeding from 2% before intervention to 55% during the intervention (Kimani-Murage et al., 2017).

In another study involving implementation of the Baby Friendly Community Initiative in rural Kenya, Kimani et al. (https://bit.ly/2OBkLEn) employed a cluster-randomized trial design involving close to 1000 mother−child pairs recruited during pregnancy. The mother−child pairs were followed-up until the child was about 6 months old. The intervention involved regular counseling and support of mothers by trained community health volunteers and health professionals on maternal, infant, and young child nutrition, as well as provision of support to mothers through the community. The study indicated the potential effectiveness of the Baby Friendly Community Initiative in promoting optimal breastfeeding and infant feeding, as well as maternal and child health outcomes in the rural setting. These findings in both urban and rural settings show the potential effectiveness of the implementation of the Baby Friendly Community Initiative through the community health strategy in promoting optimal maternal, infant, and young child nutrition practices at the community level, especially in underserved settings such as urban poor settings (Kimani-Murage et al., 2015c). Previous studies have reported that involving community health volunteers under the community health strategy can result in a doubling of the rate of initiation of breastfeeding within 1 hour and improve health facility births by 28% (Lewin et al., 2010).

Moreover, nutrition promotion on proper complementary feeding for infants and children in low-income settlements enabled children to attain minimum meal frequency, minimum dietary diversity, and minimum acceptable diet, as reported in a study conducted in rural Kenya using the Baby Friendly Community Initiative strategy (Maingi, Kimiywe, & Iron-Segev, 2018). Additionally, a Cochrane review of similar interventions implemented in food secure and insecure populations showed a significant increase in height-for-age Z scores, and a significant effect on weight gain, while a statistical difference in stunting, wasting, and underweight was only reported in food insecure regions (Lassi, Das, Zahid, Imdad, & Bhutta, 2013). Therefore Baby Friendly Community Initiative interventions have been proven to be successful in promoting both exclusive breastfeeding and complementary feeding practices. Currently, interventions are ongoing in workplaces in some SSA countries to support and promote breastfeeding to mothers since studies show that workplace support interventions to have a positive impact on continued breastfeeding (Abdulwadud & Snow, 2007).

Complementary Feeding and Micronutrient Supplementation

Complementary feeding is defined as the process that starts when breast milk alone or infant formula alone is no longer sufficient to meet the nutritional requirements of infants, and therefore other foods and liquids are needed, along with breast milk or a breast milk substitute. This process that covers the period from 6 to 24 months of age is a very vulnerable period as this is when malnutrition starts in many infants. This significantly contributes to the high prevalence of malnutrition in children under 5 years of age with the WHO estimating that two out of five children are stunted in low-income countries. The indicators of complementary feeding include the time of initiation of complementary foods, the frequency of feeding of complementary feeds, dietary diversity, and minimum acceptable diet—a composite that includes appropriate frequency of feeding and minimum dietary diversity. Globally, studies show that complementary feeding practices are far from appropriate, with a minimum acceptable diet rate of 10% in SSA (International Food Policy Research Institute, 2016). Poor dietary diversity, characterized by low consumption of animal source foods, is the main reason children do not attain adequate diets. With regards to the optimization of complementary feeding, no single intervention is ideal, and various approaches are recognized (Dewey & Adu-Afarwuah, 2008; Hossain, Choudhury, Adib Binte Abdullah, Mondal, Jackson, Walson, & Ahmed, 2017). It is imperative to support educational interventions to improve complementary feeding as caregivers need skilled support to provide adequate nutrition for their infants. Educational interventions for improving complementary feeding include providing information on the timing of initiation of solid and semisolid foods; continuation of breastfeeding after the introduction to such foods; hygiene; the diversity, quantity, consistency, and frequency of complementary foods; and feeding of children during or after illness.

On the other hand, supplementing children with commercially processed/fortified complementary foods or ready-to-use micronutrient powders or tablets as home-based supplements, and/or macronutrient-dense foods including lipid-based nutrient supplements is regarded as a more direct approach. Indirect approaches target behavioral change based on nutrition education/counseling (Hawkes, 2013). Biofortification and diet diversification and modification also represent food-based opportunities to enhance complementary feeding (Gibson, Carriquiry, & Gibbs, 2015).

Commercial food-based complementary feeds primarily consist of fortified blends of cereal and legume flours and lipid-based nutrient supplements made from peanut butter, vegetable oils, and milk powder. For instance Matsungo et al. (2017) reviewed the adherence to lipid-based nutrient supplements utilized in small quantities, and their efficacy in enhancing nutrition status and reducing related health issues in four SSA countries: Burkina-Faso, Ghana, Malawi, and South Africa. The review reported mixed results, with the ultimate conclusion that the efficacy of small quantities of lipid-based nutrient supplements improving linear growth or preventing growth faltering in infants and young children remained to be elucidated. In particular, adherence that was found to be quite high, based on reported hedonic acceptance and utilization by mothers, diminished considerably. Other limiting factors included the use of length-for-age Z-scores versus variation in height-for-age to evaluate the impact on linear growth. Overall, measuring the outcomes is often reported as being problematic for multiple nutrients, especially at the biochemical level.

The lack of significant impact has also been linked to the determination of the right amounts of nutrients to supplement. With this in mind Claudine et al. (2017) proved the importance of determining the lipid content of lipid-based nutrient supplements to supplement the food of infant and young children experiencing varying degrees of food security. Basically, they found large quantity lipid-based nutrient supplements were more efficient in food insecure children, while moderate quantity lipid-based nutrient supplements had better effects in better-off children. Paul et al. (2011) found differences in strategies among more food secure Tanzanian children versus Zimbabwean children with more economical and agricultural disadvantages. The former benefitted more from relying on home-based fortification of locally available foods, while the latter needed centrally fortified food-based supplements. This study highlighted the need to take into account agroecological contexts, since regional differences in opportunities vary across the continent and within countries.

Moreover, interventions render inconsistent results when varying nutrients are considered. Some interventions such as promoting home-gardening and increased consumption of vitamin A rich fruits and vegetables, and green leafy greens, show undeniable successes in addressing a wide range of nutrient deficiencies, for example, vitamin C, provitamin A, carotenoids, and various minerals (Zeweter, Desse, & Kaleab, 2018). On the other hand, food-based interventions remain insufficient to solve the poor consumption and bioavailability of some nutrients such as iron, zinc, and to lesser extent calcium. Importantly, these nutrients are closely linked to many health conditions such as diarrhea and anemia. They are mainly found in animal source foods, that is, milk and meat products. Hence animal source foods are believed to be the way to improve the consumption of these main problematic nutrients (primarily iron and zinc), but also protein to some extent. However, in many African regions cattle, which are the main source of animal source foods, are considered to be of great social and economic value, and thus seldom are they consumed, especially by children. Many SSA regions actually rely on carbohydrate-rich foods with limited consumption of higher protein foods.

Various researchers have tried to determine the best scenarios that could help in optimizing diets and possibly the nutritional status of infants and young children in LMICs. They have reported promising results, but also persistent difficulties in optimizing the nutritional status of infants and young children with regards to the abovementioned more alarming nutrients. Overall, they concluded that multiple interventions relying on animal source foods, such as promoting animal husbandry and/or aquaculture, could provide some opportunities in optimizing diets, although currently they are limited to meeting iron and zinc requirements in children using solely local foods (Osendarp, Broersen, van Liere, De-Regil, Bahirathan, Klassen, & Neufeld, 2016). Another study which assessed the utilization of local home-prepared foods, such as soy-prepared foods to optimize protein intake in South African children, in comparison to commercially prepared foods, found that the latter had more protein content and thus potentially more impact in enhancing nutrition status in infants and young children (Duvenage, Oldewage-Theron, Egal, & Medoua, 2013). Nevertheless, some researchers ultimately suggest that commercially prepared foods may be less sustainable than relying on local resources and already familiar techniques since they increase the dependence on external donors. In addition, commercial foods may require being hydrated, and water sanitation may thus become a concern. Briefly, this shows again the importance of environmental context and the requirement to consider more holistic approaches. In conclusion there is no one approach that can be used to solve the high malnutrition rates in SSA. A combination of various interventions should be considered. However, emphasis should be on the highly effective interventions to increase the benefits and reduce the costs.

ECONOMIC AND SOCIAL RETURNS ON INVESTMENTS OF PERSONALIZED NUTRITION INTERVENTIONS FOR WOMEN, INFANTS, AND CHILDREN

Social returns on investment is a recognized methodology used to value the impact of a program. It examines the social, economic, and environmental impact of an intervention.

Due to the scarcity of public resources for interventions, it has become increasing important to justify value for money. Approaches for valuing interventions include cost-effectiveness, cost–utility, and cost–benefit analyses. Due to assumptions on benefits attributed to projects, using cost–benefit analysis has been on a decline, prompting a need for the use of better approaches. Social returns on investment has the advantage of analyzing and computing views from multiple stakeholders (giving a wider perspective) in one monetary ratio (Banke-Thomas, Madaj, Charles, & van den Broek, 2015). As a result of using financial proxies, social returns on investment is able to assign values for the social impact of the intervention which then enables an overall valuation of monetary and nonmonetary values. In this social returns on investment evaluation, negative and unexpected impacts are also captured along with the "triple bottom line" factors (social, economic, and environment). The methods used are based upon the social returns on investment as presented in the practical guide for international cooperation (Browers et al., 2010). The social returns on investment principles are as follows:

1. involve stakeholders;
2. understand what changes;
3. value what matters;
4. include only what is material;
5. avoid overclaiming;
6. be transparent; and
7. verify the result.

Kimani-Murage et al. (2013) evaluated a home-based nutritional intervention study in urban informal settlements using the social returns on investment approach. The evaluation assessed the social value of the intervention, which involved home-based nutritional counseling of mothers during pregnancy and within 1 year after birth. The assessment, which included the nonmonetary benefits of the intervention as perceived by the study community, indicated an enormous impact. The social returns on investment study revealed that the intervention did not only impact on the nutrition of the mothers and their mothers who were the primary targets, but also had many other health, social, and economic benefits to the children, mothers, family members, and other community members. The study indicated that for each $1 spent on the intervention, there was $71 return on the investment (Goudet et al., 2016).

IMPENDING IMPLEMENTATION RESEARCH OF PERSONALIZED NUTRITION PROGRAMS FOR WOMEN, INFANTS, AND CHILDREN IN LMICS

Human Milk Banking

Human milk banking is one of the impending implementations of research that needs to be actualized in most LMICs since different infants have specific dietary needs after delivery depending on the mother–infant dyad's health status. Despite the lifesaving and other important benefits of human milk, some infants, the majority of whom are sick, preterm, or of low birth weight, have no access to their mother's own milk due to a multitude of factors such as maternal illness, death, or abandonment. These newborns are therefore much more likely to suffer from adverse consequences resulting from complications that are preventable or treatable with proven and cost-effective interventions (Boyd, Quigley, & Brocklehurst, 2007; McGuire & Anthony, 2003). The WHO has issued a global call to scale up the establishment of human milk banks for the provision of safe donor human milk for children who have no access to their mother's own milk. Access to this milk has the greatest impact on child survival, since optimal breastfeeding alone has the potential to avert an estimated 820,000 child deaths globally and improve child morbidity (Victora et al., 2016).

In Kenya a collaboration between PATH and APHRC is supporting the Ministry of Health and other stakeholders to tailor the Mother−Baby Friendly Initiative Plus model—an integrated hub for infant nutrition and survival—to the Kenyan context. Key findings from a formative feasibility assessment conducted by APHRC in collaboration with PATH, the Ministry of Health, and other partners from 2016 to 2017 in Nairobi were that human milk banking is potentially acceptable and feasible in Kenya (https://bit.ly/2R24mpq).

Over 500 human milk banks have been established in more than 37 countries around the world including Brazil, South Africa, India, Canada, Japan, and France. All follow strict protocols for the collection, pasteurization, storage, and distribution of donated milk to ensure its safety. However, the actual operational feasibility of human milk banking in Kenya has not been determined. Will people donate adequate milk? Can human milk banks actually operate in Kenya? Can the country afford the establishment and operation of human milk banks? Will caregivers make use of the banks to obtain milk for their needy babies? Will the envisaged benefits be realized? These are just some of the questions that need to be answered to help determine feasibility, effectiveness, and cost-effectiveness.

The success of an established human milk bank lies in government endorsement and supports in the promotion of breastfeeding, addressing misinformation on the safety of donated milk, kangaroo mother care, and now the ethical provision of donated human milk for infants in need. This also requires addressing the awareness needs of the public by education and assurance regarding the safety and the rigorous processes of the human milk banks so that communities would accept the use of donated human milk.

Workplace Support for Breastfeeding

Support for breastfeeding in the workplace comprises several types of benefits for employees and services such as teaching employees about breastfeeding; offering professional lactation management services and support; providing designated private space for breastfeeding or expressing milk; providing high-quality breast pumps; allowing flexible scheduling to support milk expression during work; writing corporate policies to support breastfeeding women; giving mothers options for returning to work, for example, extended maternity leave, part-time work, teleworking, and providing on-site or near-site childcare. However, women in both informal and formal employment, urban and rural settings face breastfeeding challenges as evidenced by research conducted by APHRC across six counties in Kenya (https://bit.ly/2OCE9Rt).

Research conducted in Thailand reported that implementation of the workplace breastfeeding support program significantly increased breastfeeding rates for both exclusive breastfeeding and any breastfeeding at 6 months compared to rates before implementation (Yimyam & Hanpa, 2014). Many other studies conducted in middle- and high-income countries have reported a significant improvement in breastfeeding due to the implementation of workplace support benefits as recommended by the Mother-Friendly Workplace Initiatives by the World Alliance for Breastfeeding Action. However, most LMICs have not actualized similar interventions to support workplace support in both informal and formal settings.

A recent law in Kenya mandated employers to support women to combine breastfeeding and work through providing breastfeeding/lactation spaces and facilities at the workplaces and supportive policies. To inform the implementation of this law in Kenya, APHRC in partnership with UNICEF and the Ministry of Health in Kenya are conducting implementation research in an agricultural setting in Kenya. Preliminary results, yet to be published, are promising.

Action is needed to promote workplace support by creating workplace recognition programs to honor employers who support their breastfeeding employees, as well as the provision of educational materials to employers about how to support their breastfeeding employees and establish a model lactation support program for all formal and informal employees.

CONCLUSION

This chapter has highlighted the poor maternal and child nutrition practices in LMICs. The evidence indicates that a double burden of malnutrition exists among poor people who face complex situations with regards to maternal, infant, and young child nutrition resulting from multiple challenges and risk behaviors often dictated to them by their circumstances. This situation calls for macrolevel policies and personalized interventions that take into consideration the ecological settings. Research into personalized nutrition is gaining traction, and this approach is crucial for preventing complicated and highly individualized conditions such as metabolic diseases. Micronutrient supplementation, the Baby Friendly Hospital Initiative, the Baby Friendly Community Initiative, human milk banking, and workplace support for breastfeeding are all promising initiatives to promote optimal personalized maternal and child nutrition in LMICs. Moreover, further research will continue to find ways of optimizing maternal and child nutrition as more interventions are needed to optimize personalized maternal and child nutrition, not only nutrition-specific interventions but also nutrition-sensitive interventions.

References

Abdulwadud, O. A., & Snow, M. E. (2007). Interventions in the workplace to support breastfeeding for women in employment. *Cochrane Database of Systematic Reviews* (3), CD006177.
Abu-Saad, K., & Fraser, D. (2010). Maternal nutrition and birth outcomes. *Epidemiologic Reviews*, 32(1), 5–25.
Abuya, B. A., Ciera, J., & Kimani-Murage, E. (2012). Effect of mother's education on child's nutritional status in the slums of Nairobi. *BMC Pediatrics*, 12(1), 80.

African Population and Health Research Center (APHRC). (2014). *Population and Health Dynamics in Nairobi's Informal Settlements: Report of the Nairobi Cross-sectional Slums Survey (NCSS) 2012*. Nairobi: APHRC.

Ahmed, T., Hossain, M., & Sanin, K. I. (2012). Global burden of maternal and child undernutrition and micronutrient deficiencies. *Annals of Nutrition and Metabolism, 61*(Suppl. 1), 8−17.

Akombi, B. J., Agho, K. E., Merom, D., Renzaho, A. M., & Hall, J. J. (2017). Child malnutrition in sub-Saharan Africa: A meta-analysis of demographic and health surveys (2006−2016). *PLOS ONE, 12*(5), e0177338.

APHRC. (2002). *Population and health dynamics in Nairobi Informal Settlements*. Nairobi: APHRC.

Bain, L. E., Awah, P. K., Geraldine, N., Kindong, N. P., Sigal, Y., Bernard, N., & Tanjeko, A. T. (2013). Malnutrition in sub-Saharan Africa: Burden, causes and prospects. *The Pan African Medical Journal, 15*, 120.

Banke-Thomas, A. O., Madaj, B., Charles, A., & van den Broek, N. (2015). Social Return on Investment (SROI) methodology to account for value for money of public health interventions: A systematic review. *BMC Public Health, 15*(1), 582.

Bhutta, Z. A., Ahmed, T., Black, R. E., Cousens, S., Dewey, K., Giugliani, E., ... Sachdev, H. P. (2008). What works? Interventions for maternal and child undernutrition and survival. *The Lancet, 371*.

Black, R. E., Allen, R. H., Bhutta, Z. A., Caulfied, L., de Onis, M., & Ezzati, M. (2008). Maternal and child under nutrition: Global and regional exposures and health consequences. *The Lancet, 371*, 243−260.

Blumfield, M. L., Hure, A. J., Macdonald-Wicks, L., Smith, R., & Collins, C. E. (2012). Systematic review and meta-analysis of energy and macronutrient intakes during pregnancy in developed countries. *Nutrition Reviews, 70*(6), 322−336.

Boyd, A., Quigley, C. M., & Brocklehurst, P. (2007). Donor breast milk versus infant formula for preterm infants: Systematic review and meta-analysis. *Archives of Disease in Childhood—Fetal and Neonatal Edition, 92*, F169−F175.

Browers, et al. (2010). *SROI: A practical guide for the development cooperation sector*. Available from http://bigpush-forward.net/wp-content/uploads/2011/09/sroi_practical_guide_context_international_cooperation.pdf.

Casey, P. H., Simpson, P. M., Gossett, J. M., Bogle, M. L., Champagne, C. M., Connell, C., ... Weber, J. (2006). The association of child and household food insecurity with childhood overweight status. *Pediatrics, 118*(5), e1406−e1413.

Checkley, W., Buckley, G., Gilman, R. H., Assis, A. M., Guerrant, R. L., Morris, S. S., ... Infection, N. (2008). Multi-country analysis of the effects of diarrhoea on childhood stunting. *International Journal of Epidemiology, 37*(4), 816−830.

Claudine, P., Céline, L., Thomas, R., Stéphane, D., Abdoul-Aziz, M., Lynda, W.-M., ... Rebecca, F. , G. (2017). Effect of ready-to-use foods for preventing child undernutrition in Niger: Analysis of a prospective intervention study over 15 months of follow-up. *Maternal & Child Nutrition, 13*(1).

Cox, J. T., & Phelan, S. T. (2008). Nutrition during pregnancy. *Obstetrics and Gynecology Clinics of North America, 35*(3), 369−383.

Dewey, K. G., & Adu-Afarwuah, S. (2008). Systematic review of the efficacy and effectiveness of complementary feeding interventions in developing countries. *Maternal & Child Nutrition, 4*, 24−85.

Dominguez-Salas, P., Alarcón, P., Häsler, B., Dohoo, I. R., Colverson, K., Kimani-Murage, E. W., ... Grace, D. (2016). Nutritional characterisation of low-income households of Nairobi: Socioeconomic, livestock and gender considerations and predictors of malnutrition from a cross-sectional survey. *BMC Nutrition, 2*(1), 47.

Duvenage, S. S., Oldewage-Theron, W. H., Egal, A. A., & Medoua, G. N. (2013). Home-prepared soymilk: Potential to alleviate protein-energy malnutrition in low-income rural communities in South Africa? *Health SA Gesondheid, 18*(1), Art. #721, 7 pages.

Engle, P. L., Black, M. M., Behrman, J. R., Cabral de Mello, M., Gertler, P. J., Kapiriri, L., ... Young, M. E. (2007). Strategies to avoid the loss of developmental potential in more than 200 million children in the developing world. *The Lancet, 369*(9557), 229−242.

Engle, P. L., Menon, P., & Haddad, L. (1999). Care and nutrition: Concepts and measurement. *World Development, 27*(8), 1309−1337.

Fanzo. (2012). *The nutrition challenge in Sub-Saharan Africa. UNDP—Reg Bur Africa*. Work Paper, January, pp. 1−68.

Faye, O., Baschieri, A., Falkingham, J., & Muindi, K. (2011). Hunger and food insecurity in Nairobi's slums: An assessment using IRT models. *Journal of Urban Health, 88*(Suppl. 2), S235−S254.

Fenske, N., Burns, J., Hothorn, T., & Rehfuess, E. A. (2013). Understanding child stunting in India: A comprehensive analysis of socio-economic, nutritional and environmental determinants using additive quantile regression. *PLOS ONE, 8*(11), e78692.

REFERENCES

Fotso, J.-C. (2006). Child health inequities in developing countries: Differences across urban and rural areas. *International Journal for Equity in Health, 5*, 9.

Fotso, J.-C. (2007). Urban–rural differentials in child malnutrition: Trends and socioeconomic correlates in sub-Saharan Africa. *Health & Place, 13*(1), 205–223.

Fotso, J. C., Madise, N., Baschieri, A., Cleland, J., Zulu, E., Mutua, M. K., & Essendi, H. (2012). Child growth in urban deprived settings: Does household poverty status matter? At which stage of child development? *Health Place, 18*(2), 375–384.

Gibson, R. S., Carriquiry, A., & Gibbs, M. M. (2015). Selecting desirable micronutrient fortificants for plant-based complementary foods for infants and young children in low-income countries. *Journal of the Science of Food and Agriculture, 95*(2), 221–224.

Gillespie, S., Haddad, L., Mannar, V., Menon, P., & Nisbett, N. (2013). The politics of reducing malnutrition: Building commitment and accelerating progress. *The Lancet, 382*(9891), 552–569.

Goudet, S., Wainaina, C. W., Macharia, T. N., Wanjohi, M. N., Wekesah, F. M., Muriuki, P., ... Kimani-Murage, E. W. (2016). Social Return on Investment (SROI) assessment of a Baby-Friendly Community Initiative in urban poor settings, Nairobi, Kenya. *Field Exchange* (52), 41.

Goudet, S. M., Kimani-Murage, E. W., Wekesah, F., Wanjohi, M., Griffiths, P. L., Bogin, B., & Madise, N. J. (2017). How does poverty affect children's nutritional status in Nairobi slums? A qualitative study of the root causes of undernutrition. *Public Health Nutrition, 20*(4), 608–619.

Grantham-McGregor, S., Cheung, Y. B., Cueto, S., Glewwe, P., Richter, L., & Strupp, B. (2007). Developmental potential in the first 5 years for children in developing countries. *The Lancet, 369*(9555), 60–70.

Guo, S. S., Wu, W., Chumlea, W. C., & Roche, A. F. (2002). Predicting overweight and obesity in adulthood from body mass index values in childhood and adolescence. *The American Journal of Clinical Nutrition, 76*(3), 653–658.

Hawkes, C. (2013). Promoting healthy diets through nutrition education and changes in the food environment: An international review of actions and their effectiveness. In Nutrition Education and Consumer Awareness Group, Rome: FAO. Available from www.fao.org/ag/humannutrition/nutritioneducation/69725/en.

Hector, D., King, L., Webb, K., & Heywood, P. (2005). Factors affecting breastfeeding practices. Applying a conceptual framework. *New South Wales Public Health Bulletin, 16*(4), 52–55.

Hossain, M., Choudhury, N., Abdullah, Adib Binte, Mondal, P., Jackson, A. A., Walson, J., & Ahmed, T. (2017). Evidence-based approaches to childhood stunting in low and middle income countries: A systematic review. *Archives of Disease in Childhood, 102*, 903–909.

Imdad, A., Yakoob, M. Y., & Bhutta, Z. A. (2011). Impact of maternal education about complementary feeding and provision of complementary foods on child growth in developing countries. *BMC Public Health, 11*(3), S25.

International Food Policy Research Institute. (2016). *Global Nutrition Report 2016: From promise to impact: Ending malnutrition by 2030*. Washington, DC: International Food Policy Research Institute.

Jones, G., Steketee, R. W., Black, R. E., Bhutta, Z. A., & Morris, S. S. (2003). How many child deaths can we prevent this year? *The Lancet, 362*(9377), 65–71.

Kaput, J., Kussmann, M., Mendoza, Y., Le Coutre, R., Cooper, K., & Roulin, A. (2015). Enabling nutrient security and sustainability through systems research. *Genes & Nutrition, 10*(3), 12.

Kassebaum, N. J., Bertozzi-Villa, A., Coggeshall, M. S., Shackelford, K. A., Steiner, C., Heuton, K. R., ... Lozano, R. (2014). Global, regional, and national levels and causes of maternal mortality during 1990–2013: A systematic analysis for the Global Burden of Disease Study 2013. *The Lancet, 384*(9947), 980–1004.

Kenya National Bureau of Statistics, Ministry of Health, National AIDS Control Council, Kenya Medical Research Institute, & National Council for Population and Development. (2015). *Kenya Demographic and Health Survey 2014: Key Indicators Report*. Nairobi.

Kerac, M., Blencowe, H., Grijalva-Eternod, C., McGrath, M., Shoham, J., Cole, T. J., & Seal, A. (2011). Prevalence of wasting among under 6-month-old infants in developing countries and implications of new case definitions using WHO growth standards: A secondary data analysis. *Archives of Disease in Childhood, 96*(11), 1008–1013.

Kimani-Murage, E. W., Holding, P. A., Fotso, J.-C., Ezeh, A. C., Madise, N. J., Kahurani, E. N., & Zulu, E. M. (2011a). Food security and nutritional outcomes among urban poor orphans in Nairobi, Kenya. *Journal of Urban Health: Bulletin of the New York Academy of Medicine, 88*(Suppl 2), S282–S297.

Kimani-Murage, E. W., Madise, N. J., Fotso, J.-C., Kyobutungi, C., Mutua, M. K., Gitau, T. M., & Yatich, N. (2011b). Patterns and determinants of breastfeeding and complementary feeding practices in urban informal settlements, Nairobi Kenya. *BMC Public Health, 11*, 396.

Kimani-Murage, E. W., Kyobutungi, C., Ezeh, A. C., Wekesah, F., Wanjohi, M., Muriuki, P., ... Madise, N. J. (2013). Effectiveness of personalised, home-based nutritional counselling on infant feeding practices, morbidity and nutritional outcomes among infants in Nairobi slums: Study protocol for a cluster randomised controlled trial. *Trials, 14*, 445.

Kimani-Murage, E. W., Fotso, J. C., Egondi, T., Abuya, B., Elungata, P., Ziraba, A. K., ... Madise, N. (2014a). Trends in childhood mortality in Kenya: The urban advantage has seemingly been wiped out. *Health Place, 29*, 95–103.

Kimani-Murage, E. W., Schofield, L., Wekesah, F., Mohamed, S., Mberu, B., Ettarh, R., ... Ezeh, A. (2014b). Vulnerability to food insecurity in urban slums: Experiences from Nairobi, Kenya. *Journal of Urban Health: Bulletin of the New York Academy of Medicine, 91*(6), 1098–1113.

Kimani-Murage, E. W., Muthuri, S. K., Oti, S. O., Mutua, M. K., van de Vijver, S., & Kyobutungi, C. (2015a). Evidence of a double burden of malnutrition in urban poor settings in Nairobi, Kenya. *PLOS ONE, 10*(6), e0129943.

Kimani-Murage, E. W., Wekesah, F., Wanjohi, M., Kyobutungi, C., Ezeh, A. C., Musoke, R. N., ... Griffiths, P. (2015b). Factors affecting actualisation of the WHO breastfeeding recommendations in urban poor settings in Kenya. *Maternal & Child Nutrition, 11*(3), 314–332.

Kimani-Murage, E. W., Norris, S. A., Mutua, M. K., Wekesah, F., Wanjohi, M., Muhia, N., ... Griffiths, P. L. (2015c). Potential effectiveness of Community Health Strategy to promote exclusive breastfeeding in urban poor settings in Nairobi, Kenya: A quasi-experimental study. *Journal of Developmental Origins of Health and Disease, 7*(2), 172–184.

Kimani-Murage, E. W., Griffiths, P. L., Wekesah, F. M., Wanjohi, M., Muhia, N., Muriuki, P., ... Madise, N. J. (2017). Effectiveness of home-based nutritional counselling and support on exclusive breastfeeding in urban poor settings in Nairobi: A cluster randomized controlled trial. *Globalization and Health, 13*(1), 90.

King, J. C. (2000). Physiology of pregnancy and nutrient metabolism. *The American Journal of Clinical Nutrition, 71*(5), 1218S–1225S.

KNBS. (2015). *Kenya demographic and health surveys, 2014: Key indicators*. (p. 76) Nairobi, Kenya: Kenya National Bureau of Statistics (KNBS).

Kramer, M. S., & Kakuma, R. (2012). Optimal duration of exclusive breastfeeding. *Cochrane Database of Systematic Reviews* (8), CD003517.

Kyobutungi, C., Ziraba, A. K., Ezeh, A., & Yazoumé, Y. (2008). The burden of disease profile of residents of Nairobi's slums: Results from a demographic surveillance. *Population Health Metric, 6*, 1.

Ladipo, O. A. (2000). Nutrition in pregnancy: Mineral and vitamin supplements. *The American Journal of Clinical Nutrition, 72*(1), 280S–290S.

Lanigan, J., & Singhal, A. (2009). Early nutrition and long-term health: A practical approach. *Proceedings of the Nutrition Society, 68*, 1–8.

Lassi, Z. S., Das, J. K., Zahid, G., Imdad, A., & Bhutta, Z. A. (2013). Impact of education and provision of complementary feeding on growth and morbidity in children less than 2 years of age in developing countries: A systematic review. *BMC Public Health, 13*(3), S13.

Lassi, Z. S., Salam, R. A., Das, J. K., & Bhutta, Z. A. (2014). Essential interventions for maternal, newborn and child health: Background and methodology. *Reproductive Health, 11*(Suppl. 1), S1.

Lewin, S., Munabi-Babigumira, S., Glenton, C., Daniels, K., Bosch-Capblanch, X., van Wyk, B. E., ... Scheel, I. B. (2010). Lay health workers in primary and community health care for maternal and child health and the management of infectious diseases. *Cochrane Database of Systematic Reviews, 17*(3), CD004015.

Luoba, A. I., Wenzel Geissler, P., Estambale, B., Ouma, J. H., Alusala, D., Ayah, R., ... Friis, H. (2005). Earth-eating and reinfection with intestinal helminths among pregnant and lactating women in western Kenya. *Tropical Medicine & International Health, 10*(3), 220–227.

Lutter, C. K., Daelmans, B. M. E. G., de Onis, M., Kothari, M. T., Ruel, M. T., Arimond, M., ... Borghi, E. (2011). Undernutrition, poor feeding practices, and low coverage of key nutrition interventions. *Pediatrics, 128*(6), e1418–e1427.

Madise, N. J., Ziraba, A. K., Inungu, J., Khamadi, S. A., Ezeh, A., Zulu, E. M., ... Mwau, M. (2012). Are slum dwellers at heightened risk of HIV infection than other urban residents? Evidence from population-based HIV prevalence surveys in Kenya. *Health & Place, 18*(5), 1144–1152.

Maingi, M., Kimiywe, J., & Iron-Segev, S. (2018). Effectiveness of Baby Friendly Community Initiative (BFCI) on complementary feeding in Koibatek, Kenya: A randomized control study. *BMC Public Health, 18*(1), 600.

Marangoni, F., Cetin, I., Verduci, E., Canzone, G., Giovannini, M., Scollo, P., ... Poli, A. (2016). Maternal diet and nutrient requirements in pregnancy and breastfeeding. An Italian Consensus Document. *Nutrients, 8*(10), 629.

Martorell, R. (1999). The nature of child malnutrition and its long-term implications. *Food and Nutrition Bulletin, 20*(3), 288−292.

Matsungo, T. M., Kruger, H. S., Smuts, C. M., & Faber, M. (2017). Lipid-based nutrient supplements and linear growth in children under 2 years: A review. *Proceedings of the Nutrition Society, 76*(4), 580−588.

McGuire, W., & Anthony, M. Y. (2003). Donor human milk versus formula for preventing necrotising enterocolitis in preterm infants: Systematic review. *Archives of Disease in Childhood—Fetal and Neonatal Edition, 88*(1), F11−F14.

Mutisya, M., Orindi, B., Emina, J., Zulu, E., & Ye, Y. (2010). Is mortality among under-five children in Nairobi slums seasonal? *Tropical Medicine and International Health, 15*(1), 132−139.

Mutisya, M., Kandala, N.-b, Ngware, M. W., & Kabiru, C. W. (2015). Household food (in)security and nutritional status of urban poor children aged 6 to 23 months in Kenya. *BMC Public Health, 15*(1), 1052.

Mutisya, M., Ngware, M. W., Kabiru, C. W., & Kandala, N.-b (2016). The effect of education attainment on household food security in two urban informal settlements in Kenya: A longitudinal analysis. *Food Security, 8*, 743.

Nikièma, L., Huybregts, L., Martin-Prevel, Y., Donnen, P., Lanou, H., Grosemans, J., ... Kolsteren, P. (2017). Effectiveness of facility-based personalized maternal nutrition counseling in improving child growth and morbidity up to 18 months: A cluster-randomized controlled trial in rural Burkina Faso. *PLOS ONE, 12*(5), e0177839.

Nyamasege, C. K., Kimani-Murage, E. W., Wanjohi, M., Kaindi, D. W. M., Ma, E., Fukushige, M., & Wagatsuma, Y. (2018). Determinants of low birth weight in the context of maternal nutrition education in urban informal settlements, Kenya. *Journal of Developmental Origins of Health and Disease*, 1−9. Available from https://doi.org/10.1017/S2040174418000715.

Oddy, W. H., Kendall, G. E., Blair, E., De Klerk, N. H., Stanley, F. J., Landau, L. I., & Zubrick, S. (2003). Breast feeding and cognitive development in childhood: A prospective birth cohort study. *Paediatric and Perinatal Epidemiology, 17*(1), 81−90.

Osendarp, S. J. M., Broersen, B., van Liere, M. J., De-Regil, L. M., Bahirathan, L., Klassen, E., & Neufeld, L. M. (2016). Complementary feeding diets made of local foods can be optimized, but additional interventions will be needed to meet iron and zinc requirements in 6- to 23-month-old children in low- and middle-income countries. *Food and Nutrition Bulletin, 37*(4), 544−570.

Paul, K. H., Muti, M., Khalfan, S. S., Humphrey, J. H., Caffarella, R., & Stoltzfus, R. J. (2011). Beyond food insecurity: How context can improve complementary feeding interventions. *Food and Nutrition Bulletin, 32*(3), 244−253.

Popkin, B. M., Adair, L. S., & Ng, S. W. (2012). NOW AND THEN: The global nutrition transition: The pandemic of obesity in developing countries. *Nutrition Reviews, 70*(1), 3−21.

Prentice, A. M., Ward, K. A., Goldberg, G. R., Jarjou, L. M., Moore, S. E., Fulford, A. J., & Prentice, A. (2013). Critical windows for nutritional interventions against stunting. *The American Journal of Clinical Nutrition, 97*(5), 911−918.

UNICEF. (1990). *Strategies for improved nutrition of children and women in developing countries. A UNICEF policy peview.* New York, NY: UNICEF.

UNICEF, WHO, and World Bank. (2017). *Joint child malnutrition estimates—Levels and trends* (2017 ed.). New York/Geneva/Washington, DC: UNICEF/WHO/The World Bank.

United Nations. (2015). *Transforming our world : the 2030 Agenda for Sustainable Development*, 21 October 2015, A/RES/70/1, available at: https://www.refworld.org/docid/57b6e3e44.html.

Victora, C. G., Adair, L., Fall, C., Hallal, P. C., Martorell, R., Richter, L., ... Maternal and Child Undernutrition Study, G. (2008). Maternal and child undernutrition: Consequences for adult health and human capital. *The Lancet, 371*(9609), 340−357.

Victora, C. G., Bahl, R., Barros, A. J. D., França, G. V. A., Horton, S., Krasevec, J., ... Rollins, N. C. (2016). Breastfeeding in the 21st century: Epidemiology, mechanisms, and lifelong effect. *The Lancet, 387*(10017), 475−490.

Walsh, M., & Kuhn, S. (2012). Developments in personalised nutrition. *Nutrition Bulletin, 37*(4), 380−383.

Wanjohi, M., Griffiths, P., Wekesah, F., Muriuki, P., Muhia, N., Musoke, R. N., ... Kimani-Murage, E. W. (2017). Sociocultural factors influencing breastfeeding practices in two slums in Nairobi, Kenya. *International Breastfeeding Journal, 12*, 5-5.

Whitaker, R. C., Wright, J. A., Pepe, M. S., Seidel, K. D., & Dietz, W. H. (1997). Predicting obesity in young adulthood from childhood and parental obesity. *New England Journal of Medicine, 337*(13), 869–873.

WHO. (2002). *The optimal duration of exclusive breastfeeding. Report of an Expert Consultation.* Geneva: WHO.

World Health Organization. (2009). *Global health risks: Mortality and burden of disease attributable to selected major risks*. Geneva: WHO.

Yimyam, S., & Hanpa, W. (2014). Developing a workplace breast feeding support model for employed lactating mothers. *Midwifery, 30*(6), 720–724.

Yotebieng, M., & Behets, F. (2016). Step 10: The breastfeeding support paradox—Authors' reply. *The Lancet Global Health, 4*(1), e20.

Zeweter, A., Desse, H. G., & Kaleab, B. (2018). Simulated effects of home fortification of complementary foods with micronutrient powders on risk of inadequate and excessive intakes in West Gojjam, Ethiopia. *Maternal & Child Nutrition, 14*(1), e12443.

CHAPTER 8

Modern Technologies for Personalized Nutrition

Mike Boland[1], Fakhrul Alam[2] and John Bronlund[1]

[1]Riddet Institute, Massey University, Palmerston North, New Zealand
[2]Massey University, Auckland, New Zealand

OUTLINE

Introduction	196
What Might Smart Personalized Nutrition Look Like?	196
Modern Technologies and Food Acquisition	**200**
Virtual Reality, Augmented Reality, and Food Selection	201
Smart Kitchen Appliances and Intelligent Automated Food Ordering	202
Modern Technologies, Nutrition, and Health	**202**
The Rise of eHealth and mHealth	202
Nutritional Phenotyping	203
Connected Medical Devices	204
Modern Technologies and Food Intake	**204**
Inferential Approach	205
Direct Approach	205
Modern Technologies and Energy Expenditure (Exercise)	**206**
Wearable Technology: Activity Trackers and Smart Watches	206
Modern Technologies and Food Preparation	**207**
Assistive Kitchens	208
Automated Food Preparation	208
3-D Printed Food	208
Modern Technologies and Food Composition	**209**
Labeling	209
Intelligent Packaging	209
Sensing and Analysis	210
Allergens and Other Undesirables	211
Bringing It All Together	**211**
The Intelligent Kitchen and Its Role in Personalized Nutrition	211

Food Service and Management of Personalized Nutrition	211	Food Monitoring	216
The eHealth and mHealth Environment—Toward a Personal Virtual Dietitian	212	Reliability and Consistency of Smartphone Apps	217
		Nutritional Values and Bioaccessibility	217
The Artificial Intelligence Engine That Drives Personalized Nutrition	212	**Future Perspective**	218
		Conclusion	218
A Potential Architecture of a Personalized Nutrition System	213	**References**	219
Areas That Need to be Addressed	216	**Further Reading**	222
Privacy and Security	216		

INTRODUCTION

The fusion of digital technologies with almost all real-world activities—sometimes known as the Fourth Industrial Revolution—is changing the world. It is changing how food is researched, perceived, purchased, and used by the consumer, and it has important implications for convenience, diet, and health. It has the potential to enable personalized nutrition on an unprecedented scale.

The Internet of Things (IoT) is expected to have 20 billion devices (excluding smartphones and computers) connected by 2020 (Hung, 2017). These devices enable automated purchasing of food supplies. For example, consider smart refrigerators and smart containers that know what they contain and can order resupplies online from the supermarket (e.g., Samsung Family Hub, Neo Smart Jar), apps for tablets and smartphones that can scan and reorder packaged goods (e.g., Chefling), and attachments for garbage cans that can read barcodes on packaging or recognize voice descriptions and automatically reorder the product (e.g., GeniCan). At present these are relatively simple scan and reorder systems. But coupled with nutritional data from big datasets and appropriate personal details, the possibility exists for an artificial intelligence (AI) engine to design diets, meals, and menus and tailor food purchasing to deliver personalized nutrition in new and very convenient ways. There are evolving devices, including a myriad of smartphone apps, that can recognize food items (from barcodes and from image analysis) and link to datasets for nutritional composition and provide dietary advice. Other devices can monitor eating activities from wrist movements (e.g., HAPIfork), sounds of eating, and facial muscle activity, and systems can potentially track what and when it is eaten, how well it is chewed, and even if it is enjoyed. There are emerging devices that attach to smartphones and analyze food composition using surface infrared spectroscopy (e.g., SCio), although their effectiveness is still open to question.

What Might Smart Personalized Nutrition Look Like?

We can expect that systems will soon exist that can draw on cloud-based personal health records (eHealth), stated personal food (and other) preferences, observed food preferences

INTRODUCTION 197

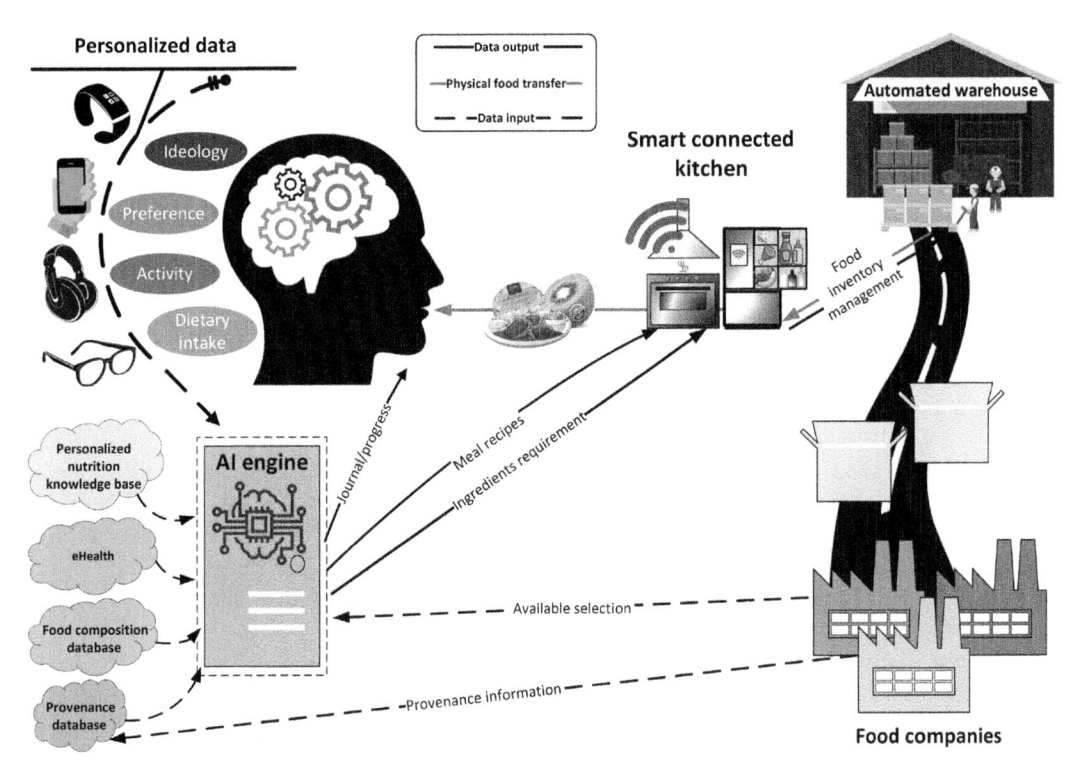

FIGURE 8.1 Schematic of the various components, food movements and data flows of an integrated smart personalized nutrition system.

and eating activities, personal energy expenditure, and observed health parameters from smart appliances (and possibly wearable devices) to guide meal planning and food purchasing using online nutrition recommendations, past food purchasing patterns, and online nutritional data about food products. We can even expect smart (assistive) kitchens that can guide us through meal preparation. This ecosystem is shown schematically in Fig. 8.1.

The reality might be that an individual would join a smart personalized nutrition scheme that would involve a one-time effort of:

- setting up an account on the Personalized Nutrition system;
- entering relevant personal and biometric data (including food, cultural, and personal preferences, etc.);
- setting health targets (e.g., for weight loss or lowering of blood pressure or managing blood glucose) if desired;
- setting up access to eHealth records and any other relevant databases (such as DNA and nutritional phenotype data, where available);
- registering personal smart devices, including smartphones, fitbits, smart bathroom scales, and wearable devices (that may include food buttons or wearable glucose meters), on the system;

B. APPLICATIONS OF PERSONALIZED NUTRITION

- registering household IoT devices, such as refrigerators, smart pantries, other smart kitchen devices; and
- potentially linkage to purchasing systems to record what has been purchased as a way of automatically managing the kitchen inventory.

This will provide the system with personal fixed and temporal data. Using this and online databases of composition of food products, together with dietary recommendations, the system will use AI to develop recommendations for diet, meal plans, and (potentially automated) food purchase. Over time the system will learn personal eating habits and preferences and adapt its recommendations. It will also record progress toward target goals and modify its dietary recommendations accordingly. Recommendations can be according to a schedule, probably by smartphone or smartwatch messaging, but may also be opportunistic: for example, if I am going out for a long walk or bicycle ride and my blood sugar is getting low, the system can alert me, through my smartphone, that there is a place nearby where I can purchase my favorite chocolate bar (or other snack) that will increase my blood sugar by the right amount.

What is needed: Most of the technology for a Smart Personalized Nutrition system as just described already exists, much of it in advanced forms, some still emerging. Diet apps and diet management systems based around smartphone communication are already widespread, and semiautomated grocery ordering systems are in use. A range of relevant smart devices with the requisite connectivity is given in Table 8.1. Some of these are more fully described later.

Parts of the ecosystem needed for personalized nutrition advice already exist. One system (DietSensor Ultimate www.dietsensor.com accessed July 2018) uses a combination of a SCio pocket NIR scanner, a smart digital scale, and a smartphone app to determine the approximate composition and weight of components in a meal and give nutritional advice. Another system (FoodSwitch www.foodswitch.com.au, accessed July 2018) is an app that scans barcodes on packaged foods and gives advice on comparable products with different nutritional values (based on manufacturers' declared composition) (Dunford et al., 2014). This app also uses crowdsourcing to update itself with new products in the supermarket.

Similarly, parts of the system needed for AI-driven food purchase and management exist. One item that seems to be missing is a smart system for home food inventory management (smart refrigerator and smart pantry—the refrigerator exists in part, the pantry does not—yet), although that will no doubt appear soon, and some prototypes have been reported. The smart kitchen concepts as shown by Miele and Ikea (Ideo, 2015; Miele, 2017) certainly assume a degree of smart food inventory management and link this to recipes and cooking instructions.

Systems exist for dietary advice, diet and menu planning, and provision of recipes, provided the inventory is known. Some weaknesses are that nutritional data are generally not available for meals served in restaurants, and that the composition of natural foods can vary considerably according to stage of growth (e.g., sugar content varies with ripeness) and conditions of growth. This can be important for functional food ingredients as well as for overall composition.

TABLE 8.1 Some Commercially Available Smart Devices That Could Support Personalized Nutrition

Name of Device	What It Does	Where to Find Out More (Web Sites Accessed July 2017)
Family hub refrigerator	Shows content of the refrigerator and can order groceries online	https://www.samsung.com/us/explore/family-hub-refrigerator/overview/
Chefling	Smartphone or tablet app—records inventory and suggests recipes	http://www.chefling.net/
Neo Smart Jar	Jar that is programmed for what it will contain, nutritional values, monitors contents, and reports/reorders via Bluetooth and an app	https://innovationessence.com/understand-pantries-accordily/
SmartPlate	Intelligent nutrition platform that uses advanced photo recognition and AI technology to identify, analyze, and track what is eaten	https://www.getsmartplate.com/ https://www.indiegogo.com/projects/smart-plate-topview-your-personal-nutritionist#/
GeniCan	Barcode scanning attachment for garbage—can reorder when you use something	https://www.genican.com/
HapiFork	Monitors eating rate and eating habits	https://www.hapi.com/product/hapifork
SCio Scanner	Near-infrared scanner smartphone attachment—gives surface composition of food	https://www.consumerphysics.com/ https://www.dietsensor.com/product/scio-scanner/
Blood Glucose Monitor	Continuously measures blood glucose levels and reports via local station or smartphone	Rodbard (2016) https://www.dexcom.com/continuous-glucose-monitoring https://freestylediabetes.co.uk/our-products/freestyle-libre
KogniChef	Prototype assistive kitchen—provides instruction and controls kitchen devices for meal preparation	Neumann et al. (2017)
VitalPatch	Monitors vital signs	https://vitalconnect.com/
Fitbit	Activity trackers and smart watches that provide health and fitness monitoring	https://www.fitbit.com/nz/home
Polar H10	Wearable (chest strap) heart rate sensor	https://www.polar.com/au-en/products/accessories/h10_heart_rate_sensor
QardioCore	Wearable (chest strap) continuous ECG monitor	https://store.getqardio.com/products/qardiocore
Cronovo	Upcoming smartwatch/fitness tracker that provides wireless connectivity and provides multiple personal health applications	http://www.cronovo.com/

Many health providers are now using patient-accessible online health systems as part of national or regional health information systems (HIS), which include records of diagnoses, treatments, test results, and prescribed drugs. These should be an important input directly into a personalized nutrition system. However, there are important privacy issues that need to be managed in this context.

The most important need is for a comprehensive data architecture that can interface with all the relevant systems, and a straightforward consumer interface that can guide the individual to provide optimal personalized nutrition—or even to do it without user intervention at all.

MODERN TECHNOLOGIES AND FOOD ACQUISITION

The 1950s saw a disruptive change in the way food is purchased. Until then there were small local grocery stores, butchers, and greengrocers, where food items were fetched by the grocer or butcher on request. Items could also be preordered by phone and either collected from the store or delivered to the home, often by a boy on a bicycle. The key to the change was allowing customers direct access to the food stores with checkouts at the door. Thus was invented the modern supermarket, which sold all kinds of food, and the selection of food items passed directly into the hands of the customer with little or no intervention from the retailer. This inevitably led to a consolidation of the food retail industry and an almost total loss of the service aspect of the industry.

Today we are on the verge of a similarly disruptive change: online ordering of almost everything has taken over from local retail outlets. Probably the most dramatic examples are in books and music—downloads are the rule and local purchase very much the exception. Food has been slower to follow, but we are on the edge of a massive change to online purchase, particularly of packaged and processed foods. Models developed by Amazon, originally for books, are being adapted for use with food items, by Amazon itself and by other players; and, as an example, the British company Ocado has developed a highly automated, completely online system for grocery retail and delivery in Andover in the UK (https://www.reuters.com/article/us-ocado-technology/ocado-courts-global-food-retailers-with-robot-army-idUSKBN1IA2BJ, accessed July 2018). It is somewhat ironic that this change will lead to something similar to the telephone order, followed by pickup or delivery that was experienced in the 1950s.

Online shopping from supermarkets has been available for nearly 20 years, but initial uptake was slow. It generally worked by having people employed as "shoppers" who put together the order—much as in the days of the local grocer—and the order could be delivered or picked up from a "pickup point." This is now changing, using the systems developed by Amazon and others (notably Ocado in the UK), whereby selections are put together and checked out in large, robotically-operated warehouses, ready for delivery. Such systems are commonplace in the supply of retail supermarkets from wholesalers. It is likely that in urban areas an Uber-type grocery delivery system will develop quickly (one example, Instacart, is already in operation in parts of the United States and Canada), and robot delivery, including delivery using drones, is already being trialed (for example Amazon Prime Air). This model will not work as easily for some fresh foods because of the variability in fresh foods and the difficulties in labeling and in handling and protection, but this can be managed in other ways, and with the trend toward purchase of fresh foods at local markets may be a separate consideration.

Variants of online grocery shopping abound. Virtual supermarkets can be as simple as displays on the wall of a subway station with barcodes that can be read by a smartphone app (such displays have been present in South Korea for many years and can be found in some airports), through to full virtual reality (VR) supermarkets as discussed below.

Another variant that has risen recently is the home-delivered meal kit. Meal kits have been in supermarkets for many years but have not been a mainstream item. Today's meal kits are often chef-designed, with balanced nutrition, and are becoming mainstream. They have not yet reached as far as personalized nutrition kits but using the principles of mass customization it should be a relatively simple step.

Virtual Reality, Augmented Reality, and Food Selection

VR enables users to feel like they are among the shop aisles without having to travel. VR-based supermarket and retail stores were considered by many as the logical successor to online shopping. E-commerce and retail giants like Alibaba (e.g., Buy +), eBay, and IKEA have trialed various VR options (Rick, 2017) and a Tesco version has been demonstrated (Pele, 2014). A few VR-based supermarkets have started operating in the last few years (e.g., a Tesco store in Berlin). The technology has also been used extensively for supermarket layout design, to gain a better understanding of shopper behavior in stores, and to test the appeal of new products with shoppers. However, the uptake of VR for shopping seems to have stagnated after the initial hype. Virtual shopping (based on QR code scans), checkoutless shop (e.g., Amazon Go), and on-demand grocery delivery (e.g., Instacart) seem to have supplanted VR.

Augmented reality (AR) blends the virtual and the real world and reconciles e-commerce with bricks and mortar stores. It facilitates the implementation of smart, interactive supermarkets, enabling the shoppers to see real-time information (product attributes, carbon footprint information, product reviews, etc.) as they move around a store. Food shopping typically involves quick decision-making. An AR-based system can help someone shop according to their dietary requirements through rapid, accurate associations between food items and dietary recommendations. Recent research has investigated an AR-based personal health assistant to aid in decision-making at grocery stores (Gutiérrez, Cardoso, & Verbert, 2017). There are AR-assisted smartphone apps for real-time, customized recommendations of healthy products that highlight products to avoid and identify suitable alternative products for various types of health concerns and general caloric intake (Ahn et al., 2015; Dunford et al., 2014). There are also operational supermarkets that use interactive tables and shelves to display augmented labels (nutritional value, presence of allergens, waste disposal instructions, etc.) on screens suspended above when a customer inspects a product (Ratti, 2018).

Smart Kitchen Appliances and Intelligent Automated Food Ordering

A smart kitchen (also known as a connected kitchen) aims to perform a variety of tasks, including ingredient recognition and grocery ordering. Image recognition, label scanning, odor recognition, and machine learning, along with wireless connectivity, underpin the smart kitchen. An ideal smart kitchen consists of connected elements that include the pantry, appliances, rubbish bin, and utensils. The fridge and the pantry or the containers (e.g., Neo Smart Jar) maintain the food/ingredient inventory, and the waste bin (e.g., GeniCan) can identify the discarded cans/packages through their barcodes and other items by voice prompts. Based on inventory level and consumption, these modules can then produce shopping lists and can even perform automated (online) orders. Some of them also track dietary consumption, offer real-time nutrition advice, and even suggest recipes based on available ingredients and their expiry dates and/or freshness level. Image processing and machine learning have reached a point where it is becoming possible to measure calorie consumption and nutrition from before and after food images (Pouladzadeh, Shirmohammadi, & Al-Maghrabi, 2014). As a result, smart utensils (e.g., SmartPlate https://getsmartplate.com/), through their apps, can perform tasks like monitoring nutrient and caloric intake and eating habits. As of now the appliances are stand-alone entities that mainly connect to their separate apps and have little or no interaction with each other. However, Smart Kitchen Platforms [e.g., Whirlpool Yummly (Min et al., 2018)] are being introduced to ensure that all aspects of the kitchen tie into a holistic system driven by an AI engine.

MODERN TECHNOLOGIES, NUTRITION, AND HEALTH

Noncommunicable diseases (NCDs) are estimated to be responsible for 70% of all deaths globally (WHO). These include cardiovascular disease, cancers, respiratory disease, and diabetes. There is a strong link between many NCDs and diet. The World Health Organization is leading a campaign to decrease the risk of NCDs. In terms of attributable deaths, the leading metabolic risk factor globally is elevated blood pressure (to which 19% of global deaths are attributed), followed by overweight and obesity, and raised blood glucose. All these factors can, in part, be managed by diet, especially when coupled with appropriate exercise. Properly designed personalized nutrition thus has the potential to reduce NCDs significantly.

The Rise of eHealth and mHealth

Twenty-first century information and communications technology has led to the possibility of widespread management of health through the internet and smart devices. "eHealth" is defined by the World Health Organization as "the use of information and communication technologies (ICT) for health."

The breadth of eHealth was acknowledged by the World Health Assembly in resolution WHA58.28 (2005): "eHealth is the cost-effective and secure use of ICT in support of health and health-related fields, including health-care services, health surveillance, health literature, and health education, knowledge and research." Nutrition has to date received little attention in the eHealth environment, but we expect eNutrition to emerge as an important component in the near future.

mHealth is a component of eHealth. The WHO Global Observatory for eHealth (GOe) has defined mHealth or mobile health as "medical and public health practice supported by mobile devices, such as mobile phones, patient monitoring devices, personal digital assistants (PDAs), and other wireless devices." mHealth usually involves the use of a mobile phone's core utility of communication by voice and short messaging service (SMS) and internet connectivity, as well as more complex applications, including the use of global positioning system (GPS) and Bluetooth technology. This can be further enhanced by interaction with large cloud-based data systems, including eHealth repositories, and by the use of sensing devices that use either the native capability of a mobile phone (such as an accelerometer) or a range of connected sensing devices as diverse as blood glucose monitors, blood pressure monitors, electrocardiographs, and even pocket-sized cardiac ultrasound units.

Online health records can be an important component of a smart personalized nutrition system, providing diagnosis information to guide diet, information on allergies to avoid foods that may contain undesired ingredients, and information about drugs to avoid adverse drug reactions (for example patients taking statins must avoid grapefruit in the diet).

Nutritional Phenotyping

Individuals can easily obtain information about their own genetic profile. With new sequencing technologies, it is now possible for anyone to have their DNA genotyped for under US$100 (23andMe DNA Saliva Collection Kit, or Ancestry.com) and several companies offer sequencing for under US$2000. These services vary according to their stated purpose and only some of these provide information with respect to known genetic polymorphisms related to health and metabolism—others being focused on heritage (AncestryDNA) or legal issues such as paternity.

The combination of the availability of individual genetic data with a detailed understanding of nutrition has led to the field of "nutrigenomics": the study of the relationship between a person's genetic makeup and their individual nutritional needs—this is discussed in depth elsewhere in this volume. While early studies in nutrigenomics suggested quick wins, with simple gene differences (single nucleotide polymorphisms, or SNPs) indicating specific dietary needs, the situation has been found to be much more complex. The focus is now on understanding "nutritional phenotypes," which take into account not only SNPs, but other genetic differences such as copy number variants of genes (CNVs), and also differences in expression of those genes that can be caused by a range of factors, including epigenetic effects, health status, lifestyle, and medications (Van Ommen et al., 2010). An individual's nutritional phenotype data (or data that go toward developing a nutritional phenotype) will be an increasingly important input to personalized nutrition AI systems.

Connected Medical Devices

There is a range of medical devices that can connect to the online cloud, usually via a smartphone, by either wired or wireless connection. Examples of these are:

- *Smart bathroom scales*: bathroom scales are among the most widely used health devices. While traditionally they allowed the users to track weight, a new breed of smart scales can track a variety of health parameters like BMI, body composition (fat mass %, water %, bone mass), and heart rate. They use wireless connectivity (e.g., Bluetooth or Wi-Fi) to work in conjunction with smartphone apps and fitness trackers. The scales predominantly rely on foot-to-foot Bioelectrical Impedance Analysis (BIA) for computing body composition information. Thus they may not be as accurate as typical medical equipment since the electrical signal does not travel across the stomach (Dehghan & Merchant, 2008) and their calibration may not be valid for all ethnic groups and ages (Wang & Hui, 2015). However, they are still useful for monitoring trends.
- *Blood glucose monitors*: both discrete and wearable blood glucose monitors are well developed and are largely used for the monitoring and management of health in diagnosed diabetics. Some of the wearable devices are capable of continuous monitoring of blood glucose—examples are Dexcom G6 and Freestyle Libre. Of these the Dexcom device can read directly using an app on most smart devices, while others have separate meters that can download to a computer or smartphone via a cable. Although these devices are intended for, and mostly used by, diabetics, there is evidence of wider use in the population (Sifferlin, 2017) and use by at-risk prediabetics may become more common.
- *VitalPatch*: the VitalPatch clinical biosensor is a small stick-on disposable patch that monitors heart rate, respiratory rate, skin temperature, body posture, and activity, and has a single-lead ECG. It connects to nearby smart devices via low-energy Bluetooth. This device is being pioneered in the United States in 2018 in "virtual hospitals" that have doctors but no patients—the patients are either living at home or in another care facility (Allen, 2017). Other countries are also proposing telemedicine systems using so-called body area networks (BANs) of wearable devices, for example, to improve health care in rural India (Nedungadi, Jayakumar, & Raman, 2018).
- An internet database recently listed 88 wearable medical devices that can measure a wide range of body functions and can connect to a variety of online systems for data logging and tracking (Vandrico, 2018).

MODERN TECHNOLOGIES AND FOOD INTAKE

An important part of diet management for personalized nutrition is monitoring what food is actually consumed by an individual, which will give a direct measure of intake of nutrients and bioactives. This is also an important input for the AI engine to learn about food preferences. In the past for individuals on strict diets, food diaries have been kept manually. This has often resulted in erratic and inaccurate records, as mostly these are filled out at a later time from memory, and there is a tendency to underestimate portion sizes (Cade, 2017; Hassannejad et al., 2017) and to forget between-meal snacks. New app-supported record keeping may improve this (Maria Bejar, Adrian Reyes, & Dolores Garcia-Perea, 2018), but fully automated record keeping (that requires no effort on the part of the consumer) is preferable and can be expected to be more reliable. New technologies will allow automatic monitoring of food intake. There are two approaches to this that are complementary—one is by inference from use of recipes, changes in food inventory in the home, and food purchases and disposals; the other is from a range of direct measurements including food image capture and analysis and the use of various on-body sensing systems to monitor eating behaviors.

Inferential Approach

A smart kitchen will be able to track whole food and ingredient use in the home through changes in inventory; and an assistive kitchen will be able to track food use through recipes and cooking activities. This will give an overview of food consumption in the home, but not how it is divided between cohabiting individuals or how much is consumed or disposed of. Plating and serving sizes can be managed by tracking weights on weight-sensitive surfaces, such as may be found in a smart kitchen (Neumann et al., 2017). Eating out of home will be managed in different ways (see later section). Snacking is a particularly important of food intake that is often missed. This could be tracked through purchasing events for out of home snacks and from inventory changes in the home.

Direct Approach

Direct approaches to monitoring diet include various forms of image analysis and a range of wearable devices. For a recent review see Hassannejad et al. (2017). There are smartphone apps that can identify with surprising accuracy what is on a plate, and wearable cameras (e-buttons) can be worn, which will take a photo of a plate and identify the components of a serving. These methods are not always accurate in identification and may prove to increase in accuracy when coupled with other contextual information that may be available, such as location (from smartphone GPS, for example, for specific types of restaurant) or known preferences (Herranz, Jiang, & Xu, 2017). The biggest weakness of image analyses is that they give only a two-dimensional image of the food, which means they are not good at estimating serving size, and they analyze only the surface of the food, which, in the case of a layered food (such as a pie), means they are of limited use. The recent development of cameras that take three-dimensional images, such as the Intel device called RealSense (https://www.intel.com/content/www/us/en/architecture-and-technology/realsense-overview.html), which is a little camera that gives mm-scale accuracy 3D surface scans, may go some way to better estimation of portion size.

Smartphones can potentially be the device of choice for diet monitoring. However, current image processing-based methods are still too resource-demanding for smartphone capability. A recent review concluded, "We believe that food image analysis is not likely to provide a general fully automated mobile stand-alone solution in the near future. Nevertheless, it can be integrated with other technologies to form comprehensive solutions and improve the monitoring system's effectiveness and accuracy" (Hassannejad et al., 2017).

Another complementary approach is the use of on-body sensors. There is a wide range of different sensors that have been developed, some available commercially. Most of these devices fall into one of three functions: detection and monitoring of chewing, detection and monitoring of swallowing, and monitoring and interpretation of hand and arm movements during eating. The form of these devices varies, ranging from simple sensors worn on a necklace or as part of clothing, through to full electroencephalograph headsets. Most of these devices are still in their infancy, especially when applied to food and eating, but more accurate and more sophisticated ways to determine what and when we eat can be expected. It should be noted that, while these devices can monitor eating activities, they are silent with respect to food composition. A recent review concluded that "normally it is not very practical to use these sensors, especially if the user needs to wear several such sensors at the same time" (Hassannejad et al., 2017).

Recently there has been research interest in using wearable sensors to detect emotional status (Hwang, Jebelli, Choi, Choi, & Lee, 2018). Such data could be useful in a personalized nutrition system to evaluate stress status or mood and tailor food selection appropriately. The emotional response to eating a food or meal could be also be used to provide data on preference, that could improve future suggestions. Several sensing approaches are being evaluated, including heart rate monitoring, galvanic skin response, image-based facial activity, and EEG (electroencephalography) (Subramanian et al., 2018), that could potentially provide inputs to a personalized nutrition system.

MODERN TECHNOLOGIES AND ENERGY EXPENDITURE (EXERCISE)

Wearable Technology: Activity Trackers and Smart Watches

There is a variety of wearable technologies available in the market that monitor energy expenditure and heart health. Physical activity trackers help measure personal metrics involved in fitness, such as number of steps walked, heart rate, quality of sleep, etc. They come predominantly in the form of wristbands (e.g., Fitbit, Mio) and smartwatches (e.g., Apple Watch, Samsung Gear, Garmin). There seems to be a fine line separating them, with the demarcation becoming quite blurry. Fitbit is the most popular brand of activity trackers with 25 million active users generating more than US$1.6 billion in revenue in 2017 (Fitbit, 2018). Other wearable technologies include chest straps (e.g., Polar H10, QardioCore), patches (e.g., BioPatch, Kenzen Patch), strips (e.g., FitLinxx AmpStrip), and shirts (e.g., Zephry Shirt). Activity trackers typically sync to smart devices and/or upload to computers using wireless connectivity. The companion apps, depending on the product, also enable the users to record and track things like food consumption, activities, weight, ECG, heart rate, and temperature; and can share the data with trainers and medical professionals. Researchers have demonstrated that the data from a wearable device and its companion smartphone app can be integrated into electronic health record systems

(Wang, Coleman, Kanter, Ummer, & Siminerio, 2018). It should be noted that since these wearable devices collect a multitude of health-related data, privacy and security controls to prevent misuse or abuse of the data are of significant concern (Subedar & El-Khatib, 2015; Zhou & Piramuthu, 2014).

While wearable devices do require certain degrees of user inputs for accurate tracking (Shen, Ho, & Srivastava, 2018), research seems to indicate that they may be suitable as physical activity monitoring platforms (Amor & James, 2017) and are reasonably accurate for estimating heart rate (Koshy et al., 2017), number of steps, distance, and sleep duration (Xie et al., 2018). Fitbits have been used in a variety of research studies targeting physical activity (Winfree & Dominick, 2017), sleep tracking (Liang & Nishimura, 2017), and effectiveness in enabling sustainable lifestyle changes (Randriambelonoro, Chen, & Pu, 2017). Fitbits have also been shown to be an accurate, reliable, and efficient tool for physicians to track the adoption and maintenance of physical activity programs (Diaz et al., 2015). However, there is some skepticism regarding their benefits for monitoring physical activity and other measures (Jakicic et al., 2016; Mishra, Nieto, & Kitsiou, 2017; Ridgers, McNarry, & Mackintosh, 2016). Research also shows that the heart rate monitoring function is more accurate at rest than during moderately active exercise and may not be suitable in helping clinicians advise their patients about health issues (Cadmus-Bertram, Gangnon, Wirkus, Thraen-Borowski, & Gorzelitz-Liebhauser, 2017). A recent study has indicated that the physical indicator measurements of smartwatches are affected by activity states and there is a need to improve their algorithms for different activity states (Xie et al., 2018). The same study also found the accuracy of measurement of energy consumption to be inadequate. It should be noted that the pace of the business sector and consumer demand outstrips science reporting and there are often noticeable gaps between the devices used in most studies and those available in the market (Ridgers et al., 2016).

Manufacturers are in a race to make medical grade monitoring available with wearable devices. A recent partnership between Fitbit and Dexcom is promising to bring continuous glucose monitoring (CGM) by integrating the popular Dexcom G5 sensor to the Fitbit Ionic. Medical equipment manufactures like Omron are poised to enter the market with their smart watch Omron HeartGuide that can provide medical grade blood pressure measurements and sleep tracking. There are also products on the horizon (e.g., Cronovo smartwatch) that can provide accurate heart rate functions along with prescribing fitness regimes based on individual physical characteristics and guiding the user through video tutorials, calorie and dietary intake tracking, and integrating these functionalities with voice-based recipes.

MODERN TECHNOLOGIES AND FOOD PREPARATION

There is a range of intelligent technologies that can be used in food preparation. This includes connected devices, such as smart kitchen scales and ovens, which are rapidly becoming widely available, through to concept assistive kitchens that can guide the user through food preparation and even an example of a completely automated kitchen. Printed foods are another automated way of preparing foods and are emerging as a real option.

Assistive Kitchens

Concept kitchens that can guide the user through the steps of preparation and cooking have been demonstrated by both Miele (Miele, 2017)—called "the invisible kitchen"—and IKEA (Ideo, 2015). These kitchens use a range of connected smart kitchen appliances, load cells, video cameras that interpret what is happening, and projectors that project images and instructions onto the kitchen bench or a screen on the wall. A working prototype of the Miele kitchen, called "Kognichef," has been fully described and demonstrated (Neumann et al., 2017). It can be expected that over the next decade, fully assistive kitchen systems will become available with the capacity to interface with personal nutrition information to guide the preparation of customized meals.

Automated Food Preparation

An automated fast food restaurant kitchen has been developed at the Massachusetts Institute of Technology (IFT, 2016) and is now in commercial operation in a Boston restaurant called "Spyce" (www.spyce.com). The restaurant is limited to stir-fry type meals served as fast food and uses a unique robotic mixer-cooker. The meals include vegetarian, vegan, and gluten-free dishes, and all dishes have a stated list of ingredients and calories (including known allergens), but full nutritional composition is not listed. It would be relatively simple to calculate nutritional value from the ingredients if actual amounts were available, thus facilitating inclusion in a personalized nutrition plan. A further step would be having the ingredients for the stir-fry being selected specifically for the customer at the time of ordering, through their personalized nutrition AI engine.

A concept two-arm robotic kitchen system has been promoted by a company called Moley and may become a reality in the future.

3-D Printed Food

Three-dimensional printing of food has been around on a small scale for some years now. Printers are mostly the same robotic systems that are used for 3-D printing of plastics, but modified so that food pastes can be printed. Early examples include printed confections like pancakes and chocolate and there are commercial bakeries and confectionaries that use 3D food printers. Current commercially available 3-D food printers (a list is available at www.aniwaa.com/food-3d-printers/) range from simple printers that children can use and learn with (e.g., PancakeBot, ZBot) to printers aimed at restaurants and bakeries (e.g., byFlow). The traveling pop-up restaurant FoodInk has been serving meals with all components (including seats and tables, and cutlery and plates as well as food) made by 3-D printing. 3-D printing allows a high degree of personalization in terms of the shape and design of a meal and its components. However, the current technology is restricted to a range of food pastes that can be used for printing. Therefore there is little scope for personalized nutritional design. As the technology improves there is potential for printing customized food with optimized nutritional content based on biometric and/or genomic data. One printer, the DeltaWasp, has an option developed with the capability of printing gluten-free foods (www.3dprint.com/166204/wasp-gluten-free-3d-printer/), and printed foods especially designed for elderly patients with dysphagia have been described (Kira, 2015). In principle, printed foods could be customized to a high degree from quite a small number of components using a mass customization approach (Boland, 2006, 2008), and the recent literature proposes personalization strategies for printed foods (Jie, Weibiao, Liangkun, Dejian, & Lien-Ya, 2017). However, most food printers have a single extruder, so custom mixtures are not readily available, and some form of personalized premix would be needed. One printer, RoVaPaste, has a dual extruder, which makes a degree of customization of composition possible, but we await more complex extrusion systems before true personalized nutrition becomes available directly through 3-D printed foods.

MODERN TECHNOLOGIES AND FOOD COMPOSITION

In any form of nutrition and diet management it is necessary to understand the nutritional composition of all foods being consumed, not only to monitor the intake of nutrients, but also to protect against intake of components that may be undesirable for an individual.

Labeling

Labeling of packaged foods, including a nutritional panel, is commonplace and mandated in many jurisdictions. Labeling generally includes a barcode that is scanned at the till when a product is purchased. This scanning identifies the product and its price for the supermarket and the purchaser, but it also has the potential to link into databases of food composition and to a home inventory system and could thus inform a personal nutrition system. The reliability of labeling with respect to composition is an important issue, as manufacturers may change the composition of a product over time for a variety of good reasons. The not-for-profit organization GS1 (www.GS1.org) maintains global standards for the GS1 barcode system and ensures the best available data are attached to the barcode, but the onus is on manufacturers to ensure all data are up to date.

Intelligent Packaging

New generation intelligent packaging (smart packaging) will do much more than just labels. Packaging will be able to sense things about the contents, environment, and history. Current sensing capabilities include (Janjarasskul & Suppakul, 2018):

- temperature sensing;
- ripeness of fruit;
- intactness of the packaging;
- range of temperature exposure (time—temperature indicators); and/or
- spoilage.

In some cases these packages or their labels are connected via RFID tags.

Smart packaging of the future will be more connected, enabling better supply chain management (e.g., supply chain visibility has been estimated to be able to save the fresh foods industry globally about US$3 billion), and inventory management in the home, in the store, and in the warehouse.

To communicate packages need to be able to broadcast—if only over a short distance. This requires a power source, which can come from local magnetic fields over a very short range (transponder type) but needs an inbuilt power source for longer range transmission (such as Bluetooth or Wi-Fi). Passive sensors can operate without power sources typically by receiving an externally transmitted signal through an antenna, modifying the signal through some functionalized material (e.g., temperature, RH, ionic strength dependence), and reflecting the signal back for interpretation (Kassal, Steinberg, & Steinberg, 2018). These technologies are attractive because they are small and do not required direct powering, however they suffer from short read distances (ranging from cm to a few m). A number of both passive and active wireless sensors are reviewed by Kassal et al. (2018) that could be implemented as wearable or smart packaging technologies.

There are issues to be overcome before truly smart packaging can become mainstream, including challenges of:

- reliability and robustness;
- price (microchips cost 10–50 cents);
- food safety in case of contact; and
- recyclability (EU regulations are under review as to whether printed electronics should be treated as e-waste).

New packaging developments using hybrid printed electronics built into the packaging or labeling are making this close to a reality and some prototypes exist (Feng, Xie, Chen, & Zheng, 2015; Javed et al., 2016). An example where intelligent connected packaging has been demonstrated is the Johnnie Walker Blue Label whisky bottle launched in 2015, which has a label with near-field communication that can communicate with a smartphone (Kite-Powell, 2015). Although there are challenges to be overcome, intelligent packaging can be expected to become increasingly available and, if widely adopted, could simplify inventory and diet management.

Sensing and Analysis

In the absence of other data about composition, and especially in cases such as fresh foods, where cultivation, growth, age, and ripeness may be considerations, other approaches are necessary. One option to obtain data on the composition of foods is the use of so-called "pocket scanners" (for example the Scio pocket scanner www.consumerphysics.com accessed July 2018), which connect to a smartphone and scan the surface of food using near-infrared reflectance spectrometry and are able to report composition. They are limited in that they can see only the surface of the food, but they have shown promise in some circumstances, such as determining the sugar content of fruit (Kaur, Kunnemeyer, & Mcglone, 2017). These devices are at an early stage of development for nutritional purposes.

Allergens and Other Undesirables

An important consideration in personalized nutrition—or for the nutrition of any individual—is total avoidance of foods or food ingredients that will cause adverse health effects. This includes substances that may cause allergic reactions and foods that may interact unfavorably with pharmaceuticals that they may be taking. Most jurisdictions have had clear regulations about labeling for possible allergens for the last decade or so. Possible allergens (usually of the 8–10 commonest classes of allergens) are required to be clearly printed on the label of packaged foods. Fresh whole foods are obvious to most as to what they are, so hidden allergens in them are unlikely to be a problem. The biggest concern of possible hidden allergens is in restaurant meals, although increasingly restaurants are identifying options that are, for example, dairy-free or gluten-free. For an AI-driven personal nutrition assistive system, it will be necessary to record any specific allergies for the individual, and to interface with package labels, images, and menus to ensure proper warnings and exclusions.

For people on long-term treatments with pharmaceuticals, there can be certain foods that are incompatible. A common example is for people on statins, which regulate cholesterol production. If these people ingest naringenin, and other phenolic compounds found in grapefruit, an adverse interaction occurs with the statins (Hare & Elliott, 2003). For this reason an AI system that guides personalized nutrition will need to have access to medical records, particularly prescribed pharmaceuticals, and take account of any necessary food restrictions.

BRINGING IT ALL TOGETHER

The Intelligent Kitchen and Its Role in Personalized Nutrition

An AI system like Kognichef or the IKEA concept kitchen can guide a cook through recipes (Neumann et al., 2017). The assistive aspect of the cooking can be tied to personalized caloric and nutritional information (Chen, Karvela, Sohbati, Shinawatra, & Toumazou, 2018). Machine learning algorithms are being developed to provide personalized recommendations based on nutritional requirements (Chen et al., 2018). The AI translates nutrient recommendations resulting from health and dietary requirements into recipes and ingredient lists. An ideal system should also accept feedback from users to fine-tune and adjust meal plans and consider cost and availability of ingredients and the individual's cooking skills.

Food Service and Management of Personalized Nutrition

While management of diet in the home can be achieved when guided by the labeling of packaged goods and the general knowledge of the composition of fresh foods, the situation for out of home eating is rather different. It has been estimated that nearly half of the world's population eats out at least once a week (Nielsen, 2016), and many of us more often than that. Understanding the composition or nutritional values for restaurant and other food service dishes is therefore important. The nutritional composition of food from the major chains of restaurants in the United States is available through the website Menustat.org, and these values are likely to be valid for those chains where they extend outside the United States, although this would need to be verified. One of the problems with nutritional values from many of these restaurants is that while the composition of dishes is known, serving sizes can vary, thus altering intake values (Niederman, Leonard, & Clapp, 2017). The situation with independent restaurants is different: being able to report and manage meal composition is beyond the means of most, both technically and in terms of compliance costs (Brown et al., 2017).

There are some other possibilities for obtaining nutritional values for restaurant foods, although they have limitations. The most commonly reported is image analysis (as discussed earlier), through photographs from a smartphone or e-button (see Hassannejad et al., 2017 for a recent review of this topic). Image analysis does not always accurately identify foods, but it can be augmented by system knowledge of the consumer's preferences or through a selection of alternatives, or from situational aspects (such as GPS location and a restaurant menu). Image analysis also has limitations in estimating portion size. Another option to obtain the composition of foods is the use of so-called "pocket scanners," as described earlier in this chapter.

The eHealth and mHealth Environment—Toward a Personal Virtual Dietitian

The concept of a virtual dietitian has been around for nearly a decade, although most of the recent focus has been on the combination of diet management apps and/or diet monitoring apps with professional advice and support. It is useful to distinguish between many services that have been touted as virtual dietitian services that are in fact really tele-dietitian or remote dietitian services (involving a registered dietitian with remote monitoring and online consultation), and a truly automated, AI-driven virtual dietitian. A fully AI-driven personal virtual dietitian has yet to be described. Such a system could be expected to use a combination of wearable sensors, such as described earlier, automated diet/food intake monitoring, activity tracking, and input from smart scales to provide continual dietary recommendations on a frequent, user-selectable basis, but also providing unsolicited warnings if a risk is detected by the system (e.g., a food allergy or drug incompatibility), probably via a smartphone.

The Artificial Intelligence Engine That Drives Personalized Nutrition

An artificial intelligence (AI) engine is required to select foods and build a menu plan given the variety of input data sources available. In addition to access to appropriate data sources, the AI engine consists of an optimization algorithm and an objective function (or target).

A range of methods have been reported in the literature for optimization, the first in 1964 using linear programming (Balintfy, 1964). Ngo et al (2016) and Mák et al. (2010) provide good reviews of the different classes of optimization or expert systems that have been applied to menu planning, including case- or rule-based reasoning, mixed integer linear programming models, genetic algorithms, and fuzzy logic. Early approaches limited the scope of the problem to enable implementation of the optimization methods, however with modern computing methods, more sophisticated and comprehensive data-driven AI approaches are being applied to menu planning (Ngo et al., 2016). More recent examples include multiple objective expert systems that seek to achieve optimal solutions on a meal, daily, and weekly food level (Mák et al., 2010), and optimization based on bioinspired algorithms such as cat swarm, wolf search (Moldovan et al., 2017), particle swarm (Chifu, Bonta, Chifu, Salomie, & Moldovan, 2017), and bacterial foraging (Hernández-Ocaña, Chávez-Bosquez, Hernández-Torruco, Canul-Reich, & Pozos-Parra, 2018).

Any optimization process needs a target function, the outcome goal that changes in diet are aimed at achieving. These targets could include weight loss, maintenance of current health status, lowering of blood pressure, precaution against dietary-related disease (such as prediabetic conditions, high blood pressure, dyslipidemia), and fitness improvement. Development of an AI engine requires formalization of these objective functions. One approach is to select recipes, foods, and portion sizes based on mass and energy balances to meet recommended daily intake (RDI) guidelines for macro- and micronutrients (Institute of Medicine, 2000). Methods exist to vary RDI to account for a specific consumer's medical history, body parameters (e.g., BMI), and level of physical activity. An alternative approach used for systems based on deep learning fuzzy or neural networks includes training of the system based on data, potentially based on dietitian-prescribed menus for specific patients or populations (Zenun Franco, 2017).

Hernández-Ocaña et al. (2018) implemented a hierarchy of four objective functions based on guidelines from Pedro Escudero, a prominent nutritionist in Latin America. These are:

- *Quantity*: that considers the energy needs of the body.
- *Quality*: that considers a balance between food groups.
- *Harmony*: that considers interactions between ingested nutrients.
- *Adequacy*: that considers the nutritional, social, and psychological needs of the user.

Chen et al (2018) reported an AI implementation named PERSON (personalized expert recommendation system for optimal nutrition). In this instance deep learning neural network models were used to present personalized meal plans based on several filtering approaches, including filtering based on individual users' genetic data and phenotypic information.

A Potential Architecture of a Personalized Nutrition System

Fig. 8.2 demonstrates a potential architecture of a Personalized Nutrition AI Engine. It is made up of five interacting levels centered around the AI engine itself (Level 3). Level 1 is a collection of information around food and ingredient availability, preparation methods (recipes), and the nutritional properties associated with them. Many countries have developed their own food compositional databases (Haytowitz & Pehrsson, 2018, Sivakumaran, Huffman, & Sivakumaran, 2018; Watanabe & Kawai, 2018), primarily

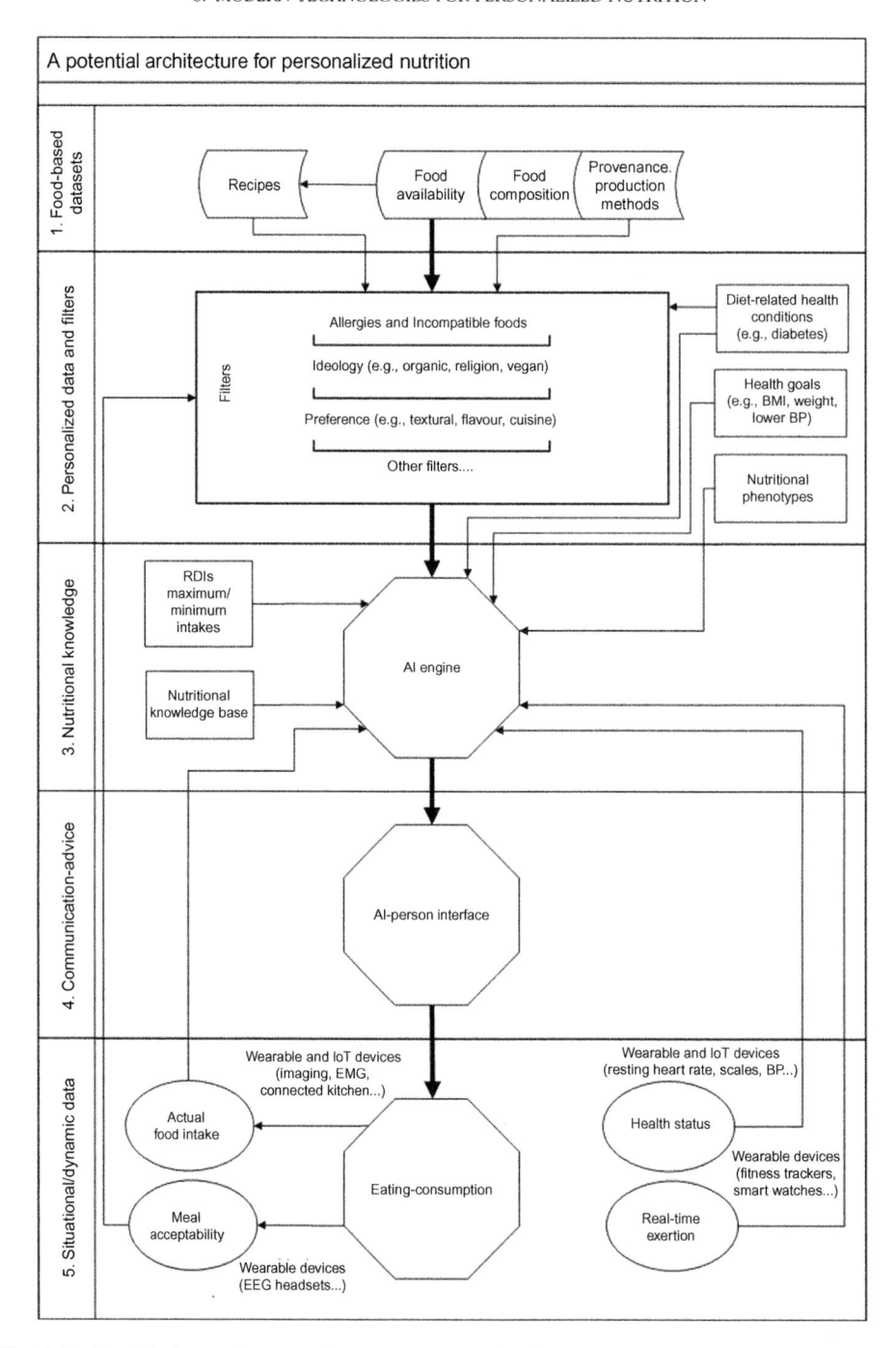

FIGURE 8.2 Possible data architecture for a smart personalized nutrition system.

B. APPLICATIONS OF PERSONALIZED NUTRITION

because growing conditions, soil types, etc. can affect nutrient levels. Differing formulations are sometimes used for global products in different markets and different reporting requirements are required by different countries. FoodCASE (Presser, Weber, & Norrie, 2018) and Food Explorer (EuroFIR - European Food Information Resource) have been developed as systems to manage the acquisition, management, and processing of multiple data sources. Additional tools such as Food Basket (EuorFIR) allow the prediction of nutrient compositions of combined and prepared foods from ingredients. These systems together with recipe databases form the set of foods from which the AI engine can potentially select.

Level 2 contains person-specific metadata, obtained either from the consumer directly or through linkage to other databases, such as medical information and genetic or phenotypic data, as discussed above. This information is relatively constant and may also include information like ideology, allergies, textural preferences, favored cuisines, medical conditions, medication, location, season, favored food suppliers, and health goals (weight loss or maintenance, fitness improvement). The overall set of available foods (from Level 1) will be reduced to a smaller subset through filtering using this information. Some foods will be eliminated completely because of a consumer's allergies, medical conditions (and treatments), or beliefs (e.g., foods containing gluten for sufferers of celiac's disease, pork products for Jewish or Muslim individuals, or animal products for vegans). Other filters may reduce (rather than eliminate) the likelihood of a food being selected (such as a preference for organic produce) or increase the chances of selection (e.g., if it is available in the pantry or refrigerator).

A range of different methods are required to communicate the outputs of the AI engine (Level 4), as discussed elsewhere in this chapter. The last level in the personalized nutrition system (Level 5) is centered around dynamic and situational data. Information on exercise done throughout the day (e.g., from a fitness tracker) may lead to modifications to the meal plans produced by the AI engine. For example, if more or less than expected exercise levels are achieved, portion size could be modified, or alternative recipes could be substituted or added. Similarly, if wearable technology or a smart kitchen system can identify actual food intake, the planned food intake for the remainder of the day can be adjusted. If mood or emotion measuring devices are used, then personalized databases on food preference could be updated as each meal is consumed. Alternative meals could potentially be substituted by the AI engine, subject to the mood measured by the EEG technology, for example, substituting a new recipe for an old favorite, or comfort food after a stressful day.

For each component of the personalized nutrition system, extra data will provide a greater level of sophistication and make the system more attractive to potential users. For example, the use of wearable technologies to track food intake will not only improve the potential accuracy of the AI engine predictions, it will reduce the manual input of data required from the end user, minimizing the overhead required to achieve tangible benefits. The screening of potential foods or ingredients by the AI engine, based on provenance considerations or flavor/textural preference, will reduce the risk of advocating recipes that don't appeal to the user and choosing to ignore advice or substitute a suboptimal meal replacement.

AREAS THAT NEED TO BE ADDRESSED

We have described a wide range of devices and datasets that could be incorporated into an AI-driven personalized nutrition support system. Before such a system can be developed and used with confidence, there are some issues that need to be addressed.

Privacy and Security

Privacy and security of personal data is a concern for everyone, particularly when health records are concerned. Increasingly, health records are kept online or in the cloud, and individuals can access their own medical records via a simple login. Any AI system for medically-supported personalized nutrition would need to be able to ensure privacy and security of these records. On most HISs, eHealth records are simply password protected and susceptible to being hacked. Biometric security is an emerging technology, and a recent announcement of heartbeat pattern being used for protection of medical records is an example of the new options that are being considered (Brown, 2017).

Food Monitoring

There are several aspects of food monitoring that need attention:

- Natural whole foods, such as fruits and vegetables, or fish and meat, can vary considerably in composition, according to genetics (varieties and breeds), methods of production, and degree of maturity or ripeness. This means that any estimate of nutritional composition will have a degree of error or uncertainty. Whether these variations are enough to matter is unclear, but certain aspects, such as the conversion of starch to sugars during the ripening of fruit and some vegetables, will be of concern to some. In this context, portable infrared scanners have shown some promise (Kaur et al., 2017).
- For packaged, processed foods, full nutritional labeling is commonplace and can generally be picked up from the product's barcode. To what extent all food products are fully compliant with their nutritional panels is unclear, but it can be expected that most will be quite accurate. Nevertheless, it is important that rigor is maintained around nutritional labeling.
- While systems can accurately determine what foods are purchased, there also needs to be an accounting of food that is wasted—either not served or left on the plate after a meal. Image analysis of the plate before and after a meal can be helpful, but systems are not well developed to account for this.
- Nutrition in cohabiting groups is an issue that needs to be addressed: most households include more than one occupant for whom food is to be prepared. In this case, meal planning will need to consider the personalized nutrition needs of all members, and simple tracking of overall consumption will not be enough to account for intakes. These issues can be managed but will need to be considered as new technologies and systems develop for personalized nutrition in the home.

Reliability and Consistency of Smartphone Apps

While there is a wide range of apps to support mHealth, diets, and nutrition, there is no regulatory framework to support the accuracy of these apps. A recent review identified more than 165,000 mobile health apps and stated:

> These apps have the potential to provide low-cost, around-the-clock access to high-quality, evidence-based health information to end users on a global scale. However, they have not yet lived up to their potential due to multiple barriers, including lack of regulatory oversight, limited evidence-based literature, and concerns of privacy and security. The future directions may consist of improving data integration into the health care system, an interoperable app platform allowing access to electronic health record data, cloud-based personal health record across health care networks, and increasing app prescription by health care providers. For consumer mobile health apps to fully contribute value to health care delivery and chronic disease management, all stakeholders within the ecosystem must collaborate to overcome the significant barriers. (Kao & Liebovitz, 2017)

There are issues around the accuracy of nutrition and diet apps too. A recent survey in Germany of three apps selected from a random sample of 100 nutrition apps from Google Play identified significant variances in the caloric values ascribed to different foods, up to 66% in one case (Holzmann, Proell, Hauner, & Holzapfel, 2017).

It is to be expected that in the near future there should be a system for quality control and/or certification and approval for such apps, and that qualified apps will be sufficiently accurate and reliable to be supported by the medical profession and integrated into health care plans.

Notwithstanding this, there is plentiful evidence that a significant proportion of consumers will start using a nutrition app, but not stick with it for more than a few weeks. (For a discussion of nutrition and fitness app uptake behaviors see Konig, Sproesser, Schupp, & Renner, 2018.) There appears to be better compliance when a dietitian is involved, or when a clinical condition (such as diabetes) is present. A stand-alone app may not be the answer for general consumers, but apps may be better used as part of a larger self-managing system.

Nutritional Values and Bioaccessibility

One of the current weaknesses of all nutritional data on foods is that reported values are for the nutrients as they are contained in the food. It has become increasingly clear over recent decades that just because nutrients are contained in a food, they are not necessarily digested or taken up into the body to the full extent they exist in the food. Moreover, it is not just the extent to which nutrients are taken up, but the rate at which they are taken up that becomes important. This has been highlighted for carbohydrates by the reporting of glycemic index, a measure especially important to diabetics (Russell et al., 2016), and more recently for protein nutrition, particularly in the elderly (Dardevet et al., 2012).

The availability of nutrients can be substantially altered by food processing and preparation that can change natural structures in food (e.g., denaturation and cross-linking of proteins and pasting of starch) to alter bioaccessibility (Nayak, Berrios, & Tang, 2014; Singh, Dartois, & Kaur, 2010). This can affect not only what is digested, but also what is left over for fermentation by the microbiota in the colon. Additionally, the fermentation activities of the microbiota can have an important effect on health: this is an emerging area that will increasingly be taken into account.

Interactions of food components during eating and digestion (food synergy) can also change digestibility—for example, fruit proteases, such as actinidin from kiwifruit, can enhance digestion of proteins (Montoya et al., 2014), and conversely tannins and other plant phenolics in the diet can cross-link proteins—and other nutrients—and make them unavailable (Velickovic & Stanic-Vucinic, 2018).

These issues are not specific to personalized nutrition but are of concern to all engaged in providing nutritional advice, and they are increasingly being taken into account when developing diets and meal plans.

FUTURE PERSPECTIVE

The automated, AI-driven management of food, meals, and overall diet outlined at the start of this chapter may seem futuristic, but it may not be as far away as one might think. We should be reminded of the quote from Bill Gates, founder of Microsoft and now one of the most influential people in the world. In his early (1995) book "The Road Ahead," written when the Internet was in its infancy, he said, "We always overestimate the change that will occur in the next two years and underestimate the change that will occur in the next ten. Don't let yourself be lulled into inaction." If the pace of change over the past two decades has been rapid, it can be expected to be even greater over the next one and we can confidently expect systems such as we have described, and even beyond that, to be commonplace within ten years. That is not to say they will be universally adopted, because the rate of change of public acceptance can be much slower than the rate of advance of technology, but the systems will be there for those who want to use them. As demographics change, with digital natives becoming the main part of the population, we can expect more rapid uptake in the future, with the consequence of substantial public health benefits through a decrease in and better management of NCDs.

CONCLUSION

There is a wide range of relatively new technologies and applications that can assist with personalized nutrition. However, a holistic system that brings them together does not yet exist. Moreover, there are severe deficiencies in some of the assistive systems, notably smartphone apps, that bring into question their accuracy, reliability, and hence usefulness in their present state. There is a need for oversight and regulation of these systems to ensure appropriateness, accuracy, and reliability of all components before any system can be relied on for dietary advice. Notwithstanding these limitations, there is good scope for at least partial systems to manage personalized nutrition, and undoubtedly new, better systems will emerge in the near future.

References

Ahn, J., Williamson, J., Gartrell, M., Han, R., Lv, Q., & Mishra, S. (2015). Supporting healthy grocery shopping via mobile augmented reality. *ACM Transactions on Multimedia Computing Communications and Applications*, 12. Available from https://doi.org/10.1145/2808207.

Allen, A. (2017). *A hospital without patients* [Online]. POLITICO. <https://www.politico.com/agenda/story/2017/11/08/virtual-hospital-mercy-st-louis-000573> Accessed 24.07.18.

Amor, J. D., & James, C. J. (2017). Validation of a commercial android smartwatch as an activity monitoring platform. *IEEE Journal of Biomedical and Health Informatics*, 22, 968–978.

Balintfy, J. L. (1964). Menu planning by computer. *Communications of the ACM*, 7(4), 255–259.

Boland, M. (2006). Perspective mass customisation of food. *Journal of the Science of Food and Agriculture*, 86, 7–9. Available from https://doi.org/10.1002/jsfa.2348.

Boland, M. (2008). Innovation in the food industry: Personalised nutrition and mass customisation. *Innovation-Management Policy & Practice*, 10, 53–60. Available from https://doi.org/10.5172/impp.453.10.1.53.

Brown, B. (2017). *Heartbeat electrical signature protects medical records* [Online]. <https://healthtechinsider.com/2017/11/27/heartbeat-electrical-signature-protects-medical-records/> Accessed 24.07.18.

Brown, T., Vanderlinden, L., Birks, A., Mamatis, D., Levy, J., & Sahay, T. (2017). Bringing menu labelling to independent restaurants: Findings from a Voluntary Pilot Project in Toronto. *Canadian Journal of Dietetic Practice and Research*, 78, 177–181. Available from https://doi.org/10.3148/cjdpr-2017-014.

Cade, J. E. (2017). Measuring diet in the 21st century: Use of new technologies. *Proceedings of the Nutrition Society*, 76, 276–282. Available from https://doi.org/10.1017/s0029665116002883.

Cadmus-Bertram, L., Gangnon, R., Wirkus, E. J., Thraen-Borowski, K. M., & Gorzelitz-Liebhauser, J. (2017). The accuracy of heart rate monitoring by some wrist-worn activity trackers. *Annals of Internal Medicine*, 166(8), 610–612.

Chen, C.-H., Karvela, M., Sohbati, M., Shinawatra, T., & Toumazou, C. (2018). PERSON-Personalized Expert Recommendation System for Optimized Nutrition. *IEEE Transactions on Biomedical Circuits and Systems*, 12, 151–160. Available from https://doi.org/10.1109/tbcas.2017.2760504.

Chifu, V., Bonta, R., Chifu, E. S., Salomie, I., & Moldovan, D. (2017). *Particle swarm optimization based method for personalized menu recommendations*. International conference on advancements of medicine and health care through technology; 12–5th October 2016, Cluj-Napoca, Romania (pp. 232–237). Cham: Springer.

Dardevet, D., Remond, D., Peyron, M. A., Papet, I., Savary-Auzeloux, I., & Mosoni, L. (2012). Muscle wasting and resistance of muscle anabolism: The "Anabolic Threshold Concept" for adapted nutritional strategies during Sarcopenia. *Scientific World Journal*, 269531. Available from https://doi.org/10.1100/2012/269531.

Dehghan, M., & Merchant, A. T. (2008). Is bioelectrical impedance accurate for use in large epidemiological studies? *Nutrition Journal*, 7, 26. Available from https://doi.org/10.1186/1475-2891-7-26.

Diaz, K. M., Krupka, D. J., Chang, M. J., Peacock, J., Ma, Y., Goldsmith, J., ... Davidson, K. W. (2015). Fitbit: An accurate and reliable device for wireless physical activity tracking. *International Journal of Cardiology*, 185, 138–140.

Dunford, E., Trevena, H., Goodsell, C., Ka Hung, N., Webster, J., Millis, A., ... Neal, B. (2014). FoodSwitch: A mobile phone app to enable consumers to make healthier food choices and crowdsourcing of national food composition data. *JMIR mHealth and uHealth*, 2. Available from https://doi.org/10.2196/mhealth.3230.

Feng, Y., Xie, L., Chen, Q., & Zheng, L.-R. (2015). Low-cost printed chipless RFID humidity sensor tag for intelligent packaging. *IEEE Sensors Journal*, 15(6), 3201–3208.

Fitbit. (2018). <https://investor.fitbit.com/press/press-releases/press-release-details/2018/Fitbit-Reports-571M-Q417-and-1616B-FY17-Revenue/default.aspx> Accessed 17.07.18.

Food Basket. http://www.eurofir.org/our-tools/foodbasket/.

Food Explorer. http://www.eurofir.org/our-tools/foodexplorer/.

Gutiérrez, F., Cardoso, B., & Verbert, K. (2017). PHARA: A Personal Health Augmented Reality Assistant to support decision-making at grocery stores. In *Second international workshop on Health Recommender Systems co-located with ACM RecSys 2017*. Como, Italy. <http://ceur-ws.org/Vol-1953/healthRecSys17_paper_7.pdf> Accessed 24.07.18.

Hare, J. T., & Elliott, D. P. (2003). Grapefruit juice and potential drug interactions. *The Consultant Pharmacist: The Journal of the American Society of Consultant Pharmacists*, 18, 466–472.

Hassannejad, H., Matrella, G., Ciampolini, P., De Munari, I., Mordonini, M., & Cagnoni, S. (2017). Automatic diet monitoring: A review of computer vision and wearable sensor-based methods. *International Journal of Food Sciences and Nutrition, 68*, 656–670. Available from https://doi.org/10.1080/09637486.2017.1283683.

Haytowitz, D. B., & Pehrsson, P. R. (2018). USDA's National Food and Nutrient Analysis Program (NFNAP) produces high-quality data for USDA food composition databases: Two decades of collaboration. *Food Chemistry, 238*, 134–138.

Hernández-Ocaña, B., Chávez-Bosquez, O., Hernández-Torruco, J., Canul-Reich, J., & Pozos-Parra, P. (2018). Bacterial foraging optimization algorithm for menu planning. *IEEE Access, 6*, 8619–8629.

Herranz, L., Jiang, S., & Xu, R. (2017). Modeling restaurant context for food recognition. *IEEE Transactions on Multimedia, 19*, 430–440. Available from https://doi.org/10.1109/tmm.2016.2614861.

Holzmann, S. L., Proell, K., Hauner, H., & Holzapfel, C. (2017). Nutrition-Apps: Quality and limitations an explorative investigation on the basis of selected Example-Apps. *Ernährungs Umschau, 64*, M260–M269.

Hung, M. (2017). *Leading the IoT*. Gartner Research. <https://www.gartner.com/imagesrv/books/iot/iotEbook_digital.pdf> Accessed 24.07.18.

Hwang, S., Jebelli, H., Choi, B., Choi, M., & Lee, S. (2018). Measuring workers' emotional state during construction tasks using wearable EEG. *Journal of Construction Engineering and Management, 144*(7), 04018050.

Ideo. (2015). *Concept Kitchen 2025* [Online]. <http://conceptkitchen2025.ideo.london/#Collaboration> Accessed 24.07.18.

IFT. (2016). MIT students invent robotic kitchen. *Food Technology, 70*, 17.

Institute of Medicine. (2000). *Dietary reference intakes: Applications in dietary assessment*. Washington, DC: National Academies Press.

Jakicic, J. M., Davis, K. K., Rogers, R. J., King, W. C., Marcus, M. D., Helsel, D., . . . Belle, S. H. (2016). Effect of wearable technology combined with a lifestyle intervention on long-term weight loss: The IDEA randomized clinical trial. *JAMA, 316*(11), 1161–1171.

Janjarasskul, T., & Suppakul, P. (2018). Active and intelligent packaging: The indication of quality and safety. *Critical Reviews in Food Science and Nutrition, 58*, 808–831. Available from https://doi.org/10.1080/10408398.2016.1225278.

Javed, N., Habib, A., Amin, Y., Loo, J., Akram, A., & Tenhunen, H. (2016). Directly printable moisture sensor tag for intelligent packaging. *IEEE Sensors Journal, 16*(16), 6147–6148.

Jie, S., Weibiao, Z., Liangkun, Y., Dejian, H., & Lien-Ya, L. (2017). Extrusion-based food printing for digitalized food design and nutrition control. *Journal of Food Engineering, 220*, 1–11. Available from https://doi.org/10.1016/j.jfoodeng.2017.02.028.

Kao, C.-K., & Liebovitz, D. M. (2017). Consumer mobile health apps: Current state, barriers, and future directions. *PM&R, 9*, S106–S115. Available from https://doi.org/10.1016/j.pmrj.2017.02.018.

Kassal, P., Steinberg, M. D., & Steinberg, I. M. (2018). Wireless chemical sensors and biosensors: A review. *Sensors and Actuators B: Chemical, 266*, 228–245. Available from https://doi.org/10.1016/j.snb.2018.03.074.

Kaur, H., Kunnemeyer, R., & Mcglone, A. (2017). Comparison of hand-held near infrared spectrophotometers for fruit dry matter assessment. *Journal of Near Infrared Spectroscopy, 25*, 267–277. Available from https://doi.org/10.1177/0967033517725530.

Kira. (2015). *EU develops PERFORMANCE 3D printed food for elderly and patients with dysphagia* [Online]. <http://www.3ders.org/articles/20151026-eu-develops-performance-3d-printed-food-for-elderly-and-patients-with-dysphagia.html> Accessed 22.06.18.

Kite-Powell, J. (2015). *Johnnie Walker Smart Bottle Debuts at Mobile World Congress* [Online]. Forbes. <https://www.forbes.com/sites/jenniferhicks/2015/03/02/johnnie-walker-smart-bottle-debuts-at-mobile-world-congress/#3a0804147ca1> Accessed 24.07.18.

Konig, L. M., Sproesser, G., Schupp, H. T., & Renner, B. (2018). Describing the process of adopting nutrition and fitness apps: Behavior stage model approach. *JMIR mHealth and uHealth, 6*(3), e55.

Koshy, A. N., Sajeev, J., Zureik, M., Street, M., Wong, M. C., Roberts, L., & Teh, A. W. (2017). Accuracy of smart watches in arrhythmias: Smarts study. *Journal of the American College of Cardiology, 69*(11 Supplement), 337.

Liang, Z., & Nishimura, T. (2017). Are wearable EEG devices more accurate than fitness wristbands for home sleep tracking? Comparison of consumer sleep trackers with clinical devices. In *2017 IEEE 6th global conference on consumer electronics (GCCE 2017)* (pp. 1–5). doi: 10.1109/GCCE.2017.8229188.

Mák, E., Pintér, B., Gaál, B., Vassányi, I., Kozmann, G., & Németh, I. (2010). *A formal domain model for dietary and physical activity counseling*. International conference on knowledge-based and intelligent information and engineering systems (pp. 607–616). Berlin: Springer, September.

Maria Bejar, L., Adrian Reyes, O., & Dolores Garcia-Perea, M. (2018). Electronic 12-Hour Dietary Recall (e-12HR): Comparison of a mobile phone app for dietary intake assessment with a food frequency questionnaire and four dietary records. *JMIR mHealth and uHealth*, 6. Available from https://doi.org/10.2196/10409.

Miele. (2017). *The invisible kitchen* [Online]. <https://theinvisiblekitchen.miele.com/> Accessed 24.07.18.

Min, W., Bao, B.-K., Mei, S., Zhu, Y., Rui, Y., & Jiang, S. (2018). You are what you eat: Exploring rich recipe information for cross-region food analysis. *IEEE Transactions on Multimedia*, 20, 950–964. Available from https://doi.org/10.1109/tmm.2017.2759499.

Mishra, A., Nieto, A., & Kitsiou, S. (2017). Systematic review of mHealth interventions involving Fitbit activity tracking devices. In *2017 IEEE international conference on healthcare informatics (ICHI)* (pp. 455–455). IEEE.

Moldovan, D., Stefan, P., Vuscan, C., Chifu, V. R., Anghel, I., Cioara, T., & Salomie, I. (2017). *Diet generator for elders using Cat Swarm Optimization and Wolf Search*. International conference on advancements of medicine and health care through technology; 12–15 October 2016, Cluj-Napoca, Romania (pp. 238–243). Cham: Springer.

Montoya, C. A., Rutherfurd, S. M., Olson, T. D., Purba, A. S., Drummond, L. N., Boland, M. J., & Moughan, P. J. (2014). Actinidin from kiwifruit (*Actinidia deliciosa* cv. Hayward) increases the digestion and rate of gastric emptying of meat proteins in the growing pig. *British Journal of Nutrition*, 111, 957–967. Available from https://doi.org/10.1017/s0007114513003401.

Nayak, B., Berrios, J. D., & Tang, J. (2014). Impact of food processing on the glycemic index (GI) of potato products. *Food Research International*, 56, 35–46. Available from https://doi.org/10.1016/j.foodres.2013.12.020.

Nedungadi, P., Jayakumar, A., & Raman, R. (2018). Personalized health monitoring system for managing wellbeing in rural areas. *Journal of Medical Systems*, 42. Available from https://doi.org/10.1007/s10916-017-0854-9.

Neumann, A., Elbrechter, C., Pfeiffer-Lessmann, N., Koiva, R., Carlmeyer, B., Ruether, S., ... Ritter, H. J. (2017). "KogniChef": A cognitive cooking assistant. *Kunstliche Intelligenz*, 31, 273–281. Available from https://doi.org/10.1007/s13218-017-0488-6.

Ngo, H. C., Cheah, Y. N., Goh, O. S., Choo, Y. H., Basiron, H., & Kumar, Y. J. (2016). A review on automated menu planning approaches. *Journal of Computer Sciences*, 12(12), 582–596.

Niederman, S. A., Leonard, E., & Clapp, J. E. (2017). Restaurant nutrition reporting and impact on surveillance. *Journal of Food Composition and Analysis*, 64, 73–77. Available from https://doi.org/10.1016/j.jfca.2017.04.011.

Nielsen. (2016). What's in our food and on our mind—Ingredient and dining-out trends around the world. The Nielsen Company. <http://www.nielsen.com/content/dam/nielsenglobal/eu/docs/pdf/Global%20Ingredient%20and%20Out-of-Home%20Dining%20Trends%20Report.pdf> Accessed 24.07.18.

Pele. (2014). Tesco Pele—Virtual Reality Experience [Online]. <https://www.youtube.com/watch?v=08S86X_5Crs> Accessed 24.07.18.

Pouladzadeh, P., Shirmohammadi, S., & Al-Maghrabi, R. (2014). Measuring calorie and nutrition from food image. *IEEE Transactions on Instrumentation and Measurement*, 63, 1947–1956. Available from https://doi.org/10.1109/tim.2014.2303533.

Presser, K., Weber, D., & Norrie, M. (2018). FoodCASE: A system to manage food composition, consumption and TDS data. *Food Chemistry*, 238, 166–172.

Randriambelonoro, M., Chen, Y., & Pu, P. (2017). Can fitness trackers help diabetic and obese users make and sustain lifestyle changes? *Computer*, 50(3), 20–29.

Ratti, C. A. (2018). Supermarket of the future. <http://www.carloratti.com/project/supermarket-of-the-future/> Accessed June 2018.

Rick, A. (2017). *The other side of singles' day: Alibaba's Virtual Reality Testing Ground* [Online]. <https://www.forbes.com/sites/augustrick/2017/11/12/the-other-side-of-singles-day-alibabas-virtual-reality-testing-ground> Accessed 20.06.18.

Ridgers, N. D., McNarry, M. A., & Mackintosh, K. A. (2016). Feasibility and effectiveness of using wearable activity trackers in youth: A systematic review. *JMIR mHealth and uHealth*, 4(4), e129.

Rodbard, D. (2016). Continuous glucose monitoring: A review of successes, challenges, and opportunities. *Diabetes Technology & Therapeutics*, 18(Suppl 2), S2-3–S2-13. Available from https://doi.org/10.1089/dia.2015.0417.

Russell, W. R., Baka, A., Bjorck, I., Delzenne, N., Gao, D., Griffiths, H. R., ... Weickert, M. O. (2016). Impact of diet composition on blood glucose regulation. *Critical Reviews in Food Science and Nutrition*, 56, 541–590. Available from https://doi.org/10.1080/10408398.2013.792772.

Shen, C., Ho, B.-J., & Srivastava, M. (2018). Milift: Efficient smartwatch-based workout tracking using automatic segmentation. *IEEE Transactions on Mobile Computing*, 17(7), 1609–1622.

Sifferlin, A. (2017). Why perfectly healthy people are using diabetes monitors. Time. New York: Time Inc. <http://time.com/4703099/continuous-glucose-monitor-blood-sugar-diabetes/> Accessed 24.07.18.

Singh, J., Dartois, A., & Kaur, L. (2010). Starch digestibility in food matrix: A review. *Trends in Food Science & Technology*, 21, 168–180. Available from https://doi.org/10.1016/j.tifs.2009.12.001.

Sivakumaran, S., Huffman, L., & Sivakumaran, S. (2018). The New Zealand Food Composition Database: A useful tool for assessing New Zealanders' nutrient intake. *Food Chemistry*, 238, 101–110.

Subedar, H., & El-Khatib, K. (2015). Privacy and security concerns for health data collected using off-the-shelf health monitoring devices.In *IEEE 11th international conference on wireless and mobile computing, networking and communications (WiMob)*, 2015 (pp. 341–348).

Subramanian, R., Wache, J., Abadi, M. K., Vieriu, R. L., Winkler, S., & Sebe, N. (2018). ASCERTAIN: Emotion and personality recognition using commercial sensors. *IEEE Transactions on Affective Computing*, 2, 147–160.

Van Ommen, B., Bouwman, J., Dragsted, L. O., Drevon, C. A., Elliott, R., de Groot, P., ... Evelo, C. T. (2010). Challenges of molecular nutrition research 6: The nutritional phenotype database to store, share and evaluate nutritional systems biology studies. *Genes Nutrition.*, 5, 189–203.

Vandrico. (2018). The Wearable Database [Online]. Vandrico Solutions Inc. <https://vandrico.com/wearables/> Accessed 22.07.18.

Velickovic, T. D. C., & Stanic-Vucinic, D. J. (2018). The role of dietary phenolic compounds in protein digestion and processing technologies to improve their antinutritive properties. *Comprehensive Reviews in Food Science and Food Safety*, 17, 82–103. Available from https://doi.org/10.1111/1541-4337.12320.

Wang, J., Coleman, D. C., Kanter, J., Ummer, B., & Siminerio, L. (2018). Connecting smartphone and wearable fitness tracker data with a nationally used electronic health record system for diabetes education to facilitate behavioral goal monitoring in diabetes care: Protocol for a Pragmatic Multi-Site Randomized Trial. *JMIR Research Protocols*, 7(4), e10009.

Wang, L., & Hui, S. S.-C. (2015). Validity of four commercial bioelectrical impedance scales in measuring body fat among Chinese children and adolescents. *BioMed Research International*, 2015, 614858. Available from https://doi.org/10.1155/2015/614858.

Watanabe, T., & Kawai, R. (2018). Advances in food composition tables in Japan-Standard Tables of Food Composition in Japan−2015. *Food Chemistry*, 238, 16–21.

Winfree, K. N., & Dominick, G. (2017). Modeling clinically validated physical activity using commodity hardware. *IEEE Journal of Biomedical and Health Informatics*, 22(2), 335–345. Available from https://doi.org/10.1109/JBHI.2017.2787461.

Xie, J., Wen, D., Liang, L., Jia, Y., Gao, L., & Lei, J. (2018). Evaluating the validity of current mainstream wearable devices in fitness tracking under various physical activities: Comparative Study. *JMIR mHealth and uHealth*, 6, e94.

Zenun Franco, R. (2017). *Online recommender system for personalized nutrition advice. Proceedings of the Eleventh ACM conference on recommender systems* (pp. 411–415). ACM, August.

Zhou, W., & Piramuthu, S. (2014). Security/privacy of wearable fitness tracking IoT devices. In A. Rocha, D. Fonseca, E. Redondo, L. P. Reis, M. P. Cota (Eds.), *Proceedings of the 2014 9th Iberian conference on information systems and technologies (CISTI 2014)*.

Further Reading

Bashiardes, S., Godneva, A., Elinav, E., & Segal, E. (2018). Towards utilization of the human genome and microbiome for personalized nutrition. *Current Opinion in Biotechnology*, 51, 57–63. Available from https://doi.org/10.1016/j.copbio.2017.11.013.

Braconi, D., Bernardini, G., Millucci, L., & Santucci, A. (2018). Foodomics for human health: Current status and perspectives. *Expert Review of Proteomics*, 15(2), 153–164. Available from https://doi.org/10.1080/14789450.2018.1421072.

Nasser, T., & Tariq, R. S. (2015). Big data challenges. *Journal of Computer Engineering and Information Technology*, 4, 3. Available from http://doi.org/10.4172/23249307(2).

Schiboni, G., & Amft, O. (2018). *Automatic dietary monitoring using wearable accessories. Seamless healthcare monitoring* (pp. 369–412). Cham: Springer.

Storey, V. C., & Song, I. Y. (2017). Big data technologies and management: What conceptual modeling can do. *Data & Knowledge Engineering*, 108, 50–67.

SECTION C

POLICY AND COMMERCIALIZATION OF PERSONALIZED NUTRITION

CHAPTER 9

Consumer Acceptance of Personalized Nutrition

Zoltán Szakály, András Fehér and Marietta Kiss
University of Debrecen, Debrecen, Hungary

OUTLINE

Introduction	226	Prevention of Diseases	238
Concept, Areas, and Applications of Personalized Nutrition	226	Health Conscious Lifestyle	238
		Consumers' Information Processing	239
		Convenience Function and Time Factor	239
Consumer Judgment of Personalized Nutrition and Nutrigenomics	228	Costs	240
		The Nature of Different Foods	240
Factors Influencing the Consumer Acceptance of Personalized Nutrition	230	Comprehensive Models of Factors Influencing the Consumer Acceptance of Genetic-Based Personalized Nutrition	241
Consumer Doubts About the Protection of Personal Data and Information (Privacy Risk)	232	Consumer Acceptance of Personalized Nutrition in Central Europe: The Case of Hungary	245
Nature of Personalized Nutrition Advice	235		
Availability and Reliability of Information	236	The Future of Personalized Nutrition	250
Interrelationships Between Genes and Nutrition	237	References	253
Demographic Factors	237		
Being Personally Affected	238		

INTRODUCTION

Efforts made to develop nutrition habits over the last few decades have not been too effective: in developed countries people still eat too much saturated fat, added sugar and salt, and not enough vegetables, fruits, and fish. As a result the prevalence of diseases related to nutrition is increasing. Worldwide noncommunicable diseases currently account for 71% of mortality (the equivalent of 41 million people each year) (WHO, 2018a), and according to the predictions of the World Health Organization, they will represent 60% of the disease burden and over 73% of mortality in 2020 (WHO, 2018b). Chronic conditions such as obesity, diabetes, and cardiovascular and malignant diseases impose an increasing burden on health care systems (Bouwman et al., 2005; Ghosh, 2014); at the same time, up to 80% of chronic diseases could be prevented through improvements in diet and lifestyle (Fallaize, Macready, Butler, Ellis, & Lovegrove, 2013). This creates the need to develop new, more effective strategies to change nutrition habits (Bouwman et al., 2005; Fallaize et al., 2013) and to move individuals toward healthier nutrition. Part of this can occur through a move from population-based nutrition guidance toward personalized nutrition (Fallaize et al., 2013). By benefiting public health, personalized nutrition reduces health care costs (Lewis & Burton-Freeman, 2010; van Trijp & Ronteltap, 2007); if adopted widely, it holds the potential to reduce them by as much as 13% (Marsh & McLennan Co., 2014). Therefore the European Commission aims to make personalized diets widely accessible by 2050 (Bock et al., 2014; EC, 2014).

CONCEPT, AREAS, AND APPLICATIONS OF PERSONALIZED NUTRITION

There are substantial interindividual variations in response to dietary interventions (Beckett, Jones, Veysey, & Lucock, 2017; de Roos, 2013; Hesketh, Wybranska, Dommels, & King, 2006) that suggest that the currently dominant "one-size-fits-all" approach is inadequate (Fallaize et al., 2013). Personalized nutrition is the answer to individual differences by attempting to adjust individual diet to specific individual and situational needs, and providing optimal customized nutrition for the individual (Boland, 2008).

The concept of personalized nutrition is, however, not without precedent, as it has been known about since the 1970s (Nizel, 1972). Based on age or particular physiological status, special nutrition recommendations for various individuals such as children, the elderly, pregnant women, athletes, etc. have existed for a long time. Beside this, people with allergic or chronic diseases (e.g., diabetes) also need special diets (de Roos, 2013; Fallaize et al., 2013; Kussmann & Fay, 2008). However, since the end of Human Genome Project in 2003 (Collins, Morgan, & Patrinos, 2003) the understanding of the complex interactions between genes and environmental factors, such as nutrition, has been improved significantly (Fallaize et al., 2013), providing a new impetus and new direction to development.

Although several researchers (e.g., Bouwman, te Molder, & Hiddink, 2008) have narrowed down the concept of personalized nutrition to recommendations of foods and/or food supplements based on an individual's whole genetic profile, personalized nutrition is not only confined to nutritional genomics (NGx) studies (Gibney & Walsh, 2013), but can also be built on phenotypic information such as blood chemistry, weight and height, or lifestyle information such as dietary intake (Boland, 2008; Fallaize et al., 2013; Rimbach & Minihane, 2009; Stewart-Knox et al., 2015).

Thus personalized nutrition has three levels (Fischer et al., 2016; Gibney & Walsh, 2013; Rimbach & Minihane, 2009): the first, least personal level is personalized (often Internet-based) nutritional advice based on individual lifestyles (including nutritional data)—this is currently the dominant approach in the marketplace. A substantial proportion of cases involve personalized nutrition based on phenotypic information (e.g., anthropometry, clinical parameters, biochemical markers of nutritional status), and it is only the third level of personalized nutrition using genomic data which is still the exception rather than a mainstream activity in the market (Ronteltap, van Trijp, Berezowska, & Goossens, 2013).

NGx includes both nutrigenomics (i.e., the effect of nutrients on gene expression) and nutrigenetics (i.e., the effect of genes on the response to nutrients, or to put it another way, the effect that genetic variation has on the interaction between nutrients and disease) (Bouwman et al., 2008; de Roos, 2013; Farhud, Zarif Yeganeh, & Zarif Yeganeh, 2010; Kang, 2012; Kussmann & Fay, 2008). Nutrigenomics studies the relationship between what we eat and how our genes, proteins, and metabolism function to affect our long-term health, while nutrigenetics studies single gene—single food components where possession of a particular genotype may confer a disadvantage that can be addressed through dietary modification (Bouwman et al., 2008). Although a distinction between nutrigenomics and nutrigenetics is often blurred by various and often conflicting definitions (for an interpretation of the distinction which varies from the one above, see e.g., Boland, 2008), and both terms are still commonly used interchangeably (Hurlimann et al., 2014), nutrigenomics is often the term widely used to cover both aspects of NGx (Boland, 2008; Nielsen & El-Sohemy, 2012; Ronteltap, van Trijp, Renes, & Frewer, 2007).

With the use of NGx, we can scientifically examine how our body interacts with various nutrients. In this way we are able to actually implement the concept of real personalized nutrition in which diet, foods, and nutrients can be adapted to the specific (lifestyle, genetic, and environmental) needs of the individual (Kussmann & Fay, 2008). This kind of personalized nutrition aims to identify genetically determined differences in how diet impacts a chronic disease in terms of food and food components, both as a cause of a disease, and as a curative agent (Komduur, Korthals, & te Molder, 2009). Thus NGx can be applied to health promotion, as well as disease prevention (Nielsen & El-Sohemy, 2012; Ronteltap, van Trijp, & Renes, 2007).

Personalized nutrition can appear as nutritional advice based on genetic information (primarily through the Internet, and known as "direct-to-consumer"—DTC), which has become an appealing business opportunity, as is confirmed by the large number of firms operating in this area (Ahlgren et al., 2013; Gibney & Walsh, 2013; Ronteltap et al., 2013), although so far they have met with little commercial success (Berezowska, Fischer, Ronteltap, Kuzneof, et al., 2014; Saukko, Reed, Britten, & Hogarth, 2010; Stewart-Knox et al., 2015). The other potential application of personalized nutrition is the production of personalized foods (Ghosh, 2010, 2014), that is, specific functional food products that are targeted to specific risk groups or even individual consumers (Roosen, Bruhn, Mecking, & Drescher, 2008). Several food ingredient companies have started investing in this area (de Roos, 2013); however, extensive commercialization of these products has not yet begun (Ronteltap, van Trijp, & Renes, 2009).

CONSUMER JUDGMENT OF PERSONALIZED NUTRITION AND NUTRIGENOMICS

Personalized nutrition is a conceptual analogue to personalized medicine (Kussmann & Fay, 2008), so genetic test-based personalized nutrition and personalized medicine share certain technologies, namely, genetic profiling is common to both of them (Stewart-Knox et al., 2015). Because of this, several of the barriers to genetic testing are, in general, also present in a NGx context (Beckett et al., 2017). Consequently, understanding attitudes toward genetic testing is relevant to understanding public acceptance of nutrigenomics, which represents the more "medicalized" level of personalized nutrition (Stewart-Knox et al., 2015).

Consumer attitudes toward genetic tests aiming to reveal the risks of a predisposition to various illnesses have already been examined by several papers; consumer acceptance of nutrigenomics-based personalized nutrition, however, has only been examined by a few (Fallaize et al., 2013; Gibney & Walsh, 2013; Stewart-Knox et al., 2015).

Studies on consumer acceptance of genetic tests—both qualitative (e.g., in the United States—Catz et al., 2005; Glenn, Chawla, & Bastani, 2012; Goldman et al., 2008; McGowan, Fishman, & Lambrix, 2010; O'Daniel, Haga, & Willard, 2010; Streicher et al., 2011; Su, Howard, & Borry, 2011; in Canada—Morin, 2009; in Australia—Hardie, 2011; Keogh et al., 2011; in the United Kingdom—Catz et al., 2005; in Switzerland—Vayena, Gourna, Streuli, Hafen, & Prainsack, 2012; in the Netherlands—Wijdenes-Pijl, Dondorp, Timmermans, Cornel, & Henneman, 2011; in Finland—Nyrhinen, Leino-Kilpi, & Hietala, 2004; in Spain and China—Catz et al., 2005; in South-Africa—Basson, Futter, & Greenberg, 2007) and quantitative (e.g., in the United States—Akinleye et al., 2011; Alford et al., 2011; Falcone, Wood, Xie, Siderowf, & Van Deerlin, 2011; Finney Rutten, Gollust, Naveed, & Moser, 2012; Gollust et al., 2012; Grant et al., 2009; Haga et al., 2013; Horn & Terry, 2012; Hull et al., 2008; Jonassaint et al., 2010; Kerath et al., 2013; McGuire, Diaz, Wang, & Hilsenbeck, 2009; Ormond et al., 2011; Perez et al., 2011; in Canada—Etchegary et al., 2010; Ries, Hyde-Lay, & Caulfield, 2010; in Australia—Taylor, 2011; Wilde, Meiser, Mitchell, Hadzi-Pavlovic, & Schofield, 2011; Wilde, Meiser, Mitchell, & Schofield, 2010; in the United Kingdom—Cherkas, Harris, Levinson, Spector, & Prainsack, 2010; in the Netherlands Henneman et al., 2013; Henneman, Timmermans, & Wal, 2006; Morren, Rijken, Baanders, & Bensing, 2007; in Sweden—Hoeyer, Olofsson, Mjörndal, & Lynöw, 2004; in Russia—Makeeva, Markova, & Puzyrev, 2009; Makeeva, Markova, Roses, & Puzyrev, 2010; in Finland—Toiviainen, Jallinoja, Aro, & Hemminki, 2003)—beside mentioning certain risk factors, often report positive attitudes in the case of the majority of consumers.

The most important motivator to have a genetic test done was the consumers' own health and the health of their family members (Akinleye et al., 2011; Cherkas et al., 2010; Glenn et al., 2012; Goldman et al., 2008; Gollust et al., 2012; Hardie, 2011; Keogh et al., 2011; McGowan et al., 2010; Streicher et al., 2011). Beside this, curiosity (Akinleye et al., 2011; Basson et al., 2007; Gollust et al., 2012; Hardie, 2011; Hull et al., 2008; Keogh et al., 2011; Makeeva et al., 2009, 2010; O'Daniel et al., 2010; Ormond et al., 2011; Streicher et al., 2011; Su et al., 2011; Vayena et al., 2012), and participation for research purposes (Glenn et al., 2012; Keogh et al., 2011; Su et al., 2011) were also important. Some respondents might prefer not to know test results unless treatment was available (Hoeyer et al., 2004; Morren et al., 2007).

Individuals whose families had certain inherited diseases showed more positive attitudes toward genetic tests (Catz et al., 2005; Wilde et al., 2011), as did men (Cherkas et al., 2010; Haga et al., 2013) and the elderly (Finney Rutten et al., 2012; Kerath et al., 2013). Moreover, there was a greater willingness to pay (WTP) when inherited diseases were present in the family's health history (Ries et al., 2010). The effect of education on attitudes toward genetic tests was mixed according to the studies (Alford et al., 2011; Catz et al., 2005; Finney Rutten et al., 2012; Jonassaint et al., 2010).

Related to genetic tests, considerable concerns were consistently raised about internet privacy, data security, data use, and data destiny; participants articulated their fears about the potential for information to be used by companies for commercial gain or to fall into the hands of insurers, employers, or government agencies (Catz et al., 2005; Etchegary et al., 2010; Glenn et al., 2012; Goldman et al., 2008; Haga et al., 2013; Henneman et al., 2013; Hoeyer et al., 2004; Horn & Terry, 2012; Keogh et al., 2011; Kerath et al, 2013; McGuire et al., 2009; Morren et al., 2007; Nyrhinen et al., 2004; Ormond et al., 2011; Ries et al., 2010; Streicher et al., 2011; Taylor, 2011; Toiviainen et al., 2003; Vayena et al., 2012; Wijdenes-Pijl et al., 2011; Wilde et al., 2010, 2011).

In contrast with the more numerous research studies examining consumer judgements related to genetic tests, only a few studies examined consumer preferences for genetic-based personalized nutrition. Based on both qualitative (Berezowska, Fischer, Ronteltap, Kuzneof, et al., 2014; Morin, 2009; Stewart-Knox et al., 2013, 2015) and quantitative studies (Ahlgren et al., 2013; Berezowska, Fischer, Ronteltap, van der Lans, & van Trijp, 2014; Berezowska, Fischer, Ronteltap, van der Lans, & van Trijp, 2015; Fischer et al., 2016; Roosen et al., 2008; Stewart-Knox et al., 2016, 2009; Szakály, Kiss, & Jasák, 2014; Szakály, Polereczki, & Kovács, 2016), we can state that consumers usually show positive attitudes toward genetic-based personalized nutrition; about one third to a half of respondents would use a service of this kind and would follow a personalized diet (Stewart-Knox et al., 2015), although there are significant international differences in this area. For example, in the research conducted by Stewart-Knox et al. (2009), among the six European countries examined the proportion of individuals who would follow a personalized diet is the highest in the United Kingdom and Italy (38.7% and 38.3%, respectively), and the lowest in Germany (13.4%).

A questionnaire survey conducted among German consumers showed a slightly more positive picture about consumer acceptance of nutrigenomics. According to this research, 45% of consumers were willing to have a nutrigenomics test done, and, in the framework of a personalized diet—depending on product types—40%—50% were willing to purchase functional foods which decrease the risk of cardiovascular diseases (Roosen et al., 2008). According to the results of a research study conducted in Sweden (Ahlgren et al., 2013), respondents showed an even more positive attitude toward personalized nutrition: 70% were willing to undergo a genetic test in order to get personalized nutrition advice. Sixty-five percent of the Swedish respondents thought that they would also follow a personalized recommendation of this kind, while 20% would be willing to do this only if they could prevent a serious disease with this diet. In contrast, based on their focus group research conducted in eight European countries, Berezowska, Fischer, Ronteltap, Kuzneof, et al. (2014) stated that the least preferred type of personalized nutrition advice was the genetic-based type, as opposed to the advice based on dietary intake and phenotypic information.

If consumer acceptance of personalized nutrition is approximated by the WTP, based on the examination by Fischer et al. (2016) conducted in eight European countries, we can state that a significant minority (20%) were not willing to pay anything, almost half of the participants would pay less for personalized nutrition advice than for a standard nutritional advice, and only 30% were willing to pay more for it—approximately 50% more on average. They would pay only a slightly higher price for the two higher level personalization variants of personalized nutrition compared to the lifestyle-only based personalized advice, which confirms the results of Berezowska, Fischer, Ronteltap, van der Lans, and van Trijp (2015). There are, however, significant differences among countries: consumers were willing to pay the least amount for this kind of service in the Netherlands and in the United Kingdom, although those who were willing to pay more than the reference price in these countries, were willing to pay the most. This can be explained by the relatively cheap or free primary health care in these countries, where consumers, however, have become accustomed to paying for additional, nonstandard health care services.

Factors influencing—both driving and hindering—consumer acceptance of nutrigenomics and personalized nutrition are discussed in detail in the next section.

FACTORS INFLUENCING THE CONSUMER ACCEPTANCE OF PERSONALIZED NUTRITION

Ultimately, consumer acceptance of personalized nutrition is determined either by consumer perception of the rational trade-off between the technology's benefits and costs, or more emotional perceptions of risk and uncertainty (Ahlgren et al., 2013; Berezowska et al., 2015; Berezowska, Fischer, Ronteltap, van der Lans, et al., 2014). In fact, the costs and benefits of personalized nutrition turned out to be of primary importance in consumer judgements (Poínhos et al., 2014; Ronteltap et al., 2009; Ronteltap, 2008; Wendel, Dellaert, Ronteltap, & van Trijp, 2013). Interestingly, determinants of consumer acceptance identified in the literature are better predictors of consumer rejection than acceptance (Frewer et al., 2011).

In this section the drivers and hindering factors of consumers' acceptance of personalized nutrition and nutrigenomics found in and identified by the literature are discussed in detail. The order in which the factors are discussed does not necessarily indicate an order of importance, but simply reflects the subjective judgement of the authors. The factors discussed here are briefly summarized in Tables 9.1 and 9.2 for better understanding.

TABLE 9.1 Summary of the Most Important Factors Driving and Hindering Consumer Acceptance of Personalized Nutrition and Nutrigenomics.

Factors Driving Consumer Acceptance	Factors Hindering Consumer Acceptance
CONSUMER DOUBTS ABOUT THE PROTECTION OF PERSONAL DATA AND INFORMATION (PRIVACY RISK)	
Ahlgren et al. (2013); Berezowska et al. (2014); Berezowska et al. (2014); Berezowska et al. (2015); Bergmann et al. (2008); Castle and Ries (2007); Catz et al. (2005); de Roos (2013); Fallaize et al. (2013); Ghosh (2009, 2010, 2014); Görman et al. (2013); Gudde (2009); Henneman et al. (2006); Hurlimann et al. (2014); Kaput (2007); Kaput and Rodriguez (2004); Komduur et al. (2009); Korthals (2011); Lévesque et al. (2008); Morin (2009); Morren et al. (2007); Nordström et al. (2013); Oliver (2005); Otlowski et al. (2012); Reilly and Debusk (2008); Ries and Castle (2008); Ronteltap et al. (2013); Ronteltap et al. (2009); Roosen et al. (2008); Stewart-Knox et al. (2009); Stewart-Knox et al. 2013; Stewart-Knox et al. (2014); Wendel et al. (2009); Wendel et al. (2013)	
"Personalized" label instead of "nutrigenomics" label	Data might end up in the hands of employers, insurance companies, or other organizations for marketing purposes, who can easily misuse them
	Lack of integrated governmental regulations
	Data can be used unethically for population planning
NATURE OF PERSONALIZED NUTRITION ADVICE	
Adams et al. (2006); Ahlgren et al. (2013); Berezowska et al. (2014); Birmingham et al. (2013); Boland (2008); Bouwman et al. (2008); Castle and Ries (2007); Cormier et al. (2014); Eaton et al. (2003); Fallaize et al. (2015); Gudde (2009); Morin (2009); Oliver (2005); Poínhos et al. (2017); Ronteltap et al. (2009); Stewart-Knox et al. (2013); Weir et al. (2010); Whelan et al. (2008)	
Online advice offers a higher level of anonymity than face-to-face advice, and is more convenient	Online advice is less reliable in terms of handling sensitive information
Face-to-face advice is more flexible, increases consumer trust and motivation through emotional support, and the risk of misuse of sensitive information is lower	"Personalized" advice is often merely common sense advice
	Health care systems are not ready to adopt nutrigenomics yet
AVAILABILITY AND RELIABILITY OF INFORMATION	
Ahlgren et al. (2013); Berezowska et al. (2014); Bottorff et al. (2002); Catz et al. (2005); Goddard et al. (2009); Gudde (2009); Mehrotra (2004); Morren et al. (2007); Nielsen and El-Sohemy (2012); Nielsen et al. (2014); Oliver (2005); Poínhos et al. (2017); Ronteltap et al. (2007); Ronteltap et al. (2007); Ronteltap et al. (2009)	
Presence of reliable, professional, and trustworthy opinion leaders	There is little easily available and easy to understand information
Transfer of complex scientific results to consumers through positively framed simple messages	Lack of agreement among, and accountability of, service providers
	Health care providers lack adequate education and enough time

(Continued)

TABLE 9.1 (Continued)

Factors Driving Consumer Acceptance	Factors Hindering Consumer Acceptance
INTERRELATIONSHIPS BETWEEN GENES AND NUTRITION	
Ahlgren et al. (2013); Boland (2008); Bouwman et al. (2005); Görman et al. (2013); Hesketh et al. (2006); Hurlimann et al. (2014); Morin (2009); Oliver (2005); Penders (2008); Ronteltap et al. (2007); Ronteltap et al. (2007)	
Increasing knowledge of the relationship between genes and nutrition	Uncertainty about the context of nutrigenomics is still relatively high
	Nutrigenomics research is costly
DEMOGRAPHIC FACTORS	
Ahlgren et al. (2013); Cohen et al. (2013); Roosen et al. (2008); Stewart-Knox et al. (2009)	
Attitudes of women toward personalized nutrition are more positive than those of men	
Attitudes of the elderly and/or the young toward personalized nutrition are more positive than those of other age groups	
Consumers in the highest income classes are willing to pay the highest price for personalized nutrition	

Consumer Doubts About the Protection of Personal Data and Information (Privacy Risk)

A fundamental trade-off in personalized nutrition lies between the benefits and the privacy risk: the higher the consumer benefit due to the more personalized recommendations available, the higher the privacy risk perceived by the consumer because of the transmission of more and more sensitive information, and vice versa. This trade-off is the main challenge facing the application of personalized nutrition (Berezowska, Fischer, Ronteltap, Kuzneof, et al., 2014; Berezowska, Fischer, Ronteltap, van der Lans, et al., 2014, 2015; Ronteltap et al., 2013; Wendel et al., 2013). Some research studies show that, according to consumers, the potential benefits of nutrigenomics outweigh its risks (Morin, 2009); moreover, according to the examinations by Hurlimann et al. (2014), Kaput (2007), and Kaput and Rodriguez (2004), nutrigenomics researchers do not perceive potential risks to be high. In contrast, health care professionals expressed more skepticism toward nutrigenomics (Morin, 2009). In spite of this, the usual tendency, at least for the time being, is that personalized nutrition as a service cannot yet achieve an acceptable balance between avoiding fears related to personal data misuse and enjoying the benefits of personalization (Ahlgren et al., 2013; Berezowska, Fischer, Ronteltap, Kuzneof, et al., 2014).

In several research studies, consumers have expressed concerns over the misuse of genetic information, and they also believe nutrigenomics raises important ethical issues (Berezowska et al., 2015; Bergmann, Gorman, & Mathers, 2008; Castle & Ries, 2007; Ghosh, 2009, 2014; Görman, Mathers, Grimaldi, Ahlgren, & Nordström, 2013; Gudde, 2009; Komduur et al., 2009; Korthals, 2011; Lévesque, Ozdemir, Gremmen, & Godard, 2008; Morin, 2009;

TABLE 9.2 Summary of the Most Important Factors Driving and Hindering Consumer Acceptance of Personalized Nutrition and Nutrigenomics.

Factors Driving Consumer Acceptance	Factors Hindering Consumer Acceptance
BEING PERSONALLY AFFECTED	
Ahlgren et al. (2013); de Vrieze et al. (2009); Fallaize et al. (2013); Joost et al. (2007); Pin (2009); Roosen et al. (2008); Stewart-Knox et al. (2009)	
If the individual has a nutrition-related disease or a risk of contracting such diseases, and if serious illnesses have been present in the family or among acquaintances, then his or her willingness to adopt personalized nutrition will be higher	Losing a person who had an extremely healthy diet to nutrition-related diseases (e.g., cancer)
PREVENTION OF DISEASES	
Frosch et al. (2005); Hunter et al. (2008); Joost et al. (2007)	
Personalized nutrition can help disease prevention	It might cause a fatalistic attitude in both directions: with positive results consumers might think "it does not matter," with negative results they might not feel the importance of healthy nutrition
HEALTH CONSCIOUS LIFESTYLE	
Ahlgren et al. (2013); Berezowska et al. (2014); Brown (2013); Cherkas et al. (2010); de Roos (2013); Elder et al. (2009); Fallaize et al. (2013); Görman (2006); Görman et al. (2013); Korthals (2011); Lustria et al. (2009); McBride et al. (2012); Nielsen and El-Sohemy (2012); Nielsen et al. (2014); Oenema et al. (2001); Ronteltap et al. (2009, 2012); Vernarelli (2012); Saukko (2013); Hurlimann et al. (2014); Henneman et al. (2006)	
Higher consumer responsibility (freedom of choice, higher level of involvement, satisfaction, and loyalty)	Higher consumer responsibility and shrinking choice options
Personalized nutrition advice is more effective than general nutrition recommendations	According to some consumers, the pursuit of a healthy diet is enough per se
CONSUMERS' INFORMATION PROCESSING	
Bergmann et al. (2008); Bouwman et al. (2008); Catz et al. (2005); de Roos (2013); Frewer et al. (2011); Gudde (2009); Morin (2009); Ronteltap et al. (2007)	
Living with a disease but being aware of the treatment	Results of nutrigenomics tests might cause anxiety
CONVENIENCE FUNCTION AND TIME FACTOR	
Berezowska et al. (2014); Fallaize et al. (2013); Fallaize et al. (2015); Ghosh (2014); Henneman et al. (2006); Makeeva et al. (2009); Nielsen and El-Sohemy (2012); Ronteltap et al. (2009); Stewart-Knox et al. (2013)	
Genotype-based personalized nutrition advice is much more enjoyable and easier to understand than general diet advice	Personalized nutrition is much more time-consuming
COSTS	
Aro et al. (1997); Berezowska et al. (2014); Cherkas et al. (2010); de Roos (2013); de Vrieze et al. (2009); Gibney and Walsh (2013); Gudde (2009); Joost et al. (2007); Morin (2009); Oliver (2005); Penders (2008); Stewart-Knox et al. (2013)	

(Continued)

TABLE 9.2 (Continued)

Factors Driving Consumer Acceptance	Factors Hindering Consumer Acceptance
Higher costs of personalized advice ensures its high quality	Fear of high costs
Costs of diseases prevented by personalized nutrition	
Personalized diet makes more efficient food purchases possible	

THE NATURE OF DIFFERENT FOODS

Bouwman et al. (2005); Coppens et al. (2006); German et al. (2004); Görman (2006); Hurlimann et al. (2014); Kutz (2006); Mehrotra (2004); Ronteltap and van Trijp (2007); Ronteltap et al. (2007); Stewart-Knox et al. (2013); Stewart-Knox et al. (2016)

	Cultural and social implications of dietary restrictions
	Everybody eats different meals, and so different meals have to be prepared for individuals in the household
	Food has begun to be "medicalized," losing its hedonic nature
	New food safety and health label regulations are required

Nordström, Coff, Jönsson, Nordenfelt, & Görman, 2013; Reilly & Debusk, 2008; Ries & Castle, 2008; Roosen et al., 2008; Stewart-Knox et al., 2013, 2015; Wendel et al., 2013). The majority of consumers feel that there is a real threat that genetic tests will lead to discrimination, i.e., a society will develop in which disabled individuals are not accepted (Henneman et al., 2006).

A survey conducted by Ahlgren et al. (2013) showed that 63% of consumers interviewed feared that data from personalized nutrition services might end up in the hands of unauthorized persons or organizations (e.g., insurance companies, employers) who can easily misuse them. American consumers are afraid of the possibility that in extreme cases insurance companies might access genetic data and, based on this data, classify individuals into various insurance categories (Fallaize et al., 2013), so that those with a health risk might be at a disadvantage. The privacy risk posed by insurance companies was confirmed by several other research studies, too (de Roos, 2013; Gudde, 2009; Morren et al., 2007; Oliver, 2005; Otlowski, Taylor, & Bombard, 2012; Reilly & Debusk, 2008; Ronteltap et al., 2009).

The role of the employer is difficult to categorize, according to Berezowska, Fischer, Ronteltap, Kuzneof, et al. (2014). It is a positive development if an employer assists their employees in developing personalized nutrition, since employees may evaluate this as a kind of care. Moreover, work may be more efficient if employee performance increases as a result of personalized nutrition. However, in theory an employer should have nothing to do with their employees' diet; moreover, an even more serious problem according to the consumers is that an employer might not promote or might even fire an employee, on the basis of the risk factors revealed by a genetic test, and that the employee will not find reemployment due to this information (Morren et al., 2007; Oliver, 2005; Otlowski et al., 2012; Reilly & Debusk, 2008; Ronteltap et al., 2009). In contrast, among British consumers Stewart-Knox et al. (2009) revealed a relatively low level of concern related to personal data handling by both insurance companies and employers.

Beside these concerns, consumers also feel that the commercial use of personal data by food companies may be problematic (Wendel et al. 2013; Wendel, Ronteltap, Dellaert, & van Trijp, 2009). Consequently, the government needs to establish an efficacious, transparent, and trustworthy regulatory framework for personalized nutrition in order to alleviate consumers' privacy concerns (Stewart-Knox et al., 2013).

Furthermore, according to some consumers, the results of genetic tests can also be used unethically by governments at a population level (e.g., for controlling population levels and regulating births, cloning, etc.) (Catz et al., 2005). Outside the United States, resistance toward new products and processes in which genes and/or cloning are involved has been strong and appears to be growing; therefore consumers are more ready to accept a product with a "personalized" label than one with a "nutrigenomics" label (Ghosh, 2010, 2014).

Nature of Personalized Nutrition Advice

When considering online or traditional face-to-face variants of personalized nutrition, there are both pros and cons. The majority of consumers prefer to have a genetic test done and receive personalized nutrition advice face-to-face (Morin, 2009), partly to avoid any misuse of sensitive information related to DNA. At the same time, personal advice might increase consumer trust and make communication easier and more flexible (Berezowska, Fischer, Ronteltap, Kuzneof, et al., 2014; Poínhos et al., 2017), as well as providing the emotional support, encouragement, and motivation needed to follow a personalized dietary plan (Stewart-Knox et al., 2013). In contrast, according to Castle and Ries (2007), DTC testing provides more privacy protection for consumers, since results are not stored in general medical notes, thus reducing third parties' access to the data. Besides anonymity, email contact offers convenience, something which is preferred by some groups (Fallaize et al., 2015; Stewart-Knox et al., 2013). However, the situation is different for those who have never been able to use the Internet properly (e.g., the elderly or individuals living in difficult financial circumstances) (Berezowska, Fischer, Ronteltap, Kuzneof, et al., 2014).

Adherence to advice is stimulated by regular progress monitoring and support (Bouwman et al., 2008; Stewart-Knox et al., 2013), especially when these are provided face-to-face (Berezowska, Fischer, Ronteltap, Kuzneof, et al., 2014). Support is also important from the consumer's direct environment, in order to engage them in the use of personalized nutrition applications (Ronteltap et al., 2009). Regarding the content of personalized nutrition services, advice on a suitable shopping list and lifestyle (together with exercise advice) is seen as a valuable extension to personalized nutrition (Berezowska, Fischer, Ronteltap, Kuzneof, et al., 2014). Some researchers mention the problem that the information is much less instructive than the companies indicate; often the consumer is merely offered common sense advice, for example, quit smoking, take exercise, and eat less unhealthy food (Ahlgren et al., 2013).

According to Oliver (2005), health care systems are not yet ready to adopt the increasingly innovative new technologies related to nutrigenomics at the required rate (Boland, 2008). Although health care professionals are aware of the possibilities of genetic tests, they only possess minimal nutrition-specific expertise, and it is not commonly used in clinical practice (Birmingham et al., 2013; Cormier et al., 2014; Weir, Morin, Ries, & Castle, 2010; Whelan, McCarthy, & Pufulete, 2008). An indicative fact is that while only about half of dietitians, nutritionists, and naturopaths knew the expression "nutrigenomics," none of the physicians or pharmacists had encountered it. This latter group also do not think themselves sufficiently qualified to give advice on nutrigenomic testing in a focus group interview (Morin, 2009). This result was also confirmed among physicians by the research of Adams, Lindell, Kohlmeier, and Zeisel (2006). A further problem can be that physicians do not have enough time to give nutrition advice in the primary care office (Eaton, McBride, Gans, & Underbakke, 2003). For the time being, however, willingness to adopt innovations is also still low among dietitians, as is their interest in nutrigenomics (Gudde, 2009).

Availability and Reliability of Information

In a focus group interview among consumers and health care professionals, Catz et al. (2005) found out that consumers who were interested and participated in genetic tests objected that it was difficult to obtain information, since there were few relevant information sources (Bottorff et al., 2002). Related to this, individuals are afraid of using tests in genetic examinations that are inappropriate (Gudde, 2009). If individuals do find adequate information and decide to go through with genetic testing after all, then interpreting the results can be a serious hurdle for them, as there is a high risk they will misunderstand the test results (Ahlgren et al., 2013). Moreover, the majority of consumers are frightened of performing these kinds of examinations at home (Berezowska, Fischer, Ronteltap, Kuzneof, et al., 2014). Thus it is very important for the consumer to consult with a competent expert, both before and after the examination (Nielsen & El-Sohemy, 2012). However, there is currently no consensus—even among personalized nutrition service providers themselves—about the relevant recommendations, and there is also a lack of accountability (Goddard et al., 2009).

To achieve public acceptance of nutrigenomics, unanimously agreed statements from expert stakeholders (e.g., dietitians and nutrition scientists) about the scientifically proven technology are also important (Berezowska, Fischer, Ronteltap, Kuzneof, et al., 2014; Ronteltap et al., 2007, 2009). According to market surveys, general practitioners are considered important actors in implementing and communicating about personalized nutrition based on genetic information (Morren et al., 2007; Poínhos et al., 2017); however, according to the results of Berezowska, Fischer, Ronteltap, Kuzneof, et al. (2014), a physician is not always considered to be a qualified expert, as he or she may lack both the expertise and the time to discuss patients' nutrition-related problems. This was also confirmed by the results of Nielsen, Shih, and El-Sohemy (2014), according to which the majority of

Canadian consumers (56%) considered dietitians to be the best source of personalized nutrition, followed by medical doctors (27%); this was supported by the results of Poínhos et al. (2017) for Poland, where dietitians and nutritionists were the preferred service providers.

It is also important that the product/service should provide clear benefits for the consumers (Ronteltap et al., 2009), and the complex scientific results should be communicated to consumers via simple messages (Mehrotra, 2004; Oliver, 2005). Framing messages positively (i.e., highlighting the health and performance enhancements at later life stages or a reduction in the risk of catching a disease) instead of offering a negative focus can also facilitate consumer acceptance (Mehrotra, 2004; Ronteltap et al., 2007).

Interrelationships Between Genes and Nutrition

Nutrigenomics is a relatively new scientific field, and although we know more and more about the relationship between genes and nutrition, there is a significant uncertainty about its role in the promotion of health (Ahlgren et al., 2013; Boland, 2008; Bouwman et al., 2005; Görman et al., 2013; Oliver, 2005; Ronteltap et al., 2007). The complexity of the interaction between nutrition and health inhibits nutrigenomics development, as does the fact that most diseases have a multifactorial and polygenetic etiology, meaning that it is very difficult to identify and target responsible genes (Ronteltap et al., 2007). Nevertheless, as long as nutritionists themselves are uncertain about the various methods of nutrigenomics, barriers to the spread of this novel method of nutrition will remain (Morin, 2009). There are, however, some research results (Hurlimann et al., 2014) that suggest researchers are often convinced that their personalized nutrition advice and the recommendations based on the results of genetic tests are unarguable, and they cannot see the real risks of this novel method.

Beside this, the high costs of genomic research also hinder the development of the field, since due to the existence of minor genetic differences very large samples are needed (Hesketh et al., 2006; Penders, 2008).

Demographic Factors

Several research studies have shown that it is primarily women who are willing to use genetic-based personalized nutrition (Roosen et al., 2008; Stewart-Knox et al., 2009). In terms of age, research results are mixed; according to Stewart-Knox et al. (2009) individuals above 65 years were more ready to accept genetic-based personalized nutrition, while according to the results of a research study conducted in Sweden (Ahlgren et al., 2013), it is mainly the young (between 16 and 45 years of age).

If consumer acceptance is measured by WTP, in terms of gender, it can be stated that men with a lower than standard WTP would pay less, while those with a higher than standard WTP would pay more than women, that is, men are more extreme in their deviation from a standard WTP. Considering individual income, in line with our expectations, those in the highest income classes are willing to pay the highest price, which suggests that this group is a promising target group for personalized nutrition; at the same time, however, this segment also has the highest health status (Cohen, Rai, Rehkopf, & Abrams, 2013).

Being Personally Affected

According to the majority of research studies, the health problems (known risk or presence of an illness) of the consumer or of his or her immediate family member(s), that is, being personally affected, play a serious role in consumers' judgement of personalized nutrition (Ahlgren et al., 2013; de Vrieze et al., 2009; Fallaize et al., 2013; Joost et al., 2007; Pin, 2009; Roosen et al., 2008; Stewart-Knox et al., 2009). For example, according to a survey conducted in several European countries (Stewart-Knox et al., 2009), individuals who would be willing to get themselves genetically tested with the aim of receiving personalized nutrition advice often had higher cholesterol levels, were more obese, and had higher stress levels than individuals who would only get themselves tested for general reasons. Consumers who were aware of the problems caused by metabolic syndrome they suffered from particularly appreciated the possibility of personalized nutrition advice (Stewart-Knox et al., 2009). On the other hand, a person who has lost a friend who had an extremely healthy diet to cancer may lose hope in healthy food (de Vrieze et al., 2009).

Prevention of Diseases

Connected to the previous point, genotypic-based personalized nutrition can be beneficial in prevention, as there are several diseases (e.g., diabetes or osteoporosis) that have an effect over a longer time period; moreover, their symptoms also appear much later, and after their appearance it is much more difficult to treat them. It is worth noting here, however, that this may also have an opposite effect; knowledge of a genetic predisposition may result in a fatalistic attitude and reduced compliance (Joost et al., 2007). Beside this, high-risk individuals have lower perceived behavioral control over their eating, and hence feel less able to change their dietary habits (Frosch, Mello, & Lerman, 2005). On the other hand, a negative result from a genetic test may result in reduced motivation as individuals become reassured that they will not develop a particular disease (Hunter, Khoury, & Drazen, 2008).

Health Conscious Lifestyle

The opportunity of self-managed health appears to have an appeal for consumers and is perceived as empowering (Ahlgren et al., 2013). A particularly important factor in the public acceptance of genetic-based personalized nutrition is if the consumer has freedom of choice in terms of undergoing nutrigenomic genetic testing (Henneman et al., 2006; Ronteltap et al., 2009). With an awareness of their genetic conditions consumers will have greater responsibility toward developing their own health (Brown, 2013; de Roos, 2013); however, according to some authors, this does not broaden consumers' choice options but reduces them (Görman, 2006; Korthals, 2011).

In their research, Nielsen et al. (2014) found that genetic information acquired during personalized nutrition advice positively affected the proper development and maintenance of one's diet and eventually one's health (Ahlgren et al., 2013; Cherkas et al., 2010). Several researchers highlighted the fact that personalized nutrition advice was more efficient in changing individual diet habits than general nutrition advice (Elder, Ayala, Slymen, Arredondo, & Campbell, 2009; Lustria, Cortese, Noar, & Glueckauf, 2009; Oenema, Brug, & Lechner, 2001; Ronteltap et al., 2013). For the consumer the benefits of personalized nutrition appear as perceived added value, which results in higher involvement, satisfaction, and loyalty toward personalized nutrition (Berezowska, Fischer, Ronteltap, Kuzneof, et al., 2014).

According to others, however, the real effect of genetic information on a change to a nutrition-related lifestyle is still uncertain (Fallaize et al., 2013; Görman et al. 2013; McBride, Bryan, Bray, Swan, & Green, 2012; Nielsen & El-Sohemy, 2012; Saukko, 2013; Vernarelli, 2012). Moreover, Fallaize et al. (2013) found that, according to some individuals, a healthy diet was more than sufficient in itself, and in addition or related to this, it was not necessary to undergo a genetic test as well.

Another type of threat is discrimination against and stigmatization of some consumers because they are not able to follow their nutrition advice, although this is not a real threat according to the majority of researchers (Hurlimann et al., 2014).

Consumers' Information Processing

According to research studies, there is a danger that the results of nutrigenomics examinations cause anxiety to those trying them (Bergmann et al., 2008; Bouwman et al., 2008; Catz et al., 2005; de Roos, 2013; Morin, 2009), and this can make them more reluctant to get themselves tested. An important question is what test participants do when they learn they will get a very serious illness sooner or later, and how they are able to live with this burden (Gudde, 2009). On the one hand, it can be beneficial, since their problems have been discovered in time with the help of genetic tests and because of this the chance to develop adequate treatment and diet will be higher. On the other hand, living with the knowledge that they are (or will be) ill can cause anxiety and depression (Ronteltap et al., 2007).

Convenience Function and Time Factor

Genotype-based advice is much more enjoyable and understandable for consumers than general dietary recommendations (Fallaize et al., 2013; Ghosh, 2014; Nielsen & El-Sohemy, 2012). In personalized nutrition advice consumers usually get exact instructions about how to develop their diet that might be convenient for them. Makeeva et al. (2009), however, highlight the drawback of this, too, since their analysis showed that 20% of Russian consumers believed participation in genetic tests was too time-consuming. Moreover, it may also require more time to comply with the requirements of a personalized nutrition plan which usually includes special ingredients every day (Fallaize et al., 2013).

Thus consumer acceptance is facilitated if the new dietary habits can be easily adapted to the consumer's daily life and the new technology can be used easily (Ronteltap et al., 2009; Stewart-Knox et al., 2013). Therefore it is important to tailor personalized nutrition to the preferences, lifestyle, and motivation of the consumer (Berezowska, Fischer, Ronteltap, Kuzneof, et al., 2014; Fallaize et al., 2015; Stewart-Knox et al., 2013), and not only to his or her nutrition, phenotypic, and genetic characteristics in a strict sense.

Costs

In sum, it can be stated that the personalized diets available in the market are much more costly than diets based on mass produced foods. This is partly due to the fact that nutrigenomics research needs larger cohorts which are inherently very expensive (de Vrieze et al., 2009; Gibney & Walsh, 2013; Joost et al., 2007; Penders, 2008), and partly due to the higher production costs of personalized products.

Genetic tests before advice are, however, effective in some senses, since the consumer can save a lot of money by avoiding diseases which will not develop in the future as a result of personalized nutrition (Aro et al., 1997). With the personalization of nutrition and the development of a proper diet the effectiveness of expenditure related to food can also be increased. This is because the risk that the consumer will purchase ingredients for a less efficient diet—which is not as effective as a personalized diet—can be decreased (de Roos, 2013; Joost et al., 2007). In contrast, in research studies by Cherkas et al. (2010), Gudde (2009), Makeeva et al. (2009), Morin (2009), Oliver (2005), and Stewart-Knox et al. (2013) it was found that a fear of the high costs of genetic tests and genetic-based nutrition advice was clearly present among consumers.

On the other hand, however, higher costs related to personalized nutrition might suggest reliability and better quality for the customer (Berezowska, Fischer, Ronteltap, Kuzneof, et al., 2014; Stewart-Knox et al., 2013).

The Nature of Different Foods

Dietary restrictions can have societal and cultural implications if individuals are advised to refrain from particular eating practices that are central to their identity because the role played by food can extend beyond nutritional aspects. Consumers' food choices are largely determined by collective values and social norms (Kutz, 2006). Meals with family and friends, religious meals and meals during cultural events largely determine the individual's willingness to follow a personalized diet (Bouwman et al., 2005). Thus when developing personalized nutrition, it is not only individual preferences, but those of family members and friends which have to be taken into account (Stewart-Knox et al., 2016).

Some experts are afraid of the negative consequences of personalized diets on family meals, since everybody has to eat different foods (Ronteltap et al., 2007); moreover, consumers are afraid of preparing different foods for each member of the household (Stewart-Knox et al., 2013). Therefore it is highly important that personalized nutrition advice should be valid in order to avoid unnecessary changes in the consumer's lifestyle. Incorrect results (or the incorrect interpretation of results) might lead to unnecessary preventative actions (Kutz, 2006).

Some research studies highlight the dangers of the medicalization of diet, and the fact that by targeting individuals and focusing on the molecular components of food and the genetic predisposition of individuals, nutrigenomics might blur boundaries between health and disease, and between food and drugs, and negatively alter consumers' social relationship to food (Görman, 2006). According to them, nutrition will be viewed as merely fuel for the body, ignoring its hedonic aspect (Ronteltap et al., 2007). In an expert interview, however, researchers highlighted that nutrigenomics will not reconfigure foods as medication or transform the conception of eating into a health hazard; following nutrition advice does not pose an additional burden on individuals, and it will not threaten their individual autonomy in daily food choices (Hurlimann et al., 2014). The question is whether consumers are willing to give up the benefits provided by the taste, fragrance, texture, and convenience of foods for their health (Mehrotra, 2004). According to German, Yeretzian, and Watzke (2004), however, they do not have to give up those values; foods should be tasty, convenient, secure, and affordable at the same time, that is, the kind of personalized foods which will be successful in the market are those which complement the attributes of existing foods with the promise of healthiness.

The new, nutrigenomics-based food products require new regulations in the fields of food safety and nutrition health labeling (Ronteltap & van Trijp, 2007). The development of nutrigenomics applications, however, is inhibited by the fact that due to the amount of regulations and procedures to be followed, getting nutrigenomics products ready for the market is an expensive and time-consuming process (Coppens, da Silva, & Pettman, 2006).

COMPREHENSIVE MODELS OF FACTORS INFLUENCING THE CONSUMER ACCEPTANCE OF GENETIC-BASED PERSONALIZED NUTRITION

In the literature some conceptual models providing a comprehensive framework for influencing factors of consumer acceptance of genetic-based personalized nutrition can be found that do not only identify those factors but also the relationships and direct and indirect effects among them. Four of these models are briefly discussed here.

Based on previous research results, Ronteltap et al. (2007) developed a conceptual framework for the consumer acceptance of technology-based food innovations. This model builds on some elements of Theory of Planned Behavior (TPB), and distinguishes between "distal" and "proximal" determinants of acceptance. Distal factors include the characteristics of the innovation, the consumer, and the social system, while proximal factors include perceived cost/benefit considerations, perceptions of risk and uncertainty, social norms, and perceived behavioral control. Distal factors influence consumers' intentions to adopt an innovation through proximal factors. A further element of the model is communication, which is represented in the model as an important means linking innovation features to consumer perceptions (Fig. 9.1).

Building on the conceptual model developed by Ronteltap et al. (2007) and on a survey conducted among Dutch consumers, Ronteltap et al. (2009) elaborated an empirical model of the relationships among factors influencing consumer preferences for personalized nutrition. The starting point was the fact that consumer acceptance of personalized nutrition is affected by consumer perceptions of personalized nutrition that are influenced by an identified set of psychological processes that determine the consumer acceptance of food innovations more generally (Fig. 9.2). This set of psychological processes consists of perceived risk and uncertainty, subjective norms (i.e., whether significant others are likely to endorse the behavior), perceived cost–benefits, and perceived behavioral control (i.e., whether a person believes he or she can actually perform the behavior necessary for acceptance). Consumer perceptions include framing (i.e., the positive or negative wording of a

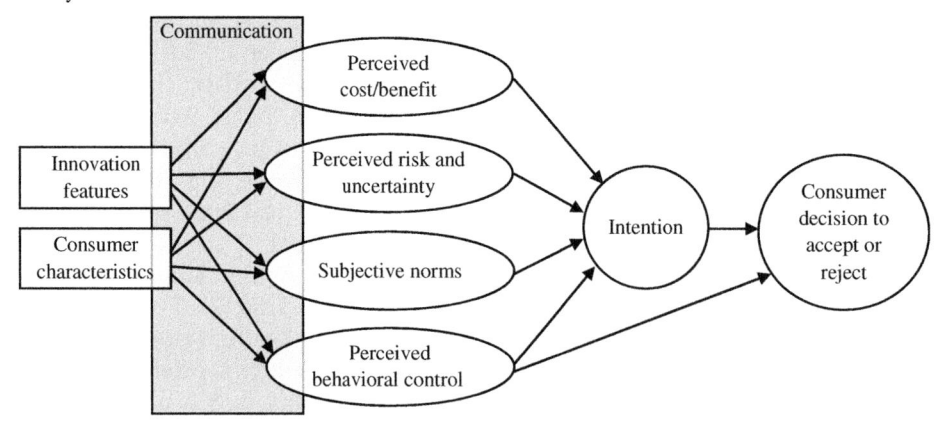

FIGURE 9.1 Conceptual framework for acceptance of technology-based food innovations. *Source: From Ronteltap, A., van Trijp, J. C. M., Renes, R. J., & Frewer, L. J. (2007). Consumer acceptance of technology-based food innovations: Lessons for the future of nutrigenomics. Appetite, 49(1), 5.*

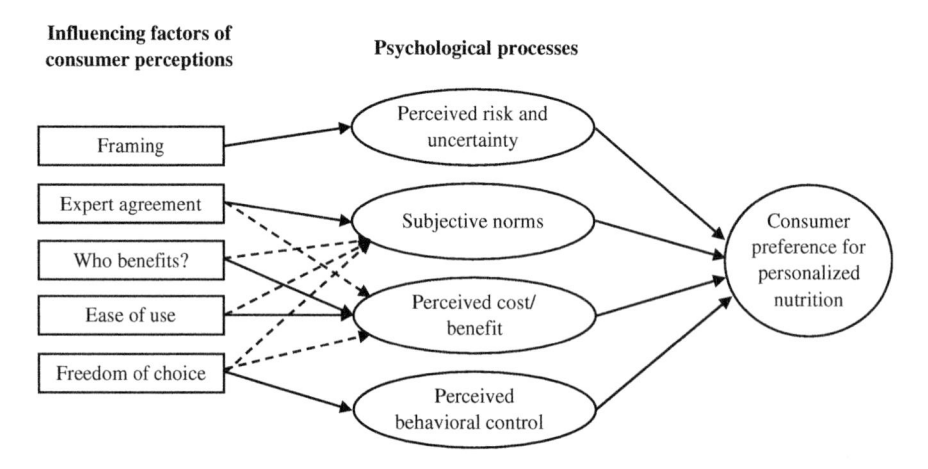

FIGURE 9.2 Model of influencing factors of consumer preference for personalized nutrition.
Notes: *Dashed arrows* indicate relationships additional to the original theoretical model revealed by the empirical analysis. *Source: Modified from Ronteltap, A., van Trijp, J. C. M., & Renes, R. J. (2009). Consumer acceptance of nutrigenomics-based personalised nutrition. British Journal of Nutrition, 101(1), 135.*

message); positive framing was expected to affect positively the consumer preference for personalized nutrition, mediated by perceived risk and uncertainty, although in the final model, framing did not contribute significantly to explaining preference. Another element of consumer perceptions is expert agreement on the feasibility and desirability of personalized nutrition; its positive effect was expected to be primarily mediated by a directive and positive subjective norm, although the authors also found a mediation effect of the perceived cost–benefit ratio. The third consumer perception item relates to the beneficiaries of personalized nutrition (i.e., the consumer, the science, or the industry, with the first two having a positive effect), which was expected to be mediated by the perceived cost—benefit ratio; however, subjective norms also played a mediating role when the consumer was the main beneficiary. The fourth element of consumer perceptions is ease of use (i.e., the extent to which personalized diets are perceived as being compatible with current food habits and easy to implement in consumers' existing lifestyles); if personalized nutrition integrates smoothly into existing eating habits, and is easy to implement in daily life, this will reduce the perceived costs. Beside this, however, ease of use was also mediated by subjective norms in the final model. Last, but not least, the extent to which consumers are free to choose whether or not to make their genetic profile available was also expected to determine consumer acceptance of personalized nutrition, mediated by perceived behavioral control. However, perceived cost—benefit considerations and, to a lesser extent, subjective norms also proved to be mediators.

Based on a survey conducted in nine European countries (Germany, Greece, Ireland, Poland, Portugal, Spain, the Netherlands, the United Kingdom, and Norway) and on some elements of the TPB, Poínhos et al. (2014) developed a model for consumer intention to adopt personalized nutrition with the use of structural equation modeling (SEM). The model proved to be highly stable across countries. According to this model, individuals with a more positive attitude toward personalized nutrition are more likely to adopt it. Attitudes toward personalized nutrition are positively influenced by the perception of benefits, perceptions of the efficacy of regulatory control to protect consumers (e.g., in relation to personal data protection), health commitment, self-reported internal health locus of control (beliefs on being able to control our own health through our own volitional behaviors), and nutrition self-efficacy (i.e., the extent to which people perceive that the adoption of personalized nutrition is achievable). Although higher perceived risk has a negative relationship with attitude, its effect is less influential than that of perceived benefit. This means that higher levels of benefit perception, perceived efficacy of regulatory control, health commitment, internal health locus of control and self-efficacy, and a lower level of perceived risk are related to more positive attitudes toward personalized nutrition, and a greater expressed intention to adopt it. Beside the indirect effects, both perceived benefits and self-efficacy exhibit a positive direct relationship with the intention to adopt personalized nutrition (Fig. 9.3).

Starting from the theoretical framework developed by Berezowska, Fischer, Ronteltap, Kuzneof, et al. (2014), Berezowska and colleagues (Berezowska et al., 2015; Berezowska, Fischer, Ronteltap, van der Lans et al., 2014) analyzed the results of an empirical survey conducted in eight European countries (Greece, Spain, the Netherlands, Ireland, the United Kingdom, Germany, Poland, and Norway) with the use of SEM. In the resulting model, consumer adoption of personalized nutrition services originated in the privacy calculus (risk—benefit trade-off) (Fig. 9.4). The model is robust and applicable across European countries. According to the model, the intention to adopt is primarily determined by perceptions of privacy risk (negative relationship) and personalization benefits (positive relationship); however, according to the empirical results, benefits have a more significant effect than risks. Perceived risk is primarily determined by perceived information control, that is, the extent to which consumers feel in control of their personal information and, with this control, are equipped to limit potential privacy risks; while

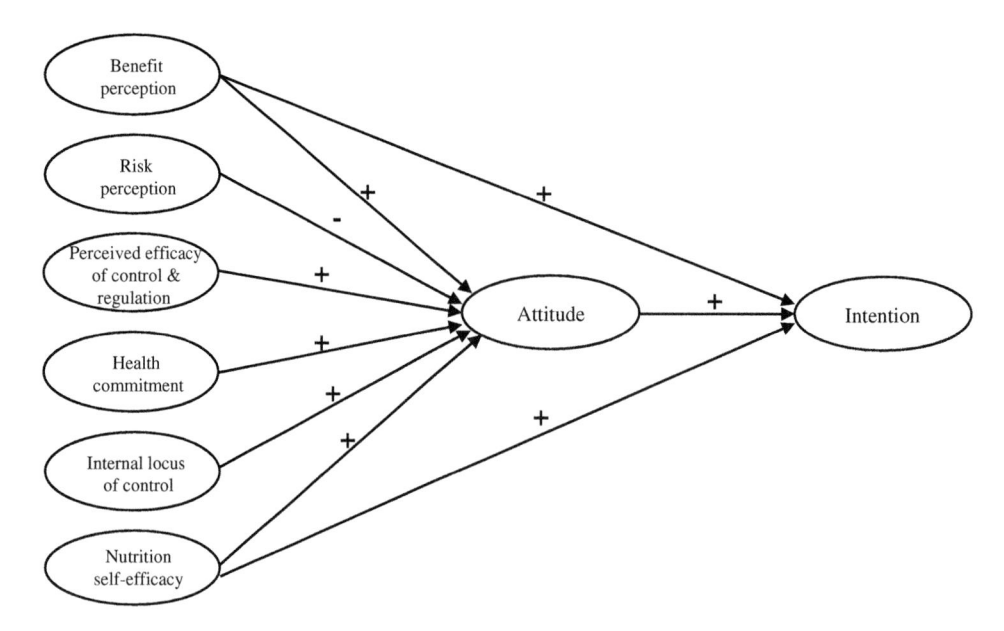

FIGURE 9.3 Model of factors influencing the intention to adopt personalized nutrition. Source: *Modified from Poínhos, R., van der Lans, I. A., Rankin, A., Fischer, A. R. H., Bunting, B., Kuznesof, S., Stewart-Knox, B. J., & Frewer, L. J. (2014). Psychological determinants of consumer acceptance of personalised nutrition in 9 European countries.* PLoS One, 9(10), e110614, 6.

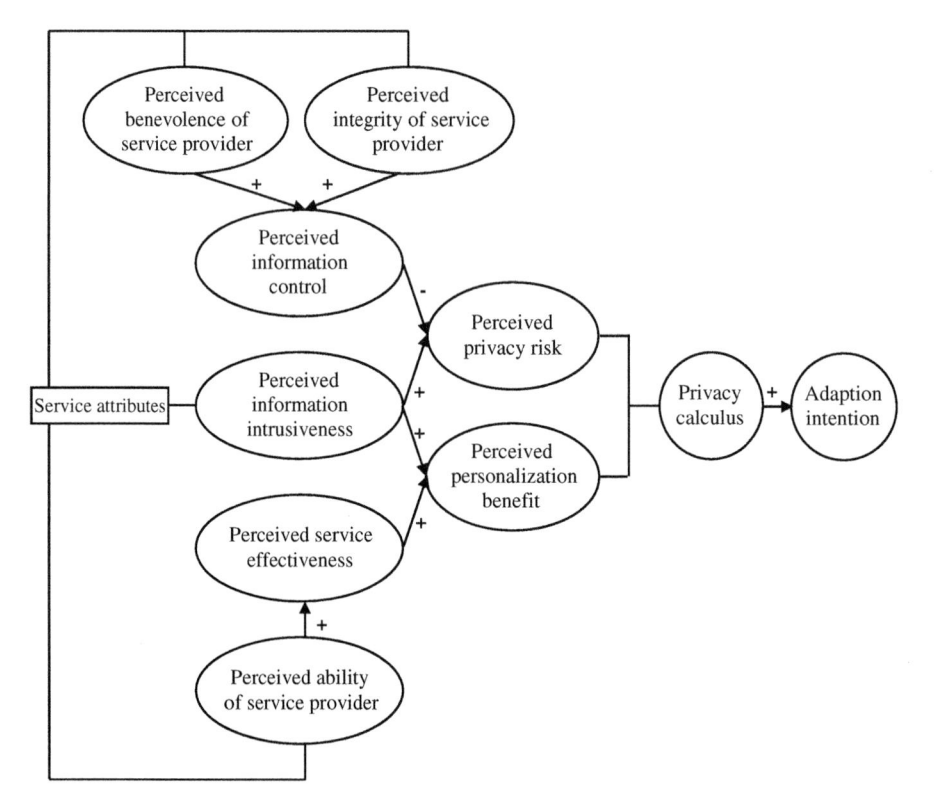

FIGURE 9.4 Model of factors influencing the intention to adopt personalized nutrition. Source: *Modified from Berezowska, A., Fischer, A. R. H., Ronteltap, A., van der Lans, I. A., van Trijp, H. C. M. (2015). Consumer adoption of personalised nutrition services from the perspective of a risk–benefit trade-off.* Genes and Nutrition, 10(6), 42, 3.

perceived benefit is mainly determined by the perceived effectiveness of the service. To a lesser extent, however, perceived identity knowledge/information intrusiveness (i.e., the extent of the personal information disclosed) influences both perceived risk and benefit, since a higher level of intrusiveness results in more advanced levels of personalization, but also in more severe consequences of possible privacy loss. Various service attributes affect information control perception (the perceived benevolence and the perceived integrity of the service provider) and perceived service effectiveness (the perceived ability of the service provider). If consumers perceive a service provider to be a person of benevolence (i.e., someone who wants to do good) and integrity (i.e., someone who adheres to sound moral and ethical principles) in terms of his or her behavioral intentions (i.e., he or she is reliable), perceived information control will be higher. Finally, the perceived ability of the service provider (i.e., competence) has a great positive effect on perceived service effectiveness.

CONSUMER ACCEPTANCE OF PERSONALIZED NUTRITION IN CENTRAL EUROPE: THE CASE OF HUNGARY

As is clear from the previous literature review, several research studies have already been conducted into consumer acceptance of personalized (mainly genetic-based) nutrition, both in Western Europe and in the United States. The number of such studies carried out in Central and Eastern Europe, however, is significantly lower. Although these countries often lag behind the more developed countries in the adoption of new technologies (Suriñach, Autant-Bernard, Manca, Massard, & Moreno, 2009), the gap is shrinking continuously. An interesting question is the current state of consumer attitudes toward and acceptance of genetic tests and genetic-based personalized nutrition in these countries, a few years after relevant research studies were performed in Western European countries and the United States. Therefore our primary research is designed to reveal consumer attitudes toward and preference for genetic tests and personalized nutrition in Hungary, based on two previous research studies (Ronteltap et al., 2009; Stewart-Knox et al., 2009). The most important results will be discussed here.

In order to achieve the set objective, a nationwide representative questionnaire-based survey was carried out involving 500 people in Hungary in 2014. Basic statistical analysis and an ordered factorial logit response model with proportional odds (OFLR-PO) were performed on survey data. The questionnaire design, the sampling, and statistical methods have been described in detail previously (Szakály et al., 2014, 2016).

After introducing the concept of personalized nutrition as described by Stewart-Knox et al. (2009) respondents declared whether the new opportunity outlined is appealing to them. Results clearly showed the fragmentation of consumers, with only 27% of them responding positively to the new opportunity; these are consumers who would happily use the service in order to preserve their health. The ratio of uncertain consumers is very high, approaching 45%, and they make up the largest group. For almost 30% of respondents personalized nutrition is not appealing at all, and so they would not use it.

Several significant relationships were found between the adoption of personalized nutrition and demographic variables, although the predictive strength of the latter is low.

In terms of gender, it can be stated that women reject the new technology at a significantly lower rate than men (24.0% and 34.2%, respectively), and there are more women (30.4%) than men (23.2%) who consider the use of genetic-based personalized nutrition as an appealing opportunity. With an increase in education levels, acceptance of the new technology also increases significantly. Beside this, the higher the monthly income of the family, the higher the likelihood that the individual considers the use of personalized nutrition appealing. Our results show that due to the novelty of the technology the majority of the consumers have not yet developed attitudes toward the concept of personalized nutrition; however, there are target groups that are interested in it, and who consider the new technology potentially to be appealing.

In terms of the potential reasons for getting genetically tested we can state that the proportions of respondents who would have a test because they want to follow a personalized diet is very low (16.0%). They are committed to preventive health behavior. Slightly more than one fourth of the respondents (28.6%) are interested in the results of the genetic test only in a general sense; 24.6% reject genetic testing outright, and 30.8% are uncertain about the new technology.

Comparing our results to those of a survey conducted in six European countries (Stewart-Knox et al., 2009) it is clear that—among the examined countries—the lowest willingness to get genetically tested was detected in Hungary. In Portugal 48.5% of respondents, in France 44.3%, and even in the country with the lowest rate (Poland) 32.9% would have a test out of general interest. The proportion of those who are willing to follow a health preserving personalized diet based on the test results is the highest in the United Kingdom and in Italy (38.7% and 38.3%, respectively). In this sense, among the countries examined by Stewart-Knox et al. (2009) only Germany has a lower rate (13.4%) than Hungary.

The willingness to have a test in order to follow a personalized diet shows some significant differences in terms of demographic background variables; however, these variables' prediction strength is no more than a low or medium level. The younger somebody is, the more open he or she is to the genetic test-based personalized nutrition. While 20.9% of 18–29 year-olds would have a genetic test done with this aim, with consumers over 60 the figure is only 5.6%. This sharply differs from the results of Stewart-Knox et al. (2009), according to which in the countries examined the acceptance of a genetic test to follow a personalized diet tends to increase with age, reaching an extremely high value in those over 65 (50.0%), and is slightly higher than our results in the case of the younger age groups (14–24 and 25–34 years old, 24.5% and 28.5%, respectively). These results suggest that commitment to preventive health behavior is a natural state of about one fifth of Hungarian youth. Beside this, an extremely high proportion of those with a higher education degree (26.7%) would have a genetic test done to develop a personalized diet, while only 8.3% of consumers with vocational training, and 13.2% of those with primary education would do the same. There is also a significant relationship between family income and willingness to have a genetic test, with a higher level of willingness to get tested among those with better financial circumstances.

Based on the answers we can state that Hungarian consumers are mistrustful and uncertain about the new technology, in spite of its obvious benefits. The not particularly positive attitudes are likely to be the result of several factors. Traditional thinking, aversion to innovations, as well as a lack of information and misconceptions about genetic tests play a role in this. The technology is so new for consumers that we could identify only a few significant differences among consumer segments, that is, consumer preferences cannot be grouped, they are highly scattered, at least in terms of demographics. It can be assumed that segmentation based on further grouping variables such as psychographic and lifestyle variables might be more successful.

Our results drove us to examine what incentives would motivate consumers to accept personalized nutrition to a higher degree. To achieve this, we used the theoretical model developed by Ronteltap et al. (2009) (Fig. 9.2), which determines consumer preferences through psychological processes induced by factors influencing consumer perceptions.

Factors influencing consumer perceptions were analyzed on the basis of 11 statements. Statements were evaluated on a 1—5 interval scale, where 1 meant "I do not agree at all" and 5 meant "I totally agree." The related results are in Table 9.3.

The most positively (4.52) evaluated factor was freedom of choice; 67.4% of consumers fully agreed with the statement that it was better if they could voluntarily choose to switch to a genetic-based personalized diet. Half of consumers (50.4%) agreed with the statement that research had to provide more clarity on the benefits and drawbacks of personalized nutrition (4.19). This can be interpreted as a proof of consumer distrust, and at the same time, can be the basis for the development of positive preferences. As a confirmation of this point, a relatively high mean value (3.87) characterizes the statement that a consensus is required among researchers about the benefits of the new technology. Consumers took a clear position on the question about the beneficiaries of personalized nutrition: they prefer if it is primarily beneficial for themselves (3.95), then for researchers (3.05), and lastly for the industry (2.88). It is also much easier for them to accept if they have to change their diet only slightly (3.83) than if they have to change it radically.

In the next step, psychologic processes induced by factors influencing consumer perceptions were analyzed, based on the logic of Fig. 9.2. The results can be found in Table 9.4.

Eighty-five percent of respondents feel that the concept of genetic-based personalized nutrition still holds a lot of uncertainty. This is related to the fact that 50% of them think the new technology risky. In sum, it can be stated that the level of perceived risk and uncertainty among Hungarian consumers is high, which may hinder the launch of the new health protective method, so reducing this is definitely a key factor. Consumers are fragmented in terms of subjective norms, too. Their responses indicate that people important to them do not necessarily switch to personalized nutrition; this is indicated by the high proportion (40.8%) of those agreeing with this statement. Forty-seven percent of consumers believe that the genetic test-based new method has more advantages than disadvantages. This is more than 10% points higher than the proportion of those stating the opposite (36.2%). In terms of the new technology it is obviously beneficial that consumers are able to control their behavior when they have to decide about the switch to personalized nutrition, that is, they feel themselves able to make a prudent decision. At the same time, however, this might indicate either a decision to purchase or not to purchase.

The descriptive statistical results introduced above can be used in marketing communications for personalized nutrition. According to the results, consumers do not distinguish between the following messages: "living in good health for longer" and "living in bad health for a shorter period." Both messages carry a positive content; if the communicator

TABLE 9.3 Analysis of Factors Influencing Consumer Perception (N = 500).

Statement	Mean	Standard Deviation	Relative Standard Deviation, %	Skewness
MESSAGE FRAMING				
Personalized nutrition makes me able to live longer in good health	3.48	1.249	35.89	−0.492
Personalized nutrition makes us able to delay the appearance of diseases, therefore we can spend a shorter period in bad health	3.49	1.190	34.09	−0.448
CONSENSUS AMONG EXPERTS				
It would be better if researchers fully agreed on the benefits of personalized nutrition	3.87	1.111	28.71	−0.798
It would be better if research made benefits and drawbacks of personalized nutrition clearer	4.19	0.986	23.53	−1.122
WHO BENEFITS?				
It would be good if the prevention of diseases by a diet adjusted to my genetic background was primarily beneficial for me	3.95	1.101	27.87	−0.990
It would be good if understanding the relationship between nutrition and genetics was primarily beneficial for the researchers	3.05	1.286	42.16	−0.152
It would be good if developing special foods based on the knowledge of the relationship between nutrition and genetics was primarily beneficial for the food industry	2.88	1.312	39.31	−0.035
EASE OF USE				
It is more beneficial if I can keep my previous diet habits to the greatest degree possible, and only have to complement my diet with some personalized foods and food supplements	3.83	1.055	27.54	−0.693
It is more beneficial if I have to change my previous diet habits. I would have to consume more of some foods and less of others. Besides this, I also have to include several new products in my diet	3.13	1.261	40.29	−0.232
FREEDOM OF CHOICE				
It is better if I can decide voluntarily whether to switch to genetic-based personalized nutrition	4.52	0.817	18.07	−1.891
It is better if genetic-based personalized nutrition was compulsory for everybody	1.91	1.274	66.70	1.070

From Szakály, Z., Kiss, M., Jasák, H., (2014). Funkcionális élelmiszerek, fogyasztói attitűdök és személyre szabott táplálkozás. *Táplálkozásmarketing*, 1(1−2), 14.

TABLE 9.4 Analysis of Psychological Processes Induced by Factors Influencing Consumer Perception (N = 500)

Statement	Agree	Do Not Agree	Do Not Know
PERCEIVED RISK AND UNCERTAINTY			
I feel that genetic-based personalized nutrition has a lot of risks	47.6	36.2	16.2
I feel that there is a lot of uncertainty around genetic-based personalized nutrition	84.8	7.4	7.8
SUBJECTIVE NORM			
People important to me will certainly switch to genetic-based personalized nutrition	39.8	40.8	19.4
PERCEIVED COST/BENEFIT			
If I weigh up the benefits and drawbacks of genetic-based personalized nutrition, I can see more benefits	47.0	36.2	16.8
PERCEIVED BEHAVIORAL CONTROL			
If personalized nutrition were really available in the future, I would be able to fully control my decision about whether to use it	86.2	7.2	6.6

Distribution of Answers, %

has to choose one of them, "health" should be placed at the center of communication. For consumers, evidence-based research results which experts thought to be trustworthy in the field (e.g., doctors, researchers) agree with are definitely important. It is not a coincidence that new health protecting products are advertised by messages which include the fact that they are "recommended by" a famous professional organization. A further important aspect is what benefits the new technology can provide and for who. Consumers "save energy"; they can only change their habits with difficulty; therefore all solutions that promise a better life quality with a minor lifestyle change can be a successful concept. Consumers show a very strong desire for freedom of choice, and the chance to make independent decisions. According to our survey, the largest difference is between a judgement involving free will and an obligation. "You decide" type messages concentrate exactly on this consumer need.

To reveal the relationships among factors influencing consumer preferences for genetic-based personalized nutrition, OFLR-PO was performed. The main results (statistically significant relationships) are summarized in Fig. 9.5.

According to our results, which are in line with those of Ronteltap et al. (2009), consumer preference for personalized nutrition is positively associated with the lack of perceived risks, positively framed health communication (in our model this has a direct, rather than an indirect, effect), expert agreement on the benefits of personalized nutrition, and freedom of choice. The subjective norm (the presence of credible opinion leaders) positively mediates the effect of expert agreement, and similarly, perceived behavioral control positively mediates the freedom of choice. Based on our analysis, we can conclude that the

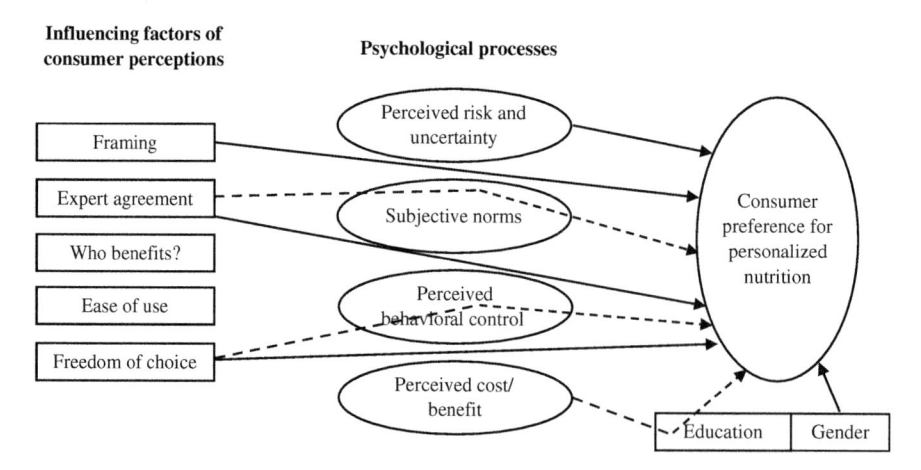

FIGURE 9.5 Extended model of consumer preference for personalized nutrition.
Notes: Nonsignificant effects have been omitted. *Dashed arrows* represent indirect effects. Source: *Based on Ronteltap, A., van Trijp, J. C. M., & Renes, R. J. (2009). Consumer acceptance of nutrigenomics-based personalised nutrition.* British Journal of Nutrition, 101(1), 135.

most important factors in consumer preference for personalized nutrition are perceived risk and uncertainty, positively framed communication about personalized nutrition, and perceived costs/benefits moderated by education level. However, unlike the results of Ronteltap et al. (2009), in our model perceived costs/benefits are not the most dominant psychological processes that determine consumer acceptance (they come second, after perceived risk and uncertainty), and subjective norms are not the second most dominant; moreover, both cost/benefit perceptions and subjective norms play a mediator role only for one consumer perception factor each. Additionally, in our model, demographic factors were also incorporated, with the result that gender has a significant direct effect on consumer preference for personalized nutrition (women show more positive preferences than men), and education has a moderating effect.

THE FUTURE OF PERSONALIZED NUTRITION

There is no consensus among experts about the development of nutrigenomics over time, nor the factors that will determine market success or failure (Ronteltap et al., 2007). It is still very unclear, in fact, how nutrigenomics will develop from fundamental research to consumer applications: whether dietary advice will be the only viable application, and/or personalized/individualized food products, or neither of these (Ronteltap et al., 2007).

Personalization efforts can only be effective if they are supported by a viable business model (Ronteltap et al., 2013). The first business area which may benefit from personalized nutrition is the area of weight management. There are already some firms today that offer personalized nutrition advice with the aim of reducing weight, building on phenotypic measurements of energy expenditure. In the future, however, as genotypic data become available, it will become possible to offer weight loss programs tailored to the genotype of each consumer. Another possible early market application of personalized nutrition is the area of food supplements. Currently food supplements are offered to the general market or a segment of the general market such as the elderly. Knowledge of the individual's genetic profile, however, means that he or she can be offered the optimal food supplement, suited to his or her metabolic profile (Gibney & Walsh, 2013).

At the beginning of the 2000s some stated that nutrigenomics had reached its commercialization stage (Muller & Kersten, 2003), and a few years later other researchers predicted that nutrigenomics would take its place in mainstream healthy nutrition within a few (10–15) years—all of us would have a list, not only of what is healthy and unhealthy based on our particular set of genes, but also in which quantities and at which intervals nutrients would have to be consumed (Boland, 2008). At the same time, the market appearance of personalized nutrition in the form of advice or food was expected to appear between 2010 and 2050 by experts in the various disciplines of nutrigenomics (including molecular biologists, food scientists, bioethicists, governmental bodies, food and biotech companies, and nongovernmental groups, especially patient representatives); their average prediction was 2020 (Ronteltap et al., 2007). Some authors (e.g., German et al., 2004) have argued that the application of nutrigenomics in the form of personalized foods holds the potential to shift the food market from a technology push into a consumer pull system, where the consumer's preference for optimal health is a major driver in food choice, and as a consequence for food production.

However, this is still not the case. Indeed, the concept of personalized nutrition has not yet brought big changes in the food industry (de Roos, 2013). This could cause trust issues among people who are not directly involved in the research, because if people heard 10 years ago that nutrigenomics would have concrete applications in about 10 years, and even today there is still no implementation, they might lose faith in the technological possibilities (Gudde, 2009).

On the one hand, of course, there are several important drivers of genetic-based personalized nutrition. Advances in nutrigenomics will undoubtedly further the understanding of the complex interplay between genotype, phenotype, and environment, which is required to enhance the development of personalized nutrition in the future (de Roos, 2013). As doctors will have increasing knowledge of nutrigenomics, mainstream acceptance will occur (Boland, 2008).

Other drivers are related to the consumer side of the market. One of them is an aging and affluent baby boom population aware of the importance of healthy nutrition to prevent or minimize the adverse effects of aging (Boland, 2008). Beside awareness, they also have the means (in terms of new technologies and financial circumstances) to fight against aging.

A further driver of personalized nutrition is the increasing awareness of consumers (in a marketing sense) of their individuality (Boland, 2008). Personalized nutrition fits well into the current marketing trend of moving the consumer–company relationship from the mass model toward a customized model (Ahlgren et al., 2013; Ronteltap et al., 2009; Sutton, 2007). Consumer goods have become increasingly personalized, particularly during the second half of the 20th century (German et al., 2004; Ghosh, 2010). Individualized products appeal to today's sophisticated consumers, and allow them to feel empowered and to stand out from the crowd. In affluent societies, all survival needs are easily met for the majority of the population. It is the "self-actualization" drivers at the higher levels that drive the consumer. Personalized nutrition is all about meeting these higher level needs in the context of nutrition (Boland, 2008).

A further driver for the development of personalized nutrition on the consumer side is that personalized nutrition may be a part of the "experience economy" (Boland, 2008). This means that affluent customers today will make purchases of goods based not only on the quality of the good, but also on the experience of the purchase (Pine & Gilmore, 1998). Beside this, the growing consumer interest in health and nutrition as a result of the fact that being slim has become a societal trend, stimulates people's interest in using nutrigenomics (Ronteltap et al., 2007).

At the same time, however, consumer acceptance of personalized nutrition is hindered by several factors, as was discussed in the earlier section "Consumer Judgment of Personalized Nutrition and Nutrigenomics." Some of them are scientific in nature, some technical, and others are related to consumer, ethical, or market issues (Ghosh, 2009; Ronteltap et al., 2009). On the one hand, on the scientific side it can be stated that examinations of the fundamental mechanisms of our genes and nutrition have revealed more and more complexity (Stewart-Knox et al., 2009): nutrition affects not only one gene but clusters of genes, and the majority of diseases can relate to more than one gene. Moreover, between nature (genetics) and nurture (environment), intermediaries exist (de Vrieze et al., 2009). Furthermore, testing products might raise ethical issues as well, since the rejection of healthy nutrition by the control group is questionable. Another problem is caused by the fact that biological differences are very small, thus examinations require large and costly samples (Hesketh et al., 2006; Penders, 2008). All this may cause a certain level of professional scepticism, which—if it persists—will mean the uptake of nutrigenomics may remain limited (Morin, 2009).

On the other hand, on the consumer side, nutrigenomics-based personalized nutrition does not fit well into the daily life of consumers; it is not yet compatible with a relaxed and enjoyable life (de Vrieze et al., 2009).

As we could see in "Consumer Judgment of Personalized Nutrition and Nutrigenomics" and "Factors Influencing the Consumer Acceptance of Personalized Nutrition" sections, the most important hindering factor for consumer acceptance of personalized nutrition may be consumers' privacy concerns. Because of consumers' benefit—risk considerations, benefits have to be emphasized, while the delivery system needs to be made secure (Stewart-Knox et al., 2015). To take up such services the information collected will require regulation (Ahlgren et al., 2013) and this is where governments have to become involved in the process as facilitators of the consumer acceptance of personalized nutrition.

A further ethical question concerns how access to personalized nutrition could be ensured for lower income classes which have a greater need for it but lack the means to adopt it. One solution might be, for example, if it were offered by employers or insurance companies instead of commercial businesses (although trust issues might emerge in these cases), or if a hybrid form is created with a combination of commercial and public services, where the basic service is provided by the national health care system, while specific implementations, such as comprehensive lifestyle advice applications to monitor progress, may be left to the market (Fischer et al., 2016).

Beside this, from a company point of view, personalized diets have proved to be more expensive than mass production (de Vrieze et al., 2009), in particularly because personalized foods are produced at an additional cost; and what is more, their marketing and distribution have to be targeted at increasingly small consumer segments, which may not be financially viable (de Roos, 2013). Beside this, personalized nutrition advice is also more expensive due to the higher research and service costs. At the same time, WTP for genetic-based personalized advice (and maybe foods) is relatively low, suggesting that nutrigenomics methods should be developed at little extra cost (Berezowska et al., 2015).

Part of the solution can be the so-called mass customization that makes efficiencies available which are normally associated with mass production, but at the same time can satisfy personalized requirements by producing individually tailored products that are developed from a range of mass-produced precursors (Boland, 2008), through adding specific ingredients to products at the very last step in the production chain (van Trijp & Ronteltap, 2007). With the use of this method, we are able to match various nutrition requirements of a wide range of individuals, that is, a widespread of personalized nutrition can be achieved (Boland, 2008), as the high costs of customization can be reduced to the level of those of mass production. Mass customization—as a kind of build to order approach—makes it possible to take the customer's specific nutritional needs (functional performance) as well as personal food preferences (sensory performance) into account (Boland, 2008). Thus with a high level of consumer involvement through codesign, consumers may derive value (Wendel et al., 2013). To achieve this, however, the business model of the food industry would need to change: instead of selling through an intermediary, it might be necessary to have one-to-one contact with the customer (Mehrotra, 2004; Ronteltap et al., 2007), otherwise customer involvement will be cumbersome.

Finally, the expertise and collaboration of all stakeholders, especially opinion leaders (scientists at universities and research institutes, food industries, consumer or patient organizations, and the government) are needed to overcome the challenges (Ghosh, 2014; Hurlimann et al., 2014; Nielsen & El-Sohemy, 2012; Ronteltap et al., 2007) mentioned above to further develop and implement a viable business model of personalized nutrition.

References

Adams, K. M., Lindell, K. C., Kohlmeier, M., & Zeisel, S. H. (2006). Status of nutrition education in medical schools. *American Journal of Clinical Nutrition*, 83(4), 941S–944S. Available from https://doi.org/10.1093/ajcn/83.4.941S.

Ahlgren, J., Nordgen, A., Perrudin, M., Ronteltap, A., Savigny, J., van Trijp, H., ... Görman, U. (2013). Consumers on the Internet: Ethical and legal aspects of commercialization of personalized nutrition. *Genes and Nutrition*, 8 (4), 349–355. Available from https://doi.org/10.1007/s12263-013-0331-0.

Akinleye, I., Roberts, J. S., Royal, C. D. M., Linnenbringer, E., Obisesan, T. O., Fasaye, G.-A., & Green, R. C. (2011). Differences between African American and white research volunteers in their attitudes, beliefs and knowledge regarding genetic testing for Alzheimer's disease. *Journal of Genetic Counseling*, 20(6), 650–659. Available from https://doi.org/10.1007/s10897-011-9377-6.

Alford, S. H., McBride, C. M., Reid, R. J., Larson, E. B., Baxevanis, A. D., & Brody, L. C. (2011). Participation in genetic testing research varies by social group. *Public Health Genomics*, 14(2), 85–93. Available from https://doi.org/10.1159/000294277.

Aro, A. R., Hakonen, A., Hietala, M., Lönnqvist, J., Niemelä, P., Peltonen, L., & Aula, P. (1997). Acceptance of genetic testing in a general population: Age, education and gender differences. *Patient Education and Counseling*, 32(1-2), 41−49. Available from https://doi.org/10.1016/S0738-3991(97)00061-X.

Basson, F., Futter, M. J., & Greenberg, J. (2007). Qualitative research methodology in the exploration of patients' perceptions of participating in a genetic research program. *Ophthalmic Genetics*, 28(3), 143−149. Available from https://doi.org/10.1080/13816810701356627.

Beckett, E. L., Jones, P. R., Veysey, M., & Lucock, M. (2017). Nutrigenetics—personalized nutrition in the genetic age. *Exploratory Research and Hypothesis in Medicine*, 2(4), 109−116. Available from https://doi.org/10.14218/ERHM.2017.00027.

Berezowska, A., Fischer, A. R. H., Ronteltap, A., Kuzneof, S., Macready, A., Fallaize, R., & van Trijp, H. C. M. (2014). Understanding consumer evaluations of personalised nutrition services in terms of the privacy calculus: A qualitative study. *Public Health Genomics*, 17(3), 127−140. Available from https://doi.org/10.1159/000358851.

Berezowska, A., Fischer, A. R. H., Ronteltap, A., van der Lans, I. A., & van Trijp, H. C. M. (2014). *Personalised nutrition: An integrated analysis of opportunities and challenges. Project acronym: Food4Me. Consumer acceptance report 2* (pp. 1−31). Wageningen University and Research Centre.

Berezowska, A., Fischer, A. R. H., Ronteltap, A., van der Lans, I. A., & van Trijp, H. C. M. (2015). Consumer adoption of personalised nutrition services from the perspective of a risk−benefit trade-off. *Genes and Nutrition*, 10(6), 42. Available from https://doi.org/10.1007/s12263-015-0478-y.

Bergmann, M. M., Gorman, U., & Mathers, J. C. (2008). Bioethical considerations for human nutrigenomics. *Annual Review of Nutrition*, 28, 447−467. Available from https://doi.org/10.1146/annurev.nutr.28.061807.155344.

Birmingham, W. C., Agarwal, N., Kohlmann, W., Aspinwall, L. G., Wang, M., Bishoff, J., . . . Kinney, A. Y. (2013). Patient and provider attitudes toward genomic testing for prostate cancer susceptibility: A mixed method study. *BMC Health Services Research*, 13, 279. Available from https://doi.org/10.1186/1472-6963-13-279.

Bock, A. K., Maragkoudakis, P., Wollgast, J., Caldeira, S., Czimbalmos, A., Rzychon, M., & Ulberth, F. (2014). *Tomorrow's healthy society − research priorities for foods and diets (Final Report)*. Luxembourg: Joint Research Centre − Foresight and Behavioural Insights Unit.

Boland, M. (2008). Innovation in the food industry: Personalised nutrition and mass customisation. *IOM*, 10(1), 53−60. Available from https://doi.org/10.5172/impp.453.10.1.53.

Bottorff, J. L., Ratner, P. A., Balneaves, L. G., Richardson, C. J., McCullum, M., Hack, T., . . . Buxton, J. (2002). Women's interest in genetic testing for breast cancer risk: The influence of sociodemographics and knowledge. *Cancer Epidemiology, Biomarkers & Prevention*, 11(1), 89−95.

Bouwman, L., Hiddink, G. J., Koelen, M. A., Korthals, M., van Veer, P., & van Woerkum, C. (2005). Personalized nutrition communication through ICT application: how to overcome the gap between potential effectiveness and reality. *European Journal of Clinical Nutrition*, 59(Suppl. 1), S108−S116. Available from https://doi.org/10.1038/sj.ejcn.1602182.

Bouwman, L., te Molder, H., & Hiddink, G. (2008). Patients, evidence and genes: An exploration of GPs' perspectives on gene-based personalized nutrition advice. *Family Practice*, 25(Suppl. 1), i116−i122. Available from https://doi.org/10.1093/fampra/cmn067.

Brown, R. C. (2013). Moral responsibility for (un)healthy behaviour. *Journal of Medical Ethics Online First*. Available from https://doi.org/10.1136/medethics-2012-100774, 11 January 2013.

Castle, D., & Ries, N. A. (2007). Ethical, legal and social issues in nutrigenomics: the challenges of regulating service delivery and building health professional capacity. *Mutation Research*, 622(1−2), 138−143. Available from https://doi.org/10.1016/j.mrfmmm.2007.03.017.

Catz, D. S., Green, N. S., Tobin, J. N., Lloyd-Puryear, M. A., Kyler, P., Umemoto, J. C., . . . Wolman, F. (2005). Attitudes about genetics in underserved, culturally diverse underserved, culturally diverse populations. *Journal of Community Genetics*, 8(3), 161−172. Available from https://doi.org/10.1159/000086759.

Cherkas, L. F., Harris, J. M., Levinson, E., Spector, T. D., & Prainsack, B. (2010). A survey of UK public interest in Internet-based personal genome testing. *PLoS One*, 5(10), e13473. Available from https://doi.org/10.1371/journal.pone.0013473.

Cohen, A. K., Rai, M., Rehkopf, D. H., & Abrams, B. (2013). Educational attainment and obesity: A systematic review. *Obesity Reviews*, 14(12), 989−1005. Available from https://doi.org/10.1111/obr.12062.

Collins, F. S., Morgan, M., & Patrinos, A. (2003). The Human Genome Project: Lessons from large-scale biology. *Science, 300*(5617), 286−290. Available from https://doi.org/10.1126/science.1084564.

Coppens, P., da Silva, F. M., & Pettman, S. (2006). European regulations on nutraceuticals, dietary supplements and functional foods: A framework based on safety. *Toxicology, 221*(1), 59−74. Available from https://doi.org/10.1016/j.tox.2005.12.022.

Cormier, H., Tremblay, B. L., Paradis, A. M., Garneau, V., Desroches, S., Robitaille, J., & Vohl, M. C. (2014). Nutrigenomics − perspectives from registered dietitians: A report from the Quebec-wide e-consultation on nutrigenomics among registered dietitians. *Journal of Human Nutrition and Dietetics, 27*(4), 391−400. Available from https://doi.org/10.1111/jhn.12194.

de Roos, B. (2013). Personalized nutrition: Ready for practice? *Proceedings of the Nutrition Society, 72*(1), 48−52. Available from https://doi.org/10.1017/S0029665112002844.

de Vrieze, J., Bouwman, L., Komduur, R., Pin, R., Ronteltap, A., Vandeberg, R., ... Penders, B. (2009). Nutrition tailored to the individual? Not just yet − realigning nutrigenomic science with contemporary society. *Journal of Nutrigenetics and Nutrigenomics, 2*(4−5), 184−188. Available from https://doi.org/10.1159/000253870.

Eaton, C. B., McBride, P. E., Gans, K. A., & Underbakke, G. L. (2003). Teaching nutrition skills to primary care practitioners. *Journal of Nutrition, 133*(2), 563S−566S. Available from https://doi.org/10.1093/jn/133.2.563S.

Elder, J. P., Ayala, G. X., Slymen, D. J., Arredondo, E. M., & Campbell, N. R. (2009). Evaluating psychosocial and behavioural mechanisms of change in a tailored communication intervention. *Health Education & Behavior, 36*(2), 366−380. Available from https://doi.org/10.1177/1090198107308373.

Etchegary, H., Cappelli, M., Potter, B., Vloet, M., Graham, I., Walker, M., & Wilson, B. (2010). Attitude and knowledge about genetics and genetic testing. *Public Health Genomics, 13*(2), 80−88. Available from https://doi.org/10.1159/000220034.

European Commission (EC). (2014). *Improving health for all European citizens. The European Union explained: Public health*. Luxembourg: Publications Office of the European Union.

Falcone, D. C., Wood, E. M., Xie, S. X., Siderowf, A., & Van Deerlin, M. (2011). Genetic testing and Parkinson disease: Assessment of patient knowledge, attitudes, and interest. *Journal of Genetic Counseling, 20*(4), 384−395. Available from https://doi.org/10.1007/s10897-011-9362-0.

Fallaize, R., Macready, A. L., Butler, L. T., Ellis, J. A., Berezowska, A., Fischer, A. R. H., ... Lovegrove, J. A. (2015). The perceived impact of the National Health Service on personalised nutrition service delivery among the UK public. *British Journal of Nutrition, 113*(8), 1271−1279. Available from https://doi.org/10.1017/S0007114515000045.

Fallaize, R., Macready, A. L., Butler, L. T., Ellis, J. A., & Lovegrove, J. A. (2013). An insight into the public acceptance of nutrigenomic-based personalised nutrition. *Nutrition Research Reviews, 26*(1), 39−48. Available from https://doi.org/10.1017/S0954422413000024.

Farhud, D. D., Zarif Yeganeh, M., & Zarif Yeganeh, M. (2010). Nutrigenomics and nutrigenetics. *Iranian Journal of Public Health, 39*(4), 1−14.

Finney Rutten, L. J., Gollust, S. E., Naveed, S., & Moser, R. P. (2012). Increasing public awareness of direct-to-consumer genetic tests: Health care access, internet use, and population density correlates. *Journal of Cancer Epidemiology*. Available from https://doi.org/10.1155/2012/309109, Article ID 309109.

Fischer, A. R. H., Berezowska, A., van der Lans, I. A., Ronteltap, A., Rankin, A., Kuznesof, S., ... Frewer, L. J. (2016). Willingness to pay for personalised nutrition across Europe. *The European Journal of Public Health, 26*(4), 640−644. Available from https://doi.org/10.1093/eurpub/ckw045.

Frewer, L. J., Bergmann, K., Brennan, M., Lion, R., Meertens, R., Rowe, G., ... Vereijken, C. (2011). Consumer response to novel agri-food technologies: Implications for predicting consumer acceptance of emerging food technologies. *Trends in Food Science & Technology, 22*(8), 442−446. Available from https://doi.org/10.1016/j.tifs.2011.05.005.

Frosch, D. L., Mello, P., & Lerman, C. (2005). Behavioral consequences of testing for obesity risk. *Cancer Epidemiology Biomarkers & Prevention, 14*(6), 1485−1489. Available from https://doi.org/10.1158/1055-9965.EPI-04-0913.

German, J. B., Yeretzian, C., & Watzke, H. J. (2004). Personalizing foods for health and preference. *Food Technology, 58*(12), 26−31.

Ghosh, D. (2009). Future perspectives of nutrigenomics foods: Benefits vs. risks. *Indian Journal of Biochemistry and Biophysics, 46*(1), 31−36.

Ghosh, D. (2010). Personalised food: How personal is it? *Genes and Nutrition*, 5(1), 51–53. Available from https://doi.org/10.1007/s12263-009-0139-0.

Ghosh, D. (2014). The drivers and consumer attitudes in the personalisation of health and nutrition. *Agro Food Industry Hi Tech*, 25(2), 48–49.

Gibney, M. J., & Walsh, M. C. (2013). The future direction of personalised nutrition: My diet, my phenotype, my genes. *Proceedings of the Nutrition Society*, 72(2), 219–225. Available from https://doi.org/10.1017/S0029665112003436.

Glenn, B. A., Chawla, N., & Bastani, R. (2012). Barriers to genetic testing for breast cancer risk among ethnic minority women: An exploratory study. *Ethnicity & Disease*, 22(3), 267–273.

Goddard, K. A., Robitaille, J., Dowling, N. F., Parrado, J., Bradley, L. A., Moore, C. A., & Khoury, M. J. (2009). Healthrelated direct-to-consumer genetic tests: a public health assessment and analysis of practices related to Internet-based tests for risk of thrombosis. *Public Health Genomics*, 12(2), 92–104. Available from https://doi.org/10.1159/000176794.

Goldman, R. E., Kingdon, C., Wasser, J., Clark, M. A., Goldberg, R., Papandonatos, G. D., ... Koren, G. (2008). Rhode Islanders' attitudes towards the development of a statewide genetic biobank. *Journal of Personalized Medicine*, 5(4), 339–359. Available from https://doi.org/10.2217/17410541.5.4.339.

Gollust, S. E., Gordon, E. S., Zayac, C., Griffin, G., Christman, M. F., Pyeritz, R. E., ... Bernhardt, B. A. (2012). Motivations and perceptions of early adopters of personalized genomics: Perspectives from research participants. *Public Health Genomics*, 15(1), 22–30. Available from https://doi.org/10.1159/000327296.

Görman, U. (2006). Ethical issues raised by personalized nutrition based on genetic information. *Genes and Nutrition*, 1(1), 13–22. Available from https://doi.org/10.1007/BF02829932.

Görman, U., Mathers, J. C., Grimaldi, K. A., Ahlgren, J., & Nordström, K. (2013). Do we know enough? A scientific and ethical analysis of the basis for genetic based personalized nutrition. *Genes and Nutrition*, 8(4), 373–381. Available from https://doi.org/10.1007/s12263-013-0338-6.

Grant, R., Hivert, M., Pandiscio, J., Florez, J. C., Nathan, D. M., & Meigs, J. B. (2009). The clinical application of genetic testing in type 2 diabetes: A patient and physician survey. *Diabetologia*, 52(11), 2299–2305. Available from https://doi.org/10.1007/s00125-009-1512-7.

Gudde, L. (2009). *Towards a successful implementation of nutrigenomics: Experts and their visions on public acceptance* (MS thesis). Enschede: University of Twente.

Haga, S. B., Barry, W. T., Mills, R., Ginsburg, G. S., Svetkey, L., Sullivan, J., & Willard, H. F. (2013). Public knowledge of and attitudes toward genetics and genetic testing. *Genetic Testing and Molecular Biomarkers*, 17(4), 327–335. Available from https://doi.org/10.1089/gtmb.2012.0350.

Hardie, E. A. (2011). Australian community responses to the use of genetic testing for personalised health promotion. *Australian Journal of Psychology*, 63(2), 119–129. Available from https://doi.org/10.1111/j.1742-9536.2011.00017.x.

Henneman, L., Timmermans, D. R. M., & Wal, G. V. D. (2006). Public attitudes toward genetic testing: perceived benefits and objections. *Genetic Testing*, 10(2), 139–145. Available from https://doi.org/10.1089/gte.2006.10.139.

Henneman, L., Vermeulen, E., van El, C. G., Claasen, L., Timmermans, D. R. M., & Cornel, M. C. (2013). Public attitudes towards genetic testing revisited: Comparing opinions between 2002 and 2010. *European Journal of Human Genetics*, 21(8), 793–799. Available from https://doi.org/10.1038/ejhg.2012.271.

Hesketh, J., Wybranska, I., Dommels, Y., & King, M. (2006). Nutrient–gene interactions in benefit–risk analysis. *British Journal of Nutrition*, 95(6), 1232–1236. Available from https://doi.org/10.1079/BJN20061749.

Hoeyer, K., Olofsson, B. O., Mjörndal, T., & Lynöw, N. (2004). Informed consent and biobanks: A population-based study of attitudes towards tissue donation for genetic research. *Scandinavian Journal of Public Health*, 32(3), 224–229. Available from https://doi.org/10.1080/14034940310019506.

Horn, E. J., & Terry, S. F. (2012). Consumer perceptions of genetic testing. *Genetic Testing and Molecular Biomarkers*, 16(6), 463–464. Available from https://doi.org/10.1089/gtmb.2012.1532.

Hull, S. C., Sharp, R. R., Botkin, J. R., Brown, M., Hughes, M., Sugarman, J., ... Sankar, P. (2008). Patients' views on identifiability of samples and informed consent for genetic research. *American Journal of Bioethics*, 8(10), 62–70. Available from https://doi.org/10.1080/15265160802478404.

Hunter, D. J., Khoury, M. J., & Drazen, J. M. (2008). Letting the genome out of the bottle – will we get our wish? *New England Journal of Medicine*, 358(2), 105–107. Available from https://doi.org/10.1056/NEJMp0708162.

Hurlimann, T., Menuz, V., Graham, J., Robitaille, J., Vohl, M.-C., & Godard, B. (2014). Risks of nutrigenomics and nutrigenetics? What the scientists say. *Genes and Nutrition*, 9(1), 370. Available from https://doi.org/10.1007/s12263-013-0370-6.

Joost, H. G., Gibney, M. J., Cashman, K. D., Görman, U., Hesketh, J. E., Mueller, M., ... Mathers, J. C. (2007). Personalised nutrition: Status and perspectives. *British Journal of Nutrition*, 98(1), 26–31. Available from https://doi.org/10.1017/S0007114507685195.

Jonassaint, C. R., Santos, E. R., Glover, C. M., Payne, P. W., Fasaye, G.-A., Oji-Njideka, N., ... Royal, C. D. (2010). Regional differences in awareness and attitudes regarding genetic testing for disease risk and ancestry. *Human Genetics*, 128(3), 249–260. Available from https://doi.org/10.1007/s00439-010-0845-0.

Kang, J. X. (2012). The coming of age of nutrigenetics and nutrigenomics. *Journal of Nutrigenetics and Nutrigenomics*, 5(1), I–II. Available from https://doi.org/10.1159/000339375.

Kaput, J. (2007). Nutrigenomics—2006 update. *Clinical Chemistry and Laboratory Medicine*, 45(3), 279–287. Available from https://doi.org/10.1515/CCLM.2007.057.

Kaput, J., & Rodriguez, R. L. (2004). Nutritional genomics: The next frontier in the postgenomic era. *Physiological Genomics*, 16(2), 166–177. Available from https://doi.org/10.1152/physiolgenomics.00107.2003.

Keogh, L., McClaren, B., Maskiell, J., Niven, H., Rutsein, A., Flander, L., ... Jenkins, M. (2011). How do individuals decide whether to accept or decline an offer of genetic testing for colorectal cancer? *Hereditary Cancer in Clinical Practice*, 9(Suppl. 1), 17. Available from https://doi.org/10.1186/1897-4287-9-S1-P17.

Kerath, S. M., Klein, G., Kern, M., Shapira, L., Witthuhn, J., Norohna, N., ... Taioli, E. (2013). Beliefs and attitudes towards participating in genetic research – a population based cross-sectional study. *BMC Public Health*, 13(1), 114. Available from https://doi.org/10.1186/1471-2458-13-114.

Komduur, R. H., Korthals, M., & te Molder, H. (2009). The good life: Living for health and a life without risks? On a prominent script of nutrigenomics. *British Journal of Nutrition*, 101(3), 307–316. Available from https://doi.org/10.1017/S0007114508076253.

Korthals, M. (2011). Coevolution of nutrigenomics and society: Ethical considerations. *American Journal of Clinical Nutrition*, 94(Suppl. 6), 2025S–2029S. Available from https://doi.org/10.3945/ajcn.110.001289.

Kussmann, M., & Fay, L. B. (2008). Nutrigenomics and personalized nutrition: Science and concept. *Journal of Personalized Medicine*, 5(5), 447–455. Available from https://doi.org/10.2217/17410541.5.5.447.

Kutz, G. (2006). *Nutrigenomic testing. Tests purchased from four websites mislead consumers*. Testimony before the special committee on aging. U.S. Senate Report GAO-06- 977T. U.S. Government Accountability Office, Washington, DC. <https://www.gao.gov/assets/120/114612.pdf> Accessed 01.07.18.

Lévesque, L., Ozdemir, V., Gremmen, B., & Godard, B. (2008). Integrating anticipated nutrigenomics bioscience applications with ethical aspects. *OMICS*, 12(1), 1–16. Available from https://doi.org/10.1089/omi.2007.0042.

Lewis, K. D., & Burton-Freeman, B. M. (2010). The role of innovation and technology in meeting individual nutritional needs. *Journal of Nutrition*, 140(2), 426S–436S. Available from https://doi.org/10.3945/jn.109.114710.

Lustria, M. L. A., Cortese, L., Noar, S. M., & Glueckauf, R. L. (2009). Computer-tailored health interventions delivered over the web: Review and analysis of key components. *Patient Education and Counseling*, 74(2), 156–173. Available from https://doi.org/10.1016/j.pec.2008.08.023.

Makeeva, O. A., Markova, V. V., & Puzyrev, V. P. (2009). Public interest and expectations concerning commercial genotyping and genetic risk assessment. *Journal of Personalized Medicine*, 6(3), 329–341. Available from https://doi.org/10.2217/pme.09.14.

Makeeva, O. A., Markova, V. V., Roses, A. D., & Puzyrev, V. P. (2010). An epidemiologic-based survey of public attitudes towards predictive genetic testing in Russia. *Journal of Personalized Medicine*, 7(3), 291–300. Available from https://doi.org/10.2217/pme.10.23.

Marsh and McLennan Co. (2014). *How much could the world save through innovative healthcare delivery models?* Oliver Wymann Health and Life Sciences <http://www.oliverwyman.com/content/dam/oliver-wyman/global/en/files/insights/health-life-sciences/2014/Jan/NYC-MKT08001-025%20global%20delivery%20models.pdf>. Accessed 28.06.18.

McBride, C. M., Bryan, A. D., Bray, M. S., Swan, G. E., & Green, E. D. (2012). Health behavior change: Can genomics improve behavioral adherence? *American Journal of Public Health*, 102, 401–405. Available from https://doi.org/10.2105/AJPH.2011.300513.

McGowan, M. L., Fishman, J. R., & Lambrix, M. A. (2010). Personal genomics and individual identities: Motivations and moral imperatives of early users. *New Genetics and Society*, 29(3), 261–290. Available from https://doi.org/10.1080/14636778.2010.507485.

McGuire, A. L., Diaz, C. M., Wang, T., & Hilsenbeck, S. G. (2009). Social networkers' attitudes toward direct-to-consumer personal genome testing. *American Journal of Bioethics*, 9(6−7), 3−10. Available from https://doi.org/10.1080/15265160902928209.

Mehrotra, I. (2004). A perspective on developing and marketing food products to meet individual needs of population segments. *Comprehensive Reviews in Food Science and Food Safety*, 3(4), 142−244. Available from https://doi.org/10.1111/j.1541-4337.2004.tb00064.x.

Morin, K. (2009). Knowledge and attitudes of Canadian consumers and health care professionals regarding nutritional genomics. *OMICS*, 13(1), 37−41. Available from https://doi.org/10.1089/omi.2008.0047.

Morren, M., Rijken, M., Baanders, A. N., & Bensing, J. (2007). Perceived genetic knowledge, attitudes towards genetic testing, and the relationship between these among patients with a chronic disease. *Patient Education and Counseling*, 65(2), 197−204. Available from https://doi.org/10.1016/j.pec.2006.07.005.

Muller, M., & Kersten, S. (2003). Nutrigenomics: Goals and strategies. *Nature Reviews Genetics*, 4(4), 315−322. Available from https://doi.org/10.1038/nrg1047.

Nielsen, D. E., & El-Sohemy, A. (2012). Applying genomics to nutrition and lifestyle modification. *Journal of Personalized Medicine*, 9(7), 739−749. Available from https://doi.org/10.2217/PME.12.79.

Nielsen, D. E., Shih, S., & El-Sohemy, A. (2014). Perceptions of genetic testing for personalized nutrition: A randomized trial of DNA-based dietary advice. *Journal of Nutrigenetics and Nutrigenomics*, 7(2), 94−104. Available from https://doi.org/10.1159/000365508.

Nizel, A. E. (1972). Personalized nutrition counseling. *American Society of Dentistry for Children*, 39(5), 353−360.

Nordström, K., Coff, C., Jönsson, H., Nordenfelt, L., & Görman, U. (2013). Food and health: Individual, cultural, or scientific matters? *Genes and Nutrition*, 8(4), 336. Available from https://doi.org/10.1007/s12263-013-0336-8.

Nyrhinen, T., Leino-Kilpi, H., & Hietala, M. (2004). Ethical issues in the diagnostic genetic testing process. *New Genetics and Society*, 23(1), 73−87. Available from https://doi.org/10.1080/1463677042000189570.

O'Daniel, J. M., Haga, S. B., & Willard, H. F. (2010). Considerations for the impact of personal genome information: A study of genomic profiling among genetics and genomics professionals. *Journal of Genetic Counseling*, 19 (4), 387−401. Available from https://doi.org/10.1007/s10897-010-9297-x.

Oenema, A., Brug, J., & Lechner, L. (2001). Web-based tailored nutrition education: Results of a randomized controlled trial. *Health Education Research*, 16(6), 647−660. Available from https://doi.org/10.1093/her/16.6.647.

Oliver, D. The future of nutrigenomics, Institute for the Future report SR−889. (2005). <http://www.iftf.org/uploads/media/SR_889_Future_of_Nutrigenomics_01.pdf>. Accessed 03.07.18.

Ormond, K. E., Hudgins, L., Ladd, J. M., Magnus, D. M., Greely, H. T., & Cho, M. K. (2011). Medical and graduate students' attitudes toward personal genomics. *Genetics in Medicine*, 13(5), 400−408. Available from https://doi.org/10.1097/GIM.0b013e31820562f6.

Otlowski, M., Taylor, S., & Bombard, Y. (2012). Genetic discrimination: International perspectives. *Annual Review of Genomics and Human Genetics*, 13, 433−454. Available from https://doi.org/10.1146/annurev-genom-090711-163800.

Penders, B. (2008). *From seeking health to finding healths: The politics of large-scale cooperation in nutrition science*. Maastricht: Maastricht Pers Universitaire.

Perez, G. K., Cruess, D. G., Cruess, S., Brewer, M., Stroop, J., Schwartz, R., & Greenstein, R. (2011). Attitudes toward direct-to-consumer advertisements and online genetic testing among high-risk women participating in a hereditary cancer clinic. *Journal of Health Communication*, 16(6), 607−628.

Pin, R. R. (2009). *Public perceptions of nutrigenomics. affect, cognition & behavioral intention*. Enschede: University of Twente.

Pine, B. J., & Gilmore, J. H. (1998). *Welcome to the experience economy*. Boston, MA: Harvard Business Review Harvard Business School Press.

Poínhos, R., Oliveira, B. M. P. M., van der Lans, I. A., Fischer, A. R. H., Berezowska, A., Rankin, A., ... de Almeida, M. D. V. (2017). Providing personalised nutrition: Consumers' trust and preferences regarding sources of information, service providers and regulators, and communication channels. *Public Health Genomics*, 20(4), 218−228. Available from https://doi.org/10.1159/000481357.

Poínhos, R., van der Lans, I. A., Rankin, A., Fischer, A. R. H., Bunting, B., Kuznesof, S., ... Frewer, L. J. (2014). Psychological determinants of consumer acceptance of personalised nutrition in 9 European countries. *PLoS One*, 9(10), e110614. Available from https://doi.org/10.1371/journal.pone.0110614.

Reilly, P. R., & Debusk, R. M. (2008). Ethical and legal issues in nutritional genomics. *Journal of the American Dietetic Association*, 108(1), 36−40. Available from https://doi.org/10.1016/j.jada.2007.10.016.

Ries, N. M., & Castle, D. (2008). Nutrigenomics and ethics interface: Direct-to-consumer services and commercial aspects. *OMICS*, *12*(4), 245–250. Available from https://doi.org/10.1089/omi.2008.0049.

Ries, N. M., Hyde-Lay, R., & Caulfield, T. (2010). Willingness to pay for genetic testing: A study of attitudes in a Canadian population. *Public Health Genomics*, *13*(5), 292–300. Available from https://doi.org/10.1159/000253120.

Rimbach, G., & Minihane, A. M. (2009). Nutrigenetics and personalised nutrition: How far have we progressed and are we likely to get there? *Proceedings of the Nutrition Society*, *68*(2), 162–172. Available from https://doi.org/10.1017/S0029665109001116.

Ronteltap, A. (2008). *Public acceptance of nutrigenomics-based personalised nutrition. Exploring the future with experts and consumers* (MS thesis).Wageningen: Wageningen University and Research Centre.

Ronteltap, A., & van Trijp, H. (2007). Consumer acceptance of personalised nutrition. *Genes and Nutrition*, *2*(3), 85–87. Available from https://doi.org/10.1007/s12263-007-0003-z.

Ronteltap, A., van Trijp, H., Berezowska, A., & Goossens, J. (2013). Nutrigenomics-based personalised nutritional advice: In search of a business model? *Genes and Nutrition*, *8*(2), 153–163. Available from https://doi.org/10.1007/s12263-012-0308-4.

Ronteltap, A., van Trijp, J. C. M., & Renes, R. J. (2007). Expert views on critical success and failure factors for nutrigenomics. *Trends in Food Science & Technology*, *18*(4), 189–200. Available from https://doi.org/10.1016/j.tifs.2006.12.007.

Ronteltap, A., van Trijp, J. C. M., & Renes, R. J. (2009). Consumer acceptance of nutrigenomics-based personalised nutrition. *British Journal of Nutrition*, *101*(1), 132–144. Available from https://doi.org/10.1017/S0007114508992552.

Ronteltap, A., van Trijp, J. C. M., Renes, R. J., & Frewer, L. J. (2007). Consumer acceptance of technology-based food innovations: Lessons for the future of nutrigenomics. *Appetite*, *49*(1), 1–17. Available from https://doi.org/10.1016/j.appet.2007.02.002.

Roosen, J., Bruhn, M., Mecking, R.-A., & Drescher, L. S. (2008). Consumer demand for personalized nutrition and functional food. *International Journal for Vitamin and Nutrition Research*, *78*(6), 269–274. Available from https://doi.org/10.1024/0300-9831.78.6.269.

Saukko, P. (2013). State of play in direct-to-consumer genetic testing for lifestyle-related diseases: Market, marketing content, user experiences and regulation. *Proceedings of the Nutrition Society*, *72*(1), 53–60. Available from https://doi.org/10.1017/S0029665112002960.

Saukko, P. M., Reed, M., Britten, N., & Hogarth, S. (2010). Negotiating the boundary between medicine and consumer culture: Online marketing of nutrigenetic tests. *Social Science & Medicine*, *70*(5), 744–753. Available from https://doi.org/10.1016/j.socscimed.2009.10.066.

Stewart-Knox, B. J., Bunting, B. P., Gilpin, S., Parr, H. J., Pinhão, S., Strain, J. J., ... Gibney, M. (2009). Attitudes toward genetic testing and personalised nutrition in a representative sample of European consumers. *British Journal of Nutrition*, *101*(7), 982–989. Available from https://doi.org/10.1017/S0007114508055657.

Stewart-Knox, B. J., Kuznesof, S., Robinson, J., Rankin, A., Orr, K., Duffy, M., ... Frewer, L. J. (2013). Factors influencing European consumer uptake of personalised nutrition. Results of a qualitative analysis. *Appetite*, *66*, 67–74. Available from https://doi.org/10.1016/j.appet.2013.03.001.

Stewart-Knox, B. J., Markovina, J., Rankin, A., Bunting, B. P., Kuznesof, S., Fischer, A. R. H., ... Frewer, L. J. (2016). Making personalised nutrition the easy choice: Creating policies to break down the barriers and reap the benefits. *Food Policy*, *63*, 134–144. Available from https://doi.org/10.1016/j.foodpol.2016.08.001.

Stewart-Knox, B. J., Rankin, A., Kuznesof, S., Poínhos, R., de Almeida, M. D. V., Fischer, A., ... Frewer, L. J. (2015). Promoting healthy dietary behaviour through personalised nutrition: Technology push or technology pull? *Proceedings of the Nutrition Society*, *74*(2), 171–176. Available from https://doi.org/10.1017/S0029665114001529.

Streicher, S. A., Sanderson, S. C., Jabs, E. W., Diefenbach, M., Smirnoff, M., Peter, I., ... Richardson, L. D. (2011). Reasons for participating and genetic information needs among racially and ethnically diverse biobank participants: A focus group study. *Journal of Community Genetics*, *2*(3), 153–163. Available from https://doi.org/10.1007/s12687-011-0052-2.

Su, Y., Howard, H. C., & Borry, P. (2011). Users' motivations to purchase direct-to-consumer genome-wide testing: an exploratory study of personal stories. *Journal of Community Genetics*, *2*, 135–146. Available from https://doi.org/10.1007/s12687-011-0048-y.

Suriñach, J., Autant-Bernard, C., Manca, F., Massard, N., Moreno, R. *The diffusion/adoption of innovation in the internal market*. Economic Papers 384, European Commission. (2009). <http://ec.europa.eu/economy_finance/publications/pages/publication15826_en.pdf>. Accessed 03.07.18.

Sutton, K. H. (2007). Considerations for the successful development and launch of personalised nutrigenomic foods. *Mutation Research*, 622(1–2), 117–121. Available from https://doi.org/10.1016/j.mrfmmm.2007.03.007.

Szakály, Z., Kiss, M., & Jasák, H. (2014). Funkcionális élelmiszerek, fogyasztói attitűdök és személyre szabott táplálkozás. *Táplálkozásmarketing*, 1(1–2), 3–17. Available from https://doi.org/10.20494/TM/1/1-2/1.

Szakály, Z., Polereczki, Zs, & Kovács, S. (2016). Consumer attitudes toward genetic testing and personalised nutrition in Hungary. *Acta Aliment*, 45(4), 500–508. Available from https://doi.org/10.1556/066.2016.45.4.6.

Taylor, S. (2011). A population-based survey in Australia of men's and women's perceptions of genetic risk and predictive genetic testing and implications for primary care. *Public Health Genomics*, 14(6), 325–336. Available from https://doi.org/10.1159/000324706.

Toiviainen, H., Jallinoja, P., Aro, A. R., & Hemminki, E. (2003). Medical and lay attitudes towards genetic screening and testing in Finland. *European Journal of Human Genetics*, 11(8), 565–572. Available from https://doi.org/10.1038/sj.ejhg.5201006.

van Trijp, J. C. M., & Ronteltap, A. (2007). A marketing and consumer behaviour perspective on personalised nutrition. In F. J. Kok, L. Bouwman, & F. Desiere (Eds.), *Personalized nutrition: Principles and applications*. Boca Raton, FL: CRC Press. https://doi.org/10.1201/9781420009170.ch14.

Vayena, E., Gourna, E., Streuli, J., Hafen, E., & Prainsack, B. (2012). Experiences of early users of direct-to-consumer genomics in Switzerland: an exploratory study. *Public Health Genomics*, 15(6), 352–362. Available from https://doi.org/10.1159/000343792.

Vernarelli, J. A. (2012). Impact of genetic risk assessment on nutritionrelated lifestyle behaviours. *Proceedings of the Nutrition Society*, 72(1), 153–159. Available from https://doi.org/10.1017/S0029665112002741.

Weir, M., Morin, K., Ries, N., & Castle, D. (2010). Canadian health care professionals' knowledge, attitudes and perceptions of nutritional genomics. *British Journal of Nutrition*, 104(8), 1112–1119. Available from https://doi.org/10.1017/S0007114510002035.

Wendel, S., Dellaert, B. G. C., Ronteltap, A., & van Trijp, H. C. M. (2013). Consumers' intention to use health recommendation systems to receive personalized nutrition advice. *BMC Health Services Research*, 13(1), 126. Available from https://doi.org/10.1186/1472-6963-13-126.

Wendel, S., Ronteltap, A., Dellaert, B. G. C., & van Trijp, J. C. M. (2009). Service value chains to support knowledge-based personalized recommendations. In A. L. McGill, S. Shavitt, & M. N. Duluth (Eds.) *NA – Advances in Consumer Research* (Vol. 36, p. 855).

Whelan, K., McCarthy, S., & Pufulete, M. (2008). Genetics and diet-gene interactions: Involvement, confidence and knowledge of dietitians. *British Journal of Nutrition*, 99(1), 23–28. Available from https://doi.org/10.1017/S0007114507793935.

WHO. (2018a). *Noncommunicable diseases*. <http://www.who.int/news-room/fact-sheets/detail/noncommunicable-diseases>. Accessed 01.06.18.

WHO. (2018b). *WHO NCD Surveillance strategy*. <http://www.who.int/ncd_surveillance/strategy/en/>. Accessed 01.06.18.

Wijdenes-Pijl, M., Dondorp, W. J., Timmermans, D. R. M., Cornel, M. C., & Henneman, L. (2011). Lay perceptions of predictive testing for diabetes based on DNA test results versus family history assessment: A focus group study. *BMC Public Health*, 11(1), 535. Available from https://doi.org/10.1186/1471-2458-11-535.

Wilde, A., Meiser, B., Mitchell, P. B., Hadzi-Pavlovic, D., & Schofield, P. R. (2011). Community interest in predictive genetic testing for susceptibility to major depressive disorder in a large national sample. *Psychological Medicine*, 41(8), 1605–1613. Available from https://doi.org/10.1017/S0033291710002394.

Wilde, A., Meiser, B., Mitchell, P. B., & Schofield, P. R. (2010). Public interest in predictive genetic testing, including direct-to-consumer testing, for susceptibility to major depression: Preliminary findings. *European Journal of Human Genetics*, 18(1), 47–51. Available from https://doi.org/10.1038/ejhg.2009.138.

CHAPTER 10

Personalized Nutrition: Making It Happen

Barbara Stewart-Knox[1], Eileen R. Gibney[2], Mariette Abrahams[1], Audrey Rankin[3], Eleanor Bryant[1], Bruno M.P.M. Oliveira[4] and Rui Poínhos[4]

[1]Department of Psychology, University of Bradford, Bradford, United Kingdom [2]UCD Institute of Food and health, University College Dublin, Dublin, Ireland [3]School of Pharmacy, Queen's University, Belfast, United Kingdom [4]Faculty of Nutrition and Food Sciences, University of Porto, Porto, Portugal

OUTLINE

Current Evidence, What it Means and How Reliable is It?	262
What is Personalized Nutrition?	262
Personalized Nutrition in Practice—Does It Work?	263
How Firm is the Science-Base for Personalized Nutrition?	265
What Does the Consumer Want From Personalized Nutrition?	266
What are the Consumer-Perceived Barriers to Uptake of Personalized Nutrition?	266
Who Should Deliver Personalized Nutrition?	269
Implementation of Personalized Nutrition in Practice: Implications for Nutrition/Health Professionals	270
What Can We Learn From Dietitians Who Have Already Adopted Personalized Nutrition?	271
What are the Challenges Faced by Nutrition Professionals in Acquiring the Skills Necessary to Bring Personalized Nutrition into Practice?	271
What is Needed to Widen Access to Personalized Nutrition in the Future?	272
Conclusions	272
References	273

CURRENT EVIDENCE, WHAT IT MEANS AND HOW RELIABLE IS IT?

The importance of diet to health is well established (Arouca et al., 2018; Bendinelli et al., 2018; Vitale et al., 2018). Different patterns of food intake are known to be linked to differing disease risks. Diets low in calcium and vitamin D, for example, are linked to increased risk of bone diseases such as osteoarthritis, and diets high in certain types of saturated fat are linked to increased risk of cardiovascular diseases (CVD) (de Souza et al., 2015; Hooper, Martin, Abdelhamid, & Davey Smith, 2015). As our knowledge of the relationship between diet and disease risk increases, so does the knowledge that considerable variation in response to food consumption exists within the population (Kirwan et al., 2016; Manach et al., 2017; Ryan et al., 2014). Whilst research investigating these variations has been ongoing for many years, in more recent times the task has been to determine the cause of these variations, and then offer advice taking an individual's variations into account. This has developed into an area of nutrition referred to as "personalized nutrition."

What is Personalized Nutrition?

As Ordovas, Ferguson, Tai, and Mathers (2018) recently commented, there is no agreed definition of personalized nutrition. Common to the many definitions that exist is a common goal, which is to use information derived from the individual(s) to deliver more specific dietary and lifestyle advice than that offered by existing standardized healthy eating guidelines (Gibney, Walsh, & Goosens, 2016). Ordovas et al. (2018) defined personalized nutrition as "an approach that uses information on individual characteristics to develop targeted nutritional advice" (Ordovas et al., 2018, p. 1), while for the purpose of the recent Food4Me project the general objective of personalized nutrition was "to maintain or improve health using genetic, phenotypic, clinical, dietary and other information to provide more precise and efficacious personalized healthy eating advice" (Grimaldi et al., 2017, p. 2). Other definitions are more specific and driven by the approach or technology used to "personalize" the information or advice being given. Nutrigenomics, for example, uses molecular tools to clarify and understand different responses to nutrient intakes, to personalize advice for an individual or stratify advice for a group (Maranhão et al., 2018; Ordovas et al., 2018).

The Food4Me project (Celis-Morales et al., 2015; Food4Me, 2015; Gibney et al., 2016; Mathers, 2017) defined personalized nutrition in terms of the manner and depth of personalization and type of data upon which the advice was based: level 1 advice based on individual dietary and anthropometric data; level 2 + advice based on individual phenotypic data; and level 3+ advice based on individual genomic data. These levels offer flexibility in delivering personalized nutrition advice, in that advice given may be based on any combination of personalized data across the levels (Celis-Morales et al., 2015) (Fig. 10.1). Taking this classification of personalized nutrition enables the level of personalization offered to be adjusted to the characteristics of the client and expertise of the provider.

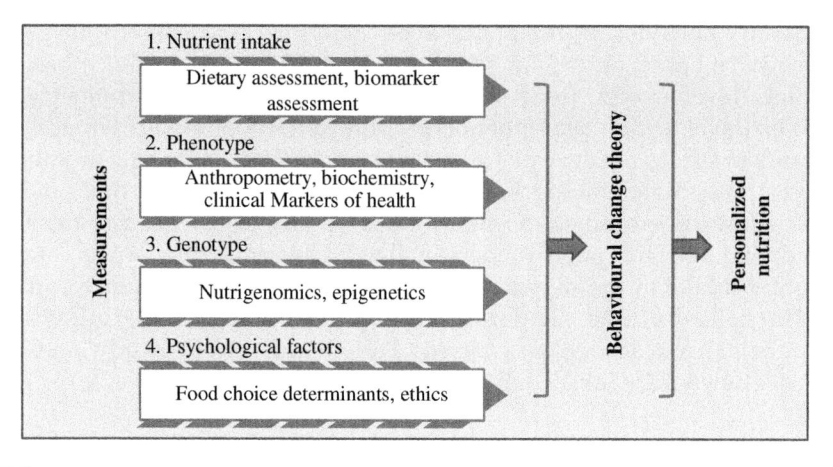

FIGURE 10.1 Personalized nutrition: definition and process.

Personalized Nutrition in Practice—Does It Work?

Regardless of how it is defined, to be able to offer personalized or tailored advice, knowledge on the drivers or causes of the variation in response to diet is required. This is not novel and has been the cornerstone of nutritional advice since the advent of dietary advice, with differing recommended intakes (DRVs) given for age, sex, and lifestyle (Mathers, 2017). Metabolomics and whole genome sequencing allow more complete characterization of an individual and their response to food consumption. With the development of these technologies, societal interest in personalized nutrition has grown (de Roos & Brennan, 2017; Mathers, 2017). Researchers strive to determine the demographic, lifestyle, psychological, phenotypic, and genetic parameters that cause or influence known variation in response to food consumption and dietary advice with the aim of more tailored and effective recommendations.

As interest in the use of personalized nutrition among consumers (Stewart-Knox et al., 2016) and the food and health industry is growing (Abrahams, Frewer, Bryant, & Stewart-Knox, 2018a), it is important to consider existing evidence of its efficacy in effecting positive dietary and/or lifestyle behavioral changes. Whilst considered the "gold standard" in study design, published randomized controlled trails (RCTs) examining the efficacy of personalized nutrition remain few. Moreover, evidence for behavior change following genetics-based advice is mixed (Fallaize et al., 2016; Frosch, Mello, & Lerman, 2005; Guasch-Ferre, Dashti, & Merino, 2018; Li, Ye, Whelan, & Truby, 2016; Nielsen & El-Sohemy, 2012, 2014; O'Donovan, Walsh, Gibney, Brennan, & Gibney, 2017; Roke et al., 2017). One of the more recent and largest RCTs to date examining the impact of personalized nutrition was conducted as part of the Food4Me project. Volunteers ($N = 1607$) were recruited across seven European countries to take part in the Food4Me internet-delivered RCT which examined whether providing personalized nutrition advice based on individual diet, anthropometry, and lifestyle, with the addition of information on phenotype and/or genotype, would promote sustained healthy changes in dietary behavior. Participants were randomized to one of four groups: (control) dietary advice based on public health eating guidelines; or advice based on baseline individual: (level 1) diet; (level 2) diet plus phenotype (anthropometry and blood biomarkers); or (level 3) diet plus phenotype plus genotype taking five diet-responsive genetic variants (*FTO*; *TCF7L2*; *ApoE4*; *FADS1*; and *MTHFR*). Changes in dietary intake, anthropometry, and blood biomarkers measured at baseline and at 3 and 6 months postintervention were examined (Celis-Morales et al., 2015). Results from the study demonstrated that the provision of personalized advice resulted in greater improvements in dietary intake in the personalized groups, compared to the control group, but the change in behavior was similar, irrespective of the type of information upon which the personalized advice was based. Full details of the study and the results can be found elsewhere (Celis-Morales et al., 2017; Fallaize et al., 2016; Livingstone et al., 2016).

Another study (Nielsen & El-Sohemy, 2014), focused specifically on gene–diet interactions (equivalent to level 3 in the Food4Me study) and investigated the short- (3-month) and long- (12-month) term effects of disclosing nutrition-related genetic information for personalized nutrition on dietary intakes of specific dietary components. Participants in the intervention group were genotyped for variants that affect caffeine metabolism (*CYP1A2*), vitamin C utilization (*GSTT1* and *GSTM1*), sweet taste perception (*TAS1R2*), and sodium-sensitivity (*ACE*). For each of these food components, participants who possessed a genotype that has been associated with increased risk of a health outcome when consuming above or below a certain daily amount, were given a "targeted" dietary recommendation. Compared to the control group, no significant changes in dietary intakes were observed at 3 months. At 12 months, however, those in the intervention group who possessed a risk version of the ACE gene (and were therefore advised to limit their sodium intake), had significantly reduced their sodium intake (mg/day) compared to the control group. Those who had the nonrisk version of ACE (and were not advised to alter their sodium intake) did not change their sodium intake compared to the control group. No differences were seen in other parameters. This implies that behavior change in response to genetic-based advice does not happen immediately, which may at least partially explain the lack of short-term differences when genetic data are used. Further in-depth research is needed to understand the psychological processes experienced by the individual subsequent to receiving genetics-based personalized advice, and to determine how this relates to behavior change.

Research results on the efficacy of personalized approaches to dietary health promotion are mixed, even when focused in specific areas such as weight loss. For instance, a study looking at the efficacy of a personalized web-based weight loss maintenance program compared to standard treatment (Collins et al., 2017) not only found no significant weight rebound from the start of weight loss maintenance up to 12 months for either group, but also no significant between-group differences in body mass index (BMI). It was therefore concluded that the addition of personalized e-feedback provided limited additional benefits compared to the standard program (Collins et al., 2017). The ANODE study, on the other hand, was a 16-week RCT in a group of patients with Type 2 Diabetes Mellitus (T2DM) and abdominal obesity who were randomized to a fully automated personalized program that provided either (1) personalized menus and a shopping list for the day, or the week, or (2) general nutritional advice (control). They found a significant improvement in dietary habits and favorable clinical and laboratory changes in the personalized nutrition group (Hansel et al., 2017).

To determine the reasons why interventions are successful or not, and to understand how best to encourage healthy dietary change, future research should consider embedding psychological measures associated with behavior change within trial designs. Results from Food4Me (Macready et al., 2018; Rankin et al., 2017) indicated that preferences for service delivery were in congruence with theories of behavior change based on Social Cognitive Theory (SCT) (Bandura, 1986). Service design and provision therefore should put the client in control, take account of individual goals and embed measures to encourage agency. This could be achieved by providing clients with regular feedback on dietary health markers and thereby enabling them to monitor their progress toward the achievement of their own preset dietary health goals (Rankin et al., 2017). Some potential consumers may prefer automated feedback, others by telephone or in person (Stewart-Knox et al., 2013). The way in which services are delivered therefore may also need to be personalized.

How Firm is the Science-Base for Personalized Nutrition?

With respect to genetic variation and personalized nutrition, whilst many genetic variants show links with nutritional factors, few have the depth and strength of evidence to support their use in personalized advice. Take the folate-metabolizing enzyme methylenetetrahydrofolate reductase (MTHFR) for example. In recent years genome-wide association studies have demonstrated a link between the gene encoding MTHFR with hypertension risk (McNulty, Strain, Hughes, & Ward, 2017). Epidemiological studies show that the 677C→T polymorphism in MTHFR is associated with increased risk of hypertension by 24%–87% and of CVD by up to 40% (McNulty et al., 2017). RCTs conducted in hypertensive patients prescreened for this polymorphism have demonstrated that riboflavin supplementation in homozygous individuals (MTHFR 677TT genotype) lowers systolic blood pressure by 6–13 mmHg, independently of the effect of preprescribed antihypertensive drugs. This has implications for personalized nutrition, given that riboflavin, targeted at those homozygous for a common polymorphism in MTHFR, may offer personalized prevention and/or treatment for hypertension.

Whilst links between genetic variants and response to specific nutrient intakes are known, use in clinical practice is not yet common (Camp & Trujillo, 2014). As the American Dietetic Association noted, "Applying nutritional genomics in clinical practice through the use of genetic testing requires that registered dietitian nutritionists understand, interpret, and communicate complex test results in which the actual risk of developing a disease may not be known. The practical application of nutritional genomics in dietetics practice will require an evidence-based approach to validate that personalized recommendations result in health benefits to individuals and do not cause harm" (Camp & Trujillo, 2014). So when can a consumer trust genetics-based personalized advice? And when should a practitioner decide to begin to offer dietetic advice based on nutrigenetic testing? As a first step to help support the interpretation of existing evidence for the provision of genotype-based dietary advice, Grimaldi et al. (2017), as part of the Global

Nutrigenetics Knowledge Network and the Food4Me project, developed a framework for assessing the scientific validity of providing personalized dietary advice based on a specific gene variant. Factors such as study design and quality, type of gene—diet interaction, the nature of the genetic variant and biological plausibility are used to calculate a scientific validity score for researchers and health care professionals that enables them to determine the level of evidence supporting the use of a specific genetic variation in the provision of gene-based personalized nutrition offerings (Grimaldi et al., 2017). This tool is dynamic and can be improved as the science develops. For personalized nutrition to happen, however, further research will be required employing large diverse samples to establish the efficacy of technology-based personalized nutrition (Ahlgren et al., 2013; Kohlmeier et al., 2016) and enable better understanding of relationships between genes, epigenetics, the microbiome, and metabolomics (Kohlmeier et al., 2016). Innovation to develop more accurate, convenient dietary assessment methods will also be needed (Kohlmeier et al., 2016).

WHAT DOES THE CONSUMER WANT FROM PERSONALIZED NUTRITION?

The Food4Me study considered not only the efficacy of personalized nutrition but also the potential market. A "bottom-up," mixed-method (qualitative and quantitative) approach was adopted to afford the European public a voice in determining best practice in the design and delivery of personalized nutrition. Focus group discussions and a survey involving members of the public took place in nine EU countries. Details of the sampling and methodology have been published elsewhere (Poínhos et al., 2014; Stewart-Knox et al., 2013).

What are the Consumer-Perceived Barriers to Uptake of Personalized Nutrition?

For clients to comply with dietary recommendations, individual differences in motivations for food choice will need to be considered in the design of personalized nutrition advice. Analysis of food choice motives using the Food Choice Questionnaire (FCQ) (Steptoe, Pollard, & Wardle, 1995) indicated that control of body weight and mood were the most important motives in determining attitude toward and intention to take up personalized nutrition (Rankin et al., 2018). The importance of body weight was unsurprising given current societal levels of obesity. That mood was important indicates a need for translational research focusing on dietary solutions to problems related to mental health and well-being. That health was not associated with intention to take up personalized nutrition could reflect a general problem in getting the general public to engage with dietary health promotion. Results also indicated that those for whom the sensory appeal and familiarity of food were important determinants of food choice were less likely to intend to take up personalized nutrition. Recommendations therefore would need to consider individual food preferences and existing habits (Stewart-Knox et al., 2016). Advice will also need to be adapted to the individual's ethnicity and the culture around diet, food, and health (Nordström, Coff, Jönsson, Nordenfelt, & Görman, 2013).

Household income (N = 1061)

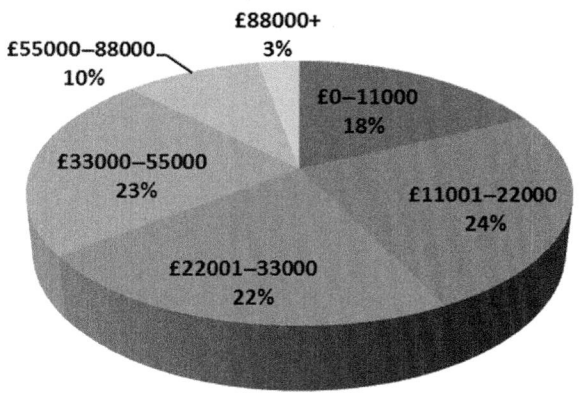

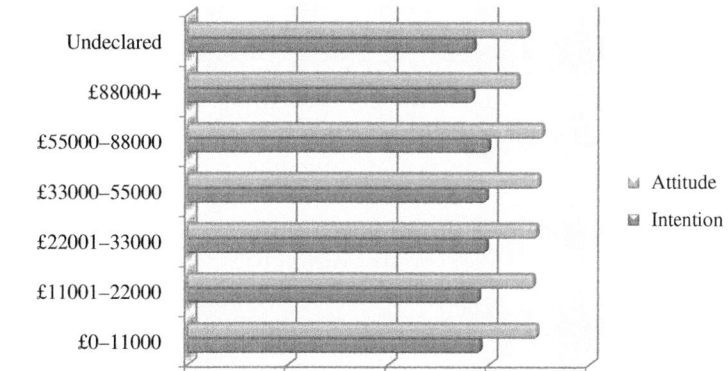

- £0–11000: 18%
- £11001–22000: 24%
- £22001–33000: 22%
- £33000–55000: 23%
- £55000–88000: 10%
- £88000+: 3%

FIGURE 10.2 Food4Me survey household income in the United Kingdom.

FIGURE 10.3 Household income in the United Kingdom and attitudes toward and intention to adopt personalized nutrition in the United Kingdom (N = 1061).

Price as a motive of food choice was found to be negatively associated with intention to take up personalized nutrition (Rankin et al., 2018). Given different economies and currencies, it was difficult to compare income between countries taking part in the Food4me survey. Results for the UK sample (Fig. 10.2), however, indicated that neither attitudes nor intention to adopt personalized nutrition differed significantly by income (Fig. 10.3) (previously unpublished results). Measures will nevertheless be needed to ensure that all sections of society, irrespective of income, are afforded the opportunity to avail of personalized nutrition in the future. To avoid catering only to the "worried wealthy" and the widening inequalities in dietary health that could ensue, provision will need to be embedded within, and offered as part of existing health services (Rankin et al., 2018; Stewart-Knox et al., 2016).

Other barriers identified by the Food4Me qualitative research were concerned with the eating context. Personalized diets may be difficult to adhere to in social situations, both within the home where the preferences of other household members may have to be considered, as well as problems encountered when eating outside the home. The Food4Me

TABLE 10.1 Barriers to Uptake of Personalized Nutrition by EU Country (N = 9381)

Country	Mean (Scale From 1 to 5)	Standard Error	Homogeneous Subsets
Norway	3.069	0.021	a
The Netherlands	3.207	0.022	b
United Kingdom	3.373	0.021	c
Portugal	3.397	0.019	c, d
Spain	3.447	0.022	c, d, e
Ireland	3.472	0.021	d, e, f
Germany	3.521	0.022	e, f, g
Greece	3.535	0.022	f, g
Poland	3.589	0.022	g

survey asked consumers to indicate (on a five-point scale) the extent to which the following contextual factors posed barriers to personalized nutrition: providing different food for family members; eating in restaurants; eating at other people's houses; eating when traveling; eating at work; being recommended foods you do not like; family rejecting personalized nutrition; friends rejecting personalized nutrition; and society rejecting personalized nutrition. Previously unpublished analysis of the Food4Me survey data (using univariate ANOVA) has indicated significant between-country differences ($P < .001$) with a moderate effect size (partial eta^2 = 0.050) in the degree to which these factors were perceived to be a barrier to personalized nutrition (Table 10.1). The "barriers toward personalized nutrition" scale had a univariate structure with good internal consistency ($\alpha = 0.883$). Of the nine countries surveyed, Norway had the lowest and the Netherlands the second lowest mean perceived barriers, indicating that these countries constitute more "ready" markets for personalized nutrition. On the other hand, Germany, Greece, and Poland had the highest means, implying there may be greater obstacles to rolling out personalized nutrition in these countries. These results imply that for a prescribed diet to be adhered to, extrinsic factors associated with the eating context (work and social life) may have to be adapted not only to the client's dietary needs, but also to their nationality and food-related culture (Fournier & Poulain, 2018; Rankin et al., 2018; Stewart-Knox et al., 2013, 2016). Meanwhile, policies directed toward supporting personalized diets in the wider societal context will be required, including the provision of incentives for restaurants, public transport providers, and employers to cater for individual dietary needs.

Among other potential barriers to compliance with personalized advice identified by the Food4Me qualitative research (Stewart-Knox et al., 2013) were those concerned with providing blood and saliva samples for testing and, as also implied by more recent qualitative research (Fournier & Poulain, 2018), fear and anxiety around receiving results. Receiving genetic information could trigger unintended adverse psychological effects such as increased anxiety levels (Meisel, Walker, & Wardle, 2012) which could lead to

TABLE 10.2 Test Anxiety by EU Country (N = 9381).

Country	Mean	Standard Error	Homogeneous Subsets
The Netherlands	1.991	0.029	a
Norway	2.097	0.027	b
Germany	2.171	0.029	b, c
Spain	2.279	0.029	c, d
United Kingdom	2.339	0.028	d
Ireland	2.477	0.027	e
Poland	2.676	0.030	f
Portugal	2.725	0.025	f
Greece	3.077	0.029	g

decreased motivation and compliance with dietary health intervention, particularly if genes are considered immutable by the individual receiving the dietary advice (Hunter, Khoury, & Drazen, 2008; Marteau et al., 2010). The Food4Me survey required responses (on a five-point scale) indicating to what degree the following procedures would make people feel anxious: taking a blood test; providing a finger-prick blood test; taking a DNA test; mailing a blood sample; mailing a DNA sample; identifying through a blood test, a disease that cannot be treated; identifying through a DNA test, a disease that cannot be treated; about the security of blood test data; and about the security of DNA test data. Previously unpublished analysis of the Food4Me survey responses indicated differences between countries with large effect size ($P < .001$; partial eta^2 = 0.112) in the degree to which the process associated with the provision of samples was perceived to cause anxiety (Table 10.2). This "test anxiety" scale had a univariate structure with very good internal consistency ($\alpha = 0.905$). The Netherlands had the lowest mean score indicating that little anxiety was perceived in providing and supplying samples for analysis. The highest mean was for Greece, followed by Portugal and Poland, indicating high anxiety associated with the process for submitting samples and receiving genetic advice, implying a need to take particular measures in these countries. There were some sex and age differences in perceived barriers to personalized nutrition and anxiety about the sampling process but with negligible effect sizes.

Taken together, the implication of these findings is that to address perceived barriers so European consumers will take up personalized nutrition, it is not a case of "one size fits all" and different approaches may need to be taken within and between European countries.

Who Should Deliver Personalized Nutrition?

Food4Me findings indicated two potential markets for personalized nutrition within Europe, one that would prefer services to be aligned with existing health provision, and another that would favor the autonomy, anonymity, and control that a commercial offering could afford (Stewart-Knox et al., 2013; Stewart-Knox et al., 2016). Accordingly, a substantial proportion of consumers surveyed indicated willingness to pay for services (Fischer et al., 2016). The potential strength of commercial markets, however, may vary by EU country. Meanwhile, commercial offerings are becoming increasingly available as well as more affordable for the consumer.

Those who took part in initial Food4Me focus groups agreed that a first step in attracting users to personalized nutrition was to build trust in providers (Stewart-Knox et al., 2013). In keeping with this, the survey results indicated that trust in service providers was associated with intention to adopt personalized nutrition (Poínhos et al., 2017). Direct-to-consumer personalized nutrition companies were rated lower on trust than government agencies, family doctors, and Departments of Health (Stewart-Knox et al., 2016). Trust in commercial providers was greater in Spain, the Netherlands, and Portugal, while those surveyed in Greece were the least trusting (Poínhos et al., 2017). According to members of the public consulted, trust in providers could be enhanced in various ways, including provision of a data protection guarantee, displaying credentials on web sites, and by ensuring that those delivering services are professionally qualified (Stewart-Knox et al., 2013). Recent EU legislation (Data Protection Act, 2018) has been implemented to better protect consumer rights with regards to information storage, sharing of information, and confidentiality. When it comes to dietary health and nutrigenomic related data, however, further legislation may be required (Fournier & Poulain, 2018). For personalized nutrition to become mainstream, these ethical and legal aspects will need to be addressed through legislation, regulation, and policy (Ahlgren et al., 2013; Kohlmeier et al., 2016). Beyond that, trust in the national Departments of Health as regulators of personalized nutrition showed high intercountry variability, implying that different agencies may need to be consulted in different EU countries (Poínhos et al., 2017).

IMPLEMENTATION OF PERSONALIZED NUTRITION IN PRACTICE: IMPLICATIONS FOR NUTRITION/HEALTH PROFESSIONALS

Best practice will entail treating clients as partners in the design and delivery of personalized dietary services. Given that test results may cause anxiety, health professionals will need to be employed to interpret results and provide counseling to the client (Ahlgren et al., 2013; Kohlmeier et al., 2016). The Food4Me survey indicated that general practitioners and dietitians were the most trusted professionals to provide personalized nutrition advice (Poínhos et al., 2017). This implies that the involvement of health professionals will be crucial to the public uptake of personalized nutrition services in the future (Stewart-Knox et al., 2016). Dietitians who have applied personalized nutrition to dietetics practice, however, tend to be those working independently in the commercial sector (Abrahams, Frewer, Bryant, & Stewart-Knox, 2017; Collins et al., 2013; Cormier et al., 2014). Adoption of personalized nutrition more broadly among the dietetics profession will be required in order to widen access beyond the commercial sector. Meanwhile, there are lessons to be learned from freelance early adopting dietitians that could expediate the process.

What Can We Learn From Dietitians Who Have Already Adopted Personalized Nutrition?

Previous research on members of the nutrition and dietetics profession (Collins et al., 2013; Oosthuizen, 2011; Whelan, McCarthy, & Pufulete, 2008) has implied that a lack of knowledge and confidence in nutritional genomics and genetics to provide personalized nutrition is a deterrent to adoption of the technology. Recent qualitative (Abrahams et al., 2018a) and survey research (Abrahams, Bryant, Frewer, & Stewart-Knox, 2018, Under Review) has focused on early-adopting registered dietitians and tapped into their experiences in the field with the aim of finding ways to encourage and enable adoption of personalized nutrition more widely in practice (Abrahams et al., 2017). Most encouraging was that the early adopting registered dietitians reported positive experiences with clients who were seen to respond well to tailored advice and able to make healthy dietary behavior changes (Abrahams et al., 2018a). This was perceived by those dietitians as meaning that they had instilled in their clients greater confidence in the technology (Abrahams et al., 2018a). As previous research would suggest (Ronteltap et al., 2007), this encouraged them further to use personalized nutrition technologies in their practice. Together this implies that exposure to new technologies and learning through practice would enable the profession to become familiar with and to develop the clients' confidence in nutrition technologies so that they begin to see them as less risky (Banet & Núñez, 1997). Widening the application of personalized nutrition therefore will require a translational focus to be included as part of continued professional development (Augustine, Swift, Harris, Anderson, & Hand, 2016; Wright, 2014).

What are the Challenges Faced by Nutrition Professionals in Acquiring the Skills Necessary to Bring Personalized Nutrition into Practice?

Among the challenges faced by dietitians in addressing the research—practice gap and applying personalized nutrition in practice are those encountered in obtaining the necessary education, training, and gaining experience (Abrahams et al., 2017; Collins, Adamski, Twohig, & Murgia, 2018; Collins et al., 2013; Li et al., 2014; Rosen, Earthman, Marquart, & Reicks, 2006; Whelan et al., 2008). Nutrition practitioners will need training, especially if personalized nutrition is to be integrated into clinical care and public health promotion (Kohlmeier et al., 2016). Early adopting registered dietitians, however, report being proactive in seeking evidence-based information on novel (including nutrigenomic) technologies and acquiring skills related to personalized nutrition (Abrahams et al., 2018a). Opportunities for training were availed through participation in training courses and attendance at conferences where dietitians could engage with the wider scientific community, exchange ideas, and impart skills (Abrahams et al., 2018, Under Review). According to the early-adopting registered dietitians, along with the acquisition of skills came a certain degree of confidence in the technologies which support the personalized nutrition approach (Abrahams et al., 2018a). The perceived importance of professional development and skills therefore is likely to be a key factor determining whether a dietitian adopts different levels of personalized nutrition.

What is Needed to Widen Access to Personalized Nutrition in the Future?

Preliminary findings (Abrahams et al., 2018b) have suggested that a short intensive course directed toward MSc nutrition and dietetics students has potential to transform perceptions and enable an understanding of tech-enabled personalized nutrition (Abrahams et al., 2018b). The Nutrition Society has recently introduced a series of popular webinars through the "Nutrition Society Training Academy" and included material on nutrigenomics (Nutrition Gazette, Summer: 2018).

Delivery of personalized nutrition services may require varied and flexible models. Those that employ a team approach can offer a skills "bank" from which advice can be sourced and support systems adapted to meet personalized client needs and preferences (Abrahams et al., 2018a). The profession will also need to move beyond the commercial model and consider ways of integrating personalized nutrition into public health nutrition (Abrahams et al., 2018a; Fallaize et al., 2015; Fischer et al., 2016; Stewart-Knox et al., 2015; Stewart-Knox et al., 2016). Meanwhile, guidance from professional organizations representing nutrition and dietetics professionals will be needed to encourage the profession in the direction of public health directed personalized nutrition (Abrahams et al., 2017, 2018; Collins et al., 2013; Li et al., 2014). An ongoing challenge, meanwhile, will be to empower and motivate people to achieve dietary goals through personalized nutrition (Kohlmeier et al., 2016).

CONCLUSIONS

Current evidence suggests that the European public are accepting and ready for personalized nutrition. Personalized nutrition, in its broadest definition, will enable practitioners to provide a range of services using different diagnostic tools made available to clients. Before personalized nutrition can be offered more widely, however, a strictly evidence-based approach will be required along with a better understanding of how individuals respond to different types of advice and delivery. Different, personalized models may be needed for the delivery of personalized nutrition. An integrated approach to the delivery of personalized nutrition will be required, which embraces individual differences in propensity for behavior change, motives for food choice, social circumstances, and financial status.

There may also be some way to go in building trust among the public. One way to improve trust would be greater involvement of the nutrition and dietetics profession. For this to happen, however, personalized approaches to dietetics will require continuing debate among the profession and inclusion as part of ongoing professional development. Some EU countries may be more amenable to personalized nutrition than others. Norway and the Netherlands, for example, appear more "ready" markets for personalized nutrition while in Greece actions may be needed to allay anxieties around biological sampling. For personalized nutrition to become mainstream, however, ethical and legal aspects will need to be addressed through legislation, regulation, and policy. This will require guidance from professional organizations representing nutrition and dietetics professionals. A possible future scenario would be for industry to work with existing health providers as well as with employers and food retailers in bringing the benefits of personalized nutrition to the wider public.

References

Abrahams, M., Bryant, E., Frewer, L.J., & Stewart-Knox B. (2018). Personalised nutrition technologies and innovations: a cross-national survey of registered dietitians, (Under Review).

Abrahams, M., Frewer, L. J., Bryant, E., & Stewart-Knox, B. (2017). Factors determining the integration of nutritional genomics into clinical practice by registered dietitians. *Trends in Food Science & Technology, 59*, 139–147.

Abrahams, M., Frewer, L. J., Bryant, E., & Stewart-Knox, B. (2018a). Perceptions and experiences of early-adopting registered dietitians in integrating nutrigenomics into practice. *British Food Journal, 120*(4), 763–776.

Abrahams, M., Frewer, L., Bryant, E., & Stewart-Knox, Tech-enabled Personalised Nutrition - evaluation of an intensive module to develop an entrepreneurial mindset and creativity skills in nutrition & dietetics students, *Complete Nutrition* 2018b, November edition.

Ahlgren, J., Nordgren, A., Perrudin, M., Ronteltap, A., Savigny, J., van Trijp, H., et al. (2013). Consumers on the internet: Ethical and legal aspects of commercialization of personalized nutrition. *Genes and Nutrition, 8*, 349–355.

Arouca, A., Michels, N., Moreno, L. A., González-Gil, E. M., Marcos, A., Gómez, S., et al. (2018). Associations between a Mediterranean diet pattern and inflammatory biomarkers in European adolescents*European Journal of Nutrition, 57*(5), 1747–1760. Available from https://doi.org/10.1007/s00394-017-1457-4, Epub 2017 Apr 18. PubMed PMID. Available from 28421282.

Augustine, M. B., Swift, K. M., Harris, S. R., Anderson, E. J., & Hand, R. K. (2016). Integrative medicine: Education, perceived knowledge, attitudes, and practice among Academy of Nutrition and Dietetics Members. *Journal of the Academy of Nutrition and Dietetics, 116*(2), 319–329.

Bandura, A. (1986). *Social foundations of thought and action: a social cognitive theory*. Englewood Cliffs, N.J: Prentice-Hall.

Banet, E., & Núñez, F. (1997). Teaching and learning about human nutrition: A constructivist approach. *International Journal of Science Education, 19*(10), 1169–1194.

Bendinelli, B., Masala, G., Bruno, R. M., Caini, S., Saieva, C., Boninsegni, A., et al. (2018). A priori dietary patterns and blood pressure in the EPIC Florence cohort: A cross-sectional study. *European Journal of Nutrition*. Available from https://doi.org/10.1007/s00394-018-1758-2, [Epub ahead of print] PubMed PMID: 29951936.

Camp, K. M., & Trujillo, E. (2014). Position of the Academy of Nutrition and Dietetics: Nutritional genomics. *Journal of the Academy of Nutrition and Dietetics, 114*(2), 299–312.

Celis-Morales, C., Livingstone, K. M., Marsaux, C. F., Forster, H., O'Donovan, C. B., Woolhead, C., et al. (2015). Design and baseline characteristics of the Food4Me study: A web-based randomised controlled trial of personalised nutrition in seven European countries. *Genes & Nutrition, 10*(1), 450.

Celis-Morales, C., Livingstone, K. M., Marsaux, C. F., Macready, A. L., Fallaize, R., O'Donovan, C. B., et al. (2017). Effect of personalised nutrition on health-related behaviour change: Evidence from the Food4me European randomized controlled trial. *International Journal of Epidemiology, 46*(2), 578–588.

Collins, J., Adamski, M. M., Twohig, C., & Murgia, C. (2018). Opportunities for training for nutritional professionals in nutritional genomics: What is out there? *Nutrition & Dietetics, 75*(2), 206–218.

Collins, J., Bertrand, B., Hayes, V., Li, S. X., Thomas, J., Truby, H., et al. (2013). The application of genetics and nutritional genomics in practice: An international survey of knowledge, involvement and confidence among dietitians in the US, Australia and the UK. *Genes & Nutrition, 8*(6), 523–533.

Collins, C. E., Morgan, P. J., Hutchesson, M. J., Oldmeadow, C., Barker, D., & Callister, R. (2017). Efficacy of web-based weight loss maintenance programs: A randomized controlled trial comparing standard features versus the addition of enhanced personalised feedback over 12 months. *Behavioral Sciences, 7*(4), 76.

Cormier, H., Tremblay, B. L., Paradis, A. M., Garneau, V., Desroches, S., Robitaille, J., et al. (2014). Nutrigenomics - Perspectives from registered dietitians: A report from the Quebec-wide e-consultation on nutrigenomics among registered dietitians. *Journal of Human Nutrition and Dietetics*, 27(4), 391–400.

Data Protection Act (DPA). (2018). Data Protection Act. <http://www.legislation.gov.uk/ukpga/2018/12/contents/enacted>. Accessed August 2018.

de Roos, B., & Brennan, L. (2017). Personalised interventions - A precision approach for the next generation of dietary intervention studies. *Nutrients*, 9(8), E847. Available from https://doi.org/10.3390/nu9080847.

de Souza, R. J., Mente, A., Maroleanu, A., Cozma, A. I., Ha, V., Kishibe, T., et al. (2015). Intake of saturated and trans unsaturated fatty acids and risk of all cause mortality, cardiovascular disease, and type 2 diabetes: Systematic review and meta-analysis of observational studies. *BMJ*, 351, h3978.

Fallaize, R., Celis-Morales, C., Macready, A. L., Marsaux, C. F., Forster, H., O' Donovan, C., et al. (2016). The effect of the apolipoprotein E genotype on response to personalised dietary advice intervention: Findings from the Food4me randomized controlled trial. *American Journal of Clinical Nutrition*, 104(3), 827–836.

Fallaize, R., Macready, A. L., Butler, L. T., Ellis, J. A., Berezowska, A., Fischer, A. R., et al. (2015). The perceived impact of the National Health Service on personalised nutrition service delivery among the UK public. *British Journal of Nutrition*, 113(8), 1271–1279.

Fischer, A. R., Berezowska, A., van der Lans, I. A., Ronteltap, A., Rankin, A., Kuznesof, S., et al. (2016). Willingness to pay for personalised nutrition across Europe. *The European Journal of Public Health*, 26(4), 640–644.

Food4Me. (2015). Personalised nutrition: Paving a way to better population health. A White Paper from the Food4me Project. European Food Information Council (EUFIC) (Eds), Belgium. <http://food4me.org/component/content/article/7-news/207-white-paper>. Accessed August 2018.

Fournier, T., & Poulain, J.-P. (2018). Eating according to one's genes? Exploring the French public's understanding of and reactions to personalized nutrition. *Qualitative Health Research*, 28(14), 2195–2207.

Frosch, D., Mello, P., & Lerman, C. (2005). Behavioral consequences of testing for obesity risk. *Cancer Epidemiology Biomarkers & Prevention*, 14(6), 1485–1489.

Gibney, M., Walsh, M., & Goosens, J. (2016). Personalised nutrition: Paving the way to better population health. In M. Eggersdorfer, K. Kraemer, J. B. Cordaro, J. Fanzo, M. Gibney, E. Kennedy, et al. (Eds.), *Good nutrition: Perspectives for the 21st century* (pp. 235–248). Basel: Karger.

Grimaldi, K. A., van Ommen, B., Ordovas, J. M., Parnell, L. D., Mathers, J. C., Bendik, I., et al. (2017). Proposed guidelines to evaluate scientific validity and evidence for genotype-based dietary advice. *Genes & Nutrition*, 12(1), 35.

Guasch-Ferre, M., Dashti, H. S., & Merino, J. (2018). Nutritional genomics and direct-to-consumer genetic testing: An overview. *Advances in Nutrition*, 9(2), 128–135.

Hansel, B., Giral, P., Gambotti, L., Lafourcade, A., Peres, G., Filipecki, C., et al. (2017). A fully automated web-based program improves lifestyle habits and Hba1c in patients with type 2 diabetes and abdominal obesity: Randomized trial of patient e-coaching nutritional support (the ANODE Study). *Journal of Medical Internet Research*, 19(11), e360.

Hooper, L., Martin, N., Abdelhamid, A., & Davey Smith, G. (2015). Reduction in saturated fat intake for cardiovascular disease. *Cochrane Database of Systematic Reviews*, 6, CD011737.

Hunter, D. J., Khoury, M. J., & Drazen, J. M. (2008). Letting the genome out of the bottle—Will we get our wish? *New England Journal of Medicine*, 358(2), 105–107.

Kirwan, L., Walsh, M. C., Celis-Morales, C., Marsaux, C. F., Livingstone, K. M., Navas-Carretero, S., et al. (2016). Phenotypic factors influencing the variation in response of circulating cholesterol level to personalised dietary advice in the Food4Me study. *British Journal of Nutrition*, 116(12), 2011–2019. Available from https://doi.org/10.1017/S0007114516004256.

Kohlmeier, M., de Caterina, R., Ferguson, L., Görman, U., Allayee, H., Pradad, C., et al. (2016). Guide and position of the international society of nutrigenetics/nutrigenomics on personalized nutrition: Part 2 - Ethics, challenges and endeavors of precision nutrition. *Journal of Nutrigenetics and Nutrigenomics*, 9, 28–46.

Li, S. X., Collins, J., Lawson, S., Thomas, J., Truby, H., Whelan, K., et al. (2014). A preliminary qualitative exploration of dietitians' engagement with genetics and nutritional genomics: Perspectives from international leaders. *Journal of Allied Health*, 43(4), 221–228.

Li, S. X., Ye, Z., Whelan, K., & Truby, H. (2016). The effect of communicating the genetic risk of cardiometabolic disorders on motivation and actual engagement in preventative lifestyle modification and clinical outcome: A systematic review and meta-analysis of randomised controlled trials. *British Journal of Nutrition*, 116(5), 924−934.

Livingstone, K. M., Celis-Morales, C., Navas-Carretero, S., San-Cristobal, R., Macready, A. L., Fallaize, R., et al. (2016). Effect of an Internet-based, personalised nutrition randomized trial on dietary changes associated with the Mediterranean diet: The Food4Me Study. *The American Journal of Clinical Nutrition*, 104(2), 288−297. Available from https://doi.org/10.3945/ajcn.115.129049.

Macready, A. L., Fallaize, R., Butler, L. T., Ellis, J. A., Kuznesof, S., Frewer, L. J., et al. (2018). Applying behavior change techniques in an Internet-based personalized nutrition intervention: The Food4Me Study. *JMIR Research Protocols*. Available from https://doi.org/10.2196/resprot.8703.

Manach, C., Milenkovic, D., Van de Wiele, T., Rodriguez-Mateos, A., de Roos, B., Garcia-Conesa, M. T., et al. (2017). Addressing the inter-individual variation in response to consumption of plant food bioactives: Towards a better understanding of their role in healthy aging and cardiometabolic risk reduction. *Molecular Nutrition & Food Research.*, 61(6), 1600557. Available from https://doi.org/10.1002/mnfr.201600557.

Maranhão, P. A., Bacelar-Silva, G. M., Ferreira, D. N. G., Calhau, C., Vieira-Marques, P., & Cruz-Correia, R. J. (2018). Nutrigenomic information in the openEHR data set. *Applied Clinical Informatics*, 9(1), 221−231.

Marteau, T. M., French, D. P., Griffin, S. J., Prevost, A., Sutton, S., Watkinson, C., et al. (2010). Effects of communicating DNA-based disease risk estimates on risk-reducing behaviours. *Cochrane Database of Systematic Reviews*, 6(10), CD007275.

Mathers, J. C. (2017). Nutrigenomics in the modern era. *Proceedings of the Nutrition Society*, 76(3), 265−275. Available from https://doi.org/10.1017/S002966511600080X.

McNulty, H., Strain, J. J., Hughes, C. F., & Ward, M. (2017). Riboflavin, MTHFR genotype and blood pressure: A personalised approach to prevention and treatment of hypertension. *Molecular Aspects of Medicine*, 53, 2−9.

Meisel, S. F., Walker, C., & Wardle, J. (2012). Psychological responses to genetic testing for weight gain: A vignette study. *Obesity*, 20(3), 540−546.

Nielsen, D. E., & El-Sohemy, A. (2012). A randomized trial of genetic information for personalised nutrition. *Genes & Nutrition*, 7(4), 290.

Nielsen, D. E., & El-Sohemy, A. (2014). Disclosure of genetic information and change in dietary intake: A randomized controlled trial. *PLoS One*, 9(11), e112665.

Nordström, K., Coff, C., Jönsson, H., Nordenfelt, L., & Görman, U. (2013). Food and health: Individual, cultural, or scientific matters? *Genes and Nutrition*, 8, 357−368.

O'Donovan, C. B., Walsh, M. C., Gibney, M. J., Brennan, L., & Gibney, E. R. (2017). Knowing your genes: Does this impact behaviour change? *Proceedings of the Nutrition Society*, 76, 182−191.

Oosthuizen, L. (2011). *Aspects of the involvement, confidence, and knowledge of South-African registered dietitians regarding genetics and nutritional genomics*. MSc, University of Stellenbosch (South Africa), South Africa [Online]. <http://scholar.sun.ac.za/handle/10019.1/6796>. Accessed 15.10.15.

Ordovas, J. M., Ferguson, L. R., Tai, E. S., & Mathers, J. C. (2018). Personalised nutrition and health. *BMJ*, 361. Available from https://doi.org/10.1136/bmj.k2173.

Poínhos, R., Oliveira, B., van der Lans, I. A., Fischer, A. R. H., Berezowska, A., Rankin, A., et al. (2017). Providing personalised nutrition: Consumers' trust and preferences regarding sources of information, service providers and regulators, and communication channels. *Public Health Genomics*, 20(4), 218−228.

Poínhos, R., van der Lans, I. A., Rankin, A., Fischer, A. R. H., Bunting, B. P., Kuznesof, S., et al. (2014). Psychological determinants of consumer acceptance of personalised nutrition in 9 European countries. *PLoS One*, 9, c110614.

Rankin, A., Bunting, B. P., Poínhos, R., van der Lans, I. A., Fischer, A. R., Kuznesof, S., et al. (2018). Food choice motives, attitude towards and intention to adopt personalised nutrition. *Public Health Nutrition*, 21(2), 2606−2616.

Rankin, A., Kuznesof, S., Frewer, L., Orr, K., Davison, J., de Almeida, M. D. V., et al. (2017). Public perceptions of personalised nutrition through the lens of Social Cognitive Theory. *Journal of Health Psychology*, 22(10), 1233−1242. Available from https://doi.org/10.1177/1359105315624750.

Roke, K., Walton, K., Klingel, S. L., Harnett, A., Subedi, S., Haines, J., et al. (2017). Evaluating changes in Omega-3 fatty acid intake after receiving personal FADS1 genetic information: A randomized nutrigenetic intervention. *Nutrients, 9*(3), 240.

Ronteltap, A., & van Trijp, H. (2007). Consumer acceptance of personalised nutrition. *Genes and Nutrition, 2*(1), 85–87.

Rosen, R., Earthman, C., Marquart, L., & Reicks, M. (2006). Continuing education needs of registered dietitians regarding nutrigenomics. *Journal of the American Dietetic Association, 106*(8), 1242–1245.

Ryan, M. F., O'Grada, C. M., Morris, C., Segurado, R., Walsh, M. C., Gibney, E. R., et al. (2014). Within-person variation in the postprandial lipemic response of healthy adults. *The American Journal of Clinical Nutrition, 97*(2), 261–267. Available from https://doi.org/10.3945/ajcn.112.047936.

Steptoe, A., Pollard, T., & Wardle, J. (1995). Development of a measure of the motives underlying the selection of food—The Food Choice Questionnaire. *Appetite, 25*(3), 267–284.

Stewart-Knox, B., Kuznesof, S., Robinson, J., Rankin, A., Orr, K., Duffy, M., et al. (2013). Factors influencing European consumer uptake of personalised nutrition. Results of a qualitative analysis. *Appetite, 66*, 67–74.

Stewart-Knox, B. J., Markovina, J., Rankin, A., Bunting, B. P., Kuznesof, S., Fischer, A. R. H., et al. (2016). Making personalised nutrition the easy choice: Creating policies to break down the barriers and reap the benefits. *Food Policy, 63*, 134–144.

Stewart-Knox, B. J., Rankin, A., Poínhos, R., Fischer, A. R. H., de Almeida, M. D. V., Kuznesof., et al. (2015). Promoting healthy dietary behaviour through personalised nutrition: A case of getting the technology right? *Proceedings of the Nutrition Society, 74*(2), 171–176. Available from https://doi.org/10.1017/S0029665114001529.

Vitale, M., Masulli, M., Calabrese, I., Rivellese, A. A., Bonora, E., Signorini, S., et al. (2018). Impact of a Mediterranean dietary pattern and its components on cardiovascular risk factors, glucose control, and body weight in people with type 2 diabetes: A Real-Life Study. *Nutrients, 10*(8), E1067.

Whelan, K., McCarthy, S., & Pufulete, M. (2008). Genetics and diet-gene interactions: Involvement, confidence and knowledge of dietitians. *British Journal of Nutrition, 99*(1), 23–28.

Wright, O. R. (2014). Systematic review of knowledge, confidence and education in nutritional genomics for students and professionals in nutrition and dietetics. *Journal of Human Nutrition and Dietetics, 27*(3), 298–307.

CHAPTER 11

Personalized Nutrition Education to the Adherence to Dietary and Physical Activity Recommendations

Liliana Guadalupe González-Rodríguez[1], José Miguel Perea-Sánchez[1], Pablo Veiga-Herreros[1] and África Peral Suárez[2]

[1]Department of Nutrition and Dietetics, Universidad Alfonso X El Sabio, Madrid, Spain
[2]Department of Nutrition and Food Science, Universidad Complutense de Madrid, Madrid, Spain

OUTLINE

Health and Nutrition Education Challenges	278
Current Dietary and Physical Activity Guidelines	280
Nutrition Recommendations	280
Dietary Guidelines	280
Physical Activity Recommendations	282
Determinants of Food Choice	283
Individual Determinants	283
Environment Determinants	285
Socioeconomics Determinants	286
Mass Media and Food Advertising	287
Personalized Nutrition Education Interventions	288
Effectiveness of Personalized Nutrition Education Intervention	290
Specific and Practical Approach	290
Determinants of Dietary Behavior Change	290
Theory-Based Interventions	292
Levels of Influence in the Food Choice and Dietary Behavior	293
Use of Appropriate Behavior Change Strategies	294

Methodology for Personalized Nutrition Education	295	Step 3. Select Theory and Clarify Philosophy	300
Nutrition Care Process Applied to Personalized Nutrition Education	295	Step 4. Indicate General Objectives	301
		Step 5. Generate Action Plans	302
Effective Interview in the Nutrition Consultation	297	Step 6. Nail Down Evaluation Plan	302
Motivational Interviewing	298	Other Aspects to Take into Account in Personalized Nutritional Education	303
Nutrition Educator Profile	299		
Nutrition Education DESIGN Procedure in the Personalized Nutrition Education	299	Conclusion	303
		References	304
Step 1. Decide Behaviors	299		
Step 2. Explore Determinants of Change	300		

HEALTH AND NUTRITION EDUCATION CHALLENGES

In the past few decades, there has been a significant increase worldwide in the prevalence and incidence of noncommunicable diseases (NCDs) both in children and adults. NCDs are the leading cause of death globally and caused 38 million (68%) of the 56 million deaths recorded in 2012 of which 16 million (40%) occurred before the age of 70 (World Health Organization, 2014) NCDs have become serious health and economic burdens all over the world. These diseases are the result of a complex interaction of multiple factors including genetic predisposition and physiological, environmental, and lifestyle factors.

Enormous changes derived from industrialization, urbanization, technological and economic development, and market globalization have dramatically modified the lifestyle of the population. These changes have led to an inadequate nutrition and health status and a sedentary life, which in turn contribute to the increase in these health problems.

Scientific evidence shows a strong relationship between lifestyle and health. In this sense, unhealthy dietary patterns, limited physical activity, lack of sleep, psychological stress, and harmful alcohol and tobacco consumption are strongly associated with the risk of disease and death, particularly from obesity, cardiovascular disease, hyperlipidemias, insulin resistance, type 2 diabetes, metabolic syndrome, hypertension, osteoporosis, Alzheimer's disease, depression, and some types of cancer (GBD 2015 Risk Factors Collaborators, 2016; Kontis et al., 2014). Nonetheless, dietary habits are considered the major modifiable determinant of the health-disease process (Carrara & Schulz, 2018).

The latest world reports on the monitoring of progress in relation to NCDs show that the progress registered has neither been uniform nor enough despite the efforts and strategies carried out by countries. The prevalence of excess body weight in adults and children is increasing worldwide independently of the measuring method or cut-points used

(Williams, Mesidor, Winters, Dubbert, & Wyatt, 2015). This is mainly due to the energy imbalance associated with an increasingly sedentary lifestyle. In this sense, studies performed in different countries show that the compliance with the dietary and physical activity guidelines is pretty low (Blanchard et al., 2009; Dijkstra, Neter, Brouwer, Huisman, & Visser, 2014; Kasten, van Osch, Eggers, & de Vries, 2017; Ortega-Anta, Jiménez-Ortega, Perea-Sánchez & Navia-Lombán, 2014; Tennant, Davidson, & Day, 2014).

Studies show that most people exceed the recommended energy, salt, sugar, fat, and saturated fat intakes, while the intake of polyunsaturated fat, particularly omega-3 fatty acids, vitamin D, vitamin K, folic acid, calcium, iron, zinc, and selenium is insufficient in a significant proportion of the population. This is because people follow diets based on a high intake of red and processed meat, refined grains, and sugar-sweetened beverages and low in vegetables, fruits, whole grains, legumes, and fish (Ortega-Anta, Jiménez-Ortega, Perea-Sánchez, & Navia-Lombán, 2014).

However, public awareness of the benefits of the adoption of a healthy lifestyle is gaining increased interest in the population, especially among young people. On the one hand, there is greater dissemination of scientific evidence indicating the benefits of following a healthy lifestyle in relation to the prevention and control of different diseases, the increase of life expectancy, and the improvement in quality of life (Schulze, Martinez-Gonzalez, Fung, Lichtenstein, & Forouhi, 2018). Coverage of the promotion of healthy habits through social media and other means is increasing every day. The mass media constantly disseminates a large amount of information about health to the population, mainly about food and nutrition. Nonetheless, in many cases this information has not enough scientific evidence to validate the beneficial properties declared regarding certain food components or their safe use for individuals, especially when it comes to the intake of dietetic supplements or some specific food. Many times the information can become contradictory, which may lead to the individual getting confused and making erroneous food decisions.

On the other hand, it has been observed that not only are awareness, knowledge, or motivation sufficient for people to have a healthy lifestyle. Much of the adult population have the intention to eat more healthily and take more exercise, but the evidence shows that few people have a sufficient intake of fruit, vegetables, legumes, and whole grain cereals in their diets or undertake sufficient physical activity. The effectiveness of food and nutrition interventions are directly impacted by compliance to the advice and nutrition plan given by health professionals (Bean et al., 2015). Nonadherence to the recommended dietary and physical activity behaviors is widespread among the population, both in the short and long term, since it represents an extremely difficult task for many people. In other words, there is an important gap between the intention of people to change their lifestyle and being able to achieve it.

All the above has led to a greater awareness of the importance of nutrition education in society. It is essential to tailor food and nutrition education interventions to promote healthy dietary habits to the different characteristics and needs of individuals and it justifies the requirement to design and apply interventions not only at the individual level, but also in schools, workplaces, and communities, with a different and more effective approach than those that have been applied until now by health care practitioners. It is also driving a demand for qualified nutrition experts.

CURRENT DIETARY AND PHYSICAL ACTIVITY GUIDELINES

The amount of energy, nutrients, and physical activity needed to maintain an appropriate nutrition and health status and to prevent diseases among the population is well established through the nutrition recommendations and dietary and physical activity guidelines.

Nutrition Recommendations

Nutrition recommendations are used by health and nutrition professionals, scientists, and policy makers in order to evaluate nutrition status and design nutrition interventions. Dietary reference intakes (DRIs) in the United States or dietary reference values (DRVs) in Europe indicate the amount of recommended intake of energy and essential nutrients to maintain health and prevent deficiencies. These recommendations are usually estimated and are provided for energy, macronutrients, water, proteins, minerals, and vitamins according to sex and life stage group, that is, children, adolescents, adults, and pregnant and lactating women.

The first nutrition recommendations were the Recommended Dietary Allowances (RDAs) published by the Food and Nutrition Board of the United States in 1941. Since their first publication they have been revised periodically, the last update for vitamin D and calcium was issued in 2011 (Institute of Medicine, 2011). During this time, many countries have elaborated these allowances according to the characteristics of their population to produce their own recommendations. The Panel on Dietetic Products, Nutrition and Allergies (NDA Panel) of the European Food Safety Authority (EFSA) in 2017 updated the DRVs for energy, carbohydrates, dietary fiber, fats, protein, water, energy, as well as 14 vitamins and 13 minerals (EFSA European Food Safety Authority, 2017).

Dietary Guidelines

Dietary guidelines are the reference framework for nutritional education. Countries have different scientific committees that work on the basis of internationally established standards based on healthy eating patterns and transfer this information to the national level in order to adapt it for the user population. These guidelines provide scientific guidance using a language easily accessible for the general population on the types of food and quantities they should consume each day and other healthy messages and positive trends with the purpose of meeting nutritional recommendations and promoting and maintaining health. These guidelines also facilitate the monitoring of a balanced diet and provide a basic framework to plan meals or daily menus.

As it is evident, the nutrition recommendations are quite difficult to understand and be applied by general population. For that reason, they are usually reduced to simple messages using tools such as food-based dietary guidelines. Dietary guidelines usually include information about the amount of servings of food groups that should be eaten. The last developed dietary guidelines, in addition to this, also include other healthy habits, such as information about the importance of an adequate hydration, the need to adapt the food intake to the physical activity in order to have a suitable energy balance, maintenance of healthy weight, the importance of adequate sleep or emotion regulation on eating habits, and the use of healthy cooking techniques for the preparation of foods. Habitually, dietary guidelines use different graphic representations (e.g., pyramids, rainbow, rhombus, etc.) or information to facilitate their comprehension (Requejo, Ortega, Aparicio, & López-Sobaler, 2007) (Fig. 11.1).

There is an international consensus on the specific dietary guidelines that should be given to the population (Fig. 11.2). Among the most common are:

- Daily consumption of bread, preferably whole grain, pasta, and/or rice.
- Consume, at least, five servings of fruits and vegetables a day.
- Consume legumes 2–3 times a week.
- Include in the diet fish, 3–4 times a week.
- Moderate the consumption of foods with added sugars such as pastries, soft drinks, snacks, prepared foods, etc.

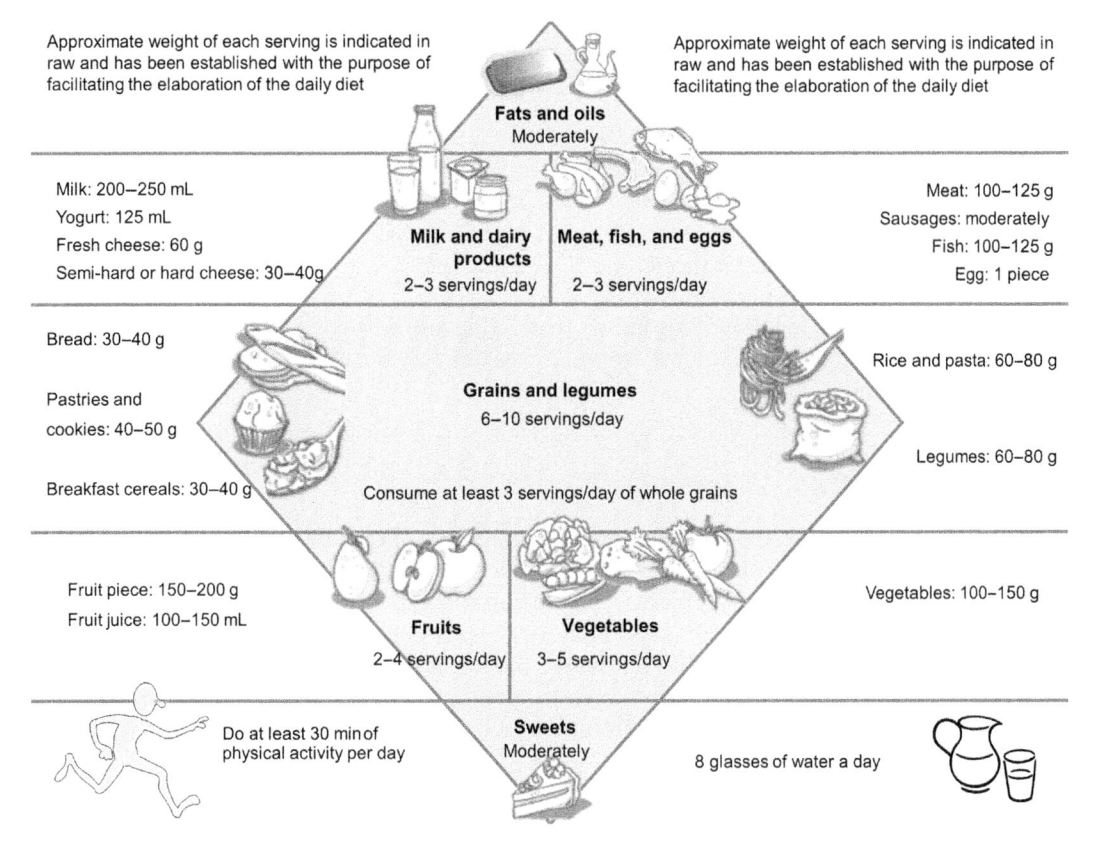

FIGURE 11.1 Food guide rhombus. Food-based dietary guideline. Source: *Adapted from Requejo, A. M., Ortega R. M., Aparicio, A., & López-Sobaler, A. M. (2007). El Rombo de la Alimentación. Madrid: Departamento de Nutrición, Facultad de Farmacia, Universidad Complutense de Madrid.*

FIGURE 11.2 Common dietary guidelines.

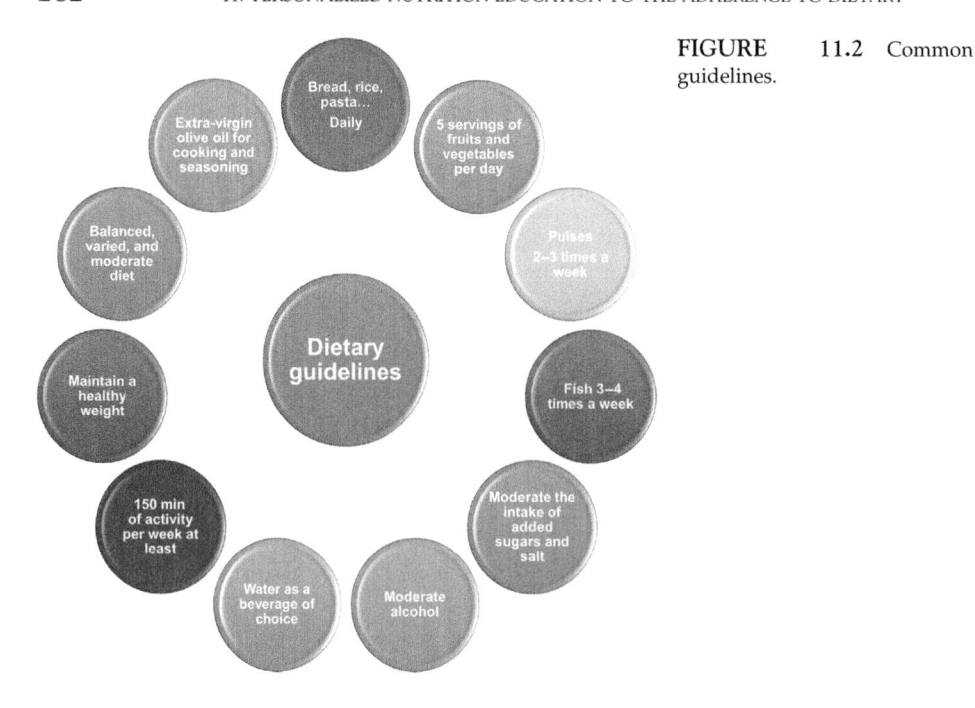

- Eat quality fat in the diet such as extra virgin olive oil.
- Moderate the consumption of foods with a composition high in salt, as well as the salt that is added to the dishes or meals.
- Drink enough water throughout the day.
- Follow a varied diet, incorporating foods from all groups.
- Do at least 150 minutes of moderate-intensity aerobic physical activity per week.
- Keep a healthy body weight.

Physical Activity Recommendations

Physical inactivity is becoming a priority in current public health policies worldwide. It is among the four leading risk factors for several diseases, such as cardio-metabolic diseases, and for general mortality (World Health Organization, 2010). Sedentary behavior is defined as "any waking behavior characterized by an energy expenditure equal or less than 1.5 Metabolic Equivalents (METs) while the individual is in a sitting, reclining or lying position" (Sedentary Behaviour Research Network, 2012). Most office work, driving a car, and sitting while watching television or using a mobile phone, tablet, and laptop are examples of sedentary behaviors.

The population is increasingly adopting a sedentary lifestyle with major consequences for health in both adults and children. Today it is very common to work in front of computer screens, to sit at desks most of time, or to stand in the same position for a long time, especially workers in the service and manufacturing sectors. Scientific literature suggests that even when individuals meet the physical activity goal levels, if they are sedentary for much of the rest of the day, they have an increased risk for cardiometabolic disease and premature death.

There are several determinants related to sedentary behavior, such as age, weight, occupation, and psychological, cognitive, and emotional factors among others. A systematic review showed that excessive time spent in sedentary behavior was associated with a more positive attitude toward this behavior and a perception of a greater social support for sedentary behavior. Conversely, having greater self-efficacy and greater intentions to reduce sedentary time was associated with lower sedentary time (Rollo, Gaston, & Prapavessis, 2016).

The World Health Organization (WHO) has set physical activity recommendations for adults, older adults, and young people, based on the available scientific evidence. The WHO indicates a minimal time of 150 minutes of moderate intensity physical activity (approximately 3–6 METs) or 75 minutes of vigorous intensity physical activity (approximately >6 METs) per week or an equal combination of both. Also, the WHO points out that to obtain greater health benefits adults should achieve 300 minutes per week of moderate intensity physical activity. Finally, it is recommended to do muscle strengthening exercises two or more days a week (World Health Organization, 2010).

In any case the nutrition attention plan of a client/patient should be based on the nutrition and physical activity recommendations but have in mind the characteristics, needs, and desires of each individual.

DETERMINANTS OF FOOD CHOICE

Food choice is a complex process and there are several determinants that influence it (Fig. 11.3). To design a personalized and effective food and nutrition education intervention, health care practitioners need a better understanding of the determinants that affect food choice and therefore dietary patterns of the population. Food choices made by people are influenced by biological mechanisms, comprising signals to the hypothalamus from the gastrointestinal tract and adipose tissue, which regulate the processes of hunger and satiety (Leng et al., 2017). However, what people choose to eat is not determined exclusively by physiological or nutritional needs, but also there are other factors that hinder the choice of food, such as the high availability of food and the presence of individual determinants (e.g., food preferences), environmental determinants (e.g., social and cultural customs), socioeconomic determinants (e.g., food prices), and mass campaigns (e.g., food packaging and labeling).

Individual Determinants

Individuals have an innate predisposition to sweet flavor, but the salty, acid, and bitter taste develops later. The preference for fat appears in childhood and as a consequence at this stage the consumption of foods with high energy density is usually increased. However, there are genetic differences in flavor sensitivity between individuals and in responses to food which may be related to the pattern of food consumption. It has been

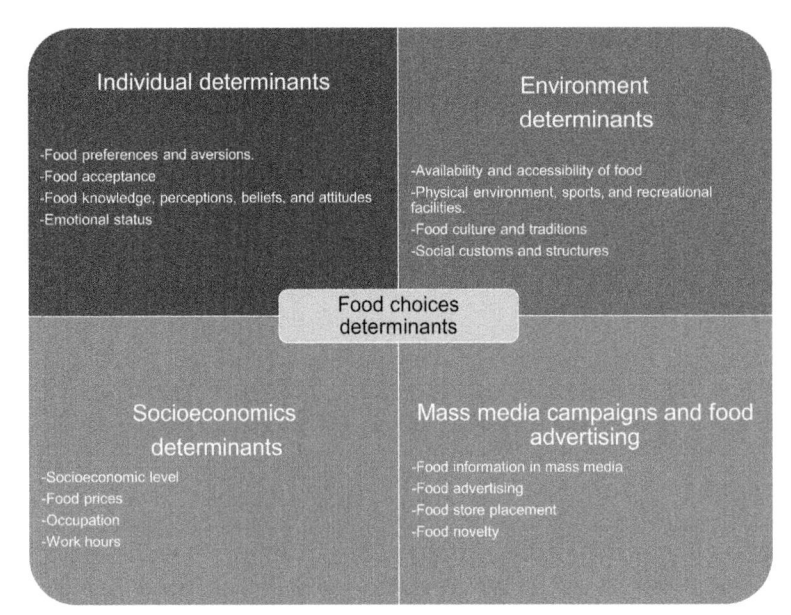

FIGURE 11.3 Food choice determinants.

described that when children make food choices, the attribute of taste is usually most important (Ha, Killian, Bruce, Lim, & Bruce, 2018).

Food acceptance is learned based on food experience. This learning could be noncognitive, physiological, or conditioned by the positive or negative consequences that individuals experience from repeated exposure to a specific food. It has been described that children have a better acceptance of certain food if their mothers consumed them during pregnancy or breastfeeding or if the food was introduced into their complementary feeding (Harris & Coulthard, 2016).

Food preferences and aversions are slowly developed through a learning process based on the repetition of food intake, familiarity, and pleasurable experiences. The food experiences in the first years of life influence the development of the dietary pattern of individuals during their whole lives. If children are exposed early to foods with a high content of fat, sugar, and salt, unhealthy preferences are likely generated. Therefore it would be desirable to try to familiarize them with foods such as whole grains, legumes, fish, eggs, vegetables, and fruits. This is very important because, although preferences for flavors can be modified by other food experiences in adulthood, in the current environment with a high supply of foods with high energy density, it is very difficult to achieve it.

Beliefs and perceptions about food can influence the choice of food, for example, the belief that a food is "natural" may motivate some people to include it in their diet. People usually associate the concept of "natural" with a beneficial effect on health because it is supposed that it has less additives or artificial ingredients (Rankin et al., 2018). Likewise, many people disregard nutrition education messages because they fail to find relevance in them, since they perceive their diet to be healthier than it is in reality.

Emotions about the possible positive or negative consequences of the consumption of certain foods interact with food experiences when foods are chosen. It is intended that food be tasty, easy to prepare, cheap, complete, and familiar, and provide emotional comfort. In this sense, in the last decades there has been a growing interest in taking into consideration aspects related with emotional eating when nutrition education interventions are being designing. Emotional eating is defined as the tendency that an individual has to regulate mood state through the consumption of unhealthy food (especially high in sugar, fat, or salt) or in an excessive amount, many times as a result of a stressful lifestyle (Mantau, Hattula, & Bornemann, 2018). This behavior often contributes to weight gain and hinders weight loss. Also, it has a negative effect on the body image, health, and self-esteem of the individual. For this reason, it is advisable to assess emotional eating in patients, through an interview or a test designed with this purpose, and address it adequately by promoting physical exercise and stress reduction, and using mindful eating and other techniques used for this purpose.

Furthermore, in the process of choosing foods, health criteria also are used by people. Nevertheless, in many cases there is a lack of knowledge of healthy patterns that in turn coexist with food misconceptions and myths. In fact, a significant percentage of the population does not know the recommended number of servings of fruits, vegetables, or cereals that should be consumed daily or the composition of energy and fat in foods.

In addition, there are an increasing number of people who lack skills in preparing and cooking healthy meals or who desire to minimize the time and physical effort to prepare them, many times due to difficulties in scheduling their daily life. This has produced the rise of the use of ready-to-eat-meals and convenience foods in the last decades, which in turn has had an important impact on diet and therefore on health.

Furthermore, evidence suggests that adequate sleep is linked to healthier eating behaviors. Children and adolescents with late bedtimes are more likely to make poorer dietary choices.

Environment Determinants

The environment is a determining factor for the development and maintenance of a healthy lifestyle. The availability and accessibility of food in developed and many of the developing countries is growing. In the same way, availability is also high in workplaces, schools, or universities, although healthy menus are not always offered. There are also food vending machines and food stores around schools with unhealthy foods high in fats, sugar, and salt, such as chips, pastries, and soft drinks, etc.

Moreover, the physical environment, sports and recreational facilities have a positive influence on the performance of outdoor activities (walks, physical exercise). The lack of these areas or public security may contribute to limit the practice of physical activity.

Culture and traditions also have a great influence on eating habits. For instance, it has been observed that many immigrants tend to maintain their food traditions in the host country, which may influence the pattern of food consumption. In this regard, local and state nutrition education policies can help these groups to have the opportunities to follow a healthy diet and active lifestyle.

Social customs can have a great influence on the choice of food and lifestyle. For example, children and adolescents may receive some pressure to consume "fast food" when they are with friends. Food can express celebration and sociability; mealtimes are perceived as an opportunity to come together and give pleasure. Celebrations, such as birthdays, weddings, dinners with friends, and work meals can generate some pressure to consume less healthy foods in excess.

Social structures may also condition eating patterns. Family has been widely recognized as a decisive factor in the food choice of its members. In this way, the learning about food choice in childhood is conditioned by observing the behavior of adults and peers, especially family members (Mura Paroche, Caton, Vereijken, Weenen, & Houston-Price, 2017). Parents play an essential role in the development of food preferences of their children. Therefore family, in addition to setting an example with healthy habits, should offer healthy foods in adequate portions, without forcing the children to eat, since it has been pointed out in the literature that highly restrictive and demanding parental controls limit the opportunities for children to practice self-regulation of energy intake (Frankel et al., 2012).

Another factor to consider is the structure of the household, since parents with children are more motivated and tend to prepare meals or snacks of higher nutritional quality than homes without children. Moreover, it has been observed that adolescents who eat with their families most days of the week have better quality diets than those who eat with their families less frequently.

Socioeconomics Determinants

The socioeconomic level also determines the dietary habits, for example, people with higher socioeconomic status in developed countries have higher quality diets and are less sedentary. Food prices may partly explain the differences in food choices and dietary habits among individuals, since ultraprocessed products with fat and sugar are cheaper than many fresh basic products in most of the developed and developing countries. One of the common consequences is that low-income people consume less fruits and vegetables than higher income people. For instance, people from the United States on average do not achieve the national goals for dietary intake, however, it has been pointed out that low-income, less educated, and ethnic minority individuals are even further away from meeting these guidelines (Strolla, Gans, & Risica, 2006).

It is well known that in lower-income households, the spending on food represents a higher percentage of their income than in higher income households. This leads them to restrict this expenditure and, consequently, to choose often foods of lower nutritional quality. In addition, it has been described that food carries a symbolic value that many times can cause dietary disparities. The socioeconomic family position shapes, in part, the meanings that parents attach to food. In a study performed with families from the United States with children aged 12–19 years old, it was shown that the differing meanings that parents attach to food influenced the distinct feeding strategies they have with their children. Parents with a low socioeconomic status use food demands as a buffer against denial of other demands of their children, while parents with a higher socioeconomic status attend most of material demands of their children and feel stronger to deny high energy density food such as candies or pastries (Fielding-Singh, 2017).

Occupation and work hours also influence the preparation of healthy meals and also can limit the practice of physical exercise. People who have long working hours find it more difficult to have healthy habits. One of the most frequently reported barriers to a healthy diet is lack of time, and this is a common reason for eating more fast food and highly processed foods, which are energy dense and nutrient poor, and fewer fresh products. For this reason, nutrition education interventions should address these aspects as well.

Mass Media and Food Advertising

Currently, information on health, nutrition, and food is widely distributed in all mass media such as television, radio, websites, and social networks. Food advertising is carried out using different strategies and methods, such as food advertising on television and the Internet, which are the most popular mass media nowadays, and using a strategic placement of products in supermarkets and food discounts among others.

Television food advertising influences food preferences and decisions and, consequently, short-term food consumption which contributes to a more unhealthy diet for people, mainly for children and youth (Bruce et al., 2016; Ha et al., 2018). There are studies that highlight the influence of food marketing trends in the population food choices, where food advertising exalts many of the functional properties of the products. Most of the content of food commercials is inconsistent with dietary guidelines. Children placed more importance on taste attributes than health attributes after watching food advertising, which suggests that food marketing may alter the psychological and neurobiologic mechanisms of food decisions in children (Bruce et al., 2016).

In this sense, it has been described that worldwide, the majority of children spend more than 2 hours per day watching television, and computer and mobile phone use especially in children is increasing significantly (Hallal et al., 2012). In addition, the results of the analysis based on children aged 6—9 years from the WHO European Childhood Obesity Surveillance Initiative have shown that the mean screen time was 2.2 hours and for television it was 1.5 hours (Bornhorst et al., 2015). Likewise accordingly with a recent systematic review on sedentary time in European children and adolescents, television time ranged from a mean value of 1—2.7 hours a day in children and 1.3—4.4 hours a day in adolescents, which is in general excessive (Verloigne et al., 2016).

Furthermore, the Internet and social network channels (e.g., Facebook, Twitter, Instagram, YouTube, or blogs) are the main sources that the population uses to obtain information about health and wellness (Klassen, Douglass, Brennan, Truby, & Lim, 2018). In this sense, people are bombarded constantly by food, often unhealthy food, dietetic supplements, and meal recipes which may led to suboptimal dietary choices.

Advertising through the media has a great persuasive power and the food industry is one of the largest advertisers, spending a large amount of money compared to the little invested in campaigns promoting a healthy lifestyle. In addition to the negative impact of sedentarism on the health of the population, the publicity to which all people are constantly exposed has a negative impact on the choice of food.

Moreover, food placement on the supermarkets shelves may promote the consumption of low nutritional value products such as sweets, chocolate, and pastries to many consumers, although the most affected are the youngest.

In addition to food advertising and placement in stores, the novelty of new products plays an important role in making certain foods more appealing than others. People are greatly interested in trying new food, especially when they "promise" a beneficial effect on health or in relation to weight control or muscle mass gaining.

PERSONALIZED NUTRITION EDUCATION INTERVENTIONS

Over the years, healthy dietary messages have been present in the health promotion and education efforts. Nevertheless, evidence shows that they have had not the expected impact upon dietary behavior and health of the population.

Nutrition education has been defined as:

> the combination of educational strategies, accompanied by environmental supports, designed to facilitate voluntary adoption of food choices and other food- and nutrition-related behaviors conducive to health and well-being and delivered through multiple venues, involving activities at the individual, institutional, community, and policy levels *Contento, 2008*.

For a long time, nutrition education interventions have been focused on changing individual behavior through direct or prescriptive education, under the premise that fostering knowledge helps to promote the dietary behavior change of individuals. It has traditionally consisted of orientations provided habitually in health services, often with an inappropriate use of some educational methods, using informative sessions and educational materials indiscriminately, in which contents are frequently based on the description and properties of food and nutrients or how food choices could have harmful consequences later in life. These contents are usually selected by the educator, having a limited or nonexistent rational analysis of causes of nutrition problems based on the characteristics of the individuals or groups. Most of the time, these nutrition education interventions are conceived and implemented by health care practitioners who are often inadequately motivated or trained in both nutrition and education (Kris-Etherton et al., 2014; Mogre, Stevens, Aryee, & Amalba, 2018). Additionally, the conventional education approach is intended to reach some specific subgroup of the general population usually based on one or more demographic characteristic shared by its members (Kreuter, Strecher, & Glassman, 1999).

Currently, this approach is considered ineffective, because it leads individuals to assume a passive attitude in the education process, ignoring the active sense that should characterize this process, on the part of both educators and learners. Furthermore, health educators indicate what individuals must do, instead of providing the information they need according to their nutrition assessment, but in a way that lets them feel free to put it into practice and not as an imposition as happens on many occasions. Likewise, often there are no discussions with the patient/client about their own outcome expectancies, motivations, facilitators, and the barriers to change their dietary behavior in order to allow them to meet their nutrition and physical activity recommendations. Although it is well known that this approach is inadequate for patients/clients to be able to modify their dietary behavior, it is still used in many places. Given that it is ineffective and that the records of diseases related to food and nutrition have not been significantly reduced, it is necessary that nutrition and health care practitioners are aware of this situation and can be properly trained.

Personalized nutrition education has been defined as:

> any combination of strategies and information intended to reach one specific person, based on characteristics that are unique to that person, related to the outcome of interest, and derived from individual assessment *Kreuter et al., 1999.*

Education in the field of food and nutrition should involve the participation of individuals using different channels to transmit the information and the collaboration of different professionals, in which emphasis should be placed on improving motivation of the individuals to facilitate the dietary behavior change and, above all, promoting the empowerment of the individual, providing all the knowledge and skills necessaries to be able to decide and make decisions assuming responsibility for their actions. Nutrition education needs to take into consideration and address many factors around the person, such as food patterns, perceptions, food preferences, beliefs, barriers, attitudes and sensory-affective, socioeconomic and environmental factors.

Although the scientific literature on the impact of personalized nutrition interventions on health is scarce, there is growing evidence that this model plays a key role in the promotion of healthy eating habits, active lifestyle, and related health behaviors (Stewart-Knox et al., 2015). Also it is receiving widespread attention in contemporary nutrition promotion because it is expected to be more effective than traditional approaches in encouraging more healthful eating. This model denotes an interesting progression for the discipline of nutrition and aims to provide tailor-made healthy eating advice adapted to food and nutritional needs and the key characteristics of the individuals considering income, race/ethnic, time available, food literacy, and preferred communication channels used by clients/patients to interact with health and nutrition professionals.

Regarding this, an intervention study pointed out that personalized nutrition education which includes the planning and practice of meal choices with the aid of a nutrition professional produced dietary behavioral and food intake changes more effectively than general instructions regarding diet in middle-aged and older type 2 diabetes outpatients and these behavioral changes were sufficient to improve clinical parameters related to diabetic conditions as well (Yang, Chung, & Lee, 2016).

Also another study performed in patients with intestinal failure demonstrated that nutritional education tailored to specific requirements and the use of a booklet with specific advice for this type of disease, significantly improved the knowledge and clinical outcomes (Culkin, Gabe, & Madden, 2009).

Personalized nutrition education should enhance short- and long-term adherence to nutrition care plans and dietary guidelines. This model facilitates dietary change by assessing patient nutrition needs and by emphasizing the state of change of the patient, self-efficacy for dietary changing, personal goal setting and the proper address of challenges and barriers that the patient may present during the process.

EFFECTIVENESS OF PERSONALIZED NUTRITION EDUCATION INTERVENTION

It seems necessary to clarify that nutrition education needs to be much more than the transference of food and nutritional knowledge to be effective. There are a number of elements that can help make personalized nutrition education effective, such as setting specific goals with the client/patient, acting on the factors that influence dietary behavior at the individual, family, and community levels through appropriate strategies based on scientific evidence (Hawkes, 2013; Whitehead, 1973).

Specific and Practical Approach

A focus on specific goals that modifies behavior dietary patterns will be useful in the long term to improve the quality of life of people and their health. For example, the goal of decreasing body weight is too nonspecific, even the goal that the patient consumes a healthy diet is still somewhat ambiguous, so the goal should focus on a pattern of behavior that involves eating more fruits, vegetables, and whole-grain cereals, and reducing the intake of high energy density foods such as pastries, snacks, etc., as well as a specific program of physical activity (Baranowski, Cerin, & Baranowski, 2009).

Determinants of Dietary Behavior Change

Nutrition education is more likely to be successful when the mechanisms underlying dietary behavior are clearly identified and acted upon. Dietary behavior change determinants are the direct targets of the nutrition education interventions. In fact, the determinants of change in dietary behavior must be addressed, although the client/patient must be involved in the dietary behavior change process, by providing them with supportive tools and adequate motivation.

Many health and nutrition professionals tend to think about nutrition knowledge and skills as the main areas to address in a nutrition education intervention. In fact, this approach has been widely used in traditional nutrition education. However, not only is education about providing information, but it is also about improving motivation and facilitating the dietary behavior change.

Nutrition Knowledge and Food Literacy

Two types of nutrition knowledge have been identified. On the one hand, critical knowledge that refers to the information and understanding about the composition of foods and their effect on health, and on the other hand, functional knowledge as a facilitator of dietary behavior change and its maintenance (Truman, Lane, & Elliott, 2017).

In most nutrition education interventions, the term knowledge refers to the communication of information about elementary data on food and nutrition, such as knowing the food groups and servings of a food-based dietary guideline, the composition of energy and nutrients of a food, the understanding and use of nutrition labeling, etc. This knowledge is the basis of food literacy, which refers to the skills needed for a healthy and responsible nutrition behavior such as reading, understanding, and judging the quality of information, as well as gathering and exchanging knowledge related to food and nutrition themes (Krause, Sommerhalder, Beer-Borst, & Abel, 2018).

Food literacy is especially important for social groups with a low level of education, since they need more help to understand and use the basic information about food and nutrition and its relationship with health. Also it is very important for those people who have to improve their health due to the presence of nutrition-related diseases. In addition, the environment of misinformation involving myths and misconceptions about food and nutrition, which is present in media and social networks can create problems for those who wish to eat a healthy diet or follow a healthy lifestyle (Carbone & Zoellner, 2012).

The term food literacy also includes the facilitating knowledge of the dietary behavior change that in practice consists of putting this information into practice, for which the nutrition professional must help the patient in a way that enables him or her to develop that skill, overcoming the difficulties that arise. This includes practical skills like shopping and preparing a determined dish from a recipe, planning menus that contribute to a balanced diet, or how to store and preserve food properly. Although it can also refer to the decision-making involved in purchasing healthy foods, organic foods, or choosing a suitable menu or restaurant when eating out. Despite both types of knowledge being necessary, they are also unlikely in themselves to significantly improve the dietary behavior of patients, if they are not empowered, motivated, or ready to take action.

Scientific evidence shows mixed results on interventions that involve changes in food literacy and their impact on nutrition recommendations compliance. One study performed in women showed that higher levels of food literacy was associated with more self-control, less impulsiveness, and higher intake of fruits, vegetables, and fish (Poelman et al., 2018). In addition to this, a recent systematic review showed a significant positive association between food literacy and dietary adherence and other nutrition behaviors such as dietary quality and variety in the general adult population. Conversely, a significant negative association or nonsignificant associations have been observed in several studies that involved participants who suffered some nutrition-related diseases that suggests other approaches most be considered for patients (Ajzen, Joyce, Sheikh, & Cote, 2011; Carrara & Schulz, 2018; Zoellner et al., 2011). Additionally, other systematic review concluded food literacy may play a key role in the dietary intake of adolescents. It was observed that adolescents with greater food knowledge and those who frequently helped to prepare food had healthier dietary intakes (Vaitkeviciute, Ball, & Harris, 2015).

Psychosocial Influences as Determinants of Action and Behavior Change

In addition to knowledge, there are other motivational influences and facilitators for dietary behavior change. One of those determinants is food beliefs, defined as the mental acceptance of a particular concept that is arrived at from external evidence, facts, observation, or personal experience. That is, this belief represents how a person perceives that their action regarding something will bring about a certain result, for example, that physical activity reduces the risk of diabetes. These beliefs have motivational power because individuals come to believe, or find convincing scientific reasons, why to make a particular food choice or physical activity, such as eating more fruits and vegetables or foods produced in a more sustainable way, or eating related behaviors with the control of diabetes or breastfeeding (Fishbein, 2010).

Attitudes are defined as the degree to which an individual evaluates a particular behavior favorably or unfavorably. That is, attitudes reflect the emotional state of an individual toward the targeted behavior and have a strong impact on their motivational state to perform a specific action, leading to behavioral intention. Evidence suggests that attitudes are among the most important factors determining intentions to execute behaviors according to the theory of planned behavior (Rankin et al., 2018).

Additionally, nutritional information that is communicated and the way in which it is communicated must be taken into account, since such information can be especially powerful when it is communicated in the form of a group activity or presented visually in a motivational way, considering the emotional and rational side of the client/patient, in order to stimulate and develop thinking convictions. The dietary behavior change definitely requires the emotional and cognitive commitment of people.

For instance, an adolescent who suffers from type 2 diabetes should change their dietary habits and increase their physical activity. However, he or she does not change or is not even interested because at that time in their life, their priority is to look good and to be popular with their classmates, so they do not respond to the information given to improve their lifestyle. Therefore the communication strategy must be changed and must include other reasons that are more important to them. In addition to the information on food and control of the disease, it can be pointed out that positive and immediate benefits such as energy to do things with your colleagues successfully can be obtained. All these considerations help to recognize that individuals internalize the beliefs, norms, and values of their culture, and that they are powerful in people's lives and become the determinants of their own behavior. Therefore, nutrition educators must know the context surrounding their lives, recognize the individual differences that exist between them and the different interpretations they can make in the situations that are presented to them, in order to design the most appropriate and personalized intervention(Thomson & Ravia, 2011).

The most effective way to help people make changes in their dietary practices is to identify the determinants of their current diets, as well as the determinants that can potentially produce behavioral changes and then develop strategies to address these determinants. These determinants operate in the context of family, community, and culture, and their identification is most effective when carried out in a personalized way.

Theory-Based Interventions

Designing and implementing theory-based nutrition education interventions may facilitate dietary behavior changes and maintenance of these changes for longer periods of time. These theories can be helpful in improving the understanding of behavior change determinants of people.

Researchers have identified perceptions and internal experiences as the main determinants of behavior and the motivation for change of people. In addition, it has been described that an important determinant is the belief of the people in the outcome expectancies related to their behavior and the "value" that that outcome represents for them.

For instance, consuming foods rich in calcium would avoid suffering from osteoporosis (outcome expectancy) and also would allow them to have better mobility in old age (value of the result). The determinants, expected outcomes, and values statistically predict behavior and explain why people do what they do. Another example that illustrates this theory: "if I follow a healthy diet and do exercise (outcome expectancy) my children will also have a healthy lifestyle" (value of result). Determinants are related to behavior in a predictable way and help understand why people do what they do and how they can change. In nutrition education interventions, the theory predicts and/or explains dietary behaviors or behavior change (Brug, Oenema, & Ferreira, 2005). These determinants or predictors of the behavior change include, besides beliefs, other elements such as perceptions of risk or illness, self-efficacy, self-confidence, barriers, etc., as well as knowledge and skills.

The effectiveness of the use of the theories is based on the fact that they provide an explanation of the health behavior or behavior change of an individual by identifying its determinants. Furthermore, they help to design the intervention components and the most appropriate strategies and guide the evaluation of the impact of the intervention (Diep, Chen, Davies, Baranowski, & Baranowski, 2014).

Levels of Influence in the Food Choice and Dietary Behavior

Nutrition education interventions are effective when they address the multiple levels of influences on food choice and dietary behavior. These include influences at the individual, family, social, and community level, and the physical environment (green areas, supermarkets, etc.), social structures, and health promotion policies (Whitehead, 1973). The long-term adherence to a dietary behavior depends on whether individuals can fit the new behavior into their daily lives, whether there is social support, and whether material conditions or social structures are adequate. Therefore, interventions in nutrition education should take into account the individual, interpersonal, and environmental or social level. The individual level focuses on experience with food, food preferences, and the enjoyment of food, as well as beliefs, attitudes, values, functional knowledge, skills, perceived social and cultural norms, or life experience. The interpersonal level focuses on family, friends, colleagues, interactions with health professionals, cultural norms and practices, social role, and social networks. The environment is determined by municipalities and communities and focuses on the availability and access to healthy foods, sports facilities, green areas, and other healthy environments in schools or workplaces (Hawkes, 2013; McNulty, 2013).

Other factors that should be taken into account in nutrition education interventions are working with parents or families to address their children's health problems (e.g., overweight or obesity) or to help their children to develop healthy eating and physical activity behaviors (eat more fruits and vegetables, less screen time). In these cases, parents' motivation, skills related to food, and the promotion of healthy habits of children must be worked on in order to have a positive impact on their children's behavior (Hingle et al., 2012).

Another noteworthy aspect is the duration and intensity of the intervention, since it must be sufficient to improve effectiveness. Studies suggest that nutrition education that provides sufficient duration and intensity is more likely to be effective. Sometimes this must be maintained, even for years, to achieve relevant results (Khambalia, Dickinson, Hardy, Gill, & Baur, 2012). In addition, patients often have a poor attention span, which in short interventions represents a problem, so a coordinated and systematic approach using several levels and intervention channels could increase effectiveness. For example, nutrition education interventions may include group sessions considering the individual's own characteristics, information on paper or provided by email, the use of social networks, mobile phone activities, etc.

Use of Appropriate Behavior Change Strategies

Nutrition education intervention is more likely to be successful when you use appropriate strategies based on a theory and evidence to address the determinants of dietary behavior change. To do this, an adequate evaluation must be carried out, which includes the available objective information, desires related to achieve certain health and nutrition goals, and needs that the client/patient or group have, taking into account the family, cultural, and community context. All this will help to establish the goals and to select the most appropriate strategies for dietary behavior change. It may be necessary to use several strategies in order to help change one or more behavioral determinants. Therefore, the behavior change process must be faced realistically and consider the difficulty that presents and be aware that people may need a long time to get results, so it is important to be prudent in the expectations of positive results.

On the other hand, nutritional education to change the behavior of the individual must be addressed by improving motivation, facilitating action (knowledge, skills, etc.), and promoting the most appropriate environmental supports (Norman, Abraham, & Conner, 2000).

Motivation to Change

Achieving and maintaining dietary behavior changes are a multifaceted process including contemplation, awareness, and motivation for the change. Motivation helps individuals in all phases of the dietary behavior change. Initially, people may not be prepared to face the difficulties or barriers of change, likewise, motivation is needed to stay adhered to the indicated dietary pattern. In any case, thoughts, beliefs, and attitudes or feelings can predict the success or failure of the behavior change. Therefore the nutrition professional must take into account all those aspects that motivate the change, enhancing the perceived benefits and minimizing the barriers encountered by the patient. For this the professional must promote the contemplation and awareness of individuals who lack the understanding of the consequences of their behaviors and improve the motivation to act (Lacey & Street, 2017).

Action Plan for Dietary Behavior Change

When people decide to take action to improve their health, an action plan must be agreed upon based on previously established goals. The intervention plan should help the individual's good intentions to be translated into concrete actions. The action plan goals should be focused on initiating the action and maintaining it over time. Therefore it is not enough to tell them what action they should take, but the patient should be helped by training them in all the practical and technical aspects that facilitate the change of an undesirable behavior and the adherence to new guidelines such as information about food composition, food purchasing skills, planning healthy menus, adequate food servings, preparation of meals, etc. The success of action planning will improve the patient's skills in managing their food environment and increase their self-regulation and self-efficacy, which in turn will increase motivation and the effectiveness of the intervention (van Osch et al., 2009).

Environmental Support to Achieve Behavior Changes

Environmental support is important during the behavior change process. This support should include personal support from family members, friends and colleagues, community, institutional, and political support that can be translated into healthy food environments, green areas and leisure areas that invite sports and physical exercise, all in an environment of security.

In addition, of the mentioned strategies, it is important to highlight the importance of how nutrition education is taught. In this sense activities are more effective when they are attractive, well organized, and meaningful. Educators are more effective when they are enthusiastic about what they are presenting, and are seen as credible, warm, respectful, and sensitive to the cultures and social environments of the patient.

METHODOLOGY FOR PERSONALIZED NUTRITION EDUCATION

In general, the development of a nutritional education intervention needs planning that begins with the knowledge of the nutritional situation of the individual (nutritional assessment in the nutrition consultation) or collective (nutritional assessment of a group) to establish the diagnosis of the situation and to be able to intervene effectively, as described in the nutritional care process (Writing Group of the Nutrition Care Process/Standardized Language Committee, 2008a). However, change should be based on the freedom of the individual and should be prepared to address it as described in the stages of change of the transtheoretical model (Prochaska & DiClemente, 1982). Furthermore, in order to do so, qualified and trained professionals should be available to facilitate patient behavior change. Likewise, dietary advice should be based on scientific evidence.

Nutrition Care Process Applied to Personalized Nutrition Education

The nutritional care process (NCP) is a systematic methodology for solving nutrition problems that nutrition professionals use when analyzing and making decisions about nutrition-related practices. It is designed for use with clients/patients, groups, and communities of all ages and health or illness conditions (Writing Group of the Nutrition Care Process/Standardized Language Committee, 2008a).

NCP consists of four interrelated and connected phases that involve nutritional assessment, nutrition diagnosis, nutritional intervention, and nutritional monitoring and evaluation. Each phase provides information to the next and may cause a review of the previous steps of the process and reevaluation, adding or reviewing the diagnosis or the nutritional intervention, modifying or adjusting the goals intervention, and monitoring certain indicators (Writing Group of the Nutrition Care Process/Standardized Language Committee, 2008a). NCP or a similar methodology should be applied in any nutrition education intervention in order to solve nutrition education problems individually.

Nutrition Assessment

The nutritional evaluation is responsible for identifying problems related to nutrition and their causes. In general, as the level of assessment increases so does the degree of individualization of the nutrition education intervention. It is carried out at the individual level through an interview that usually comprises information about food and nutrition related history, which includes data on dietary or supplements intake, physical activity, and knowledge, beliefs, attitudes, and dietary behaviors. It also entails anthropometric measurements, biochemical data, medical tests, and procedures with nutrition-focused physical findings, which involve physical appearance, swallowing function or appetite, and the client history that includes occupation, educational level, cultural and religious beliefs, etc. (Writing Group of the Nutrition Care Process/Standardized Language Committee 2008a, b).

Nutritional Diagnosis

The professional reviews all the available information obtained from the client/patient and compares it with the reference or comparative standard. Nutritional diagnosis must be clear and concise, specific for each client/patient, limited to the problems of the individual, related to the etiology, and based on the signs and symptoms of the evaluation data. This step of the nutrition care process is essential for the setting up of a proper nutrition education intervention (Writing Group of the Nutrition Care Process/Standardized Language Committee, 2008a).

Nutrition Intervention

The aim is to resolve a nutrition problem such as inadequate dietary behavior by planning and implementing an appropriate nutritional intervention. The action plan should include goal setting, designed with the intention of changing certain dietary behavior, and reducing diseases risk factors, environmental conditions, or health state. Furthermore, it should be tailored to the needs, priorities based on the diagnosis, outcomes expectancies, and available and needed resources of the individual. In addition, the selection of the specific intervention strategies defining time, frequency of care, and monitoring should be implemented by communicating the nutritional care plan to the patient, modifying it when necessary (Writing Group of the Nutrition Care Process/Standardized Language Committee, 2008a).

Monitoring and Evaluation

Monitoring and outcome evaluation should determine the progress obtained and if the outcome expectancies are met. Strategies must be reviewed and modified in accordance with the response to the education intervention (Writing Group of the Nutrition Care Process/Standardized Language Committee, 2008a). In this step, information should be collected on the barriers and strengths that patients have had during the process of change in order to work through them with the patient and address them properly.

Effective Interview in the Nutrition Consultation

In the nutritional consultation, the interview is the usual technique to evaluate the dietary habits of the interviewee, his/her origins, lifestyle, and related information to know the nutritional status of the patient and the problems he/she presents in order to set realistic intervention goals and to identify possible alternatives to reach the required change.

Nutrition and health professionals need to have excellent communication skills in order to communicate with client/patient (Berman & Chutka, 2016). Among the conditions that facilitate the interview are to clearly define the purpose, to listen properly, to establish confidence and an understanding relationship, to avoid interruptions, to provide psychological intimacy, to have an appropriate physical environment, to have emotional objectivity, to consider the personal context of the interviewee, and to limit the note-taking or to explain why they are needed.

The interview can be divided for study into three stages: opening, body, and closing.

- The *opening of the interview*, the professional should dedicate a few minutes to establish a cordial relationship with the patient, as well as to introduce him/herself (name, work position). The patient should then be asked about the purpose of the interview, giving the patient the first opportunity to speak in order to create a positive atmosphere. It is essential for a nutrition educator to establish and maintain eye contact and listen actively to the client/patient from the opening to the closure of the interview.
- The *body of the interview* aims to obtain as much information as possible about all aspects of the problem of the patient. Particularly, to know the dietary history and explore attitudes, barriers, beliefs, thoughts, emotions, past success histories, and any other aspects of interest. In order to do this, asked questions should be appropriate, open-ended, and understandable by the client/patient. It is recommended that questions must be planned and ordered in advance. An interview guide is often useful since it prevents the forgetting of any indispensable detail. Also, it is desirable to give sufficient time for the patient to answer all questions.
- The *closing of the interview* is usually short, but should not be hasty. The nutrition professional should always bring an appropriate closure to the interview. It should be reviewed the purpose of the interview, summarizing the agreed intervention goals and the action plan with client/patient. Ask if he or she has any questions or concerns and set up the next appointment. End with a positive note and gratitude.

Motivational Interviewing

The approach that should be used in the interview or nutrition consultation to help the patient overcome the faced obstacles in order to achieve and maintain the change to an adequate diet and a healthy lifestyle should be based on understanding, motivation, and support.

In this sense, the interview in the initial phases should foster motivation and free decision-making, and in later phases seek to empower the client/patient through training in knowledge and skills related to food and nutrition, as well as self-regulation or self-control skills. In this respect, the motivational theory of Rogers (Rogers, 1942) was pioneering in indicating that a nondirective patient-centered approach should be used, so that it is the patient who directs the flow of conversation.

For his/her part, the nutrition professional must explore the point of view of the patient in the context of his/her daily life by creating a favorable climate in the patient–consultant relationship, by being empathic, and by seeking to reduce ambivalence and increase readiness to change. The features that characterize this approach are the radical trust in the patient, the rejection of the managerial role of the consultant, avoiding excessive staring, and the recommendations and advice generated unilaterally by the consultant.

All this will result in improved self-esteem and self-management, which will enhance the capabilities of the patient. As conditions of this approach, it is established that in the relationship with the patient, his/her conflicts and contradictions must be respected without judgment or disapproval, provocation of anxiety with comments that could be directed to the most vulnerable aspects of the patient must be avoided, and the professional must be congruent and honest in the relationship with the patient and show concern and understanding, both verbally and nonverbally.

Likewise, Miller and Rollnick (1991) propose that the consultant should guide the patient about food and other lifestyle habits that the patient want to change, but also, he/she should be able to make feel the patient comfortable to talk about the positive and negative aspects of the behavior change. Furthermore, the consultant must establish a collaboration with the client since it is he/she who knows himself/herself, his/her environments and situations surrounding his/her life. Once the determinants of behavior and behavior change have been explored, the evocation should be used to provide ideas for the patient to consider the problem, but always taking into account the autonomy of the patient, so that decisions are left to the patient in spite of the fact that the professional may have other preferences or opinions. Once the decisions have been taken and the goals have been set, the consultant must support and train the patient to achieve the desired results.

It has been pointed out that motivational interviewing may increase the adherence to nutrition interventions. For instance, a study performed in adolescents showed that motivational interviewing enhanced adherence to an obesity intervention (Bean et al., 2015). This theory has been shown to be very useful in this age group since adolescents are in a transition age in which frequently they experiment feelings of ambivalence. On the one hand, they seek autonomy but on the other hand, reject authority, which may interfere in the adherence of the guidelines prescribed by the health practitioner (Bean et al., 2015).

Nutrition Educator Profile

The educator must have some essential characteristics to increase the possibilities that the client/patient will be able to accomplish the dietary behavior change. Personalized nutrition education should be effectively applied by qualified nutrition professionals. Also, they should be competent in communication skills, such as interpersonal communication skills, nonverbal communication, professional values, and counseling skills, given that communication is the main method by which the nutrition professional conducts their practice.

The educator needs training, experience, and professional skills as well as being specialized in nutrition education. Moreover, credibility in nutrition is a very important aspect that the educator must own due to the amount of information available in the social environment and the presence of pseudo-professionals of nutrition. Additionally, educators should base their practice on integrity and have ethical behavior. They should be consistent in their actions and demonstrate empathy, respect, and sincere interest in the emotional needs of the patient. Also they should be able to establish and maintain a relationship of trust with the patient that facilitates good communication, since the client/patient will feel more confident in expressing any idea or emotion about their expectations, goals, motivations, facilitators, barriers, or fears, without thinking that he is being judged or feeling uncomfortable. Finally, the educator should be able to guide the client/patient with arguments showing the positive aspects and the difficulties of the dietary change behavior (Berman & Chutka, 2016).

NUTRITION EDUCATION DESIGN PROCEDURE IN THE PERSONALIZED NUTRITION EDUCATION

The design of effective strategies of personalized nutrition education requires a systematic and planned process that facilitates the nutrition professional to design the nutritional care of the patient and also it enhances patient adherence to dietary and exercise guidelines. A systematic stepwise behaviorally-focused and theory-based process is the Nutrition Education DESIGN procedure (Contento, 2015). This process entails six steps:

Step 1. Decide Behaviors

The specific behavior goal must be set and be agreed between the consultant and the client/patient. The identification of the stage or disposition for behavior change of a person is important in order to decide on an appropriate behavioral approach and to design an effective intervention. The stages of the transtheoretical model of change can be adopted to personalize education for dietary behavioral change (Prochaska & DiClemente, 1982). This model or theory considers the stages of precontemplation, contemplation, preparation, action, maintenance, and completion.

At the precontemplation stage, the patient is unaware of the existence of a problem or denies it and therefore the patient does not see the need for change. It is often characterized by a history of failure and a lack of confidence in the ability of the patient to make changes. At the contemplation stage the patient considers making changes in the future and improves his attitude to receive information. The pros and cons of change are raised and ambivalence appears (positive and negative thoughts and/or emotions toward someone or something). During the preparation stage, changes are planned and the ambivalence in favor of change is resolved; even the patient usually begins to make some behavioral changes. At the action stage, the agreed action plan (changes in dietary habits and lifestyle) is put into practice. It is important to encourage self-management and self-control. Furthermore, social support is desirable in order to avoid relapses. The maintenance stage begins 6 months after desired behavioral changes have been made, so new behaviors are performed automatically. At this stage, the presence of relapses are less frequent. Finally, the completion stage is not usually defined for behavioral changes related to dietary habits.

There is evidence that the transtheoretical model of change has been useful when it has been used in personalized interventions to improve health outcomes. It has been related to the improvement of the consumption of vegetables and fruits, the increase of physical exercise, the management of emotional distress, the control of weight, and the decrease of the consumption of sugar drinks (Cook, O'Leary, & Allman-Farinelli, 2018; Johnson et al., 2008; Saeidi, Mirzaei, Mahaki, Jalali, & Jalilian, 2018). Understanding the stages and processes of dietary and physical activity behavior change may yield essential information for augmenting adoption, adherence, and relapse prevention.

Step 2. Explore Determinants of Change

The understanding and addresses of the determinants will help the client/patient to be successful at changing toward their behavior goal. The exploration of change determinants attempts to understand the possible knowledge, skills, motivations, facilitators, and barriers of the patient in their environmental context.

Exploring the determinants of behavior change shows the preconceived ideas of the patient, as well as the beliefs and attitudes that are potential motivators of change (e.g., staying healthier and fit), and knowledge and skills the patient possesses and may facilitate the change process (e.g., knowing how to prepare healthy meals, or knowing the recommended food servings).

Particularly, it is about identifying the relevant personal, psychosocial, and environmental determinants or precursors of the observed behavior, as well as identifying the facilitators and barriers the client/patient may find in the process and that may impede or encourage behavior change, such as the degree of environmental support available to help patients achieve the proposed goals. In addition, it helps to identify the additional skills and competence needed to achieve the consensual goals and the development of the action plan directed to the needs and desires of the patient.

Step 3. Select Theory and Clarify Philosophy

Selecting the right theory helps to organize the set of actions related to dietary behavior change. The exploration of determinants usually indicates whether the individual is aware of the problem that represents his/her behavior or if he/she is motivated to act, or requires skills or other resources for training. All of this will facilitate the approach to the desired behavior change, minimizing as much as possible the time and effort dedicated to it.

There are motivation theories that may be useful for raising awareness, promoting active contemplation, and improving patient motivation, in order to help to resolve ambivalence and facilitating decision-making and action. They provide guidance on the design of messages and activities that increase motivation and awareness for action. Examples of these theories are the health belief model, theory of planned behavior, theory of self-determination, etc.

On the other hand, translating motivations and intentions into action is difficult for individuals, so it is important to empower them by building the capacity to perform actions related to changing desired eating behaviors. Specific knowledge and skills about food and nutrition, including food choice, purchase, and preparation, are often useful. In addition, self-regulatory skills of possible undesirable behaviors are important to act according to the stated targets. In this sense, the social cognitive theory, theories of self-efficacy and self-regulation, and the theory of self-determination can be used for this purpose (Bandura, 2004; Schwarzer & Renner, 2000).

In most cases, nutrition education looks for the inclusion of motivational activities and the facilitation of action, which can be used together during the intervention. In this sense, the theory of planned behavior, social cognitive theory, and the approach to the health action process, among others, may be very useful.

In general, there are common determinants of the different theories that have been shown to be important motivators of food and nutrition-related behavior or determinants of changing dietary behavior:

- Outcome expectancies (including perceived benefits and negative results or pros and cons of the change).
- Attitudes and feelings toward behavior change.
- Perception of the risk of the current behavior.
- Food preferences (sensory properties and affective attributes).
- Perceived social and personal norms (often derived from cultural norms)
- Perceived self-efficacy or control in performing specific behaviors.

Likewise, it has also been seen that the elements that compose the different theories are useful to improve motivation and to facilitate action capacity:

- Self-efficacy.
- Perceived behavioral control.
- Self-regulation and self-direction skills, including goal setting and self-monitoring.
- Specific behavioral abilities related to food and nutrition: skills in food preparation or physical activity, and critical behavioral assessment skills.

Step 4. Indicate General Objectives

The general educational plan objectives should be reached by consensus with the patient and should guide the entire intervention. In addition, educational objectives can be agreed upon for each individual session. These are the specific objectives and guide the development of specific activities in that session. Furthermore, the goals must be measurable, realistic and achievable, relevant, and time-limited (Marzano & Kendall, 2007).

In general, the objectives must be oriented toward encouraging a change in behavior, increasing motivation, or enabling the patient to take action. Therefore, they should be based on the analysis of the determinants of the observed behaviors. An example of a motivational objective is to make the patient see the risk posed by excessive and habitual consumption of salty snacks, which increases the risk of heart disease. On the other hand, an example of a tool to train in knowledge may be that the patient makes a record of 24 hours of his/her diet and compares it with the recommended rations of the different food groups of a food guide and thus observes the possible deviations of his diet in relation to the recommendations.

Step 5. Generate Action Plans

In order to establish the action plan, the general and specific objectives as well as the determinants of the behavior of the client/patient must be analyzed. The action plan will be derived from this analysis. This plan will comprise an organized sequence of activities that encourage motivation and empowerment for behavior change. The educational strategies that help motivation are related to activities that show the perception of the risk or benefits of a certain behavior, as well as those activities that show how to overcome barriers or promote self-efficacy. On the other hand, educational strategies tending to facilitate action are linked to the training of skills related to the food environment and those related to self-regulation. The activities must be designed in an interesting and relevant manner in accordance with the characteristics of the patient in order to achieve behavioral change according to the established objective (Michie et al., 2013).

Step 6. Nail Down Evaluation Plan

Evaluation is an important component of nutrition education planning in order to see if the designed and applied intervention achieved the set objectives. The information drawn from the evaluation is useful for improving the planning and implementation of future nutrition education interventions. In addition, evaluation can be effective as a motivating tool for the patient, even if not all of the established goals have been met, as it can point to changes that need to be made to improve the effectiveness of the intervention.

Two main types of evaluation can be distinguished: process and outcomes evaluations. The evaluation of the process analyzes whether the action plan is being implemented according to the design carried out. It allows the early detection of existing or potential problems, such as barriers to achieve the dietary habits modification, and permits the making of changes to improve the nutrition education intervention. Whereas the outcome evaluation is conducted at the end of the intervention and provides information on changes achieved. Both are intended to provide knowledge for the development of the intervention and its effectiveness and as far as possible to improve the nutritional education provided to the patient (Institute of Medicine, 2007).

OTHER ASPECTS TO TAKE INTO ACCOUNT IN PERSONALIZED NUTRITIONAL EDUCATION

A relapse in terms of nutrition is the return to previous eating and physical activity behaviors and is very frequent among those patients that are under nutritional treatment. Given this, nutrition professional must forewarn clients to watch for this possibility and prepare them as to how they should handle this situation. The patient should be provided with the knowledge and skills to be able to identify the situations or triggers that prompt their lapse or relapse, such as a party, where everyone overeats or pecks tempting foods, vacations, or tense moments at work, etc. When a lapse or relapse have taken place, it is necessary to guide clients through the frustration of a relapse into a renewed commitment to their healthy eating and activity behaviors, reflecting on what circumstances, thoughts, and feelings preceded the lapse or relapse and considering that every mistake should be seen as a learning opportunity, not as a personal failure.

In addition, short- and long-term adherence to the prescribed pattern or dietary behavior change is associated with long-term benefits in health interventions. To facilitate patient adherence to the dietary guidelines, nutrition professionals need to increase their knowledge and training in personalized nutrition education based on the patient-centered counseling model, since it provides an effective approach for intervening with patients to promote dietary change behavior and long-term adherence.

In general, adherence to desired dietary patterns or physical activity patterns tend to decrease over time. In this sense, evidence on this subject shows different alternatives to promote long-term adherence (Middleton, Anton, & Perri, 2013).

- Maintain patient care for long periods of time in a personal manner, by telephone or via Internet.
- Provide problem solving or relapse prevention skills by enabling patients to overcome barriers that interfere with adherence to desired behavior.
- Encourage social support from family and friends.
- Make flexible recommendations that fit the wishes of the patient, his or her lifestyle, and time availability.
- Self-monitoring of adherence to recommendations, weight evolution, or other noted behaviors.

CONCLUSION

Nutrition education interventions should be carried out in a personalized manner in accordance with the factors that influence food decisions and the determinants of changing dietary behavior of the individual. Interventions need to address many factors, such as dietary patterns, food preferences and aversions, perceptions, attitudes and beliefs toward food, motivators, facilitators, and barriers for behavior change, and psychological, socioeconomic, and environmental factors.

An effective strategy of personalized nutrition education requires a systematic and planned process that facilitates nutrition professionals to design the nutritional care of the patients and also enhances the compliance of the dietary and physical activity guidelines by the population.

There are different theories, methods, and tools that can be useful in this process. However, it would be desirable to gain more information about their impacts on adherence in the short and long term, and also to develop other methods to guide health professionals to empower individuals to achieve their personal and health goals.

Personalized nutrition education represents a challenge for health care services and its application is crucial for contributing to the prevention and control of nutrition-related diseases. It should be applied by qualified professionals, and as a result, there is an imperative to train health professionals in this approach in order to be able to design and apply effective individual education strategies to help individuals to change their lifestyles.

References

Ajzen, I., Joyce, N., Sheikh, S., & Cote, N. G. (2011). Knowledge and the prediction of behavior: The role of information accuracy in the theory of planned behavior. *Basic and Applied Social Psychology*, *33*(2), 101−117.

Bandura, A. (2004). Health promotion by social cognitive means. *Health Education & Behavior*, *31*(2), 143−164.

Baranowski, T., Cerin, E., & Baranowski, J. (2009). Steps in the design, development and formative evaluation of obesity prevention-related behavior change trials. *International Journal of Behavioral Nutrition and Physical Activity*, *6*, 6, 6-5868-6-6.

Bean, M. K., Powell, P., Quinoy, A., Ingersoll, K., Wickham, E. P., III, & Mazzeo, S. E. (2015). Motivational interviewing targeting diet and physical activity improves adherence to paediatric obesity treatment: Results from the MI Values randomized controlled trial. *Pediatric Obesity*, *10*(2), 118−125.

Berman, A. C., & Chutka, D. S. (2016). Assessing effective physician-patient communication skills: "Are you listening to me, doc?. *Korean Journal of Medical Education*, *28*(2), 243−249.

Blanchard, C. M., Fisher, J., Sparling, P. B., Shanks, T. H., Nehl, E., Rhodes, R. E., et al. (2009). Understanding adherence to 5 servings of fruits and vegetables per day: A theory of planned behavior perspective. *The Journal of Nutrition Education and Behavior*, *41*(1), 3−10.

Bornhorst, C., Wijnhoven, T. M., Kunesova, M., Yngve, A., Rito, A. I., Lissner, L., et al. (2015). WHO European Childhood Obesity Surveillance Initiative: Associations between sleep duration, screen time and food consumption frequencies. *BMC Public Health*, *15*, 442, 442-015-1793-3.

Bruce, A. S., Pruitt, S. W., Ha, O. R., Cherry, J. B. C., Smith, T. R., Bruce, J. M., et al. (2016). The influence of televised food commercials on children's food choices: Evidence from ventromedial prefrontal cortex activations. *Journal of Pediatrics*, *177*, 27−32.e1.

Brug, J., Oenema, A., & Ferreira, I. (2005). Theory, evidence and Intervention Mapping to improve behavior nutrition and physical activity interventions. *International Journal of Behavioral Nutrition and Physical Activity*, *2*(1), 2, 2-5868-2-2.

Carbone, E. T., & Zoellner, J. M. (2012). Nutrition and health literacy: A systematic review to inform nutrition research and practice. *Journal of the Academy of Nutrition and Dietetics*, *112*(2), 254−265.

Carrara, A., & Schulz, P. J. (2018). The role of health literacy in predicting adherence to nutritional recommendations: A systematic review. *Patient Education and Counseling*, *101*(1), 16−24.

Contento, I. R. (2008). Nutrition education: Linking research, theory, and practice. *Asia Pacific Journal of Clinical Nutrition*, *17*(Suppl 1), 176−179.

Contento, I. R. (2015). *Nutrition education: Linking research, theory, and practice* (3rd ed.). Sudbury, MA: Jones & Bartlett.

Cook, A. S., O'Leary, F., & Allman-Farinelli, M. (2018). The relationship between process use and stage of change for sugary drinks. *Journal of Human Nutrition and Dietetics*, *31*(5), 697−703.

Culkin, A., Gabe, S. M., & Madden, A. M. (2009). Improving clinical outcome in patients with intestinal failure using individualised nutritional advice. *Journal of Human Nutrition and Dietetics*, *22*(4), 290−298, quiz300-1.

Diep, C. S., Chen, T. A., Davies, V. F., Baranowski, J. C., & Baranowski, T. (2014). Influence of behavioral theory on fruit and vegetable intervention effectiveness among children: A meta-analysis. *Journal of Nutrition Education and Behavior*, 46(6), 506–546.

Dijkstra, S. C., Neter, J. E., Brouwer, I. A., Huisman, M., & Visser, M. (2014). Adherence to dietary guidelines for fruit, vegetables and fish among older Dutch adults: The role of education, income and job prestige. *Journal of Nutrition, Health and Aging*, 18(2), 115–121.

EFSA (European Food Safety Authority). (2017). *Dietary reference values for nutrients: Summary report*. EFSA Supporting Publication, e15121.:92.

Fielding-Singh, P. (2017). A taste of inequality: Food's symbolic value across the socioeconomic spectrum. *Sociological Science*, 4, 424–448.

Fishbein, M. A. I. (2010). *Predicting and changing behavior: The reasoned action approach* (1st ed.). New York: Psychology Press.

Frankel, L. A., Hughes, S. O., O'Connor, T. M., Power, T. G., Fisher, J. O., & Hazen, N. L. (2012). Parental Influences on children's self-regulation of energy intake: Insights from developmental literature on emotion regulation. *Journal of Obesity*, 2012, 327259.

GBD 2015 Risk Factors Collaborators. (2016). Global, regional, and national comparative risk assessment of 79 behavioural, environmental and occupational, and metabolic risks or clusters of risks, 1990–2015: A systematic analysis for the Global Burden of Disease Study 2015. *The Lancet*, 388(10053), 1659–1724.

Ha, O. R., Killian, H., Bruce, J. M., Lim, S. L., & Bruce, A. S. (2018). Food advertising literacy training reduces the importance of taste in children's food decision-making: A Pilot Study. *Frontiers in Psychology*, 9, 1293.

Hallal, P. C., Andersen, L. B., Bull, F. C., Guthold, R., Haskell, W., Ekelund, U., et al. (2012). Global physical activity levels: Surveillance progress, pitfalls, and prospects. *The Lancet*, 380(9838), 247–257.

Harris, G., & Coulthard, H. (2016). Early eating behaviours and food acceptance revisited: Breastfeeding and introduction of complementary foods as predictive of food acceptance. *Current Obesity Reports*, 5(1), 113–120.

Hawkes, C. (2013). *Promoting healthy diets through nutrition education and changes in the food environment: An international review of actions and their effectiveness*. Rome: Nutrition Education and Consumer Awareness Group, Food and Agriculture Organization of the United Nations. Available from www.fao.org/ag/humannutrition/nutritioneducation/69725/en/.

Hingle, M., Beltran, A., O'Connor, T., Thompson, D., Baranowski, J., & Baranowski, T. (2012). A model of goal directed vegetable parenting practices. *Appetite*, 58(2), 444–449.

Institute of Medicine. (2007). *Progress in preventing childhood obesity: How do we measure up?* Washington, DC: The National Academies Press.

Institute of Medicine. (2011). *Dietary reference intakes for calcium and vitamin D*. Washington, DC: National Academic Press.

Johnson, S. S., Paiva, A. L., Cummins, C. O., Johnson, J. L., Dyment, S. J., Wright, J. A., et al. (2008). Transtheoretical model-based multiple behavior intervention for weight management: Effectiveness on a population basis. *Preventive Medicine*, 46(3), 238–246.

Kasten, S., van Osch, L., Eggers, S. M., & de Vries, H. (2017). From action planning and plan enactment to fruit consumption: Moderated mediation effects. *BMC Public Health*, 17(1), 832, 832-017-4838-y.

Khambalia, A. Z., Dickinson, S., Hardy, L. L., Gill, T., & Baur, L. A. (2012). A synthesis of existing systematic reviews and meta-analyses of school-based behavioural interventions for controlling and preventing obesity. *Obesity Reviews*, 13(3), 214–233.

Klassen, K. M., Douglass, C. H., Brennan, L., Truby, H., & Lim, M. S. C. (2018). Social media use for nutrition outcomes in young adults: A mixed-methods systematic review. *International Journal of Behavioral Nutrition and Physical Activity*, 15(1), 70, 70-018-0696-y.

Kontis, V., Mathers, C. D., Rehm, J., Stevens, G. A., Shield, K. D., Bonita, R., et al. (2014). Contribution of six risk factors to achieving the 25×25 non-communicable disease mortality reduction target: A modelling study. *The Lancet*, 384(9941), 427–437.

Krause, C., Sommerhalder, K., Beer-Borst, S., & Abel, T. (2018). Just a subtle difference? Findings from a systematic review on definitions of nutrition literacy and food literacy. *Health Promotion International*, 33(3), 378–389.

Kreuter, M. W., Strecher, V. J., & Glassman, B. (1999). One size does not fit all: The case for tailoring print materials. *Annals of Behavioral Medicine*, 21(4), 276–283.

Kris-Etherton, P. M., Akabas, S. R., Bales, C. W., Bistrian, B., Braun, L., Edwards, M. S., et al. (2014). The need to advance nutrition education in the training of health care professionals and recommended research to evaluate implementation and effectiveness. *American Journal of Clinical Nutrition, 99*(5 Suppl), 1153S–1166SS.

Lacey, S. J., & Street, T. D. (2017). Measuring healthy behaviours using the stages of change model: An investigation into the physical activity and nutrition behaviours of Australian miners. *BioPsychoSocial Medicine, 11*, 30, 30-017-0115-7. eCollection 2017.

Leng, G., Adan, R. A. H., Belot, M., Brunstrom, J. M., de Graaf, K., Dickson, S. L., et al. (2017). The determinants of food choice. *Proceedings of the Nutrition Society, 76*(3), 316–327.

Mantau, A., Hattula, S., & Bornemann, T. (2018). Individual determinants of emotional eating: A simultaneous investigation. *Appetite, 130*, 93–103.

Marzano, R., & Kendall, J. (2007). *The new taxonomy of educational objectives* (2nd ed.). Thousand Oaks, CA: Sage Publications.

McNulty, J. (2013). *Challenges and issues in nutrition education*. Rome: Nutrition Education and Consumer Awareness Group. Food and Agriculture Organization of the United Nations. Available from www.fao.org/ag/humannutrition/nutritioneducation/en/.

Michie, S., Richardson, M., Johnston, M., Abraham, C., Francis, J., Hardeman, W., et al. (2013). The behavior change technique taxonomy (v1) of 93 hierarchically clustered techniques: Building an international consensus for the reporting of behavior change interventions. *Annals of Behavioral Medicine, 46*(1), 81–95.

Middleton, K. R., Anton, S. D., & Perri, M. G. (2013). Long-term adherence to health behavior change. *American Journal of Lifestyle Medicine, 7*(6), 395–404.

Miller, W. R., & Rollnick, S. (1991). *Motivational interviewing: Preparing people to change addictive behavior*. New York: Guilford Press.

Mogre, V., Stevens, F. C. J., Aryee, P. A., Amalba, A., & Scherpbier, A. J. J. A. (2018). Why nutrition education is inadequate in the medical curriculum: A qualitative study of students' perspectives on barriers and strategies. *BMC Medical Education, 18*(1), 26, 26-018-1130-5.

Mura Paroche, M., Caton, S. J., Vereijken, C. M. J. L., Weenen, H., & Houston-Price, C. (2017). How Infants and young children learn about food: A systematic review. *Frontiers in Psychology, 8*, 1046.

Norman, P., Abraham, C., & Conner, M. (2000). *Understanding and changing health behaviour: From health beliefs to self-regulation*. Amsterdam: Harwood Academic Publishers.

Ortega-Anta, R. M., Jiménez-Ortega, A. I., Perea-Sánchez, J. M. Navia, & Lombán, B. (2014). Nutritional imbalances in the average Spanish diet; barriers to improvement. *Nutricion Hospitalaria, 30*(Suppl. 2), 29-35-35.

Poelman, M. P., Dijkstra, S. C., Sponselee, H., Kamphuis, C. B. M., Battjes-Fries, M. C. E., Gillebaart, M., et al. (2018). Towards the measurement of food literacy with respect to healthy eating: The development and validation of the self perceived food literacy scale among an adult sample in the Netherlands. *International Journal of Behavioral Nutrition and Physical Activity, 15*(1), 54, 54-018-0687-z.

Prochaska, J., & DiClemente, C. (1982). Transactional therapy: Toward a more integrative model of change. *Psychotherapy: Theory, Research & Practice, 19*(3), 276–288.

Rankin, A., Bunting, B. P., Poinhos, R., van der Lans, I. A., Fischer, A. R., Kuznesof, S., et al. (2018). Food choice motives, attitude towards and intention to adopt personalised nutrition. *Public Health Nutrition, 21*(14), 2606–2616.

Requejo, A., Ortega, R., Aparicio, A., & López-Sobaler, A. (2007). *El Rombo de la Alimentación*. Madrid: Departamento de Nutrición, Facultad de Farmacia, Universidad Complutense de Madrid.

Rogers, C. R. (1942). The use of electrically recorded interviews in improving psychotherapeutic techniques. *American Journal of Orthopsychiatry, 12*(3), 429–434.

Rollo, S., Gaston, A., & Prapavessis, H. (2016). Cognitive and motivational factors associated with sedentary behavior: A systematic review. *AIMS Public Health, 3*(4), 956–984.

Saeidi, A., Mirzaei, A., Mahaki, B., Jalali, A., & Jalilian, M. (2018). Physical activity stage of change and its related factors in secondary school students of Sarableh City: A perspective from Iran. *Open Access Macedonian Journal of Medical Sciences, 6*(8), 1517–1521.

Schulze, M. B., Martinez-Gonzalez, M. A., Fung, T. T., Lichtenstein, A. H., & Forouhi, N. G. (2018). Food based dietary patterns and chronic disease prevention. *BMJ, 361*, k2396.

Schwarzer, R., & Renner, B. (2000). Social–cognitive predictors of health behavior: Action self-efficacy and coping self-efficacy. *Health Psychology, 19*(5), 487–495.

Sedentary Behaviour Research Network. (2012). Letter to the editor: Standardized use of the terms "sedentary" and "sedentary behaviours". *Applied Physiology, Nutrition and Metabolism, 37*(3), 540–542.

Stewart-Knox, B., Rankin, A., Kuznesof, S., Poinhos, R., Vaz de Almeida, M. D., Fischer, A., et al. (2015). Promoting healthy dietary behaviour through personalised nutrition: Technology push or technology pull? *Proceedings of Nutrition Society, 74*(2), 171–176.

Strolla, L. O., Gans, K. M., & Risica, P. M. (2006). Using qualitative and quantitative formative research to develop tailored nutrition intervention materials for a diverse low-income audience. *Health Education Research, 21*(4), 465–476.

Tennant, D. R., Davidson, J., & Day, A. J. (2014). Phytonutrient intakes in relation to European fruit and vegetable consumption patterns observed in different food surveys. *British Journal of Nutrition, 112*(7), 1214–1225.

Thomson, C. A., & Ravia, J. (2011). A systematic review of behavioral interventions to promote intake of fruit and vegetables. *Journal of the American Dietetic Association, 111*(10), 1523–1535.

Truman, E., Lane, D., & Elliott, C. (2017). Defining food literacy: A scoping review. *Appetite, 116*, 365–371.

Vaitkeviciute, R., Ball, L. E., & Harris, N. (2015). The relationship between food literacy and dietary intake in adolescents: A systematic review. *Public Health Nutrition, 18*(4), 649–658.

van Osch, L., Beenackers, M., Reubsaet, A., Lechner, L., Candel, M., & de Vries, H. (2009). Action planning as predictor of health protective and health risk behavior: An investigation of fruit and snack consumption. *International Journal of Behavioral Nutrition and Physical Activity, 6*, 69, 69-5868-6-69.

Verloigne M, Loyen A, Van Hecke L, Lakerveld J, Hendriksen I, De Bourdheaudhuij I, et al. (2016). Variation in population levels of sedentary time in European children and adolescents according to cross-European studies: A systematic literature review within DEDIPAC. *Internationa Journal of Behavioral Nutrition and Physical Activity, 13*:69, 69-016-0395-5.

Whitehead, F. E. (1973). Nutrition education research 1. In G. H. Bourne (Ed.), *World review of nutrition and dietetics* (pp. 91–149). Basel: Karger.

Williams, E. P., Mesidor, M., Winters, K., Dubbert, P. M., & Wyatt, S. B. (2015). Overweight and obesity: Prevalence, consequences, and causes of a growing public health problem. *Current Obesity Reports, 4*(3), 363–370.

World Health Organization. (2010). *Global recommendations on physical activity for health*. Geneva: World Health Organization.

World Health Organization. (2014). Global status report on noncommunicable diseases 2014. Attaining the nine global noncommunicable diseases targets; a shared responsibility. Available from http://apps.who.int/medicinedocs/documents/s21756en/s21756en.pdf.

Writing Group of the Nutrition Care Process/Standardized Language Committee. (2008a). Nutrition care process and model part I: The 2008 update. *Journal of the American Dietetic Association, 108*(7), 1113–1117.

Writing Group of the Nutrition Care Process/Standardized Language Committee. (2008b). Nutrition care process part II: Using the International Dietetics and Nutrition Terminology to document the nutrition care process. *Journal of the American Dietetic Association, 108*(8), 1287–1293.

Yang, S. H., Chung, H. K., & Lee, S. M. (2016). Effects of activity-based personalized nutrition education on dietary behaviors and blood parameters in middle-aged and older type 2 diabetes Korean outpatients. *Clinical Nutrition Research, 5*(4), 237–248.

Zoellner, J., You, W., Connell, C., Smith-Ray, R. L., Allen, K., Tucker, K. L., et al. (2011). Health literacy is associated with healthy eating index scores and sugar-sweetened beverage intake: Findings from the rural Lower Mississippi Delta. *Journal of the American Dietetic Association, 111*(7), 1012–1020.

CHAPTER 12

Personalized Expert Recommendation Systems for Optimized Nutrition

Chih-Han Chen and Christofer Toumazou
IEEE, Imperial College London, London, United Kingdom

OUTLINE

Introduction	309	Conclusion and Outlook	335
Nutrients and Genes Correlation Data	311	Acknowledgment	336
Scalable Food Categorization	313	References	336
Personalized Recommendation System	327	Further Reading	338
Framework Personalized Expert Recommendation System for Optimized Nutrition	334		

INTRODUCTION

Deoxyribonucleic acid (DNA) is known to be the key to unlocking the understanding of the functioning, reproduction, and development of all living organisms. In order to improve the knowledge of such an important molecule, scientists spare no effort in studying, experimenting, and sharing their discovery through publications. On the other hand, the DNA test service has emerged on the market, providing consumers access to their DNA patterns. However, due to the high complexity and large volume of information, the knowledge of the field is rarely applied in our daily life. Aiming to apply the knowledge of genetic innovation to the market, our research focuses on developing an expert system that can provide optimized food decisions to consumers.

Expert systems have been expected as a solution for better production quality and diet choices in the food industry since 1998 (Linko, 1998). Together with the advancement of "big data" technology, systems that can cope with high variety, volume, and velocity are bringing success to business (McAfee, Brynjolfsson, Davenport, Patil, & Barton, 2012), science, and health care (Hansen, Miron-Shatz, Lau, & Paton, 2014). A recommendation system aiming to scale with big data through MapReduce has led to the birth of many applications, such as product recommendation (Linden, Smith, & York, 2003), music recommendation, and health recommendation (Huang et al., 2015). In this project, a system is proposed combining existing algorithms to construct a practical application for grocery product recommendation. The included algorithms cover the task of data categorization, data analysis, and decision recommendation. A deep neural network (DNN) model is applied to deal with data categorization due to its outstanding performance regarding the complexity of data with noise. Furthermore, a novel model is invented to cover data analysis, while decision recommendation is optimized with a genetic algorithm (GA).

The scalability of the models within all systems requires the ability to deal with unknown data (Adomavicius & Tuzhilin, 2005), which is typically measured through model generalization. In the area of health care, the introduction of deep learning analysis, or particularly DNNs is believed to be the reason why recommendation expert systems have improved over recent years (Huang et al., 2015). Neural networks aiming to simulate neuron behavior started from utilizing existing devices with the development of programming frameworks, before evolving into circuit implementation. Technology companies such as Microsoft and Google have published their open source research tools with the ability to commendably satisfy the simulation of neural networks on CPUs or GPUs. They allow researchers to focus more on designing network structures and applications (Seide, 2017). Due to the needs of higher accuracy and better performances while solving problems occurring during scaling with neuron sizes, the research on neural network systems has expanded to FPGA programming and is expected to be fully implemented in circuits down to the device level (Schneider, 2017). Some recent research publications have shown such interest in expansion, including memristor-based neural networks solving finite time synchronization problems or neural-type networks finite time stability problems (Chen, Li, Peng, Yang, & Li, 2017; Zheng et al., 2017).

From the application perspective, personalized health care and diets have gained great attention with the rise of nutrigenetics studies. It is believed that all molecules involved in the human metabolism are controlled directly or indirectly by genes and therefore the health of individuals can be optimized through personalized dietary advice (Hyman, 2006; Phillips, 2013). Direct-to-consumer (DTC) genetic services have emerged (Bloss, Schork, & Topol, 2011) with the invention of cost-effective genetic detection tests (Toumazou et al., 2013), which have led to the high expectations of relevant applications. Some surveys show that up to 50% of subjects are willing to receive genetic tests and follow the personalized suggestions (Cherkas, Harris, Levinson, Spector, & Prainsack, 2010). However, most of the services provide complicated information to the consumers and lead to the gap between the personal genetic information and the adherence to a personalized diet. In order to provide meaningful and straightforward solutions, a novel expert system is proposed in this project, which aims to personalize grocery shopping through product suggestions based on genetic phenotype. Other research work on systems for dietary decisions and the personalization of health advisories can be found in some recent publications. For example, a system that also targets providing decision support for food (Anselma, Mazzei, & De Michieli, 2017). However, instead of using genetics as input, they focus on the temporal decision for diets through optimizing reasoning. Another similar topic is the so-called medical education system, which provides personalized suggestions through individual characteristics and health objectives (Quinn, Bond, & Nugent, 2017). In our work, we focus on the temporal decision of comparison between a grocery product and all other products within the same food category. Furthermore, we aim to perform personalization through correlating the nutrition facts of grocery products and generating recommendations. The system is built based with the aim of processing two datasets: the genetic data and the grocery data. The genetic data relate to phenotypes influencing the consumption ability of the five main nutrition factors, which are energy, fat, protein, sugar, and salt. They are used to perform simulations of all possible combinations. The genetic data collection of any customer is static and assumed to remain the same over time. On the other hand, the grocery data is designed to be dynamic and varies with continuous data collection.

In our project, in order to correlate the two datasets and generate recommendations, a framework covering the process of data collection, data categorization with DNN, and the grocery product recommendation generation is proposed. The proposed expert recommendation system framework consists of four main components:

1. A word embedding and padding model is introduced for converting text data into generalized vectors to deal with data variety, unknown grocery product names, and mitigate the out-of-vocabulary problem.
2. A DNN model for product categorization is covered to cope with the complex features and sequence logics of the grocery product vectors. The selected model can perform categorization tasks with good accuracy.
3. A decision recommendation model is designed to take the categorization results, analyze nutritional data, and optimize the suggestion provided to the consumer with the designed fitness score and GA.
4. An operational state machine is included with the aim to control the state and retrain models of each component during updates of training data.

In this chapter, the correlation between nutrients and genes is described, prior to discussing the problem of data categorization and introducing the word embedding method, as well as various modeling and experiment results. Thereafter, solving the product recommendation problem through building a recommendation model is denoted. The recommendation model involves grocery shopping decisions that consider behavior, personal phenotype data, and nutrient value based on different food categories. Finally, the framework of personalized expert recommendation system for optimized nutrition (PERSON) is covered with a detailed description of the state machine. The contribution of this project includes the novel architecture of the PERSON based on genetic phenotype, the utilization of a DNN for grocery product categorization, and the implementation of a recommendation system using a GA.

NUTRIENTS AND GENES CORRELATION DATA

In recent years, nutrition research has moved their research focus from epidemiology and physiology to nutrigenetic molecular studies. This is caused by recent improvements in the understanding of interactions between nutrition, cellular, organ, tissue, and body homeostasis. To study how genetic variation affects the response to nutrients, the field of nutrigenetics is growing along with increasing interest in personalized health and diets. Nutrigenetics aims to apply the information of genetics to the optimization of a person's health (Fenech et al., 2011; Kohlmeier, 2012).

Observation of the variation of DNA between individuals is the basis for distinguishing the differences and the need for personalization in nutritional advice. The most common way of observing the variation is to study single nucleotide polymorphisms (SNPs), which are the differences in the DNA sequence between different humans of the four genome patterns, adenine (A), thymine (T), cytosine (C), or guanine (G). SNPs are known to influence how a person absorbs and metabolizes nutrients and are frequently used to find evidence to confirm the assumptions which form the basis of nutrigenetic sciences (Daniel & Klein, 2013; Fenech et al., 2011).

Scientists experiment on humans in order to correlate the candidate genes and nutritional aspects. An indication of the correlation is usually concluded as positive or negative based on the own collected evidence (Mariman, 2006). The candidate genes are usually selected by the study of bioinformatics, where statistical analysis is applied to find risky genes. Apart from the genome, nutrigenetic analysis also considers the proteome, metabolome, and transcriptome (Fenech et al., 2011).

The concept of nutrigenetics can be traced back to the 1980s, when companies first commercialized the ideas in their products. Ten years later, the Human Genome Project sequenced the whole DNA sequence of the human genome, which opened up a new area of studies (Neeha & Kinth, 2013). This new area allows the possibility of more detailed investigations, finding and defining the use of vitamins and minerals, which in turn can be expanded to aid the prevention of diseases such as obesity and type-2 diabetes (Ghoshal, Pasham, Odom, Furr, & McGrane, 2003; Raj, Sundaram, Paul, Deepa, & Kumar, 2007).

To further confirm the interests and potential markets in the real world, trials are conducted. As an example, a research team randomly separated participants into intervention groups and control groups. The intervention groups received genotype-based personalized dietary advice and the control groups received general dietary advice. The end result of this trial was that the genetic-based advice was considered to be very useful and accepted by both genders aged between 20 and 35 (Nielsen & El-Sohemy, 2012). Another example is a trial that focused on the impact of consumer behavior in dietary and DTC genetic testing, which concludes the interests positively (Bloss et al., 2011).

In order to practically link genetics to nutrition or nutritional related diseases, the first step is to look at the available data that help us to form useful linkage information. The key information that is derived from genetics is called genotype data, while phenotype data is used to link to nutrition. Phenotype refers to the observable characteristic of an organism in biology, which follows the expression of genetic code, the genotype, and environmental factors (Churchill, 1974). Environmental factors are defined differently based on various practical situations but usually are directly correlated with genotypes. For instance, an environmental factor can be defined as individual sugar intake frequency when our genotype is focusing on sugar metabolism. Such a relationship was first proposed by Wohelm in 1911 (Johannsen, 2014), and extended later by many researchers

TABLE 12.1 An Example of the Genotypes of RS5400

Genotype	Magnitude	Summary
(C; C)	0.1	Normal sugar consumption
(C; T)	1.7	Significantly higher sugar consumption
(T; T)	1.8	Significantly higher sugar consumption

(Angers, Castonguay, & Massicotte, 2010). Summarizing the concept proposed by most research, the general relationship is expressed as Eq. (12.1):

$$G + E + GE \approx P \qquad (12.1)$$

where G represents the genotype, P represents the phenotypes, E represents the environment factor, and GE represents the interaction between G and E.

Genotype data can be downloaded from SNPedia with corresponding papers sourced from Pubmed, which contains continuously updated new research results and publications (Chen, Karvela, Sohbati, Shinawatra, & Toumazou, 2018). An example of the genotypes of rs5400 from SNPedia is shown in Table 12.1. The genotype rs5400 is a gene location with three different expressions regarding three different levels of sugar consumption.

In our project, the designed mapping of the gene–nutrient relationship is described in the section of this chapter titled "Personalized Recommendation System", where the mapping is represented as a matrix and used as the basis for nutritional recommendations.

The recommendation of nutrition is done through an action of suggesting different food products. With different suggestions, the aim is to increase the probability of a customer choosing a product that is nutritionally better for him/her based on the genetic test result G. This is only practical and meaningful if the comparison of the products is done within the same category of food (Chen et al., 2018). For example, we do not want to compare a bar of chocolate to an apple, instead we want to compare chocolate to other similar sweets. Hence, the categorization of food product data is very important to this project.

SCALABLE FOOD CATEGORIZATION

Considering food data, a method has been proposed to categorize food data based on their names. The whole procedure has the following steps: accessing food data from web, the generalization of the representation of the food name from text to numeric form, and training the machine learning classifier to perform categorization.

In the first step, the aim is to access all available data on the internet. This is challenging due to the fact that structured data regarding food products are kept within providers' databases. However, most of the information is available on the World Wide Web in an encoded and unstructured format and can be accessed by almost anyone. In order to analyze and make use of this information, downloading and extracting it using information extraction (IE) is an essential step.

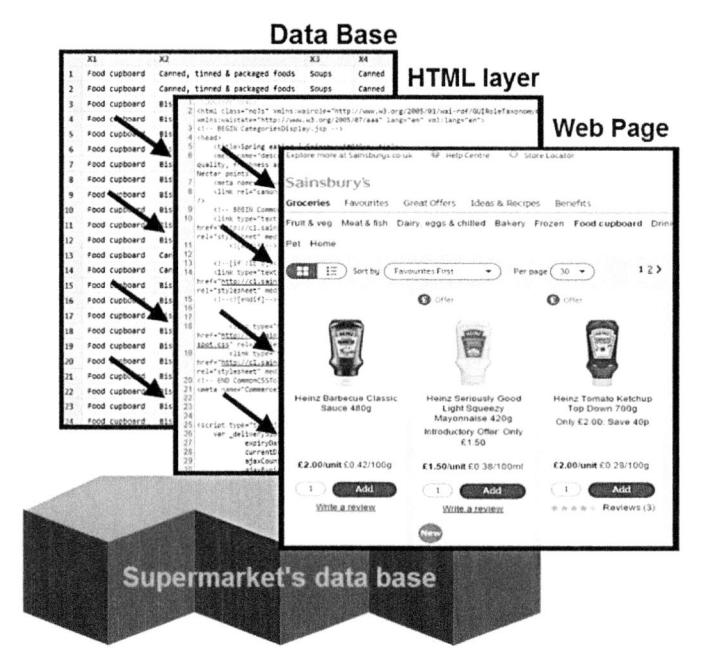

FIGURE 12.1 An example of a grocery database server.

A web page is a document that can be accessed using a web browser on the World Wide Web. Information about this document is presented on a monitor based on the source code, which is usually written in HTML, PHP, and JavaScript for the purpose of coordinating with the web resources and database elements, such as tables, images, interactive functions, etc., see Fig. 12.1.

A database normally contains a huge amount of information about different products. When a new web browser is opened, it retrieves the source code of the web page from the web server by request using Hypertext Transfer Protocol (HTTP). Then the web browser converts the source code (HTML layer) into a nice presentable web page, which links all the tables, images, and information with layouts and functions.

A procedure implementating data collection is called a wrapper. The data collection wrapper design is a highly active research area in the field of the Semantic Web, which can be found in many research papers.

A wrapper is a program for data extraction, which can be classified into three types (Liu & Agarwal, 2005):

1. A manual approach requires a programmer, supervising the program to find the data extraction patterns by observing the web page and the source code;
2. Wrapper induction is an approach that is semiautomatic and it requires manual labeling, training templates, or extraction rules to apply machine learning technique; and
3. Automatic extraction is an unsupervised approach without manual labeling being involved, which can scale up the coverage of sites for data extraction.

With a designed wrapper, there are two main types of data that can be extracted (Liu & Agarwal, 2005; Su, Wang, Lochovsky, & Liu, 2012):

1. A group of data that is described in a similar format, HTML tags, and rendered in a contiguous region;
2. A list of data presented in subtrees and under the same parent node with similar repetition of HTML tag structures.

For example, a method called IEPAD discovers repetitive patterns by matching HTML tag strings and creating a tree structure of the extracted data (Chang & Lui, 2001). In order to reduce computation and improve accuracy of the extracted data, an approach called DEPTA was proposed considering not just the source code but also visual information with an alignment technique (Chang & Lui, 2001; Zhai & Liu, 2006).

A good example of automatic extraction was proposed in 2015, which was implemented in a architecture containing four main steps (Chu, Hsu, Lee, & Tsai, 2015):

1. It transforms a web page into a document object model (DOM) tree structure, a cross-platform, and language-independent convention for presenting HTML.
2. Data path matching (DPM) is used to identify the similarity of structure of the subtrees within the DOM structure. This method takes the place of the conventional complex tree distance measure algorithms to discover the similarity of the codes of the data path.
3. After the similar subtrees are found, the unimportant data will be deleted and the observation of overlapping is done followed by the merge of the section.
4. Path-code-string alignment technique is introduced to align corresponding data items, which transform records into HTML tag strings and measure their minimum distance between characters.

Inspired by the above four steps procedures, the data collection procedure is designed specifically for food product data sets. This procedure contains five main steps. First, the HTML document should be received from the web server. Second, the document should be syntactically parsed and converted into meaningful texts based on HTML tags or stop signs of sentences written in natural language. After identifying HTML tags and their functions within text strings, the third step converts HTML objects into a tree model, where each subtree consist of texts from the start to the end HTML tags. Then texts within each subtree are compared and grouped in terms of their sentence structures and similarity of words, while key entities such as the name of a food company or a product are recorded. The group with the most key entities is identified as the most important section. Finally, texts from the most important section are extracted and key information such as names of the products, image links, and nutrition tables are recorded. Since the fact that different products are presented in the same format on the supermarket website, extraction rules for products are manually designed and extraction procedures are executed smoothly with high accuracy.

Once a data table with uniform resource identifiers (URI) of each product's details and images is generated, a nutritional table can be extracted and images can be downloaded from its provider. Fig. 12.2 presents such a procedure. Collected data are stored in a local SQL database and each data point is assigned with a unique ID relating to the name, image, and nutritional table of its corresponding product.

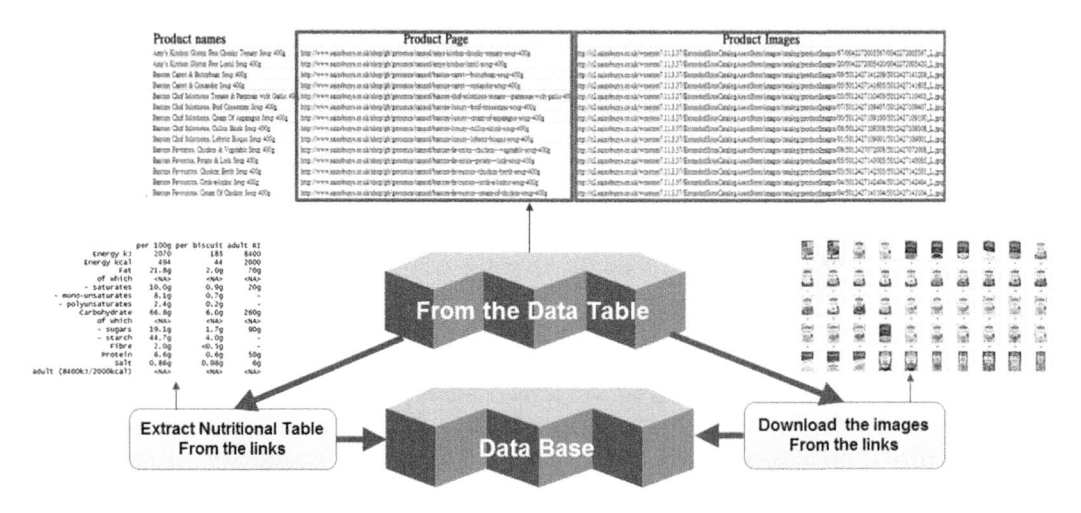

FIGURE 12.2 Data collection with the extracted uniform resource identifiers table.

After the names, image, and nutritional data are extracted, data curation takes place, which involves identification, transformation, and normalization. The nutritional table is treated as the input of this stage, in which the identification of the nutritional factors, measurement method, and units are processed. In the identification block, there are three main objectives. The first is to identify the nutritional factor, which can later be treated as the target of transformation. The second is to identify the measurement method, which helps to understand the format of transformation for later execution. The third is to identify the units, which helps in preparing the step of normalization. The nutritional tables of different products are transformed based on the nutritional factor and method of measurement into a collection table. Furthermore, units are normalized for the ease of later numerical analysis.

With the downloaded names of food products and with the aim of training models that are capable of recognizing the category, the name text is converted into numbers based on semantics with a technique called word embedding.

Word embedding represents words in distributed numerical vectors. It has been proven to perform better on word similarity tasks and word analogy/analysis tasks in deep learning studies (Mikolov, Sutskever, Chen, Corrado, & Dean, 2013). General methods such as bag-of-words models are insufficient on some basic tasks like classifying short texts (Sriram, Fuhry, Demir, Ferhatosmanoglu, & Demirbas, 2010), since they ignore orders and semantic relations between words. Word embedding with neural networks is a more advanced model because it preserves semantic types and syntactic relations. In addition, converting words into vectors with real numbers from one dimension per word to a continuous vector space guarantees the low dimensionality of vectors (Sriram et al., 2010). Vectors within the word embedding space have similar semantic relations (Mikolov et al., 2013), which allows the improvement on clustering tasks in natural language processing (NLP).

A common choice for generating word embedding is called the continuous skip-gram model, which consists of an input, a projection, and an output layer. The input layer takes in each current word and predicts a range of words located before and after the current word. Increasing the range of words improves the quality of word embedding but causes an expansion of computational load. In a case study, 100 billion words are taken from Google News to train our skip-gram word embedding model. The word embedding vector space has 300 dimensions and covers 3 million unique words (Sriram et al., 2010). In order to allow visualization, the word vector space is projected down to two dimensions using dimensionality reduction techniques such as t-distributed stochastic neighbor embedding (s-SNE) (Maaten & Hinton, 2008). Fig. 12.3 shows the visualization result. Entities with similar semantic types are clustered resulting in different regions for classification.

At this stage, the food data is extracted from the web and converted into numeric vectors. In the next section the categorization problem and the applied model for the solution will be described.

The problem that targeting objects classification, recognition, differentiation, and understanding is called categorization (Lefebvre & Cohen, 2005). To solve the problem of categorization, the objects are grouped into categories based on some purposes; this usually forms relationships of ideas or meanings of the categories and objects. The task of solving categorization problems plays an important role in computer science and can be found in many fields, such as natural language prediction, inference, decision processes, etc. (Frey, Gelhausen, & Saake, 2011).

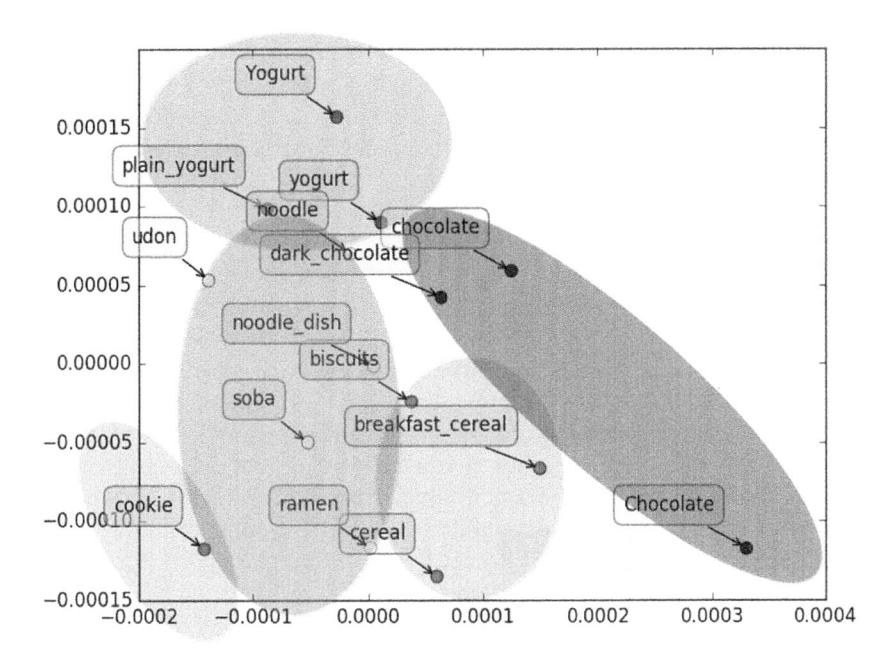

FIGURE 12.3 The two-dimensional plot of product name vector.

Machine learning is an important field in computer science that provides solution for the classification problem. It is essential to build a supervised model to solve the classification problem. The general procedure of building a supervised model begins with separating the available data into a training set and a testing set, and then setting a strategy to find the architecture of the model that performs the classification (Swain & Sarangi, 2013). The model will be trained through observing the training data set, making decisions, and receiving punishment if the decision is incorrect. In each observation the data set can be treated as a set of quantifiable properties, which are technically referred to as variables or features. Considering our project as an example, the food products' names are converted into vectors in space through word embedding, as shown previously in Fig. 12.3. The vectors contain multiple numbers that represent the values of axis in different dimensions. The space location that stores these numbers corresponds to the variables or features.

To build the model architecture, a strategy has to be defined through specifying a optimization procedure and a mathematical form of the problem. Once the model is found, it is treated as a classifier that compares observations by means of similarity. The strategy here uses what in the field of mathematics is called an algorithm, which also can be thought of as an implemented mathematical function that maps input data to a category (Cooke, 2011).

The ability of a classifier to adapt to the unknown future data is of most interest once the model is built and trained. This is done through examining the model with a testing data set. This property and the result depend highly on the characteristics and the representation of the data. The procedure of measuring this property is called evaluation. Measuring precision and recall are popular approaches, while simply performing an accuracy test is the most common way to evaluate a model (Rossi, Lipsey, & Freeman, 2003).

This experiment started with a relatively simple classifier called a linear predictor function. This type of classifier is frequently applied and can be adapted to a large number of algorithms for a categorization problem. The function can be expressed as shown in Eq. (12.2), where X_i is the value from instance i of the input feature vector and W_k is the weight to each k output category vector.

$$score(X_i, k) = W_k \cdot X_i \tag{12.2}$$

The $score(X_i,k)$ is the score for assigning input instance i to category k. The prediction is done by selecting the one with the highest score. An algorithm with this basic setup is referred to as a linear classifier. This type of classifier is known to work well with high dimensional vectors, and takes less time to train. This fits with our experiment since it has input product name vectors with 300 dimensions, a high dimensional vector problem (Yuan, Ho, & Lin, 2012). However, looking at the projected location of different food names in groups in Fig. 12.3, it is obvious that a linear classifier will have limited performance due to the shape of clusters and the nonlinearity within the dimensions of data.

To improve performance, we implemented a different classifier called a support vector machine (SVM) because of a trick called kernel function that can detect nonlinearity within dimensions of data. The SVM model represents data as points in space and targets the separation of data points through creating gaps between categories. When facing a new data point, it will predict the point category based on the side of the gap that the point location lands. When dealing with nonlinear classification, SVM can apply the kernel trick. The trick maps its input data into another dimensional feature space, and allows the algorithm to fit the model in the transformed feature space. Note that the transformed feature space is in higher dimensions, which increases the generalization error of the model.

To build a SVM model, one starts by setting up hyperplanes. The definition of any hyperplane is defined as a set of input X_i following Eq. (12.3) (Cortes & Vapnik, 1995).

$$W_k \cdot X_i - b = 0 \tag{12.3}$$

where the weight W_k is now treated as a normal vector to the hyperplane, X_i is the input data, and the bias b refers to the offset of the hyperplane. This hyperplane is an important basis for SVM to create a boundary that performs the classification task (Ben-Hur, Horn, Siegelmann, & Vapnik, 2001). There are two ways for an SVM to classify data, which are called the hard margin approach and the soft margin approach. The applied approach depends on whether the data is linearly separable or nonlinearly separable. For the case of linearly separable, the hard margin approach is applied, where parallel hyperplanes are set. The parameters such as weight W_k and bias b are tuned with the aim of maximizing the distance of the hyperplanes and still keeping the data on the correct side. As an example, Eq. (12.3) can be used to express a two-category-SVM as shown in Eqs. (12.4) and (12.5) (Boser et al., 1992, July).

$$W_k \cdot X_i - b = 1 \tag{12.4}$$

$$W_k \cdot X_i - b = -1 \tag{12.5}$$

For a two-category SVM, Eq. (12.4) is used to classify any data point for label 1 and Eq. (12.5) is used to classify any data point for label -1. For any tuning process of weight W_k and bias b, it is aimed to keep all data points with label $y_i = 1$ above the boundary defined by the hyperplane of Eq. (12.4) and all data points with label $y_i = -1$ below the boundary defined by the hyperplane of Eq. (12.5). See Eqs. (12.6) and (12.7).

$$W_k \cdot X_i - b \geq 1 \quad \text{for } y_i = 1 \tag{12.6}$$

$$W_k \cdot X_i - b \leq -1 \quad \text{for } y_i = -1 \tag{12.7}$$

Another objective of our tuning process is to maximize the distance of the two hyperplanes which can be expressed as the value of $\frac{2}{\|W_k\|}$. This also means the optimization process targets minimizing $\|W_k\|$, while keeping Eqs. (12.6) and (12.7) true. Note that during the process of optimization the max-margin hyperplane is tuned by input X_i which these inputs are referred as the support vectors.

For the case of nonlinearly separable data, the soft-margin approach is applied in the SVM. A common way of applying the soft-margin SVM is to introduce the hinge loss function as shown in function (12.8).

$$\max(0, \ 1 - y_i(W_k \cdot X_i - b)) \tag{12.8}$$

In Eq. (12.8), y_i is the target data label which takes note of feature input X_i data. In the setup of a two-category-SVM, the function of (12.8) is zero if the data X_i is located on the correct side of the margin and outputs a value when the data X_i is located on the incorrect side. The value for data X_i located on the wrong side is proportional to the distance from the defined margin.

With the introduction of the hinge loss function in function 8, the objective function can be set up with the aim of minimizing function (12.9).

$$\left[\frac{1}{n}\sum_{i=1}^{n}\max(0,\ 1-y_i(W_k \cdot X_i - b))\right] + \lambda\|W_k\|^2 \qquad (12.9)$$

where n is the total number of input data, and the parameter λ is used to determine the consideration of margin size. When the parameter λ is small, the soft-margin SVM will behave similarly to the hard-margin SVM.

In the above paragraphs, the linear classification of SVMs has been introduced. In order to improve the accuracy of nonlinear classification, the kernel trick is introduced (Aizerman, Braverman, Emmanuel, & Rozonoer, 1964). The kernel trick targets the data points projecting into another dimension with a projection kernel function $\phi(X_j)$ as shown in function (12.10).

$$k(X_i,\ X_j) = \phi(X_i) \cdot \phi(X_j) \qquad (12.10)$$

And the weight vector is transformed into function (12.11).

$$W_k = \sum_{i=1}^{n} c_i y_i \phi(X_i) \qquad (12.11)$$

With the functions (12.10) and (12.11), the objective function is set up to maximize function $\mathbf{f}(c_i)$ for $i = 1$ to n and is expressed in (12.12).

$$\mathbf{f}(c_1, c_2 \ldots c_n) = \sum_{i=1}^{n} c_i - \frac{1}{2}\sum_{i=1}^{n}\sum_{j=1}^{n} y_i c_i (\phi(X_i) \cdot \phi(X_j)) y_j c_j \qquad (12.12)$$

This is under the constraints of $\sum_{i=1}^{n} c_i y_i = 0$ and $0 \leq c_i \leq \frac{1}{2n\lambda}$. The coefficient c_i is obtained with the above objective functions and $\mathbf{b}$ is solved with Eq. (12.13).

$$b = W_k \cdot \phi(X_i) - y_i = \left[\sum_{k=1}^{n} c_k y_k \phi(X_k) \cdot \phi(X_i)\right] - y_i \qquad (12.13)$$

using the collected coefficients c_i and b. The model can be expressed to classify new points with function (12.14).

$$Classification = sgn(W_k \cdot \phi(X_i) - b) \qquad (12.14)$$

SVM works well with relatively small data sets; particularly because it considers the whole picture and generates global optimum solutions. However, when dealing with complex large data sets SVM has limited performance compared to DNNs particularly for the study of natural language such as text data processing (Jozefowicz et al., 2016; Sutskever, Vinyals, & Quoc, 2014).

In the experiment of this project, the extracted food data sets from the web are relatively large and contain text such as food names, which led us to extending our research into applying DNNs models.

DNNs are extensions of artificial neural networks, which are computing models taking the inspiration of biological neural networks in animal brains (Olshausen & Field, 1996). The artificial neurons are connected and free to transmit signals from one to another, while each neuron processes the signal that is received and sends the result to the output.

The artificial neural networks are formed by structures called artificial neurons. An artificial neuron has an internal state that is mathematically called the activation function and produces an output based on the activation function, input, and another element called the weights (McCulloch & Pitts, 1943). The weights are the key components for performing a process called learning, which tunes the values of weights according to the detection of error between the produced output and the target output (Amari, 1990; Zell, 1994).

Setting up a single neuron with label k input X_i, a weight vector W_k and a bias vector b_k see Eq. (12.15).

$$net_k = W_k \cdot X_i + b_k \tag{12.15}$$

This equation aims to mimic the behavior of a neuron receiving signal X_i and summarizes its current status value as net_k. The status value is sent through an activation function f and output signal $y_{i,k}$ as shown in Eq. (12.16).

$$y_k = f(net_k) \tag{12.16}$$

In the general learning rule, the action of learning is through modifying the weight vector W_k see Eq. (12.17).

$$W_k^{t+1} = W_k^t + \Delta W_k^t \tag{12.17}$$

Here t is the current time step and $t+1$ is the next time step, the weight of the next time step W_k^{t+1} is obtained through the sum of the weight of current time step W_k^t and the modification vector ΔW_k^t. This modification vector is derived from the learning signal e_k^t, which is a function of current weight W_k^t, current input X_k^t, and target vector T_k^t, see Eq. (12.18).

$$e_k^t = f(W_k^t, X_k^t, T_k^t) \tag{12.18}$$

In other words, this learning signal is measured based on how far away the output signal y_k^t is to target vector T_k^t, given W_k^t and X_k^t. Finally the ΔW_k^t is obtained with Eq. (12.19), where η is a defined learning rate.

$$\Delta W_k^t = \eta e_k^t X_k^t \tag{12.19}$$

When the learning signal is consistently low and the training is completed, Eqs. (12.15) and (12.16) are used to perform classification, see Eq. (12.20).

$$Classification = y_k = f(W_k \cdot X_i + b_k) \tag{12.20}$$

DNNs are artificial neural networks with multiple layers, which allows the expression of complex nonlinear relationships to be modeled (Aizerman et al., 1964). The more complicated the features of input data are, the more layers of DNN are required to be applied in our experiment in order to improve the accuracy for classification. However, variation of DNNs architectures can sometimes be a good alternative to simply scaling on layers.

DNNs have two widely used architectures: convolutional neural networks (CNNs) and recurrent neural networks (RNNs).

CNNs have many variations and are part of feed-forward neural networks that are frequently used for computer vision and NLP tasks (Collobert et al., 2011; Kalchbrenner, Grefenstette, & Blunsom, 2014; Kim, 2014). The basic form of CNN consists of one or more convolutional layers, a pooling operation, and fully connected layers (LeCun, Bottou, Bengio, & Haffner, 1998). To understand CNNs operation, we first use a single layer CNN model and scale the number of layers for experiments. A single layer CNN consists of a convolutional layer, a kernel function, a max pooling operation, and a fully connected layer, see Fig. 12.4.

Following the word embedding method introduced in the previous section, the food product names are converted into numerical vectors or word vectors $x_{i,j}$, where i represents the identification of the data we are looking at and j refers to word identification. For example, if we are looking at the word vector of "Milk" of "Milk Giant Chocolate" with the product id "5," the notation is presented as $x_{2,5}$. Note that for presenting a whole name of products we can simplify the notation with Eq. (12.21), where p is the number of words of a product.

$$X_i = x_{i,j} \quad for \quad j = 1, \ldots p \tag{12.21}$$

The kernel window takes a predefined number of inputs, which are multiplied by a set of weight W^{kernel} plus a kernel bias b_c, and shifted to a new location. After shifting to a new location, the window will take another set of inputs but multiply them with the same weight W^{kernel}. For example, setting up the predefined number of input words as 5, the kernel window as 2, and shift location length as 1, the kernel function can be expressed as Eq. (12.22), where $T = p - 1$.

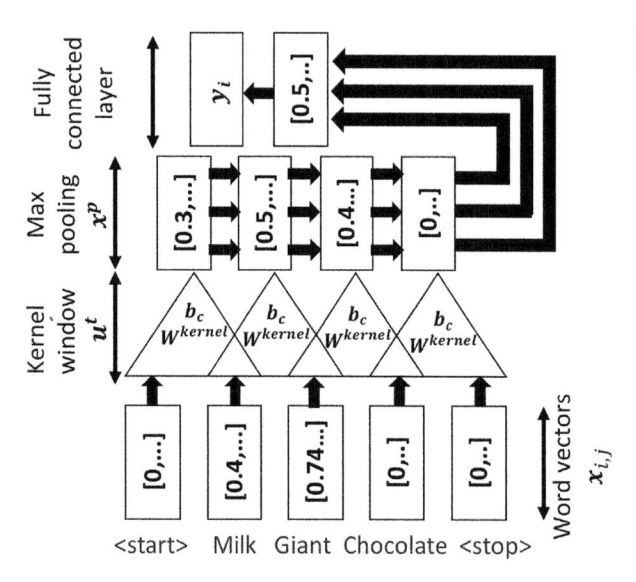

FIGURE 12.4 The architecture of the convolutional neural network model.

$$u^t = W^{kernel}X^t_{window} + b_c \quad \text{where} \quad t = 1, 2, \ldots T. \tag{12.22}$$

For the case of $t = 1$, see Eq. (12.23).

$$u^1 = W^{kernel}X^1_{window} + b_c = W^{kernel}_1 x_{<start>} + w^{kernel}_2 x_{milk} + b_c \tag{12.23}$$

For the case of $t = 2$, see Eq. (12.24).

$$u^2 = W^{kernel}X^2_{window} + b_c = w^{kernel}_1 x_{milk} + w^{kernel}_2 x_{Giant} + b_c \tag{12.24}$$

The size of W^{kernel} can be scaled based on the defined size of the windows. The max pooling operation takes u^t as the input and executes element-wise max value selection, see Eq. (12.25).

$$x_p = \left[\max_{1 \leq t \leq T} u^t_1, \max_{1 \leq t \leq T} u^t_2, \ldots \max_{1 \leq t \leq T} u^t_p\right]^{Transpose} \tag{12.25}$$

This operation aims to take the maximum value of each element location of all output vectors of the previous stage. As an example, looking at the first element of each u^t as shown in Fig. 12.4, the value can be obtained with Eq. (12.26).

$$\max_{1 \leq t \leq T} u^t_1 = \max[0.3, 0.5, 0.4, 0] = 0.5 \tag{12.26}$$

Finally, the output y_i can be defined with Eq. (12.27).

$$y_i = f(W^{FullyConnected} x_p + b_f) \tag{12.27}$$

With a similar operation to simple artificial neural networks, the fully connected layer takes x_p as the input, multiplies it with a weight $W^{FullyConnected}$, summed with a bias b_f, and wraps it with an activation function f. The output y_i is a vector that is used to perform the classification for input x_i of the i-th product.

CNNs have excellent performance for extracting features from different positions and learning relationships between positions and features by max pooling (Tai, Socher, & Manning, 2015). However, they are not designed to handle sequence data or to capture long-term dependencies. Unlike CNNs, RNNs are specialized for sequential modeling, resulting in good performance in the learning of word dependencies (Sainath, Vinyals, Senior, & Sak, 2015). Due to the significant importance of word dependency of different products in our project, RNNs are applied for food product categorization.

Traditional RNNs have simple structures such as a single hyperbolic tangent layer, shown in Fig. 12.5A. For a standard RNN model with a long chain of repeating components, vanishing gradients for parameter updates is an important issue during the training process, which has been solved by the introduction of a long short-term memory recurrent neural network (LSTM-RNN) (Hochreiter & Schmidhuber, 1997). A memory subcell located at the center of the LSTM-RNN cell removes or adds information through designed gates, shown in Fig. 12.5B. Eqs. (12.28)–(12.33) describe the operation of a single LSTM cell.

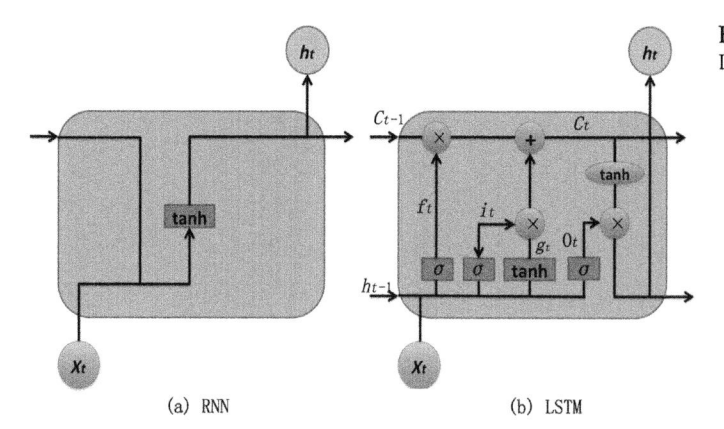

FIGURE 12.5 Basic RNN and LSTM structures.

$$f_t = \sigma(W_f[h_{t-1}, x_t] + b_f) \tag{12.28}$$

$$i_t = \sigma(W_i[h_{t-1}, x_t] + b_i) \tag{12.29}$$

$$o_t = \sigma(W_o[h_{t-1}, x_t] + b_o) \tag{12.30}$$

where x_t is the input vector to the LSTM-RNN cell at current time step t, and h_{t-1} is the vector from the previous hidden layer state. These two vectors are put together with a forget gate weight matrix W_f, an input gate weight matrix W_i, and an output gate weight matrix W_o. The weighted vectors are added up with the biases of the same gate types: $W_f[h_{t-1}, x_t]$ is summed with the forget gate bias b_f, $W_i[h_{t-1}, x_t]$ is summed with the input gate bias b_i, and $W_o[h_{t-1}, x_t]$ is summed with the output gate bias vector b_o. These summed results are inputs of sigmoid activation functions and form the outputs of three gates: forget gate output vector f_t, input gate output vector i_t, and output gate output vector o_t. In other words, each gate consisting of a sigmoid layer and a point-wise multiplication operator outputs a value between 0 and 1. The decision of whether to pass the information or not is decided by these output values.

$$g_t = \tanh(W_g[h_{t-1}, x_t] + b_g) \tag{12.31}$$

$$C_t = f_t \odot C_{t-1} + i_t \odot g_t \tag{12.32}$$

$$h_t = o_t \odot \tanh(C_t) \tag{12.33}$$

Eq. (12.31) describes the actual input information. Similar to Eqs. (12.28)–(12.30), h_{t-1} and x_t are put together with the input weight matrix W_g. Then the hyperbolic tangent activation function takes the sum of the weighted result and input bias b_g and generates the input stage g_t. In Eq. (12.32), the internal current state coefficient C_t is the sum of the forget gate output vector f_t multiplied by the previous state C_{t-1} and the input gate output vector i_t multiplied by the input state g_t. In Eq. (12.33), the hidden layer output state h_t is the result of the activation of C_t multiplied by the output gate vector o_t. The hidden layer output state h_t is the output of the LSTM-RNN cell and the recurrent input of the same cell in the next step.

LSTM can be used to learn complicated information such as capturing semantic dependencies in a sequence of words. The nature of product names is complex due to their various importance in different orders. For instance, dark chocolate is a type of chocolate with an additional information of dark, while chocolate biscuit is a type of biscuit with an additional information of chocolate. The word chocolate represents different types of information in different scenarios, indicating that different sequences cause words to play different roles.

A single layer LSTM-RNN already has deep architectures because it is a feed-forward neural network with a recurrent connection that loops multiple layers sharing the same parameters. However, single layer LSTM-RNN has limited features since input information is processed by a single nonlinear layer through multiple time instants before producing outputs. Deep LSTM-RNNs consist of multiple layers of LSTM. They have properties of processing information both through time and layers, where parameters are better used based on the distribution of meaning over spaces of multiple layers (Huang, Cao, & Dong, 2016; Sak, Senior, & Beaufays, 2014).

Fig. 12.6 shows the architecture of a deep LSTM (DLSTM) model for classifying product names. The input product name are converted into word vectors through word embedding and padded into the maximum length of all input data. At each time instance i, a word vector is fed into the DLSTM as the input x_i. LSTM cells output values to hidden layer h_j at each layer of the DLSTM, where j is the number of layers of LSTM-RNN. Finally, the last hidden layer is connected to a softmax layer described in Eq. (12.35), where u_g is the output of the fully connected layer before the softmax function, and G is the number of the prediction of the classification label.

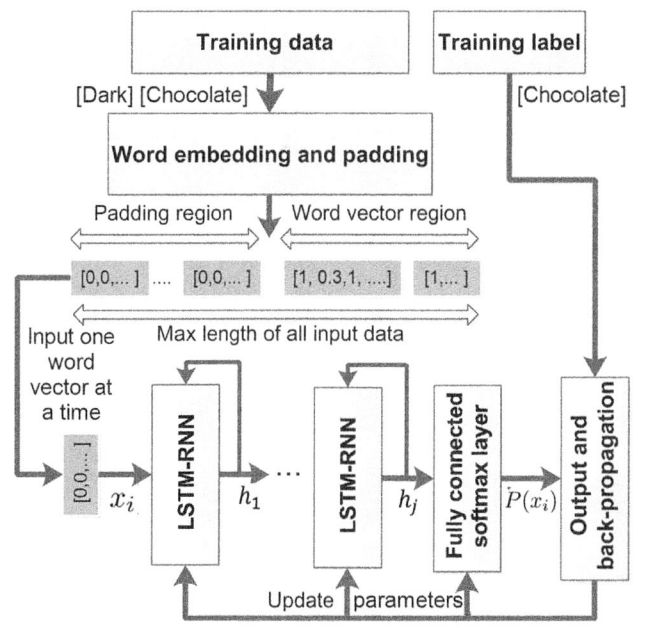

FIGURE 12.6 The architecture of the DLSTM model.

$$h_j \odot W_s = u_g \qquad (12.34)$$

$$P(x_i) = \frac{e^{u_g}}{\sum_{g=1}^{G} e^{u_g}} \qquad (12.35)$$

$$l = -\frac{1}{n}\sum_{i}^{N}\sum_{k}^{C} P_k^d(x_i)\log(P_k(x_i)) \qquad (12.36)$$

The LSTM model is trained with cross-entropy over the training data. In Eq. (12.36), l represents the loss vector, $P_k(x_i)$ is used to denote the distribution of the model prediction, and $P_k^d(x_i)$ is the distribution of the inputs. N is used to describe the total number of training data and C is the number of classification labels. The Adam method is used to achieve the stochastic optimization and update all parameters in each layer of DLSTM-RNN (Kingma & Ba, 2014).

In order to present the performance of the DLSTM-RNN model described in Fig. 12.6, it is incorporated into three databases for product name classification:

1. A consumer contributed database, Open Food Facts: it is a global package food database covering 135,891 products worldwide in February 2017 (Facts, 2016).
2. A government organized database provided by the United States Department of Agriculture (USDA): it is a Public and Private Partnered organized database, which aims to provide support to the development of consumer applications. It contained 184,022 US products in February 2017 (U. database, 2017).
3. A corporation created database from Tesco: Tesco is a British grocery retailer having branches in different countries as well.

Data from Tesco supermarket was gathered from both on-product labels and public Tesco supermarket websites. 23,518 food products of interests were collected in October 2016, including product names and nutrition facts tables (Grocery, 2016). The applied DLSTM model was tested with the three databases and used the best performing data sets to compare the introduced two architectures of DNNs.

Product names from the three datasets were used as the input of our DLSTM-RNN model. In order to compare the differences between databases and categories, only some of the common categories were chosen to participate in our experiments: cereals, biscuits, cookies, yogurts, chocolates, rice, noodle and pasta. Due to the complexity of common subgroups of the Open Food Facts dataset and Tesco dataset, categories were further grouped into cereals & biscuits & cookies, yogurts, chocolates, rice & noodle & pasta.

After removing some corrupted data, the actual number of products participating in our experiments were 942 from the Open Food Facts database, 9126 from the USDA database and 2012 from the Tesco database. Each product consists of a category tag, a name, and a nutrition facts table. Each database was separated randomly into 60% training data and 40% testing data. Random permutation cross-validation was used and the accuracy of product classification by the DLSTM-RNN model is shown in Table 12.2. It showed good improvement with more layers of LSTM-RNNs. The Tesco database obtained a high accuracy because of their organized sequence orders, which normally are brand names, flavors, and food names. Meanwhile most Open Food Facts data and USDA data follow random orders. Some data from the Open Food Facts database do not cover the full name of

TABLE 12.2 The Performance of DLSTM Models

	Open Food Facts	USDA	Tesco
1-Layer LSTM	41.8%	40.3%	81.2%
2-Layer LSTM	41.9%	45.2%	83.8%
3-Layer LSTM	42.1%	46.2%	84%

TABLE 12.3 Accuracy of DNN Structures Comparison

	LSTM	CNN
1-Layer	81.2%	72.2%
2-Layer	83.8%	72.8%
3-layer	84.0%	72.0%

products since they were created manually. Only a maximum of three layers of DLSTM-RNNs were undertaken in the experiment because the cross-validation method is time-consuming for deep learning models.

Both CNNs and LSTM-RNNs are popular architectures of DNNs. We compared the performance of these two models based on the Tesco data set with 60% training data and 40% testing data. The results are shown in Table 12.3, and show that LSTM-RNN outperforms CNNs. The reason is that CNNs are not able to capture the semantic dependencies of word sequences. Multiple layers of CNNs cannot improve the accuracy.

PERSONALIZED RECOMMENDATION SYSTEM

A recommendation system predicts or optimizes the decisions of a user. This field comes under the study of information filtering systems which look into the methods of removing unwanted information using automated or semiautomated approaches before presentation to an application or a user. The main goal of the field is to manage information overload and increase the ratio of semantic signal-to-noise.

Another perspective of the idea of filtering is the aim of helping people to dedicate their time and find the most valuable information. Nowadays with our limited time, decisions are made to read, listen, and view nonoptimally, which leave noninteresting, nonvaluable, or even false information to fill our surroundings. This situation means there is an increased importance of filters in systems and the applications of decisions, such as in search engines on the internet. These filters are designed as a key component in systems to organize and structure information that results in correct and understandable information.

It is important to find the criteria before setting up a recommendation system. To do this, first the available knowledge about the target information is gathered. This knowledge is used to derive some concepts that allow for a better understanding of the task of information filtering. In the case of product filtering, it is aimed at reducing or eliminating nutritionally and genetically worse product decisions. Generally the content of a learning system consists of providing solutions to a defined set of tasks, the ability to undergo assessment of criteria that measure performance to the solutions of the target problem, and outputting the knowledge which is used by the system to determine even better solutions. These general concepts about filtering may not find a globally best solution towards optimizing a recommendation system through filtering information but usually find a locally optimal solution. However, they provide a good reference for designing systems that learn in their use cases. The automation of such processes is frequently discussed in the fields of statistics, data mining, pattern recognition, and machine learning.

The design process of the system of a personalized recommendation system covers a comparison of the input profile information about users and the options of decisions, where the reference characteristics of both decisions and user profiles are observed through building a model. The model is trained through an optimization process which involves choosing a target and an algorithm. In this section, the recommendation process is covered with a description of the model and a selected algorithm, called the GA.

After categorizing the food products and storing their nutritional information, the next step is to design a personalized recommendation system to give recommendations of products based on users' genotypes. In order to achieve this, a threshold matrix is introduced which is used to link genes and food nutritional data. The values within the threshold matrix are decided based on phenotypic information corresponding to genotypic information—which is the users' DNA.

For demo purposes, each personal data point is expressed as a nutrition threshold matrix $T_{(l,n)}$, which maps to a different genetic phenotype for metabolism. Following Eq. (12.1), three ability levels are considered for phenotypes: good, medium, and bad. To simplify our equation, a direct mapping $G \approx P$ is considered. In order to actually connect this relation with grocery data, the threshold table $T_{(l,n)}$ is used to represent the strength of abilities to consume different nutrients. In a real-world environment, G is actually the outcome pattern of a person's genetic test, and the corresponding P has a direct one to one mapping to $T_{(l,n)}$. Table 12.4 shows such a relation between P and $T_{(l,n)}$. In the case of considering an environmental factor, adding **E** and **GE** into the matrix is simply creating more threshold types to extend Table 12.4.

TABLE 12.4 Direct Mapping of P to $T_{(l,n)}$ of a Grocery Category

	n = Energy	n = Fat	n = Salt	n = Sugar	n = Protein
l = **Good**	$P_{Good,Energy}$ → $T_{High,Energy}$	$P_{Good,Fat}$ → $T_{High,Fat}$	$P_{Good,Salt}$ → $T_{High,Salt}$	$P_{Good,Suagr}$ → $T_{High,Sugar}$	$P_{Good,Protein}$ → $T_{High,Protein}$
l = **Medium**	$P_{Medium,Energy}$ → $T_{Medium,Energy}$	$P_{Medium,Fat}$ → $T_{Medium,Fat}$	$P_{Medium,Salt}$ → $T_{Medium,Salt}$	$P_{Medium,Sugar}$ → $T_{Medium,Sugar}$	$P_{Medium,Protein}$ → $T_{Medium,Protein}$
l = **Bad**	$P_{Bad,Energy}$ → $T_{Bad,Energy}$	$P_{Bad,Fat}$ → $T_{Bad,Fat}$	$P_{Bad,Salt}$ → $T_{Bad,Salt}$	$P_{Bad,Sugar}$ → $T_{Bad,Sugar}$	$P_{Bad,Protein}$ → $T_{Bad,Protein}$

In our experiment, $T_{(l,n)}$ is a matrix of variables, which update their values by optimizing the fitness score of the model with the GA. Our personalized nutrition recommendations can be directly linked to the value within $T_{(l,n)}$. These values within the matrix are treated as nutritional value boundaries, where n represents different nutrients, varying from 1 to **M**, and l is the level of boundary for each nutrient, varying from 1 to **L**. For demo purposes, five nutrients (**M** = 5) are considered and three levels (**L** = 3): energy, fat, salt, sugar, and protein; high, medium, and low threshold.

$T_{(l,n)}$ is the input of our decision model, where the GA is applied for optimizing recommendations. The designed decision model observes two different behaviors of food choices: one follow recommendations given by our model and the other makes random decisions. The GA is set to optimize grocery-shopping recommendation by maximizing the observation of improvements of nutrition consumptions before and after recommendations are given.

The model is built starting from the design of filtering functions, shown in Eq. (12.37). The input of the filter $p_n^{i_c}$ is the product nutrient value, where i_c is the product identity number of grocery category c, varying from 1 to the total number of products I_c in category c.

$$H_{l,n}^c(P_n^{i_c}) = \begin{cases} 1 & \text{if } p_n^{i_c} \leq T_{l,n}^c \\ 0 & \text{if } p_n^{i_c} > T_{l,n}^c \end{cases} \tag{12.37}$$

The filter function is designed to be low pass, meaning the filter outputs 1 when the threshold value $T_{l,n}^c$ is larger than the product nutritional value $P_n^{i_c}$, and outputs 0 when the opposite condition occurs (Chen et al., 2018).

Eq. (12.38) represents the decision process when suggesting a product. The output of a decision is either 1 or 0, which is the multiplication result of a series of outputs of filters. When a product passes through a sequence of filters, it receives a positive decision (1) when all the nutritional factors are lower than the assigned thresholds of a certain person and receives a negative decision (0) when they are not. Note that here **M** is 5 since there are five nutritional factors for the filters.

$$D_l(p_n^{i_c}) = \prod_{n=1}^{M} H_{l,n}^c(p_n^{i_c}) \tag{12.38}$$

After scanning through all the products, the total number of the suggested products s_l^c within a category c can be expressed as Eq. (12.39).

$$s_l^c = \sum_{i_c=1}^{I_c} D_l(p_n^{i_c}) \tag{12.39}$$

The average of the nutritional values of suggested products $a_1^{n,l}$ can be obtained by Eq. (12.40) and the average of all nutritional values of all products a_2^n can be obtained by Eq. (12.41).

$$a_1^{n,l} = \sum_{i_c=1}^{I_c} \frac{p_n^{l_c} \odot D(p_n^{l_c})}{s_l^c} \tag{12.40}$$

$$a_2^n = \sum_{i_c=1}^{I_c} \frac{p_n^{l_c}}{I_c} \qquad (12.41)$$

In order to achieve realistic results, a simple behavior model is introduced, based on the Gaussian function, shown in Eq. (12.42). This model can be used to simulate the probability of a person following the suggestion when he/she receives recommendations from our system. It is assumed that the maximum value of probability happens when half of the total products are recommended. The probability decreases when more than half of the total products are recommended because the customer might psychologically doubt that the system does not filter any products. Similarly, the probability also decreases when less than half of the total products are recommended because the customer might be frustrated at having fewer options. Some other assumptions of the behavior model can also be included to fit the real-world data based on future surveys.

$$Q_l^c = F\left(\frac{s_l^c}{I_c}\right) = 1 - 0.5 \times e^{-\frac{\left(\frac{s_l^c}{I_c} \times 0.5\right)^2}{4.6^2}} \qquad (12.42)$$

Finally, two scenarios are compared to demonstrate our improvements. The first scenario considers when consumers are given a recommendation, which is the sum of the total consumption of nutrients following and not following recommendations from our system. The former can be obtained through the multiplied results of the sum of probabilities of following the suggestion and the average nutrition value of suggested products. The latter can be obtained by the remaining probabilities multiplied by the average nutrition value of all products. The second scenario considers when consumers are not given any recommendation and have no preference of any products, and this is the average of the nutrition values of all products, shown in Eqs. (12.43) and (12.44).

$$v_1^{n,l} = a_1^{n,l} \times Q_l^c + a_2^n \times (1 - Q_l^c) \qquad (12.43)$$

$$v_2^n = a_2^n \qquad (12.44)$$

The difference between these two scenarios is the reduced consumption $r_{n,l}$ of nutrition n with the nutrition threshold boundary l, see Eqs. (12.45) and (12.46).

$$r_{n,l} = v_2^n - v_1^{n,l} \qquad (12.45)$$

$$r_n = \sum_{l=1}^{L} \frac{r_{n,l}}{L} \qquad (12.46)$$

In order to consider all nutrients, for $n = 1,2,...,5$, or in other words, energy, fat, salt, sugar, and protein, the fitness score f is defined based on the sum of the normalized form of reduced consumption of nutrition z_n, see Eqs. (12.47) and (12.48).

$$Z_n = \frac{r_n}{a_2^n} \qquad (12.47)$$

$$f = \sum_{n=1}^{M} Z_n \qquad (12.48)$$

The introduction of our designed model is completed, in the following paragraphs the background of the GA and how it is applied to optimize the introduced model will be briefly described. The introduced product recommendation model introduced previously aims to maximize the fitness score f with a given input threshold matrix $T_{(l,n)}$. Since the nutrients of products within each categories varied randomly, uncertainty becomes quite significant when choosing the algorithm for our model optimization. The idea of stochastics can be used to describe our problem; this targets the problem of tuning high dimensional random variables, which involves setting up objective functions, constraints, optimization methods, and iteration (Adler & Taylor, 2009; Spall, 2003).

A GA is a type of evolutionary algorithm inspired by the process of natural selection, which is often used for stochastic optimization. It makes use of bioinspired operations such as mutation, crossover, and selection (Mitchell, Crutchfield, & Das, 1996). Starting from a set of population solutions, the algorithm aims to optimize them by changing their properties. Their properties are encoded as actual numbers representing various expressions of genes (Whitley & Yoo, 1995).

The process of optimization in GA is called evolution. This process first generates individuals randomly and then iterates individuals' gene patterns during bioinspired operations. Each iteration generates a set of populations called a new generation. During iteration, the fitnesses of individuals are evaluated by the fitness scores, which are derived from predefined functions. Stochastic selections of fit individuals are chosen to proceed into the next iteration and generate a new generation (Whitley & Yoo, 1995). The algorithm requires a few parameters to be set up before execution:

1. Population size (P) is the total number of individuals to survive in each generation.
2. String length (L) is the length of genes of each individuals.
3. Probability of crossover (P_c) is the main control of the frequency that the bioinspired crossover operation take place.
4. Probability of mutation (P_m) is the main control of the frequency that the bioinspired mutation operation is executed.
5. Fitness function (f) is the function to measure the fitness of individuals.
6. Termination criteria (T) is used to define when the algorithm ends.

After setting up the above parameters, GA follows the procedure shown in Fig. 12.7. The first generation is defined randomly using parameters P and L. Then the first generation is evaluated by the fitness function f. During the process of selection, individuals with higher fitness scores are treated as parent populations, providing genes to generate new individuals using bioinspired operations such as crossover and mutation with probabilities P_c and P_m. Next both parents and new individuals are sent back to the evaluation process while some individuals are removed. The number of removed individuals is equal to the total population minus the predefined parameter P (Whitley & Yoo, 1995).

In our project, the fitness score f is designed as a measurement for the difference between nutritional intake average after receiving recommendations, which is the objective

FIGURE 12.7 GA procedure.

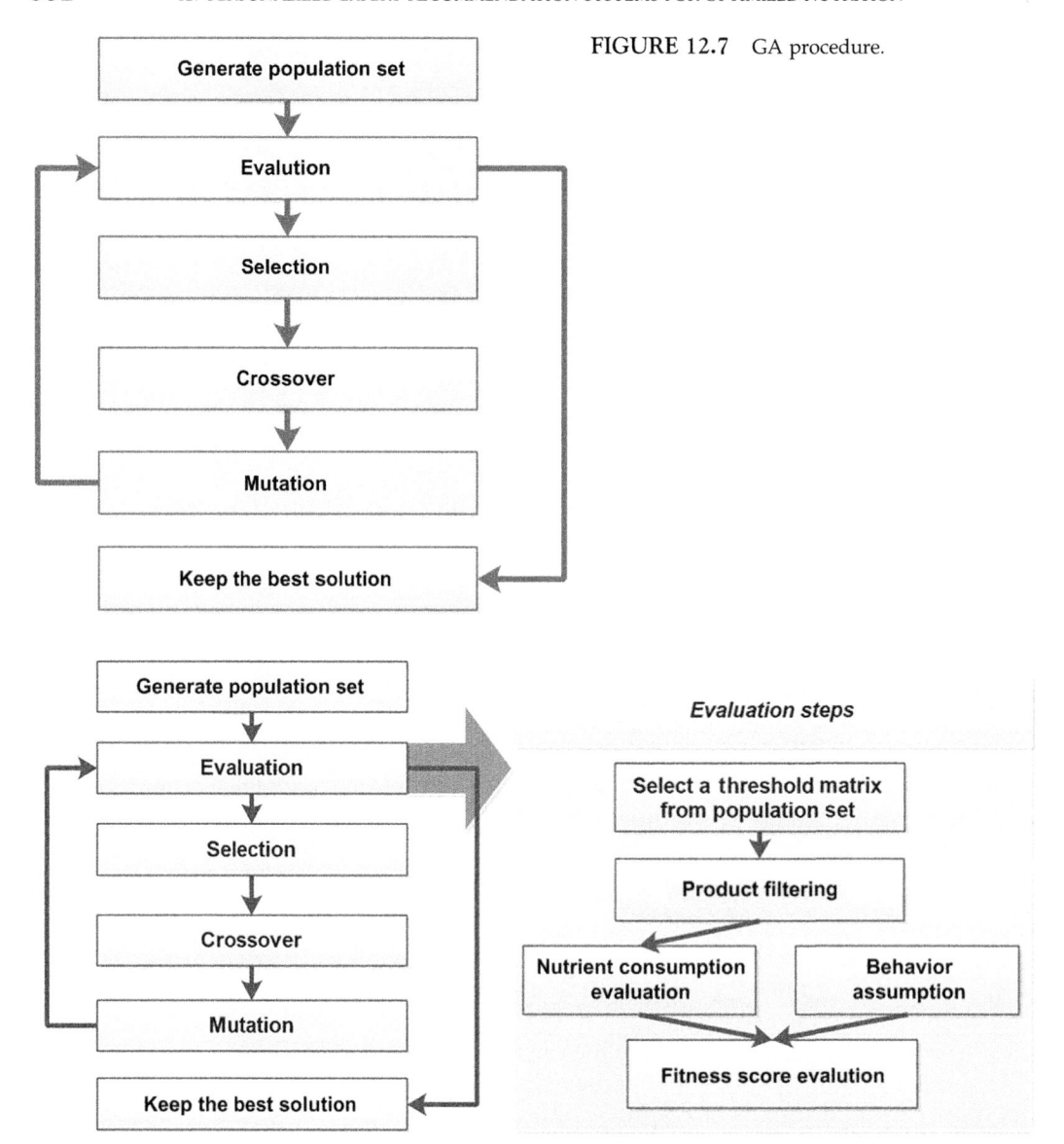

FIGURE 12.8 The procedure of recommendation optimization with GA.

for optimization. GA is applied because of its prominent performance in stochastic optimization. GA is set up with the input variable $T^C_{l,n}$ of grocery category C under the constraint that $T^C_{1,n} > T^C_{2,n} > T^C_{3,n}$ or in other words $T^C_{High,n} > T^C_{Medium,n} > T^C_{Low,n}$.

Fig. 12.8 shows the procedure of recommendation optimization of our model with GA. While generating the population, random sets of threshold matrices are initialized. Then they are fed into the evaluation step one by one, where the recommendation model follows Eqs. (12.37)–(12.48). This process is shown on the right side of Fig. 12.8. The

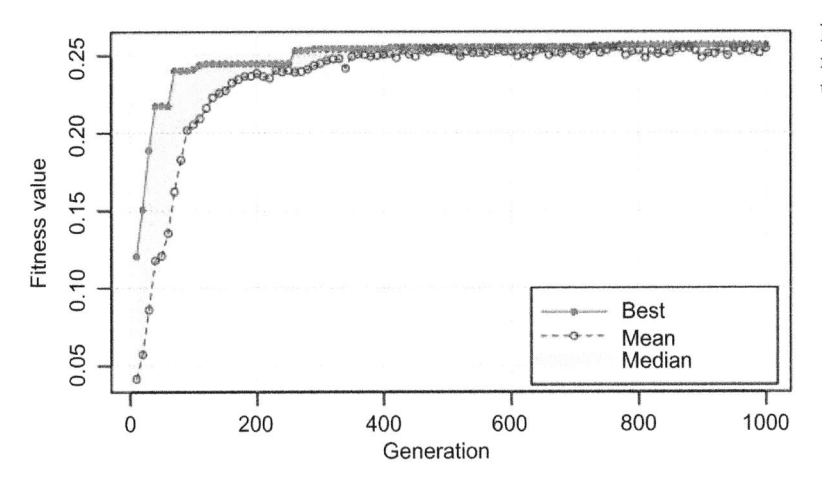

FIGURE 12.9 The optimization of fitness score using the genetic algorithm.

evaluation steps consist of selecting a sample threshold matrix from population sets, product filtering with Eqs. (12.37)–(12.38), nutrient consumption evaluation following Eqs. (12.39)–(12.41), and fitness score evaluation with the behavior assumption described in Eqs. (12.42)–(12.48). After evaluating the fitness scores of all threshold matrices in the population sets, these scores are compared and threshold matrices with the higher scores are selected. Those nonselected matrices are removed. Then random pairs of selected threshold matrices are formed and the parameters of randomly selected locations are swapped during the crossover procedure. Next, some locations of selected matrices are modified with a low probability during the mutation procedure. Finally, the new population sets of threshold matrices are sent back to the evaluation step for the next iteration (Chen et al., 2018).

In our experiment, the categorized food product data is fed to the decision recommendation models, and the GA has been set up to maximize the fitness score with 1000 iterations of the databases introduced in "Scalable Food Categorization" section.

Fig. 12.9 shows the optimization of the fitness score where the value is saturated at iteration 410 and the maximum fitness score stays at 0.2568. It is assumed that the decision of product consumption has the same weight: 100 g. The improvement is measured through how much less of a nutrient is consumed, comparing the scenario of a decision made with the personalized suggestion and without. It is found that the reductions of nutrition intake do not show a significant difference between the three databases introduced in "Scalable Food Categorization" section, however the values between the different categories are comparable.

In Table 12.5, the improvement for each nutrient from the different categories is the average of the experiment outcome based on the three databases. The category rice & noodle and pasta has a much higher reduction for energy intake, while fat, sugar, and protein show a lower reduction, since most of the products have either a low value or zero value of these nutrients. The category chocolate produces a greater improvement for salt, while the category biscuits & cereal and cookie provides a greater improvement for fat. The possible key nutrition that causes differences in diets can be presented through the relatively greater improvement described above.

TABLE 12.5 Average Reduction of Consumption in Result of Following the Expert System Recommendation

Per 100 g of the Product	Biscuit & Cereal and Cookie	Chocolate	Yogurt	Rice & Noodle and Pasta
Energy	61.2 kJ	68 kJ	63 kJ	200 kJ
Fat	3.5 g	1.64 g	1.58 g	0.38 g
Sugar	5 g	5.6 g	5.82 g	0.3 g
Salt	0.101 g	0.29 g	0.07 g	0.1 g
Protein	1.12 g	1.16 g	1.18 g	0.5 g

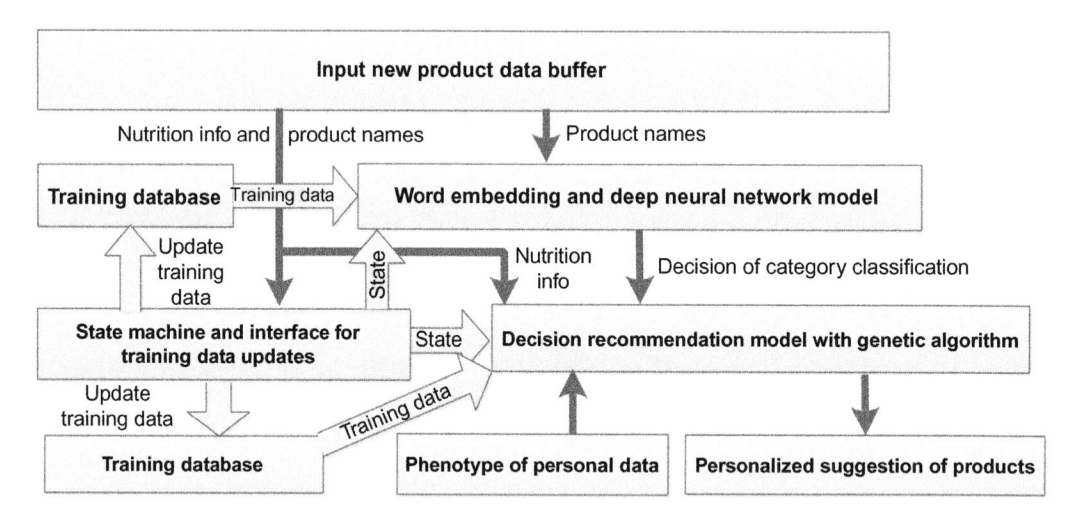

FIGURE 12.10 The architecture of the personalized expert recommendation system for optimized nutrition (PERSON).

FRAMEWORK PERSONALIZED EXPERT RECOMMENDATION SYSTEM FOR OPTIMIZED NUTRITION

In the previous sections, the models for scalable data categorization and personalized recommendations are introduced. In this section the operation, framework structure, and their interaction are described. The top level block diagram of the system is shown in Fig. 12.10. The whole system operates in two states: training state and recommendation provider state. Each block operates individually as:

1. Input new product data buffer: the top of the figure shows the input data buffer, which temporally stores the new product information.
2. State machine and interface for training data updates: the block receives new product information including the nutrition fact tables and the product names. The training data is selected and updated with the operation of human experts through an interface.

The state machine switches to training state during the training updates and sends the state signal to all other blocks.
3. Training database: the block receives updates from the state machine block and stores the updated data based on expert-decided categories.
4. Word embedding and DNN model block: the block is controlled by the state machine. It receives data from the training database during the state of training and performs category classification to the new product names with the DLSTM model when the state is switched to the recommendation provider.
5. Decision recommendation model: this block also operates based on the state signal, which receives training data and sets up the nutrition threshold matrix using the GA introduced in "Personalized Recommendation System" section.

In the state of recommendation provider, the decision recommendation model provides a personalized suggestion of products based on the phenotype of the personal data, the category classification outcome of the DNN model and the corresponding nutrition facts information. The output is a list of filtered products based on a set of threshold $T_{l,n}$ that maps to the phenotype $P_{l,n}$.

During operations for application, lists of grocery products are constantly updated to the system through the input of new product data buffers. Then the products will be categorized into groups by the word embedding and DNN model block. Product filtering and recommendation processes are carried out in the decision recommendation model block. Each consumer can receive their personalized product recommendation list through uploading their phenotype/genotype dataset from the decision recommendation model. Note that the word embedding and DNN model block and the decision recommendation model can be retrained to fit the new grocery data with a higher accuracy of categorization through switching the state and manually giving labels to the new product data.

CONCLUSION AND OUTLOOK

A potential architecture of a personalized expert recommendation system for optimized nutrition (PERSON) with the direct recommendation of products based on individual genes is proposed in this chapter. The general concept of machine learning for the categorization problem is discussed in "Scalable Food Categorization" section, while DLSTM is applied as our grocery product categorization model, and its performance is compared with that of CNNs. In "Personalized Recommendation System" section, the model for product suggestion is introduced, how our problem relates to stochastic problems is discussed, and a brief concept of the GA is introduced. With the optimized model, the categorized grocery products are compared to their own group and recommended to the consumer with different filters based on the individual's genetic phenotype. It is demonstrated that the interpretation of genetic data can be simplified through the application of nudging daily decisions such as grocery shopping.

The contribution of this project includes a novel architecture of the expert system, utilization of DLSTM for the first time on grocery product categorization, and the implementation of a new recommendation system with the GA. Further work such as improving the categorization accuracy can be done through the generalized word embedding on grocery related articles and modification of the introduced DNN model. Furthermore, a big data framework, the consideration of ingredients, and the correlation of genetics to nutrients data are potentially to be covered in future research.

Acknowledgment

This project is supported by DNAnudge Ltd and is under supervision of Prof. Christofer Toumazou at Imperial College London. I also would like to thank Dr. Maria Karvela, Dr. Mohammadreza Sohbati and Dr. Thaksin Shinawatra for the help and inspiration.

References

Adler, R. J., & Taylor, J. E. (2009). *Random fields and geometry.* Springer Science & Business Media.

Adomavicius, G., & Tuzhilin, A. (2005). Toward the next generation of recommender systems: A survey of the state-of-the-art and possible extensions. *IEEE Transactions on Knowledge and Data Engineering, 17*(6), 734–749.

Aizerman, Mark A., Braverman., Emmanuel, M., & Rozonoer, Lev I. (1964). Theoretical foundations of the potential function method in pattern recognition learning. *Automation and Remote Control., 25*, 821–837.

Amari, S.-I. (1990). Mathematical foundations of neurocomputing. *Proceedings of the IEEE, 78*(9), 1443–1463.

Angers, B., Castonguay, E., & Massicotte, R. (2010). Environmentally induced phenotypes and DNA methylation: How to deal with unpredictable conditions until the next generation and after. *Molecular Ecology, 19*(7), 1283–1295.

Anselma, L., Mazzei, A., & De Michieli, F. (2017). An artificial intelligence framework for compensating transgressions and its application to diet management. *Journal of Biomedical Informatics, 68*, 58–70.

Ben-Hur, A., Horn, D., Siegelmann, H. T., & Vapnik, V. (2001). Support vector clustering. *Journal of Machine Learning Research, 2*(Dec), 125–137.

Bloss, C. S., Schork, N. J., & Topol, E. J. (2011). Effect of direct-to-consumer genomewide profiling to assess disease risk. *New England Journal of Medicine, 2011*(364), 524–534.

Boser, B. E., Guyon, I. M., & Vapnik, V. N. (1992). A training algorithm for optimal margin classifiers. *Proceedings of the fifth annual workshop on computational learning theory* (pp. 144–152). ACM.

Chang, C. H., & Lui, S. C. (2001). IEPAD: Information extraction based on pattern discovery. *Proceedings of the 10th international conference on World Wide Web* (pp. 681–688). ACM.

Chen, C., Li, L., Peng, H., Yang, Y., & Li, T. (2017). Finite-time synchronization of memristor-based neural networks with mixed delays. *Neurocomputing, 235*, 83–89.

Chen, C. H., Karvela, M., Sohbati, M., Shinawatra, T., & Toumazou, C. (2018). PERSON—Personalized Expert Recommendation System for Optimized Nutrition. *IEEE Transactions on Biomedical Circuits and Systems, 12*(1), 151–160.

Cherkas, L. F., Harris, J. M., Levinson, E., Spector, T. D., & Prainsack, B. (2010). A survey of UK public interest in Internet-based personal genome testing. *PLoS One, 5*(10), e13473.

Chu, Y. C., Hsu, C. C., Lee, C. J., & Tsai, Y. T. (2015). Automatic data extraction of websites using data path matching and alignment. *2015 Fifth international conference on digital information processing and communications (ICDIPC)* (pp. 60–64). IEEE.

Churchill, F. B. (1974). William Johannsen and the genotype concept. *Journal of the History of Biology, 7*(1), 5–30.

Collobert, R., Weston, J., Bottou, L., Karlen, M., Kavukcuoglu, K., & Kuksa, P. (2011). Natural language processing (almost) from scratch. *Journal of Machine Learning Research, 12*(August), 2493–2537.

Cooke, R. L. (2011). *The history of mathematics: A brief course.* John Wiley & Sons.

Cortes, C., & Vapnik, V. (1995). Support-vector networks. *Machine Learning, 20*(3), 273–297.

Daniel, H., & Klein, U. (2013). Nutrigenetik: Genetische varianz und effekte der ernährung. *Biofunktionalität der Lebensmittelinhaltsstoffe* (pp. 7–16). Berlin: Springer.

Facts O. F. (2016, October 10). *Open food facts website* [Online]. Available from <http://world.openfoodfacts.org/who-we-are>.

Fenech, M., El-Sohemy, A., Cahill, L., Ferguson, L. R., French, T. A. C., Tai, E. S., ... Buckley, M. (2011). Nutrigenetics and nutrigenomics: Viewpoints on the current status and applications in nutrition research and practice. *Journal of Nutrigenetics and Nutrigenomics*, 4(2), 69–89.

Frey, T., Gelhausen, M., & Saake, G. (2011). Categorization of concerns: A categorical program comprehension model. *Proceedings of the 3rd ACM SIGPLAN workshop on Evaluation and usability of programming languages and tools* (pp. 73–82). ACM.

Ghoshal, S., Pasham, S., Odom, D. P., Furr, H. C., & McGrane, M. M. (2003). Vitamin A depletion is associated with low phosphoenolpyruvate carboxykinase mRNA levels during late fetal development and at birth in mice. *The Journal of nutrition*, 133(7), 2131–2136.

Grocery, T. (2016, October 15). *Tesco groceries website* [Online]. Available from <http://www.tesco.com/groceries/>.

Hansen, M., Miron-Shatz, T., Lau, A., & Paton, C. (2014). Big data in science and healthcare: A review of recent literature and perspectives. *Yearbook of Medical Informatics*, 9(21), 26.

Hochreiter, S., & Schmidhuber, J. (1997). Long short-term memory. *Neural Computation*, 9(8), 1735–1780.

Huang, M., Cao, Y., & Dong, C. (2016). Modeling rich contexts for sentiment classification with lstm. Available from arXiv preprint. arXiv:1605.01478.

Huang, T., Lan, L., Fang, X., An, P., Min, J., & Wang, F. (2015). Promises and challenges of big data computing in health sciences. *Big Data Research*, 2(1), 2–11.

Hyman, M. (2006). *Ultrametabolism: The simple plan for automatic weight loss*. Simon and Schuster.

Johannsen, W. (2014). The genotype conception of heredity. *International Journal of Epidemiology*, 43(4), 989–1000.

Jozefowicz, R., et al. (2016). Exploring the limits of language modeling. Available from arXiv preprint. arXiv:1602.02410.

Kalchbrenner, N., Grefenstette, E., & Blunsom, P. (2014). A convolutional neural network for modelling sentences. Available from arXiv preprint. arXiv:1404.2188.

Kim, Y. (2014). Convolutional neural networks for sentence classification. Available from arXiv preprint. arXiv:1408.5882.

Kingma, D., & Ba, J. (2014). Adam: A method for stochastic optimization. In *Proceedings of the 3rd international conference for learning representations* (pp. 1–15).

Kohlmeier, M. (2012). *Nutrigenetics: Applying the science of personal nutrition*. Academic Press.

LeCun, Y., Bottou, L., Bengio, Y., & Haffner, P. (1998). Gradient-based learning applied to document recognition. *Proceedings of the IEEE*, 86(11), 2278–2324.

Lefebvre, C., & Cohen, H. (2005). *Handbook of categorization*. Elsevier.

Linden, G., Smith, B., & York, J. (2003). Amazon. com recommendations: Item-to-item collaborative filtering. *IEEE Internet Computing*, 7(1), 76–80.

Linko, S. (1998). Expert systems what can they do for the food industry? *Trends in Food Science & Technology*, 9(1), 3–12.

Liu, H., & Agarwal, N. (2005). *Blogosphere: Research issues, tools and applications* (Vol. 1, pp. 33–41). Computer Science and Engineering Arizona State University.

Maaten, L. V. D., & Hinton, G. (2008). Visualizing data using t-SNE. *Journal of Machine Learning Research*, 9(v), 2579–2605.

Mariman, E. (2006). Nutrigenomics and nutrigenetics: The 'omics' revolution in nutritional science. *Biotechnology and Applied Biochemistry*, 44(3), 119–128.

McAfee, A., Brynjolfsson, E., Davenport, T. H., Patil, D., & Barton, D. (2012). "Big data," The management revolution. *Harvard Business Review*, 90(10), 61–67.

McCulloch, W. S., & Pitts, W. (1943). A logical calculus of the ideas immanent in nervous activity. *The Bulletin of Mathematical Biophysics*, 5(4), 115–133.

Mikolov, T., Sutskever, I., Chen, K., Corrado, G. S., & Dean, J., 2013. Distributed representations of words and phrases and their compositionality. In *Advances in neural information processing systems* (pp. 3111–3119).

Mitchell, M., Crutchfield, J. P., & Das, R. (1996, May). Evolving cellular automata with genetic algorithms: A review of recent work. In *Proceedings of the first international conference on evolutionary computation and its applications (EvCA'96)* (Vol. 8).

Neeha, V. S., & Kinth, P. (2013). Nutrigenomics research: A review. *Journal of Food Science and Technology*, 50(3), 415–428.

Nielsen, D. E., & El-Sohemy, A. (2012). A randomized trial of genetic information for personalizednutrition. *Genes & Nutrition*, 7(4), 559.

Olshausen, B. A., & Field, D. J. (1996). Emergence of simple-cell receptive field properties by learning a sparse code for natural images. *Nature, 381*(6583), 607.

Phillips, C. M. (2013). Nutrigenetics and metabolic disease: Current status and implications for personalised nutrition. *Nutrients, 5*(1), 32–57.

Quinn, S., Bond, R., & Nugent, C. (2017). Ontological modelling and rulebased reasoning for the provision of personalized patient education. *Expert Systems, 34*(2), 1–27.

Raj, M., Sundaram, K. R., Paul, M., Deepa, A. S., & Kumar, R. K. (2007). Obesity in Indian children: Time trends and relationship with hypertension. *National Medical Journal of India, 20*(6), 288.

Rossi, P. H., Lipsey, M. W., & Freeman, H. E. (2003). *Evaluation: A systematic approach*. Sage Publications.

Sainath, T. N., Vinyals, O., Senior, A., & Sak, H. (2015). Convolutional, long short-term memory, fully connected deep neural networks. *2015 IEEE international conference on acoustics, speech and signal processing (ICASSP)* (pp. 4580–4584). IEEE.

Sak,, H., Senior, A. W., & Beaufays, F. (2014). *Long short-term memory recurrent neural network architectures for large scale acoustic modeling* (pp. 338–342). Interspeech.

Schneider, D. (2017). Deeper and cheaper machine learning [top tech 2017]. *IEEE Spectrum, 54*(1), 42–43.

Seide, J. (2017). Keynote: The computer science behind the microsoft cognitive toolkit: An open source large-scale deep learning toolkit for windows and linux. In *2017 IEEE/ACM international symposium on code generation and optimization (CGO)* (p. xi),. IEEE.

Spall, J. (2003). *Introduction to stochastic searchand optimization: Estimation, simulation and control.* (34, pp. 54–58). Wiley.

Sriram, B., Fuhry, D., Demir, E., Ferhatosmanoglu, H., & Demirbas, M. (2010). Short text classification in twitter to improve information filtering. *Proceedings of the 33rd international ACM SIGIR conference on Research and development in information retrieval* (pp. 841–842). ACM.

Su, W., Wang, J., Lochovsky, F. H., & Liu, Y. (2012). Combining tag and value similarity for data extraction and alignment. *IEEE Transactions on Knowledge and Data Engineering, 24*(7), 1186–1200.

Sutskever, I., Vinyals, O., & Le, Q. V. (2014). Sequence to sequence learning with neural networks. *Advances in Neural Information Processing Systems*.

Swain, S., & Sarangi, S. S. (2013). Study of various classification algorithms using data mining. *International Journal of Advanced Research, 2*(2), 110–114.

Tai, K. S., Socher, R., & Manning, C. D. (2015). Improved semantic representations from tree-structured long short-term memory networks. *Proceedings of the 53rd annual meeting of the Association for Computational Linguistics and the 7th international joint conference on natural language processing* (pp. 1556–1566). ACL.

Toumazou, C., Shepherd, L. M., Reed, S. C., Chen, G. I., Patel, A., Garner, D. M., ... Athanasiou, P. (2013). Simultaneous DNA amplification and detection using a ph-sensing semiconductor system. *Nature Methods, 10*(7), 641–646.

U. database. (2017, January 14). US department of agriculture, agricultural research service, nutrient data laboratory. USDA branded food products database [Online]. Available from http://ndb.nal.usda.gov.

Whitley, D., & Yoo, N. W. (1995). *Modeling simple genetic algorithms for permutation problems, . Foundations of genetic algorithms* (Vol. 3, pp. 163–184). Elsevier.

Yuan, G. X., Ho, C. H., & Lin, C. J. (2012). Recent advances of large-scale linear classification. *Proceedings of the IEEE, 100*(9), 2584–2603.

Zell, A. (1994). *Simulation Neuronaler Netze [Simulation of neural networks]* (in German) (Chapter 5.2, 1st ed.). Addison-Wesley, ISBN 3-89319-554-8.

Zhai, Y., & Liu, B. (2006). Structured data extraction from the web based on partial tree alignment. *IEEE Transactions on Knowledge and Data Engineering, 18*(12), 1614–1628.

Zheng, M., Li, L., Peng, H., Xiao, J., Yang, Y., & Zhao, H. (2017). Finitetime stability analysis for neutral-type neural networks with hybrid timevarying delays without using lyapunov method. *Neurocomputing, 238*, 67–75.

Further Reading

Bengio, Y. (2009). Learning deep architectures for AI. *Foundations and Trends in Machine Learning, 2*(1), 1–127.

Cariaso, M., & Lennon, G. (2011). SNPedia: A wiki supporting personal genome annotation, interpretation and analysis. *Nucleic Acids Research, 40*(D1), D1308–D1312.

Index

Note: Page numbers followed by "*f*" and "*t*" refer to figures and tables, respectively.

A

ACCE. *See* Analytical and Clinical Validity, Clinical Utility and Ethics (ACCE)
Accelerometer, 203
Activation function, 321
Active wireless sensors, 210
Activity trackers, 206–207
AD. *See* Alzheimer disease (AD)
Adenine (A), 312
Adequacy, 213
Adherence to nutritional intervention, 21–22
Adipose tissue, 283
Adiposity, 156
Adolescent nutrition, 172–174
Aerobic training, 157
African Population and Health Research Center (APHRC), 173–176
Agrigenomics, 12
AHEI-2010. *See* Alternate Healthy Eating Index 2010 (AHEI-2010)
AI. *See* Artificial intelligence (AI)
Air-displacement plethysmography (BodPod), 138
Algorithm, 318
Alibaba, 201
Allergens, 208, 211
Alternate Healthy Eating Index 2010 (AHEI-2010), 143
Alternate Mediterranean Diet (AMED), 143
Alzheimer disease (AD), 89–90
Amazon Prime Air, 200–201
AMED. *See* Alternate Mediterranean Diet (AMED)
American Dietetic Association, 265–266
American Society of Nutrition (ASN), 18
332-amino acid protein, 156–157
Amyloid beta (Aβ), 89–90
Analytical and Clinical Validity, Clinical Utility and Ethics (ACCE), 37
Analytical validity, 37
AncestryDNA, 203
Animal
  husbandry, 186
  models, 94
Anthropometric
  dynamics, 171
  indices, 139
Antioxidants, 93
APHRC. *See* African Population and Health Research Center (APHRC)
Apolipoproteins (APOs), 156
  ApoE, 71
Aquaculture, 186
AR. *See* Augmented reality (AR)
Artificial intelligence (AI), 196
  AI-based approach, 21–22
  engine, 212–213
Artificial neural networks, 321
Artificial neurons, 321
ASN. *See* American Society of Nutrition (ASN)
Assistive kitchens, 208
Associated comorbidities, 145–146
Attitude(s), 117, 292
  attitude–behavior relationship, 106–107
  attitudinal dimensions measurement of food-related cognitive dissonance, 120
  object-centered research conceptualization, 120
Augmented reality (AR), 201
Automated food preparation, 208
Automatic extraction, 314–315
Aβ. *See* Amyloid beta (Aβ)

B

B class vitamins, 86–87
Baby Friendly Community Initiative, 183–184
Bacteria(l)
  adaptation, 85
  cell-to-cell communication, 85
  in personalized nutrition
    dysbiosis of gut microbiota detrimental to general health, 88–95
    future perspectives, 95
    GI tract microbiome establishment, 82–88
Bacteroides, 84–85
  B. fragilis, 92
Bacteroidetes, 84–85
Bag-of-words models, 316
Balanced diet, 153
BANs. *See* Body area networks (BANs)
Bariatric surgery, 158
Behavior(al)
  change strategies, 294–295
    action plan for dietary, 294–295
    environmental support to achieving, 295
    motivation to change, 294
  in personalized nutrition, 13–16
  strategies, 149–150

INDEX

Belief disconfirmation paradigm, 121–122
Beverages, 142–143
BG. *See* Blood glucose (BG)
BIA. *See* Bioelectrical impedance analysis (BIA)
Bifidobacterium, 63, 85
Big data, 19–22, 309–310
Bimuno, 92–93
Bioaccessibility, 217–218
Bioactive compounds, 11
Bioelectrical impedance analysis (BIA), 204
Bioinformatics, 24
Biological
  plausibility, 44
  variability
    foodomics, 10–11
    genes, 7–9
    gut microbiota, 9–10
    "omics" repertoires and systems biology approaches, 11–13
Biomarkers, 11
Blood glucose (BG), 55
  monitors, 204
Bluetooth technology, 203
BMI. *See* Body mass index (BMI)
Body area networks (BANs), 204
Body mass index (BMI), 8, 138
Brain
  health, 89–90
  subgingival microbiome management by diet to brain protection, 93–94
Bread types, 66–67
Breastfeeding, 171, 179–182, 180f
  workplace support for, 188–189
Business model development, 24

C

C677T gene polymorphism, 8
Caffeine metabolism, 264
Carbohydrate, 55, 57
Cardiovascular diseases (CVD), 34, 40, 55–56, 138, 174–175
Causative variants, 46
CBT. *See* Cognitive behavioral therapy (CBT)
CDT. *See* Cognitive dissonance theory (CDT)
Centers for Disease Control and Prevention, 146, 148
Ceteris paribus, 118–120
CGM. *See* Continuous glucose monitoring (CGM)
Chewing style, 64–65
Children, 226
  feeding practices in urban poor settings, 179–182
  in LMICs, 187–189
  nutrition, 174
  nutritional status, 175–179
  personalized nutrition, 174–187
    interventions to addressing child undernutrition, 182–186
Cholesterol, 174–175
Circadian biological clock, 71
Classical Mendelian inheritance, 8
Clinical utility, 34–35, 37–39
  primary prevention in high-risk groups, 39–40
  randomized controlled trials, 39
  secondary prevention in subjects with pathology, 40–41
Closed-loop system, 66
Clostridium, 63
  C. butyricum, 91–92
Cloud-based data systems, 203
Cloud-based personal health records (eHealth), 196–197
Cluster(ing), 21–22
  analysis, 6–7
  cluster-randomized controlled trial, 183–184
CNNs. *See* Convolutional neural networks (CNNs)
CNVs. *See* Copy number variants (CNVs)
Cognitive behavioral therapy (CBT), 158
Cognitive dissonance
  arousal, 121
  dietary recommendations and attitude–behavior relationship, 106–107
  FCD conceptual framework, 116–124
  locating in overall scheme of food and nutrition research, 124–127
Cognitive dissonance theory (CDT), 107
  and changing food attitudes/behaviors, 110–115, 111t
  in food and nutrition, 107–116
  and health/nutrition messages on food, 108–110
  need for unified CDT in food and nutrition, 115–116
Commensal
  bacteria, 88
  microbes, 81–82, 87
Commercial food-based complementary feeds, 185
Communication
  skills, 299
  strategies, 14, 292
Community-based intervention strategy, 183
Complementary feeding, 179–182, 184–186
Complexity, 17
Comprehensive lifestyle interventions, 149
Computer-tailored interventions, 150
Connected kitchen. *See* Smart kitchen
Connected medical devices, 204
Consumer
  from personalized nutrition, 266–270

consumer-perceived barriers to uptake, 266–269, 268t
  delivering, 269–270
 trust in personalized nutrition services, 15–16
Consumer acceptance of personalized nutrition, 230–241, 231t, 233t. *See also* Modern technologies for personalized nutrition
 areas, and applications, 226–227
 availability and reliability of information, 236–237
 in Central Europe, 245–250, 248t, 249t, 250f
 comprehensive models, 241–245, 242f, 244f
 consumer judgment, 228–230
 consumers' information processing, 239
 convenience function and time factor, 239
 costs, 240
 demographic factors, 237
 future, 250–253
 health conscious lifestyle, 238–239
 interrelationships between genes and nutrition, 237
 nature, 235–236
 nature of different foods, 240–241
 personally affected consumer, 238
 prevention of diseases, 238
 privacy risk, 232–235
Continuous glucose monitoring (CGM), 69, 207
Continuous skip-gram model, 317
Convenience function, 239
Convolutional neural networks (CNNs), 321–323, 322f, 327
Copy number variants (CNVs), 203
Core cognitive dissonance theory, 117–118
Cost-effective genetic detection tests, 310–311
Creative Commons Attribution License, 13–14
Credibility in nutrition, 299
Culturable bacterial-based dietary products, 82
CVD. *See* Cardiovascular diseases (CVD)
Cytosine (C), 312

D

DA. *See* Data assimilation (DA)
DASH. *See* Dietary Approach to Stop Hypertension (DASH)
Data assimilation (DA), 60
Data management software, 69
Data path matching (DPM), 315
Data Protection Act, 270
Decision recommendation model, 311, 335
Decision tree approach, 6–7
Deep LSTM model (DLSTM model), 325–326, 325f
 performance, 327t
Deep neural network model (DNN model), 309–310, 321–322
 model block, 335

 model for product categorization, 311
 structure accuracy comparison, 327t
Demographic factors, 237
Deoxyribonucleic acid (DNA), 309
 observation of variation with individuals, 312
Depression, 90–91, 142
Depressive mental health disorders, dysbiosis in, 90–91
DEPTA, 315
DEXA. *See* Dual X-ray absorptiometry (DEXA)
DHA. *See* Docosahexaenoic acid (DHA)
Diabetes mellitus (DM), 20–21, 58, 70, 150, 174–175
Diet(ary), 56, 71, 262–264
 action plan for dietary behavior change, 294–295
 adapting, 5
 advice, 153–157
 associated comorbidities, 145–146
 behavior change determinants, 290–292
  nutrition knowledge and food literacy, 290–291
  psychosocial influences as action and, 291–292
 diagnosis criteria, 138–139
 diet-responsive genetic variants, 263–264
 dietary factors, 142–143
 effects on human health, 9
 epidemiology, 139–141, 140f
 factors, 4, 142–143
  dietary patterns, 143
  factors associated with obesity, 144–145
  nutrients, foods, and beverages, 142–143
  sedentarism and physical activity, 144
  sleep habits, 144
 fiber, 92–93
 future approaches, 151
 genetic factors, 142
 guidelines, 280–283, 282f
  nutrition recommendations, 280
 habits, 21–22
 health promotion, 264–265
 IBS management by, 94
 interventions, 226
 levels of influence in dietary behavior, 293–294
 management systems, 198
 mental health management by, 94–95
 monitoring, 205–206
 plus phenotype, 263–264
 polyphenols, 12
 psychological factors, 142
 recommendations, 106–107
 requirements, 201
 subgingival microbiome management by, 93–94
Dietary Approach to Stop Hypertension (DASH), 143
Dietary behavior
 action plan for dietary behavior change, 294–295

Dietary behavior (*Continued*)
    determinants of dietary behavior change, 290–292
    levels of influence in, 293–294
Dietary reference intakes (DRIs), 280
Dietary reference values (DRVs), 263, 280
Dietitians, 271
Direct attributional reasoning, 109
Direct-to-consumer approach (DTC approach), 15, 227, 310–311
DLSTM model. *See* Deep LSTM model (DLSTM model)
DLSTM-RNN model, 326–327
DM. *See* Diabetes mellitus (DM)
DNA. *See* Deoxyribonucleic acid (DNA)
DNN model. *See* Deep neural network model (DNN model)
Docosahexaenoic acid (DHA), 47–48
Document object model (DOM), 315
Downstream processes, 11
DPM. *See* Data path matching (DPM)
DRIs. *See* Dietary reference intakes (DRIs)
Drug therapy, 158
DRVs. *See* Dietary reference values (DRVs)
DTC approach. *See* Direct-to-consumer approach (DTC approach)
Dual X-ray absorptiometry (DEXA), 138
Dysbiosis, 83–84
    in depressive mental health disorders, 90–91
    of gut microbiota detrimental to general health, 88–95
    in IBS, 88–89
    IBS management by diet, 94
    in mental health disorders, 91–92
    mental health management by diet, 94–95
    microbial intervention, 92
    oral biofilm dysbiosis and brain health, 89–90
    prebiotics, 92–93
    subgingival microbiome management by diet to protecting brain, 93–94
    symbiotic oral/gut biofilms for normal brain function, 90
Dysphagia, 208–209

E

E-commerce, 201
Eating behavior, 64–66
    e-coaching, 22
    meat-eating behavior, 124–125
eBay, 201
EBSCOhost, 59
Economic and social returns on investments, 186–187
Educators, 288–289
EEG. *See* Electroencephalography (EEG)
"Effect magnitude", 44

EFSA. *See* European Food Safety Authority (EFSA)
EGAPP. *See* Evaluation of Genomic Applications in Practice and Prevention (EGAPP)
eHealth, 202–203
    environment, 212
    records, 216
Electroencephalography (EEG), 206
Emotions, 22, 285
Energy, 172
    balance, 280–281
        balance-related behaviors, 144
    expenditure, 206–207
    homeostasis, 145–146
Environment(al)
    determinants, 283, 285–286
    factors, 147–149, 226, 312–313
    support to achieving behavior changes, 295
Environmentalism, 117
Enzyme lactase, 35–36
Epigenetics, 12, 265–266
Essential vitamins, 95
Ethnic diversity, 70
European Food Information Resource (EuroFIR), 213–215
European Food Safety Authority (EFSA), 43, 280
Evaluation, 318
    plan, 302
Evaluation of Genomic Applications in Practice and Prevention (EGAPP), 43
Evidence assessment
    framework for, 43–46
    in nutrigenetics, 36–37
Evolution, 331
Excess weight gain, 144–146
Exercise, 157, 206–207
Experience economy, 252
Expert system, 309–311

F

FADS.. *See* Fatty acids desaturase gene (*FADS*)
Fasting metabolic profile, 66–67
Fat mass and obesity-associated gene (FTO), 142
    polymorphisms, 157
Fatty acids desaturase gene (*FADS*), 9
FCD. *See* Food cognition dissonance (FCD)
FCQ. *See* Food Choice Questionnaire (FCQ)
Fermentable oligo-, di-, monosaccharides, and polyols diet (FODMAP diet), 94
FFQs. *See* Food Frequency Questionnaires (FFQs)
Fiber content, 57
Filter function, 329
FINGEN study, 16–17
Firmicutes, 87–88

Fitbit, 206–207
FN3KRP gene. *See* Fructosamine 3 kinase-related protein gene (*FN3KRP* gene)
FODMAP diet. *See* Fermentable oligo-, di-, monosaccharides, and polyols diet (FODMAP diet)
Food and Drug Administration, 171
Food choice, 283–288, 284f
  environment determinants, 285–286
  individual determinants, 283–285
  levels of influence in, 293–294
  mass media and food advertising, 287–288
  socioeconomics determinants, 286–287
Food Choice Questionnaire (FCQ), 266
Food cognition dissonance (FCD), 116–124, 119f
  in public health and nutrition research, 121–124
  in research, 120–121
Food Frequency Questionnaires (FFQs), 23–24
Food Standards Agency (FSA), 36–37
Food-based dietary guidelines, 280–281, 281f
Food-related cognition, 117
  cognitive discrepancy, 116–117
  cognitive dissonance, 127
Food-related dissonance, 116–117
Food4Me
  pan-European study, 5–7, 14, 24
  project, 262–263, 265–266, 267f
  qualitative research, 267–268
FoodCASE, 213–215
Foodomics, 10–11
Foods, 142–143, 279
  acceptance, 284
  acquisition, 200–202
  advertising, 287–288
  CDT in, 107–116
  components, 218
  composition, 209–211
    allergens and undesirables, 211
    intelligent packaging, 209–210
    labeling, 209
    sensing and analysis, 210
  consumption, 105–106, 285
  environments, 147
  explorer, 213–215
  food attitudes/behaviors, CDT and changing, 110–115, 111t
  food/nutrient availability, 154
  intake, 204–206
    direct approach, 205–206
    inferential approach, 205
  literacy, 290–291
  monitoring, 216
  nature, 240–241
  and nutrition research, 124–127
  preferences and aversions, 284
  preparation, 207–209
    assistive kitchens, 208
    automated food preparation, 208
    3-D printed food, 208–209
  selection, 201
  service and management of personalized nutrition, 211–212
  synergy, 218
Forkhead box P3 (Foxp3), 87–88
Fourth Industrial Revolution, 196
FPGA programming, 310
Fructosamine 3 kinase-related protein gene (*FN3KRP* gene), 9
FSA. *See* Food Standards Agency (FSA)
Functional food, 10–11
Functional immune system, 82
Fundamental trade-off in personalized nutrition, 232
Fusarium venenatum, 85–86

G

GA. *See* Genetic algorithm (GA)
Gamma-aminobutyric acid (GABA), 83
Gastrointestinal tract (GI tract), 81–82, 283
  microbiome establishment, 82–88
    bacteria adaptation, 85
    evolution shaped and protected continuity, 83–85
    probiotics, 85–86
  symbiotic microbiome
    for immune system, 87–88
    for micronutrients, 86–87
Gaussian function, 330
GE. *See* Grammatical evolution (GE)
Gene X diet interactions, 44–45
  scientific validity assessment of putative, 46–48, 48t
Gene-focused approach, 5
Gene–diet interaction, 38–39, 264
Genes, 7–9, 237, 265–266
  correlation data, 311–313
  factor, 226
Genetic
  factors, 138, 142
  polymorphisms, 7
  profiling, 228
  testing, 14–15, 70, 228–229
  variant/variation, 35–36, 42
    nature of, 45–46
    types, 46
Genetic algorithm (GA), 328–329, 331
  optimization of fitness score using, 333f
  recommendation optimization with, 332f
Genetic risk score (GRS), 7–8

344 INDEX

Genetic-based personalized nutrition, 237–238, 245–246
   consumer acceptance of, 241–245
Genome stability, 154
Genomics to systems biology, 7–13
Genotype, 70–72, 250–251
   data, 312–313
   genotype-based advice, 239
   genotypic-based personalized nutrition, 238
   of RS5400, 313t
Genotype-based dietary advice
   components of PN, 42–43
   evidence assessment in nutrigenetics, 36–37
   framework for evidence assessment, 43–46
   GNKN guidelines, 43
   guidelines to evaluating scientific validity for, 34–35
   nutrigenetics, 35–36, 41
   nutrigenomics, 35–36
   requirements to assessment, 37–38
   scientific validity assessment of putative gene X diet interaction, 46–48, 48t
   utility and randomized controlled trials, 38–41
   validating personal nutrition, 41–42
Geometric Framework for Nutrition (GFN), 22
Ghrelin, 144
GI tract. See Gastrointestinal tract (GI tract)
Global epidemiology of maternal malnutrition, 172
Global Nutrigenetics Knowledge Network (GNKN), 35, 43, 265–266
Global Observatory for eHealth (GOe), 203
Global positioning system (GPS), 203
Global values, 127
Glucose, 57
   glucose-specific cost function, 69
Glucose responses, 41–42, 57, 72–73
   methods for, 57–58
      fiber content, 57
      glycemic index, 57
      meal carbohydrate content, 57
      physical activity, 58
   results
      eating behavior, 64–66
      genotype, 70–72
      GM, 61–64
      personalized nutrition, 59–61, 61f
      phenotype, 66–70
      physical activity, 72–73
   search strategy, 59
   selection process and data extraction, 59
   variability in, 58
Glycated hemoglobin (HbA1c), 68
Glycemic index, 57

Glycemic responses, 61
Glycosylated hemoglobin (HbA1c), 56
GM. See Gut microbiota (GM)
GNKN. See Global Nutrigenetics Knowledge Network (GNKN)
GOe. See Global Observatory for eHealth (GOe)
Google, 310
GPS. See Global positioning system (GPS)
Grading of Recommendations Assessment, Development, and Evaluation (GRADE), 43
Grammatical evolution (GE), 69
Grocery shopping behavior, 148
GRS. See Genetic risk score (GRS)
Guanine (G), 312
Gut colonizing commensal bacteria, 83
Gut microbiota (GM), 9–10, 61–64, 81–82

H

Habitual sleep duration, 144
HAPA. See Health action process approach (HAPA)
Harmony, 213
Hazard Ratio (HR), 39–40
HbA1c, 69–70
HBM. See Health belief model (HBM)
Health, 202–204
   behaviors, 149
   care systems, 226
   connected medical devices, 204
   conscious lifestyle, 238–239
   health-disease process, 278
   health-related data, 206–207
   health/nutrition messages on food, 108–110
   and nutrition education challenges, 278–279
   nutritional phenotyping, 203
   recommendation, 309–310
   rise of eHealth and mHealth, 202–203
   services and clinical interventions, 150–151
   utility, 34–35
Health action process approach (HAPA), 106
Health belief model (HBM), 106
Health information systems (HIS), 200
Healthy Eating Index, 14
HGI. See High glycemic index (HGI)
High glycemic index (HGI), 68
HIS. See Health information systems (HIS)
Home inventory system, 209
Home-based nutritional intervention study, 187
Home-delivered meal kit, 201
Homozygotes, 8
Host enzymes, 83
Household factor, 181
Household level factors, 178

HPA axis. *See* Hypothalamic–pituitary–adrenal axis (HPA axis)
HR. *See* Hazard Ratio (HR)
HTML document, 315
HTTP. *See* Hypertext Transfer Protocol (HTTP)
Human biology, 58
Human genome, 7
Human Genome Project, 5, 226
Human gut microbiome, 84–85, 95
Human Microbiome Project, 81–84
Human milk banking, 187–188
Hungary case, 245–250
Hyperglycemia, 55–56
Hyperhomocysteinemia, 8
Hyperphosphorylated tau protein, 89–90
Hyperplane, 319
Hypertext Transfer Protocol (HTTP), 314
Hypocrisy, 122–124
Hypothalamic leptin–melanocortin system, 156
Hypothalamic–pituitary–adrenal axis (HPA axis), 83
Hypothesized cognitive dissonance mechanism, 118–120

I

iAUC. *See* Incremental area under curve (iAUC)
IBS. *See* Irritable bowel syndrome (IBS)
ICT. *See* Information and communication technologies (ICT)
IDF. *See* International Diabetes Federation (IDF)
IE. *See* Information extraction (IE)
IEPAD. *See* Information extraction based on pattern discovery (IEPAD)
IKEA, 201, 208, 211
Imbalanced microbiomes, 90
Immune system
  function, 142
  GI tract symbiotic microbiome for, 87–88
In vivo animal models, 91–92
Inadequate nutrient intake during pregnancy and preconception, 173
Inappropriate/inadequate feeding practices, 181–182
Incremental area under curve (iAUC), 65
Indirect interaction, 45
Individual determinants, 283–285
Industrial revolution, 144
Industrialization, 278
Infant and young child feeding practices (IYCF), 174
Infants
  in LMICs, 187–189
  personalized nutrition for, 174–186
    child nutritional status, 175–176
    complementary feeding and micronutrient supplementation, 184–186
    factors affecting nutrition status of children, 176–179
    factors influencing child feeding practices, 179–182
    personalized nutrition interventions, 182–186
    promotion of optimal breastfeeding, 183–184
  personalized nutrition interventions for, 186–187
Inferential approach, 205
Inflammophilic environment, 85
Information and communication technologies (ICT), 202
Information availability, 236–237
Information extraction (IE), 313
Information extraction based on pattern discovery (IEPAD), 315
Informed consent, 24
Institute of Medicine (IOM), 36–37
Insulin, 57, 64–65
Insulin receptors (ISR), 156
Insulin sensitivity (IS), 58
Integrative personal omic profiling (iPOP), 18
Intelligent automated food ordering, 202
Intelligent kitchen and role in personalized nutrition, 211
Intelligent packaging, 209–210
Inter-FCDp. *See* Interattitudinal, food-related cognitive discrepancy (Inter-FCDp)
Inter-FD. *See* Interattitudinal, food-related dissonance (Inter-FD)
Interattitudinal, food-related cognitive discrepancy (Inter-FCDp), 117–118
Interattitudinal, food-related dissonance (Inter-FD), 117–118
INTERMAP study, 12
Intermediate interaction, 45
International Diabetes Federation (IDF), 139
International Food Policy Research Institute (2016), 170
International Society for Advancement of Kinanthropometry (ISAK), 139
International Society of Nutrigenetics/Nutrigenomics (ISNN), 23
Internet database, 204
Internet of Things (IoT), 196
Intra-FCDp. *See* Intraattitudinal, food-related cognitive discrepancy (Intra-FCDp)
Intra-FD. *See* Intraattitudinal, food-related dissonance (Intra-FD)
Intraabdominal fat, 139
Intraattitudinal, food-related cognitive discrepancy (Intra-FCDp), 117–118
Intraattitudinal, food-related dissonance (Intra-FD), 117–118
Intraattitudinal structure, 117
Intrauterine growth restrictions, 176

Inventory management, 210
IOM. *See* Institute of Medicine (IOM)
IoT. *See* Internet of Things (IoT)
iPOP. *See* Integrative personal omic profiling (iPOP)
Irritable bowel syndrome (IBS), 83, 90f
   dysbiosis in, 88–89
   management by diet, 94
IS. *See* Insulin sensitivity (IS)
ISAK. *See* International Society for Advancement of Kinanthropometry (ISAK)
ISNN. *See* International Society of Nutrigenetics/Nutrigenomics (ISNN)
Isocaloric protein supplements, 174
ISR. *See* Insulin receptors (ISR)
IYCF. *See* Infant and young child feeding practices (IYCF)

K
K-means, 5–6
K-nearest neighbors (K-NN), 5–6
Ketoacidosis, 56
Kynurenine acid, 92

L
Labeling, 209
Lacto fermentation process, 85–86
Lactobacillus brevis, 93–94
Lactobacillus probiotics, 63
Lactobacillus reuteri, 93–94
LD. *See* Linkage disequilibrium (LD)
Learning, 321
Leptin, 144
LGI. *See* Low glycemic index (LGI)
Lifestyle interventions, 149–150, 153
Linear classifier, 318
Linear predictor function, 318
Linkage disequilibrium (LD), 45
   with known causative variant, 46
Lipid-based nutrient supplements, 185
Lipopolysaccharide (LPS), 89–90
Lipoprotein lipase (LPL), 71
Lipoprotein profiles, 6–7
LMICs. *See* Low-and middle-income countries (LMICs)
Long short-term memory (LSTM structures), 324f, 325–326
Long short-term memory recurrent neural network (LSTM-RNN), 323–324, 327
Long-term adherence, 289
Low glycemic index (LGI), 68
Low-and middle-income countries (LMICs), 171
   human milk banking, 187–188
   workplace support for breastfeeding, 188–189
LPL. *See* Lipoprotein lipase (LPL)
LPS. *See* Lipopolysaccharide (LPS)
LSTM structures. *See* Long short-term memory (LSTM structures)
LSTM-RNN. *See* Long short-term memory recurrent neural network (LSTM-RNN)

M
Machine learning (ML), 19–22, 318
   algorithms, 211
Malnutrition, 93, 174–175
Market globalization, 278
Mass customization, 253
Mass media, 287–288
Mastication, 64–65
Maternal and adolescent nutrition, 172–174
Maternal level education, 177–178
Maternal malnutrition, global and regional epidemiology of, 172
Maternal nutrition during pregnancy, 173–174
Maternal nutritional status, 172
MC4R. *See* Melanocortin 4 receptor (MC4R)
Meal, 55
Meal carbohydrate content, 57
"Meat paradox", 114–115
MedDiet. *See* Mediterranean diet (MedDiet)
Medical education system, 310–311
Medical genetic test, 37
"Medicalized" level, 228
Mediterranean diet (MedDiet), 8, 39–40, 143
Melanocortin 4 receptor (MC4R), 156
Mental health
   dysbiosis in, mental health disorders, 91–92
   management by diet, 94–95
Metabolic
   diseases, 171
      management, 20–21
   fingerprinting, 12
   phenotyping approach, 67
   surgery, 158
Metabolic Equivalents (METs), 282
Metabolic syndrome (MetS), 56, 142–143
Metabolome, 11
Metabolomics, 12, 263, 265–266
Metabotyping approach, 5–7
Metaomics approaches, 10, 24
Methylenetetrahydrofolate reductase (MTHFR), 8, 45–46, 265
METs. *See* Metabolic Equivalents (METs)
MetS. *See* Metabolic syndrome (MetS)
mHealth, 202–203
   environment, 212
Microbial intervention, 92
Microbiome, 41–42, 265–266
   microbiome-based parameters, 9

INDEX

Micronutrient
  deficiencies, 153, 173–174
  GI tract symbiotic microbiome for, 86–87
  supplementation, 184–186
Microorganisms, 9
Microsoft, 310
Miele kitchen, 208
Mixed-method approach, 266
ML. *See* Machine learning (ML)
Modern technologies for personalized nutrition, 144. *See also* Consumer acceptance of personalized nutrition
  AI engine, 212–213
  eHealth and mHealth environment, 212
  and energy expenditure, 206–207
  and food acquisition, 200–202
  and food composition, 209–211
  and food intake, 204–206
  food monitoring, 216
  and food preparation, 207–209
  food service and management of personalized nutrition, 211–212
  future perspective, 218
  intelligent kitchen and role in personalized nutrition, 211
  nutrition, and health, 202–204
  nutritional values and bioaccessibility, 217–218
  potential architecture of personalized nutrition system, 213–215
  privacy and security, 216
  reliability and consistency of smartphone apps, 217
  smart kitchen appliances and intelligent automated food ordering, 202
  smart personalized nutrition, 196–200
  virtual reality, augmented reality, and food selection, 201
Moley, 208
Monogenic disorders, 8
Monogenic obesity disorders, 156
Mother-Friendly Workplace Initiatives, 189
Mother–Baby Friendly Initiative Plus model, 188
Mother–child dyad, 180–181
Motivation(al)
  to behavior change, 294
  interviewing, 298
  theory, 298
Motor-based transport systems, 144
MTHFR. *See* Methylenetetrahydrofolate reductase (MTHFR)
MTNR1B-rs1387153 variant, 71–72
Multicomponent interventions, 150
Multiple objective expert systems, 212–213
Music recommendation, 309–310

N

National Institute for Health and Care Excellence (2014), 151
Natural language processing (NLP), 316
Nature of different foods, 240–241
Nature of personalized nutrition advice, 235–236
NCDs. *See* Noncommunicable diseases (NCDs)
NCP. *See* Nutritional care process (NCP)
NDA Panel. *See* Panel on Dietetic Products, Nutrition and Allergies (NDA Panel)
Neural networks, 310, 316
Neurotransmitter precursors, 91
New generation, 331
NGx. *See* Nutritional genomics (NGx)
NHS. *See* Nurses' Health Study (NHS)
NLP. *See* Natural language processing (NLP)
Noncommunicable diseases (NCDs), 4, 174–175, 202, 226, 278
Nurses' Health Study (NHS), 142–143
Nutraceutical food, 10–11
Nutrients, 142–143. *See also* Micronutrient
  availability, 154
  correlation data, 311–313
  nutrient–genotype interactions, 155
Nutriepigenomics field, 12
Nutrigenetics, 5, 16–17, 34–36, 41, 70, 154, 227, 312
  evidence assessment in, 36–37
  validity, 24
Nutrigenomics, 5, 12, 35–36, 70, 72, 154, 227, 236–237, 262
  consumer judgment of personalized nutrition and, 228–230
  field, 203
  nutrigenomics-based food products, 241
Nutrimetabolomics, 12
Nutrimetabonomics, 12
Nutriproteomics, 12
Nutrition education, 288, 290. *See also* Personalized nutrition education
  design procedure in personalized, 299–302
    decide behaviors, 299–300
    evaluation plan, 302
    exploring determinants of change, 300
    generating action plans, 302
    indicating general objectives, 301–302
    selecting theory and clarifying philosophy, 300–301
  interventions, 293–294
    development, 295
    effective interview in nutrition consultation, 297
    motivational interviewing, 298
    nutrition educator profile, 299
Nutrition Society Training Academy, 272

Nutrition(al), 12, 19, 202–204, 226, 237, 303. *See also* Personalized expert recommendation system for optimal nutrition (PERSON)
  aids, 95
  assessment, 288–289
  backlash, 108–109
  CDT in, 107–116
  communication, 108–109, 121–122
  data, 227
  educator profile, 299
  effective interview in nutrition consultation, 297
  factors, 57
  information, 292
  interventions, 173
  knowledge, 290–291
  nutrition-specific interventions, 182–183
  nutrition/health professionals, 270–272
    in acquiring skills, 271–272
    dietitians, 271
    widen access to personalized nutrition, 272
  panel, 209
  phenotyping, 203
  recommendations, 280
  requirements during pregnancy and preconception, 172
  research, 34–35
  status of children, 176–179
  values, 217–218
Nutritional care process (NCP), 295
  applying to personalized nutrition education, 295–297
    monitoring and evaluation, 297
    nutrition assessment, 296
    nutrition intervention, 296
    nutritional diagnosis, 296
Nutritional genomics (NGx), 226–227

O

Obesity, 138, 170
  associated comorbidities, 145–146
  diagnosis criteria, 138–139
  dietary factors, 142–143
  epidemiology, 139–141, 140f
  future approaches, 151
  genetic factors, 142
  prevention obesity strategies, 146–151
  psychological factors, 142
  treatment, 151–158
    bariatric and metabolic surgery, 158
    CBT, 158
    components, 153–158
    dietary advice, 153–157
    objectives, 151–152
    pharmacological support, 158
    physical activity, 157–158
OECD. *See* Organisation for Economic Co-operation and Development (OECD)
OFLR-PO. *See* Ordered factorial logit response model with proportional odds (OFLR-PO)
OGTT. *See* Oral glucose tolerance test (OGTT)
OLTT. *See* Oral lipid tolerance test (OLTT)
"Omics"
  repertoires, 11–13
  technologies, 18–19, 153–154
Omron HeartGuide, 207
One-size-fits-all diet approach, 4
Online
  health records, 203
  nutrition recommendations, 196–197
  shopping, 200–201
Open Food Facts, 326–327
Operational state machine, 311
Optimal breastfeeding promotion, 183–184
Optimal nutrition-targeted interventions, 182
Optimal personalized nutrition, 200
Optimization algorithm, 212
Oral biofilm dysbiosis, 89–90
Oral glucose tolerance test (OGTT), 67
Oral lipid tolerance test (OLTT), 67
Ordered factorial logit response model with proportional odds (OFLR-PO), 245
Organisation for Economic Co-operation and Development (OECD), 138
Osteoarthritis, 262
Outcomes evaluation, 302
Overweight, 138, 141, 152f, 170, 175–176. *See also* Obesity
Oxytocin, 94–95

P

P-Values, 44
Panel on Dietetic Products, Nutrition and Allergies (NDA Panel), 280
Passive sensors, 210
Path-code-string alignment technique, 315
Patient-accessible online health systems, 200
PCOS. *See* Polycystic ovary syndrome (PCOS)
PCPs. *See* Personalized care plans (PCPs)
PDAs. *See* Personal digital assistants (PDAs)
Periodontal
  disease, 89, 93–94
  pathogens, 82–83
Periodontitis, 95
Peroxisome proliferator-activated receptor (PPAR), 156
PERSON. *See* Personalized expert recommendation system for optimal nutrition (PERSON)

Personal data point, 329
Personal digital assistants (PDAs), 203
Personal health utility, 34–35, 37–38
Personalization of diet, 4–5
Personalized care plans (PCPs), 70
Personalized diabetes
　prediction mechanism, 69–70
　treatment, 70
Personalized diet, 58, 240
Personalized expert recommendation system for optimal nutrition (PERSON), 213, 311
　architecture, 334f
　framework, 334–335
　nutrients and genes correlation data, 311–313
　scalable food categorization, 313–327
Personalized health care and diets, 310–311
Personalized interventions to promote maternal nutrition, 173–174
Personalized label, 235
Personalized modeling engine, 60
Personalized nutrition (PN), 4, 34, 36–37, 58–61, 61f, 153, 226–227, 262–263, 263f
　adapting diet, 5
　areas, and applications, 226–227
　behavior role, limitations, and ethical issues, 13–16
　biological variability, 7–13
　components, 42–43
　consumer from personalized nutrition, 266–270
　consumer judgment of nutrigenomics and, 228–230
　current evidence, 262–266
　delivering, 269–270
　economic and social returns on investments, 186–187
　educational intervention, 174
　firm, 265–266
　future, 250–253
　　big data and machine learning, 19–22
　　future needs, 23–25
　　knowledge to practice, 16–17
　　"omic" technologies, 18–19
　implications for nutrition/health professionals, 270–272
　levels, 23f
　nature of personalized nutrition advice, 235–236
　personalized nutrition for infants and children, 174–186
　in practice, 263–265
　by prediction, 20f
　programs for women, infants, and children in LMICs, 187–189
　services, 243–245
　strategies to delivering personalized dietary advices, 5–7, 6f

　system, 197, 200
　validating, 41–42
　for women, 172–174
Personalized nutrition education, 303. *See also* Nutrition education
　current dietary and physical activity guidelines, 280–283
　design procedure, 299–302
　determinants of food choice, 283–288
　health and nutrition education challenges, 278–279
　intervention effectiveness, 290–295
　　determinants of dietary behavior change, 290–292
　　levels of influence in food choice and dietary behavior, 293–294
　　specific and practical approach, 290
　　theory-based interventions, 292–293
　　use of appropriate behavior change strategies, 294–295
　interventions, 288–289
　methodology for, 295–299
　NCP applying to, 295–297
Personalized recommendation system, 327–333
Phenolic compounds, 211
Phenotype/phenotyping, 66–70, 312–313
　assessments, 42
　nutritional, 203
　in PN, 67–68
Phenylketonuria, 8
Physical activity, 57–58, 72–73, 144, 157–158
　behaviors, 279
　guidelines, 280–283
　recommendations, 282–283
PMT. *See* Protection motivation theory (PMT)
PN. *See* Personalized nutrition (PN)
Pocket scanners, 210, 212
Polycystic ovary syndrome (PCOS), 146
Polyunsaturated fatty acids (PUFA), 9
Pooled panel data regression model, 69–70
Porphyromonas gingivalis, 89–90, 92
Posteriori methods, 143
Postprandial glucose responses (PPGRs), 59–60, 67
Postprandial glycemic responses, 68
Postprandial hyperglycemia, 55–56
Posttranslational modifications (PTMs), 11
PPAR. *See* Peroxisome proliferator-activated receptor (PPAR)
PPARγ2 encodes transcription factor (PPARγ2), 157
PPGRs. *See* Postprandial glucose responses (PPGRs)
Prebiotics, 83, 92–94
Precision Nutrition 4.0 approach, 12–13, 13f
Preclustered personalized regression model, 69–70
Prediabetes, 56
PREDIMED project, 39–40

Pregnancy
    maternal nutrition during, 173–174
    and preconception
        inadequate nutrient intake during, 173
        nutritional requirements during, 172
Prevention obesity strategies, 146–151
    behavioral strategies, 149–150
    environmental factors, 147–149
    support of health services and clinical interventions, 150–151
Preventive health behavior, 246
Primary prevention in high-risk groups, 39–40
Privacy
    risk, 232–235
    and security, 216
Probiotic fermented milk (kefir), 63–64
Probiotics, 85–86, 94
Process evaluation, 302
Product recommendation, 309–310
Protection motivation theory (PMT), 106
Protein, 172
    abundance, 45
    DRVs for, 280
    expression, 154
    hyperphosphorylated tau, 89–90
    PPAR-γ2, 157
Proteome, 11
Proteomics, 12
Psychobiotics, 94
Psychological factors of obesity, 142
Psychosocial influences as action and behavior change determinants, 291–292
Psyllium, 93
PTMs. *See* Posttranslational modifications (PTMs)
Public acceptance, 15
    of genetic-based personalized nutrition, 238
    of nutrigenomics, 228
Public dietary recommendations, 7
Pubmed, 313
    database, 59
PUFA. *See* Polyunsaturated fatty acids (PUFA)

Q
Quality, 213
Quantitative IS check index (QUICKI), 71
Quantity, 213
Quorn, 85–86
Quorum Sensing, 85

R
Randomized controlled trails (RCTs), 36, 39, 63, 263–264
Randomized double-blinded placebo-controlled clinical trial, 63–64
Randomized PREDIMED study, 8
Recommended daily intake (RDI), 213
Recommended Dietary Allowances (RDAs), 280
Recurrent neural networks (RNNs), 321–323, 324f
Regional epidemiology of maternal malnutrition, 172
Regulatory cells (T$_{reg}$), 87–88
Reinforcement learning, 19
Reliability
    of information, 236–237
    of smartphone apps, 217
Riboflavin, 40, 86–87, 172, 265
RNNs. *See* Recurrent neural networks (RNNs)
rs328CC homozygotes, 71

S
s-SNE. *See* t-distributed stochastic neighbor embedding (s-SNE)
Scalable food categorization, 313–327
Schaedler flora, 87–88
Science-base for personalized nutrition, 265–266
Sciencedirect database, 59
Scientific validity, 34–35, 37, 44
    assessment of putative gene X diet interaction, 46–48, 48t
        convincing, 46
        not demonstrating, 47–48
        possible, 47
        probable, 47
Secondary prevention in subjects with pathology, 40–41
Sedentarism, 144, 287
Sedentary Behaviour Research Network (2012), 282
Selective Exposure Self-and Affect-Management model (SESAM model), 110–113
"Self-actualization" drivers, 251–252
Self-justification, 110–113
Self-measured blood glucose (SMBG), 69
Semantic Web, 314
Sensing and analysis, 210
Sensors
    on-body sensors, 206
    passive, 210
    wearable, 206
Serotonin, 83, 90
SESAM model. *See* Selective Exposure Self-and Affect-Management model (SESAM model)
Short messaging service (SMS), 203
Short-chain fatty acids, 88
Short-term adherence, 289
Single-nucleotide polymorphisms (SNPs), 7–8, 35–36, 38, 46, 203, 312
Skepticism, 207
Sleep habits, 144
SMART. *See* Specific, Measurable, Attainable, Relevant, and Timely (SMART)

INDEX

Smart bathroom scales, 204
Smart kitchen, 198, 205, 215
   appliances, 202
     scales and ovens, 207
Smart packaging, 209
Smart personalized nutrition, 196–200, 199t
Smart watches, 206–207
Smartphone(s), 196, 205–206
   app, 198
     reliability and consistency of, 217
   messaging, 198
   operating system, 42
SMBG. *See* Self-measured blood glucose (SMBG)
SMS. *See* Short messaging service (SMS)
Snacking, 66, 205
SNPedia, 313
SNPs. *See* Single-nucleotide polymorphisms (SNPs)
Social
   customs, 286
   inequality, 149
   returns on investments of PN interventions, 186–187
Sociodemographic factors, 144–145
Socioeconomic determinants, 283, 286–287
Sodium-sensitivity, 264
Soft-margin SVM, 319
Sophisticated statistical approaches, 21–22
Specific, Measurable, Attainable, Relevant, and Timely (SMART), 151
"Spyce" (automated fast food restaurant kitchen), 208
SSA. *See* Sub-Saharan Africa (SSA)
SSB. *See* Sugared-sweetened beverages (SSB)
Steady-state plasma glucose diet (SSPG diet), 71
Strengthening the Reporting of Genetic Association Studies (STREGA), 43
Stress hormones, 91–92
Sub-Saharan Africa (SSA), 170
Subgingival microbiome management by diet, 93–94
Subordinate attitude object, 117
Sugared-sweetened beverages (SSB), 142
Superordinate attitude object, 117
Superorganisms, 9
Supervised learning, 19
Supply chain management, 210
Support vector machine (SVM), 318–319
   linear classification, 320
   works with relatively small data sets, 320
Support vectors, 319
Surface infrared spectroscopy, 196
Surgery, 158
SVM. *See* Support vector machine (SVM)
Sweet taste perception, 264
Symbiotic oral/gut biofilms for normal brain function, 90
Systems
   biology approaches, 11–13
   flexibility, 12–13

T

677 T allele, 40
t-distributed stochastic neighbor embedding (s-SNE), 317
T1DM. *See* Type 1 diabetes mellitus (T1DM)
TAS2R38 receptor, 35–36, 38
TCF7L2 genetic variant, 39–40
Technology-based food innovations, 241, 242f
Tesco supermarket, 326
Test anxiety, 268–269, 269t
Theory of planned behavior (TPB), 106, 241
Theory of reasoned action (TRA), 106
Theory-based interventions, 292–293
Therapeutic applications of nutrition, 36
3-D printed food, 208–209
Thymine (T), 312
Time factor influencing consumer acceptance of PN, 239
Time-series prediction model, 69–70
TPB. *See* Theory of planned behavior (TPB)
TRA. *See* Theory of reasoned action (TRA)
Traditional diet, 85
Traditional fermented foods, 85
Transcriptomics, 12
Traveling pop-up restaurant FoodInk, 208–209
Tripartite model, 117–118
"Triple bottom line" factors, 186–187
Tryptophan, 91
Two-category-SVM, 319
Type 1 diabetes mellitus (T1DM), 62
Type 2 diabetes mellitus (T2DM), 39, 55–56, 67–68, 138

U

Uber-type grocery delivery system, 200–201
Uncontrolled hyperglycemia, 56
Undernutrition, 173–176
   in children, 170–171
     conceptual framework of perceived causes of, 178f
     nutrition-related diseases, 174–175
UNICEF model, 176–177, 178f
Unified CDT in food and nutrition, 115–116
Uniform resource identifiers (URI), 315
   data collection with, 316f
United States Department of Agriculture (USDA), 326–327
Univariate ANOVA, 267–268
Universal Eating Monitor, 66
Unsupervised learning, 19
Urban poor settings, child feeding practices in, 179–182
Urbanization, 278
URI. *See* Uniform resource identifiers (URI)
USDA. *See* United States Department of Agriculture (USDA)

V

Variability in glucose responses, 58
Variables, 318
Virtual dietitian, 212
Virtual hospitals, 204
Virtual reality (VR), 201
Virtual supermarkets, 201
VitalPatch clinical biosensor, 204
Vitamin B, 95
Vitamin C, 93, 264
Vitamin D, 95
Vitamin E, 93
VR. *See* Virtual reality (VR)

W

Waist circumference (WC), 139
Wearable CGM device, 68–69
Wearable technology, 42, 206–207
Whole genome sequencing, 263
Willingness to pay (WTP), 229
Women
  in LMICs, 187–189
  PN for, 172–174
    global and regional epidemiology, 172
    inadequate nutrient intake, 173
    interventions, 186–187
    nutritional requirements, 172
    personalized interventions to promoting maternal nutrition, 173–174
Word embedding, 335
  and padding model, 311
Workplace supporting for breastfeeding, 188–189
World Health Organization (WHO), 4, 138, 170–171, 202, 226, 278, 282–283
World Wide Web, 313–314
Wrapper, 314–315
  induction, 314
WTP. *See* Willingness to pay (WTP)

CPI Antony Rowe
Eastbourne, UK
August 26, 2019